ELECTROTHERAPY EXPLAINED

Principles and Practice

Fourth Edition

For Elsevier:

Publisher: Heidi Harrison
Development Editor: Siobhan Campbell
Project Manager: Morven Dean
Design: Andy Chapman
Illustration Buyer: Gillian Murray

ELECTROTHERAPY EXPLAINED

Principles and Practice

Val Robertson PhD, BAppSc(Physio), BA(Hons)
Professor, University of Newcastle, Australia; Northern Sydney/Central Coast Health, Australia

Alex Ward PhD
Senior Lecturer, Department of Human Physiology and Anatomy, La Trobe University, Australia

John Low BA(Hons), FCSP, DipTP
Formerly Acting Principal, School of Physiotherapy, Guy's Hospital, London, UK

Ann Reed BA, MCSP, DipTP
Formerly Senior Lecturer, Department of Health Sciences, University of East London, UK

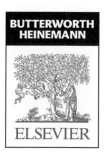

BUTTERWORTH
HEINEMANN

ELSEVIER

EDINBURGH LONDON NEW YORK OXFORD PHILADELPHIA ST LOUIS SYDNEY TORONTO 2006

BUTTERWORTH
HEINEMANN
ELSEVIER

An imprint of Elsevier Limited

First published 1990
Second edition 1994
Third edition 2000
Fourth edition 2006

ISBN-10: 0 7506 8843 2
ISBN-13: 978-0-7506-8843-7

British Library Cataloguing in Publication Data
A catalogue record for this book is available from the British Library.

Library of Congress Cataloging in Publication Data
A catalog record for this book is available from the Library of Congress.

Note
Neither the Publisher nor the Authors assume any responsibility for any loss or
injury and/or damage to persons or property arising out of or related to any use
of the material contained in this book. It is the responsibility of the treating
practitioner, relying on independent expertise and knowledge of the patient, to
determine the best treatment and method of application for the patient.

Printed in China

The Publisher's Policy is to use Paper manufactured from sustainable forests.

Contents

Foreword

The fourth edition of the text, *Electrotherapy Explained* authored by Val Robertson, Alex Ward, John Low and Ann Reed is an excellent update of the classic Low and Reed book used by countless health science students and clinicians over the years and throughout the world including in the UK, Europe, Africa, India and Australasia. The title is a true reflection of the content.

The text, which has always covered both electrotherapy and physical agents, has undergone a structural and philosophical revision that incorporates the large body of scientific theory and evidence that has been published since the last edition of the book. The two new authors, Drs. Robertson and Ward are long time collaborators who have contributed substantially to the scientific literature in their studies of ultrasound, and kHz frequency alternating current. Their imprint is clearly evident in the revision.

The underlying physiology and biophysics are clearly and extensively reviewed for each intervention. Evidence for the effectiveness of the interventions is presented where available. "Evidence-based medicine (EBM) is the integration of best research evidence with clinical expertise and patient values" (Sackett et al., 2000). The authors have used the five steps of EBP in their description and analysis of the electrotherapy and physical agents interventions described in the book. For each intervention, they convert the practice problem into an answerable question, systematically retrieve the best evidence available, critically appraise the evidence for validity, clinical relevance, and applicability, describe the application of results in practice and evaluate outcomes of performance. Where evidence is lacking, they discuss reason why and inform the readers of what needs to be done in the future to validate the practices described. Finally, they have reinforced one of the historic strengths of this text in their complete and clear descriptions of the application of the modalities.

This new edition of Electrotherapy Explained is contemporary, complete and well written. It will be a terrific addition to the libraries of clinicians and will continue to serve as an excellent text for health science clinicians and students.

Lynn Snyder-Mackler, PT, ScD, FAPTA
Professor Department of Physical Therapy
Academic Director, Graduate Program in Biomechanics and
Movement Sciences
University of Delaware
Newark, Delaware, USA

Preface to the fourth edition

Explaining electrotherapy is every bit as needed now as it was when the first edition of this book was published in 1990. Electrotherapy still has the problems identified in the preface to the first edition as confusions with 'traditional naming systems, jargon and didactic statements which have perhaps not always been justified by reason or research'. Didactic statements are still made for some modalities for which there is too little evidence either from first principles in biophysics or physiology or from clinical studies. Ironically at the same time other modalities languish as they are currently unpopular despite demonstrated benefits. A new book was needed to keep on explaining electrotherapy and electrophysical agents (EPAs). While the physical agents used clinically are much the same, the uses and the equipment change quite quickly. For example, batteries are technically more advanced and electronic devices, including electrotherapy equipment, are much smaller and more sophisticated than even 5 years ago. Microprocessor control allows a much wider range of selection and control of treatment parameters. At the same time, our electrotherapy knowledge base has expanded and continues to expand.

The new edition of 'Electrotherapy Explained' is designed to explain electrotherapy to both current and future users. The user group is widening and now includes more dentists, veterinary surgeons, physiotherapists, podiatrists, hand therapists, medical practitioners and many other clinicians who are alert to the benefits of using EPAs.

The content and the arrangement of chapters in this edition have changed and two new authors have been added. What has not changed is the focus on explaining how different modalities work and on presenting relevant clinical and biophysical and physiological evidence. In some instances the evidence might suggest that an EPA is not as effective as assumed by clinicians. In other instances it may be more effective than generally recognized or assumed. In several chapters it is made clear that there are considerable gaps between theory, clinical practice and demonstrated clinical effectiveness. We have indicated this where we are aware of gaps and the reader will hopefully recognize the thinness of research reported in some sections and draw their own conclusions.

The aim of this book is not simply to deliver judgement on the merits of different electrophysical agents. If it did, it would be dated far too quickly, given the rapid rate at which new research evidence is accumulated. Rather it seeks to evaluate electrophysical agents in terms of both:

- biophysical principles and
- clinical evidence of effectiveness.

This means that the reader is left to deliver judgement and make choices. The 'Gold Standard' is whether there is both a well-established biophysical basis and a body of clinical evidence demonstrating the effectiveness of a particular modality. In other words, whether there is a likelihood of effectiveness, based on established biophysical and physiological principles and whether there is documented empirical evidence.

Failing this the clinician must make a value judgement based on available evidence.

- If there is some clinical evidence but no biophysical/ physiological explanation, the modality could be given provisional acceptance.
- If there is a sound biophysical/ physiological basis for claims of clinical effectiveness, the modality might be given provisional acceptance, subject to clinical evaluation.
- If the claims of clinical effectiveness by proponents (clinicians or manufacturer sales representatives) are contradicted by biophysical/ physiological reasoning, the modality should not be accepted unless there is sound clinical evidence.

Having been subject to the above tests, a clinical modality must then be judged by other standards. Factors such as the simplicity of application and the capital investment and maintenance costs are important considerations in selecting a modality.

The new co-authors of this book, Val Robertson and Alex Ward have worked closely with John Low and Ann Reed to continue the tradition established by the first edition of 'Electrotherapy Explained': to present the biophysical and physiological evidence for each modality and summarize the relevant clinical evidence so that clinical decisions are well informed. A central intention of this book continues to be encouragement of understanding the underlying science. To this end the CD accompanying the text now includes both 'Physical Principles Explained' by Low and Reed and "Biophysical Bases of Electrotherapy' by Ward.

We dedicate this book to students of electrotherapy; past, present and future.

Val Robertson, Alex Ward, John Low and Ann Reed
July 2005

Preface to the first edition

Electrotherapy has tended to be a subject confused by traditional naming systems, jargon and didactic statements which have perhaps not always been justified by reason or research. In this book we have attempted to demystify electrotherapy for the physiotherapy student.

We have tried to give a fairly complete coverage of the field describing the most common modalities known to us to be employed by physiotherapists. Our intention is to explain how these modalities work and their effects upon the patient. We have used a different approach to some electrotherapy texts. In the initial chapter of each section we have tried to lay the foundations of the principles of modern electrotherapy, because we feel that a thorough understanding of these principles will ultimately lead to safer and more effective clinical practice. Therefore, the book builds up from the basics without, we hope, sacrificing accuracy to give a description of the types of energy available to the therapist. We have classified treatments of the same kind together so that the book is divided into sections devoted to electrical, mechanical, thermal and radiation energy.

The nature, production, effects and uses on the body tissues of each modality are explained and illustrated with what we hope is a reasonably comprehensive range of references to support the points made. With the very welcome involvement of physiotherapists in research, we hope to give undergraduates access to the vast amount of literature upon which they are encouraged to base their final clinical intervention. For postgraduates and practitioners our aim is to stimulate a vigorous search for answers.

We are well aware of the inherent dangers in explaining 'how things work' and in an attempt to communicate our ideas easily we may have been deliberately less precise than we could have been in some instances. We have tried to use the words that would convey the most meaning in the hope that a thorough understanding of even the more difficult concepts might be reached. Perhaps some of the ideas we offer will ultimately be shown to be too simple or just plain wrong, but we console ourselves that even these explanations can lead to debate and serve as a stepping stone to greater accuracy. Many treatments that have faded from use over the years are now returning in an appropriately modern guise, with new rational explanations. One such example is the use of low-frequency electrical stimulation following the development of the pain gate theory.

Rather than producing a step-by-step guide to technique, we have aimed for a description of the principles, the modalities and practical applications of their use. We believe that if the modality is well understood there can be a wide variation in acceptable technique and treatment within the confines of safe and effective practice.

After many years of teaching electrotherapy we both felt the need to attempt such a book. For our omissions and failings we apologize. However, our sincere hope is that we will have made electrotherapy more comprehensible for some which, in turn, will raise the standards of safe and effective treatment for our patients – the aim of us all.

John Low and Ann Reed, 1990

Introduction

Searches for 'electrotherapy' on the world wide web produce over a quarter of a million hits. This indicates something of the importance of electrotherapy. The number of manufacturers' sites found suggests it might be a financially rewarding market and the breadth of topics, a multifaceted area of interest to many. Some sites focus on equipment and the types of electrotherapy used to treat pain, some on veterinary electrotherapy products, others provide references and information on different types of electrophysical agents (EPAs) and how and when they are used. Considered together, the web sites on electrotherapy represent a wide range of countries, many different types of equipment, a large range of uses of electrotherapy and a treatment approach of relevance to those treating humans and animals.

The aim of this book is to present the most commonly used EPAs along with the biophysical principles which affect how they are applied and the potential effects they can have on a living body. The different modalities will all be discussed in terms of the relevant biophysical principles as well as their clinical effects. Where available, evidence of the therapeutic effectiveness and any known dangers and contraindications will also be presented together with the principles for applying each type of energy. The content of this book is also intended to provide a basis for evaluating and assessing other, new, modalities as they come onto the market.

WHAT IS ELECTROTHERAPY?

The term 'electrotherapy' is relatively recent and has a range of meanings. Earlier names for clinically used electrophysical agents include 'electrotherapeutics' (Neiswanger, 1912) and 'medical electricity' (Cumberbatch, 1939). This second term was consistent with the early focus on using electric currents for patient treatment. The view of the human body as containing electrical energy, which distinguished it from dead, inanimate matter, was advocated by Galvani (1780) and subscribed to by many. This view is reflected in literature, such as in the classic novel 'The Frankenstein Monster' where the man-creature that Doctor Frankenstein has assembled from parts of exhumed

A later development was the use of electrostatic fields for patient treatment (Geddes, 1984). Such treatment was impressive: arcs of electric discharge between the patient and electrodes, hairs standing on end and glowing tubes emitting coloured light as the current flowed. One could argue, at least that the placebo response would be significant!

1

human corpses is brought to life by the electrical energy of captured lightning bolts. It is perhaps not surprising, then, that the application of electric current was believed by some to be a means of enhancing or supplementing the natural energy of the human body and which could therefore be used for the treatment of disease and injury.

Nowadays the term 'electrotherapy' generally has a broader meaning that usually includes assessment despite the word suggesting it should only include treatment or therapy. Present day uses of the term in regions such as Europe and the Antipodes mean treatment or assessment using one of a range of modalities including electrical stimulation, ultrasound, different methods of heating and cooling, shortwave diathermy and clinically used electromagnetic radiation such as infrared and light therapies including ultraviolet and laser. In other countries, such as the USA, electrotherapy is another word for assessment or treatment using electrical stimulation. The other types of electrophysical agents are then typically called 'physical agents'. Whatever the definition, the aim of this book is to provide a basis for understanding the broader range of electrophysical agents.

Here the terms 'electrotherapy' and 'electrophysical agents' (EPAs) will be used interchangeably to indicate any forms of treatment or assessment conducted using an electrophysical agent which can be applied externally to the human body. This means a range of topics will be considered from electrical stimulation to ultraviolet radiation exposure as used to produce a beneficial outcome for a human or animal patient. Some types of EPAs are also used internally such as implanted electrical stimulators like gastric or cardiac pacemakers. While these uses will be mentioned the focus is on the external applications to the skin rather than within a body cavity or part.

Summary

- Electrotherapy is widely used with human and animal clients.
- Definitions of 'electrotherapy' differ throughout the world.
- Electrotherapy includes the following for treatment or assessment:
  - electrical stimulation
  - biofeedback
  - ultrasound
  - superficial heating including infrared
  - cooling
  - shortwave diathermy
  - microwave
  - phototherapy including laser
  - ultraviolet radiation.

EXOGENOUS ENERGY AND THE SKIN

An underlying premise of all EPAs is that external or exogenous applications of energy can beneficially alter physiological processes. Those processes can be normal ones: for example where ultrasound or a type of heating is applied to promote the healing of tissue following a tear, a sprain or strain. Similarly, ice or a form of cooling is applied to limit the secondary damage that can follow the normal bleeding and production of oedema in damaged tissue. Or, the healing processes may have been delayed and the EPA is used to increase the rate to a more usual level: for example, electrical stimulation with some types of wounds. Other types of EPAs are used to supplement normal learning and relearning: biofeedback and electrical stimulation can be used this way. Many EPAs are also used to reduce pain of different types and from different sources.

The skin is a barrier to all forms of exogenously applied energy. The extent to which it is an effective barrier depends on the properties of the skin itself and on the type of EPA applied and the mode and parameters of the application. The skin is not a homogeneous structure throughout the body. In some locations it is deeper and has strong fibrous connections with the underlying tissues as over the calcaneum and gluteal muscles. In other areas it is very thin, such as over the tibia, patella or malleoli or a spinous process. In some locations it is quite extensible, such as over the dorsal surface of the hand but on the palmar surface it is relatively fixed. These types of differences in skin in different locations all have implications for users of EPAs.

The relation of skin to the underlying structures and their depth can be even more important. The thickness and depth of underlying structures affects how much energy can reach deeper structures. The penetration of different forms of heating, cooling, ultrasound and electric current for example, are all affected by depth but in different ways. Skin is also altered by many different disease processes as well as by ageing and the current nutritional and medical status of the person or animal. All of these factors can potentially alter its response to different energy forms such as heat or light or electrical stimulation and the extent to which they are transmitted through it.

The type of skin in some animals is quite different from that in humans. It is often much looser and the response to an EPA can be different. By contrast, the skin of pigs has a similar structure and the underlying soft tissues a similar distribution to that of humans. This difference can be important in laboratory studies of different modalities and their likely clinical effectiveness. The amount of hair on an area in animals and humans can also alter the transmissivity of some types of energy. In summary, many properties of skin can affect the outcomes of applying all types of exogenous energy.

CHAPTER OUTLINES

Most chapters in the present book have a similar, but not identical, layout to previous editions. Chapter 2, for example, discusses topics from a biophysical perspective. This includes nerve structure and function and the response of the body to inflammation and trauma. The focus is not on modalities and how they affect the body and when they should or should not be used. Instead, chapter 2 provides details of some of the physiological processes that can be altered or affected and, in so doing, some of the boundary conditions when using electrotherapy. These issues are discussed further in later chapters where directly relevant.

Chapters 3 to 6 investigate the different aspects of clinically used electrical stimulation. These chapters start with a general overview in chapter 3 of electrical stimulation and how to use it. The more complex theory underlying some of the differences between pulsed and alternating currents is the focus in chapter 4. Chapters 5 and 6 both discuss some of the major clinical uses of electrical stimulation, from treatment to assessment. The major difference between the chapters is that chapter 5 focuses on motor stimulation using electrical stimulation. This means that a large range of uses and ways of stimulating innervated and denervated muscles is explored. How applying stimulation works, suitable parameters and what is known of the clinical effectiveness is discussed. Chapter 6 uses a similar approach but the focus is on the use of electrical stimulation for sensory stimulation, particularly for pain control. Other sections in chapter 6 focus on iontophoresis and other uses of electric current. The category 'other uses' is broad and includes some well known and understood uses and some for which the physiological underpinnings are weaker.

Safety is an issue associated with the use of electrical stimulation and many other types of EPAs. Infection control and electrical safety are among the factors that can affect safety. These and other equally important topics are discussed in chapter 7 along with the concepts of risk and contraindications.

Chapter 8 investigates the many types of biofeedback available and how they are used. A large part of this chapter considers the use of electromyographic (EMG) feedback. The reason is, it is commonly used and increasingly becoming more practical and reliable. The advantages and disadvantage of using biofeedback and when it might be preferred to electrical stimulation that produces a motor response is also considered.

Ultrasound is the focus in chapter 9, both therapeutic and diagnostic. The biophysical properties of ultrasound are described and their implications discussed along with what is currently known of its therapeutic effectiveness. Some of the methodological issues in answering such questions are discussed as well as recent research suggesting new directions for users to consider when selecting this modality. The last part of this chapter has brief overviews of longwave ultrasound, sonophoresis and diagnostic ultrasound.

Chapter 4 differs from later chapters on electrical stimulation in that, unlike them, the focus is on laboratory research and theory and not clinical research and therapeutic effectiveness.

Chapter 10 is connected with chapters 11 and 12 as all discuss some aspects of heating or cooling. Chapter 10 outlines the uses of heating or cooling and how they affect the body. Chapter 11 develops the information on superficial heating and discusses commonly used methods; similarly in chapter 12 but the topic is cooling.

Chapter 13 is stand-alone. It describes shortwave therapy, which involves the application of high-frequency alternating electric or magnetic fields to the body.

Chapters 14 and 15 are related. Chapter 14 describes the fundamentals of electromagnetic radiation. A particular type of electromagnetic radiation, microwave, is the topic of chapter 15. This topic received relatively poor press with the introduction of microwave ovens and is now little used clinically, despite clear evidence of its depth effectiveness.

The types of EPAs based on electromagnetic radiation in the visible and near visible parts of the spectrum provide the content for chapter 16. Specifically, infrared, visible light and lasers are discussed in this chapter together with their actual or proposed modes of action and their known levels of therapeutic effectiveness.

The final chapter, chapter 17, concerns ultraviolet (UV) radiation. While UV is clinically used much less often in many countries than previously, the chapter is important. UV continues to be used and there is a risk that fewer clinicians are able to use it effectively. The other potential risk is that users are not always aware of the extent of current knowledge on the dangers and long-term risks associated with using ultraviolet radiation, from equipment in tanning salons to the larger, more powerful clinical machines.

> Microwave diathermy was introduced following World War II. Radar transmitters, operating at a frequency of 2.54 GHz were found to be effective for deep heating of tissue and they were quickly adopted by clinicians. Later it was established that lower microwave frequencies are more beneficial (chapter 15).

GENERAL STRUCTURE OF MOST CHAPTERS AND COMMON ISSUES

The structure of most chapters is similar. Most focus on an EPA and present a structured development of its features and how and why it might be used clinically. The following points are used in most chapters to develop the topic.

Biophysical principles

In most chapters the first section concerns what is known of the physics of a type of energy. This is developed into the biological implications; how from first principles it might affect the living body. In most the focus is on humans but, with some provisos related to hair structure, type of skin, and tissue depth, it can equally well relate to animals which can be and are treated with the same EPAs.

The known physics, biophysics and physiology related to the modality can provide the clinician with the basis for making a considered judgement in the absence of adequate clinical evidence.

> Laboratory studies using animals can provide evidence of potential clinical significance. This is particularly important when clinical studies have not been carried out or where confounding variables make the clinical findings ambiguous.

Therapeutic and clinical effectiveness

First principles suggest that without empirical evidence of effectiveness there can be little justification for using a modality. Despite this, for many of the commonly used modalities there is little evidence other than anecdotal of beneficial effects. Sometimes this is easily understood as the evidence is unlikely to be collected as the modality, such as infrared, has a limited adjunctive role. In other instances, there is a clear need for high quality research involving patients being treated with an appropriate condition that is expected to respond to a particular EPA. Irrespective of the quality and types of evidence available, the known evidence regarding the therapeutic and clinical effectiveness is discussed for each modality covered in the present book. In some instances reasons for the lack of evidence are also discussed, such as the problems in evaluating ultrasound with ongoing issues of transducer calibration and of knowing the actual dosage levels at the affected site in treated tissue.

> More often than not the conclusion of a systematic review is that 'there is insufficient high-quality research to justify the use of this modality. There is an urgent need for high quality controlled clinical trials'. This offers little assistance in clinical decision making.

This book is not and does not attempt to provide systematic reviews of all modalities discussed. One reason is that there is too little high quality clinical research on many topics. Also, systematic reviews cannot provide guidance in specific circumstances as is well known (Petticrew, 2003). A goal of this book is to enhance the understanding of clinicians of all types of EPAs. That requires more explanations and a broader research base than systematic reviews alone can provide. The absence of a clinical evidence base does not mean a lack of evidence (Petticrew, 2003). With EPAs the issue is what should be included as evidence. Even if appropriate clinical trials and systematic reviews exist, relevant evidence also includes laboratory studies and evidence from biophysics or other basic sciences. Where the hard science and the clinical evidence agree, a convincing evidence base exists. Where the clinical evidence is inconclusive but a sound biophysical basis exists, the modality can be given provisional approval. Where the clinical evidence is inconclusive and no sound biophysical basis exists, the modality should be given provisional disapproval, meaning that the modality should not be used but that this view could change if appropriate evidence were forthcoming.

Principles of use

The many and varied problems that can be effectively treated by an EPA mean that their selection requires a knowledge of first principles. No book could cover all possible contingencies, so this book presents the principles a user needs to consider to optimize the outcome and to minimize any existing risks. Similarly, this book could not describe or illustrate all types and brands of EPA equipment currently used clinically in all countries throughout the world. Consequently, the focus is on explaining the principles of use and the factors to consider with each EPA. This is designed to provide potential users with a flexible basis for understanding and mastering specific items of equipment they may have now or obtain in the future.

The principles are considered in most chapters in a range of appropriate headings from the following listing:

Patient

Once a therapist has completed an assessment and selected a modality, they need to discuss the options with the patient. The treatment principles therefore typically include advice on explanations and warnings, positioning, instructions, examination and testing of the area to be treated. The aim is to ensure valid consent is obtained and that electrotherapy is used only how and when it is appropriate and all known risks are identified prior to treatment. In addition, any preparation of the area being treated such as cleaning the skin or testing some aspect of cutaneous sensation or blood flow is discussed when appropriate. The therapist also has an obligation to use appropriate methods of ensuring the privacy of the patient. Such ethical conduct is an essential component of professional practice.

Preparation and testing of apparatus and examination

This includes collecting and assembling the items and parts of equipment needed. When appropriate, visual checks should be made of electrodes, leads, cables, plugs, power outlets, switches, controls, dials and indicator lights. In addition, the output of some machines such as ultrasound units and stimulators should be checked, as described in the relevant chapters. The equipment must be set up so as to minimize risk and promote patient comfort during treatment and to minimize the exposure of the operator to the output of the modality being used.

Application

Depending on the modality, checking throughout an application is required to ensure safety. This is covered in the relevant chapters and advice given regarding the frequency and types of advisable checks.

Termination of treatment

On termination of treatment the area treated should be examined to identify if expected effects such as superficial vasodilation have occurred and any unexpected effects such as a burn. If appropriate, an explanation is given of what to expect after treatment, instructions regarding future treatments, and what should be done between treatments. Written instructions should also be given if, for example, the patient is taking home a stimulator.

Recording

An accurate record of all the parameters of treatment including region treated, technique, dosage and the resultant effect must be made each time. This is for assessment purposes, to meet legal requirements and sometimes to facilitate treatment audits. In addition, details of the advice and warnings given prior to treatment should be recorded.

Further details of applications are provided by many national professional bodies. These are designed to meet local conditions of practice as well as conforming with internationally agreed standards for using EPA equipment.

Contraindications and dangers

When contraindications and the different dangers or levels of risk are presented each is done so with an attempted justification. Sometimes this is easy. Some EPAs should never be used under certain circumstances. For example, an application of electrical current or shortwave or microwave diathermy through an implanted electronic device is always contraindicated. The probability of damage is sufficiently high and the outcome sufficiently disadvantageous to the patient that using these modalities is never justified. By contrast, some 'contraindications' are repeatedly advised as the possible implications of an adverse outcome are sufficiently important that use of the modality is rarely justified. A typical example of this would be the application of many different types of EPAs through the lower abdominal region of a pregnant or possibly pregnant woman because of the possible effects on a fetus. Although the risk is very small, almost any possible risk of adverse effects is sufficient to warrant contraindication.

Other so-called 'contraindications' are often based on historical misinformation that, repeated for long enough, is granted accepted status. One such example is the claim that ultrasound over an epiphysis should be a contraindication. As in the example of a pregnant woman, although the risk is very small, even improbable in a conscious child, this treatment is possibly better avoided. This is discussed in chapter 9.

An issue that also has to be considered is the use of multiple modalities either sequentially or concurrently. While not addressed in individual chapters, clinicians must be aware that this can change the level of risk of using a particular modality. If, for example, a treatment that alters sensory awareness is applied, a modality that relies on accurate sensory feedback cannot safely be used concurrently. It can be applied sequentially if sufficient time is allowed between applications, otherwise the risk is increased to an incalculable level by the addition of a second modality.

Summary of factors affecting the choice of an EPA

The choice of whether to use an EPA and which particular one is not always obvious. In some instances the known benefits of an EPA may be clearly identified and well accepted and in others it is not. Similarly, the risks of applying some EPAs are necessarily higher and must be evaluated by a clinician with appropriate training in their use and an understanding of the underlying physical principles.

Before applying an EPA the following questions should be considered:

- What outcome is intended? An intended outcome may be immediately obvious such as pain relief with heat or cooling and others, such as strengthening using electrical stimulation, may take weeks to be evident.
- Can using this EPA produce or assist in producing this outcome? Different EPAs can produce a similar outcome. For example, heat, cooling and electrical stimulation are all used for pain relief. However, the circumstances under which each is optimally effective can be quite different. The decision as to which to use and when requires an appropriately trained clinician with experience in patient evaluation as well as a thorough knowledge of EPAs.
- Is use of the selected EPA safe in the circumstances? Almost all effective treatment interventions have some attendant risks. Most types of electrotherapy have relatively low levels of risk if appropriate precautions are taken (excluding issues such as the presence of indwelling electronic devices and reduced cutaneous circulation). The risks are generally specific to the type of energy being applied and no treatment should be considered without a thorough knowledge of how each affects the body and possible consequent risks.
- What is the best treatment option in terms of patient and/or therapist time, and other costs such as initial capital and ongoing maintenance costs? This arises particularly with shortwave diathermy with its high initial capital costs and requirement for intensive supervision of treatment. Another example is the time-cost for a patient of the long-term use of electrical stimulation of denervated muscles. In this case there may be no alternative so the costs can be justified if there is the likelihood of a beneficial outcome. Where pain and discomfort are concerned, alternatives to electrotherapy, such as active exercise or mobilization using manipulation or massage, may be more effective long term for strengthening or pain reduction. However, these also raise issues of time, costs and compliance. Consequently, decisions regarding the use of any form of treatment imply the need for well-informed patients and clinicians.

Similarly with electrical stimulators: different types are all claimed to be effective for, for example, pain control, muscle strengthening, oedema reduction and muscle re-education. The important question is whether machine type A is better than machine type B for a specific clinical condition.

EPA users should confine themselves to using modalities for which they have both sufficient and current relevant theory and practical skills to be competent. Usually electrotherapy is part of an overall treatment plan which is selected and modified on the basis of repeated examination and assessment.

EVALUATING EPAS

The Cochrane Collaboration is a foundation set up to foster review and analysis of existing research into clinical interventions.

There are different sets of criteria for evaluating new and existing treatments. Even if the Cochrane Collaboration and equivalent collections of clinical research contained many meta-analyses and systematic reviews of the use of EPAs, methods for evaluating new equipment and treatment methods would still be needed. With the lack of existing methodologically rigorous studies on many topics in electrotherapy, the need is even more obvious.

The following list of five criteria includes modified versions of four of the five that Sullivan proposed and used to evaluate three different types of electrical stimulation treatments (Sullivan, 1999). They are altered here to ensure the appropriateness for of all types of electrotherapy, including electrical stimulation, ultrasound and the many other forms from heating to ultraviolet radiation. The fifth was added to counter an obvious issue in evaluations of some EPAs. The criteria included are broader than those adopted by the Cochrane Collaboration but are perhaps of more practical value.

Criterion 1. The underlying theory justifying the use of an EPA must be sound and supported by appropriate biophysical, anatomical and physiological evidence.

Criterion 2. How a modality is used or applied should be based on appropriate biophysical, anatomical and physiological evidence.

Criterion 3. Evidence of potential risks should be ascertained prior to initial uses and data should subsequently be actively collected and reviewed by proponents and independent researchers.

Criterion 4. Evidence of beneficial outcomes that justify the use of EPAs may be sought from the general scientific literature and must be sought in the clinical. Clinical studies should include people who have the condition for which a benefit is claimed. The methodologies used, while ideally randomized controlled trials, will also include other studies such as quality cohort studies, series of cases, single subject experimental designs and case studies.

Criterion 5. In clinical trials patient selection should relate to the expected effects of a modality and the outcomes should be assessed using relevant outcome measures.

The role of biophysical evidence is the first important difference in this list from that of Sullivan. Evidence supporting the use of most types of EPAs comes initially from studies using the methods and knowledge base of physics. For EPAs the effect of a particular energy on biological events is also pivotal, hence the need for biophysical evidence to be considered. The aim should be to obtain a dose–response curve or similar for each type of modality. Without this type of evidence it is difficult to identify appropriate levels of dosages for different tissues (types and pathologies). As well, other considerations such as the anatomy and physiology of the human or animal to which the modality is to be applied must also be considered.

The inclusion of the need for independent researchers in the process of identifying possible risks (side-effects) and outcomes is another difference. In the past some clinical and non-clinical trials reporting favourable outcomes have been sponsored by manufacturers or others who potentially might benefit. Unless replications of the method, conducted by independent researchers, produce similar results, beneficiary-related evidence should never be accepted as sufficient. It is necessary during the development process but not sufficient to justify the purchase or continuing use of the equipment. With the existing bias to publication of positive findings, this can be a difficult condition to meet. This same bias has another potential adverse implication: their over-representation in systematic reviews and meta-analyses (Sutton et al., 2000).

In an ideal world all EPAs would be investigated using well-designed randomized controlled trials with sufficient subjects to identify any real effects. The reality is that randomized controlled trials are not always possible with a clinical population. Obtaining sufficient homogeneous subject populations to identify an effect is a general problem, as has long been evident in the relatively limited existing clinical literature (Robertson, 1995). Using a randomized controlled trial can also limit the type of information obtained. For example, if compliance is a possible issue there is little scope for obtaining qualitative information if the trial is strictly controlled. A risk is that the literature has limited clinical relevance. If, however, a broader range of methodologies is accepted as providing valid sources of information, clinically relevant and valid material can be collected. For example, a series of cases can add considerably to our knowledge about a particular modality including the boundary conditions of use. Subsequently, researchers may investigate relevant aspects of the question using a randomized controlled trial if possible. Hopefully also replications are conducted.

The inclusion of clinical trials involving patients for whom the treatment is intended is most desirable. The results of in vitro research, for example, are difficult to extrapolate to clinical usage because of the problem of knowing how the in vitro dosage relates to dosages in clinical practice. Ultrasound at an intensity of $1\,W\,cm^{-2}$ applied to cells in a dish, which might have a volume of $2\,mL$ will produce very different effects if the same cells are part of a tissue with a volume of, for example, $200\,mL$. And it is not simply a case of adjusting the intensity in proportion to the tissue volume, as the distribution of energy in a particular volume will vary. Biophysical analysis can bridge the knowledge gap but demonstrated clinical effects avoid the possibility of errors in extrapolation.

Similarly, the findings of studies involving the treatment of experimentally induced pain, particularly if positive, should be replicated

A problematic example is laser therapy. Biophysical evidence indicates that any physiological effects must be superficial yet claims are made that deeper effects can be produced. A physiological basis for the depth effectiveness of laser therapy is lacking. The research findings are mixed and generally inconclusive. Identifying a biologically probable and plausible mechanism is important especially when improbable statistical relationships are identified between the use of a modality and an outcome (Cromie et al., 2002).

Replications should either be systematic, in which parts of the method are modified to extend knowledge of a topic, or direct replications which might, for example, use a larger subject population if a previous study found an effect which did not demonstrate statistical significance.

using a patient population because conditions such as pain can be markedly altered by context (see chapter 6). While studies using university or college students may allow better control of confounding variables, because these subjects do not meet the same criteria as a relevant patient population, the clinical significance of the results are still open to question. Subsequent clinical studies are needed to explore the generalizability of a finding. Does it apply, for example, to older patients as well as to younger? Does the presence of specific co-morbidities alter the expected outcomes?

Research into EPAs must also take into account the possibility of a placebo contribution from often impressive looking equipment. In itself a positive outcome from an inert treatment is quite acceptable but this does not advance the argument for using a particular modality in the future. Clinical trials need to account for, exclude or minimize the possibility of a placebo effect as part of the process of identifying a dose–response relationship for a modality and an explanation of why it works.

The fifth criterion proposed above relates to selecting appropriate types of patients for clinical trials and using relevant outcome measures. Many modalities are used to promote healing. A relevant question concerns the extent to which the timeframe for healing can be reduced. If there are no neurological, metabolic, vascular, immunological or other such impediments there is an onus on those recommending an EPA to show how its use will expedite repair. This is particularly so when few outcome measures could identify small changes, such as a half-day benefit, in an expected 7-day process. By contrast, with pathologically slowed healing, demonstrating a change in the rate of expected healing should be considerably easier. An integral part of this is identifying a plausible mechanism by which the modality affects the outcome. For example, methods of increasing blood flow, such as sensory level electrical stimulation, might increase the rate of healing of chronic ulcers by stimulating the autonomic nervous system and increasing the local blood flow if the area has normal or near normal sensory innervation.

Evidence that by itself should generally not be viewed as sufficient is that produced by a manufacturer or salesperson. Both have a vested interest in sales and should not be expected to be able to present a balanced argument and overview of all the supporting and non-supporting literature. The effects of 'positive only' reporting and a lack of scrutiny of the methodology of published research can lead to clinical adoption of suspect modalities. For example, the use of lasers increased in parts of Europe during the 1990s but without a commensurate level of methodologically adequate supporting evidence from systematic reviews or individual clinical studies (Cambier and Vanderstraeten, 1997). Extending this and including Sullivan's fifth criterion suggests that the proponents of new equipment and advocates of new uses of existing equipment should always be prepared actively to seek independent scientific and critical evaluations. To ensure independence such evaluations must not involve subsidization

> Clinical evidence of effectiveness, a demonstrated dose–response relationship and a sound biophysical and physiological explanation together provide the best rationale for using a particular modality.

> This last point, independence, can be difficult as research, traditionally government funded, is increasingly being outsourced in many countries. This can affect both what is funded and what is published and hence reduce the opportunities for truly independent research.

or other active assistance beyond that available to any other re-searcher or user.

ISSUES IN OBTAINING EVIDENCE

An issue that affects the quality of evidence for some modalities concerns dosage. Evidence that equipment has been adequately calibrated is not always provided, particularly with ultrasound equipment. Even if provided, the stability of the output is uncertain in some machines. Other issues affect the reliability of related evidence. How energy is provided clinically can require very specific descriptors such as the speed of movement of an applicator (if ultrasound) and the area to which it is applied (many modalities including ultrasound, heating, cooling and electrical stimulation) or the ambient temperature to ensure replicability. This is not always achievable in a clinical trial and the results of laboratory trials, as noted above, although more easily controlled, often cannot be directly extrapolated to clinical conditions.

COMPARISONS

Comparisons of different types of treatment approaches are important. One such study compared the outcomes from using electrical stimulation or a medication to treat osteoarthritis of the knee (chapter 6). Others have investigated the role of cooling following orthopaedic surgery (chapter 12), microwave with primary dysmenorrhoea following the usual medical treatments (chapter 15), and the contributions of ultraviolet radiation and photosensitizers to changes in psoriasis (chapter 17). This type of approach permits cost–benefit analyses of treatments as the benefits can be identified and the relative cost levels evaluated.

Considerably more comparisons between different EPAs and of EPAs and other types of treatments are needed. For example, which type of deep heating is optimal and when: shortwave diathermy, microwave diathermy or MHz frequency ultrasound. Similarly, without further research it is only conjecture that a hot pack is a simpler, cheaper form of heating than 45 kHz ultrasound (chapter 9). Without such studies it is hard to establish the conditions under which a particular type of treatment is optimal and, generally, when an EPA is preferred to the other options.

THE FUTURE FOR EPAS

Two major factors will affect the future of electrotherapy: research on the topic and future technological advances. Without considerably more research that is methodologically acceptable and relevant there is a risk that users will limit their use of EPAs. The focus on 'evidence-based practice' has grown considerably over the past decade. While the principles are usually now core concepts in entry-level education of clinicians, there is also an increasing recognition that the criteria used to define acceptable evidence are far too restricted. Such restricted evidence alone cannot be used to make sound clinical decisions (Guyatt et al, 2005). Similarly, systematic reviews cannot provide guidance in specific circumstances, as is well known along with the idea that the absence of answers does not mean a lack of evidence (Petticrew, 2003).

It is important that graduate clinicians continue to have sufficient depth and breadth of knowledge to be effective and discriminating users of a range of EPAs and they should also conduct clinical research. This could only improve our knowledge of which EPAs are clinically effective and under what conditions and what the risks are.

Technological advances that will be important for users of EPAs include the increasing miniaturization and concurrent sophistication of electronic hardware. Also, the development of increasingly adaptable software that can alter the output in response to a patient's input will have a major impact. So, too, will the increasing the storage capacity of batteries and decreasing the size of electronic devices.

All in all, the future of EPAs lies in the hands of researchers, clinicians and technological developers. More research is needed to identify when using an EPA is effective, more well-informed and effective clinicians are needed, using and researching their uses of EPAs, as is increasingly better and more reliable equipment. If this is the direction for the future it bodes well for users of EPAs.

References

Cambier, D., Vanderstraeten, G. (1997). Low level laser therapy: the experience in Flanders. Eur J Phys Med Rehabil, **7**, 102–105.

Cromie, J., Robertson, V., Best, M. (2002). Occupational health in physiotherapy: general health and reproductive outcomes. Aust J Physiother, **48**, 287–294.

Cumberbatch, E. (1939). Essentials of Medical Electricity, 8th edn. London: Henry Kimpton.

Geddes, L. (1984). A short history of the electrical stimulation of excitable tissue including therapeutic applications. Physiologist, Supplement, **27**, s1–s47.

Guyatt, G., Cook, D., Haynes, B. (2005). Evidence based medicine has come a long way. Br Med J, **329**, 990–991.

Neiswanger, C. (1912). Electrotherapeutical practice, 18th edn. Chicago: Ritchie & Company.

Petticrew, M. (2003). Why certain systematic reviews reach uncertain conclusions. Br Med J, **326**, 756–758.

Robertson, V. (1995). A quantitative analysis of research in physical therapy. Phys Ther, **75**, 313–322.

Sullivan, J. (1999). Evaluating new treatments in electrotherapy. In R. Nelson, K. Hayes, D. P. Currier (eds), Clinical Electrotherapy, 3rd edn, pp. 449–487. Stamford: Appleton & Lange.

Sutton, A., Duval, S., Tweedie, R. et al. (2000). Empirical assessment of effect of publication bias on meta-analyses. Br Med J, **320**, 1574–1577.

Background biophysics and physiology

Electrophysical agents have a long and interesting history and many uses were discovered long before the underlying biophysical and physiological processes were understood. Thus electrical stimulation was used well prior to any real understanding of the nervous or musculoskeletal systems. Historically, the discovery of many physical phenomena has led to exploration of their effects on the human body. Sometimes the results have been productive, as evidenced by the range of electrophysical agents available today. Sometimes such exploration has proved to be an electromedical cul-de-sac (for example, the discovery of magnetism and the subsequent pursuit of the possible benefits of magnets for healing).

The aim of this chapter is to provide a biophysical and physiological basis for the electrophysical agents which are commonly used clinically. This is to aid the understanding of clinically useful modalities and to explain why some treatments are likely to be useful and others unlikely to be so. It also provides a basis for evaluating the potential usefulness of new modalities as they are introduced into the market, as indicated in chapter 1. In the absence of adequate clinical evidence, a test must be carried out to investigate whether any claimed benefits are biophysically and physiologically plausible. If the clinical evidence does not yet exist but the physiological basis of the intervention is sound, the therapist can have much more confidence than if the clinical evidence is lacking or there is no sound physiological or biophysical basis. The emphasis in this chapter is on the hard science rather than clinical studies. Individual chapters provide more detail on some specific issues, where directly relevant.

An issue of central importance in electrotherapy is how electrophysical agents can affect the target tissue. One aspect of this, the skin as a barrier, was mentioned in chapter 1. The other aspect is that the human body is homeostatic, i.e. it resists any physiological change from predetermined values. Thus, for example, body temperature is controlled, as is the neural activity of the autonomic nervous system. Yet the aim of electrotherapy intervention is to change the body's activity or response to existing injury.

Homeostasis relies on physical structures (e.g. the skin) and neurological activity affecting the behaviour of tissues and organs to resist change. The physiological response to electrophysical agents is markedly influenced by the skin. It is the barrier which separates the organism from its external environment. It resists heat flow, the flow of electric current and the transmission of electromagnetic radiation. The response to an electrophysical agent is also determined by the organs and organ systems of the body. Thus if a particular treatment modality produces tissue heating, homeostatic mechanisms respond to reduce the heating. Any understanding of the clinical effects of a particular modality must be set against a backdrop of physiological homeostatic mechanisms.

THE SKIN AS A BARRIER

The skin is the largest organ of the human body with an area, in the adult, of about $2\,m^2$. It serves a number of important roles:

- as a first line of defence against infection. Very few microorganisms can penetrate the skin and various skin glands secrete antimicrobial molecules.
- to protect against water loss. The significance of the skin's role in restricting water loss is seen in burn victims who need intravenous fluid replacement if the area of skin loss is large.
- as a key element of the body's temperature regulation mechanism. Heat gain and loss are controlled by blood flow in the skin and immediate subcutaneous tissue and also by perspiration. This is discussed further in chapter 10.
- to shield deeper tissue from electromagnetic radiation, in particular, infrared, visible and ultraviolet radiation. This is discussed further in chapters 16 and 17.
- to protect against mechanical injury of the underlying soft tissues.

Subcutaneous tissue

The tissues under the skin include the blood and lymphatic vessels, the fat, muscles, bones, nerves, and a range of organs ranging from sensory to digestive and excretory. An important feature of these for users of electrophysical agents is that their function can be affected despite the homeostatic mechanisms which invariably operate. In the following we consider cells, tissues and organs with a focus on properties which help to explain the effects of electrophysical agents.

CELLS

A particular feature of cells is that, although they are electrically neutral, the outside of the cell is positively charged while the inside is equally negative. This is because of two factors: (i) the concentration of potassium ions, [K$^+$], inside the cell is high and (ii) the membrane is relatively permeable to K$^+$ ions. All human cells have a higher concentration of potassium ions inside. For sodium ions the situation is reversed: the concentration of Na$^+$ inside the cell is low and outside is much higher. A sodium/potassium pump in the cell membrane uses energy to actively move sodium ions out and potassium ions in to maintain the imbalance.

Because the membrane is quite permeable to K$^+$ ions but relatively impermeable to Na$^+$ ions or most negative ions, K$^+$ ions diffuse out, down their concentration gradient and the outside of the membrane becomes positively charged. K$^+$ ions do not take negative ions with them as most of the negative intracellular ions are too large to be able to cross the membrane. Thus a potential difference is established across the membrane. The outside is positively charged and the potential difference or voltage across the membrane is typically 70 mV or so. The inner surface of the membrane remains negative to the outer under most, but not all, circumstances.

Similar charge differences exist across the membranes surrounding the intracellular organelles, such as the endoplasmic reticulum, Golgi apparatus and nucleus. Mitochondria require hydrogen ions (H$^+$) to be in a higher concentration outside the inner mitochondrial membrane in order for the mitochondrion to be able to synthesize ATP. Thus cells have a net positive charge on their membranes due to K$^+$ ion movement, while mitochondria have a net positive charge on their membranes due to outward movement of H$^+$ ions. (For an extensive and valuable description of the electrical features of cells and cellular activity, see Charman (1990b,c).)

As already noted, the difference of potential across a normal cell membrane at rest, known as the resting membrane potential, has the inside of the cell negative relative to the outside. The potential varies in the cells of different tissues, being anything between −60 and −90 mV. In nerves and smooth muscle fibres it is usually about −70 mV, for skeletal muscle cells −80 mV and for glial cells −90 mV (Bray et al., 1986). This electrical potential – as it were an 'electrical pressure' – across the cell membrane is due to the fact that such membranes are much more permeable to K$^+$ than to Na$^+$. The Na$^+$/K$^+$ pump ejects three ions of sodium for every two of potassium that it takes in. The result of both mechanisms is a deficiency of positive charges inside the cell compared to the outside, hence the membrane potential.

This sodium-potassium (Na$^+$/K$^+$) 'pump' uses active transport to move these ions against their passive gradients. Potassium ions also move out of the cell by passive diffusion.

As well as the Na$^+$ and K$^+$ pump, the concentration of Ca^{2+} inside the cell is maintained at a much lower level than outside by an important Ca^{2+} pump mechanism. In both cases adenosine triphosphate (ATP) supplies the energy needed.

The resting membrane potential of nerves

Neurons consist of a cell body and several extensions which convey the nerve impulses to and from the cell body. As with other cells, a resting membrane potential is present across the membrane of the cell body. The same membrane potential exists across the whole length of

Figure 2.1 The resting membrane potential is principally determined by passive diffusion of potassium ions and active transport of sodium and potassium ions (the sodium/potassium pump).

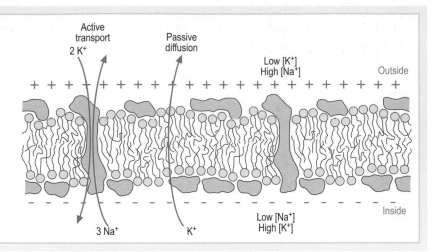

In many tissues the individual cells are connected by gap junctions which allow some electrical conduction between cells. This does not occur in skeletal muscle or nerve tissue (Finean et al., 1978).

the processes, the nerve fibres, which are extensions of the plasma membrane. The longest extension is usually called the axon.

As already stated, the resting membrane potential is ultimately due to active transport (the Na^+/K^+ pump) and to the difference in permeability to Na^+ and K^+. These ideas are illustrated in Figure 2.1. The situation is like that of a ship at sea in which the lower parts are below the water level but contain air able to pass freely in and out, like K^+. The seawater, like Na^+, is kept out by the hull and the small amount that does leak in is easily removed by the bilge pumps, an active transport mechanism. Thus different compounds – air and seawater – are separated by the ship's hull; due to the greater density of water a pressure difference is developed across the hull. If the hull is holed, water will rush in with great force because of the pressure difference, but if the hole is then quickly blocked the small quantity of additional water is ultimately removed by the bilge pumps to restore the situation.

THE NERVE IMPULSE OR ACTION POTENTIAL

The nerve impulse is a wave of electrochemical activity which passes along the nerve fibre using energy already stored as part of the membrane potential. It is a reversal of the membrane potential from −70 to +30 mV which occurs very briefly – taking about 1 ms – and spreads along the fibre without decrement. It is also called an action potential.

The impulse is initiated by depolarization – an alteration of the balance of charges – of the fibre membrane due to chemical disturbance at a synapse or receptor or to some other disturbance such as an electrical pulse. Depolarization means that the potential difference across the membrane is reduced from the −70 mV of the resting membrane. However, the impulse is only triggered when the membrane is depolarized by about 10–15 mV (i.e. to about −55 mV). Once this threshold is reached the impulse, or action potential, is generated automatically (Figure 2.2) and spreads along the nerve fibre at a rate that is characteristic of the particular fibre. If the impulse is initiated normally it will pass only in one (orthodromic) direction (distally if an efferent nerve and proximally if an afferent). If the middle of a nerve fibre is artificially stimulated two impulses will travel away from the point of stimulation, one in each direction, orthodromic and antidromic (opposite to the anatomical direction for that nerve fibre). This is shown in Figure 2.3. Whether antidromic stimulation has any physiological effect (either positive or negative) is unknown.

The effect of depolarization beyond the threshold level is to cause the membrane to become much more permeable to Na^+ by opening special channels or gates. Na^+ rushes through these channels into the fibre causing an abrupt and rapid local reversal of membrane polarity (-70 to $+30$ mV, Figure 2.4a), after which the Na^+ channels close. Depolarization also causes K^+ channels to open but the response of the K^+ channels is slower. Consequently, the rush of Na^+ into the fibre is soon stemmed and there is a loss of K^+ from the fibre. In this way the membrane repolarizes again (Figure 2.4b). Once the process is started, rapid depolarization followed by repolarization occurs automatically. A period of hyperpolarization follows (Figure 2.4c), during which time the K^+ channels are closing and the membrane takes several milliseconds to return to the normal resting state.

The voltage-gated sodium ion channels operate by an alteration of their protein configuration in response to varying local electrical potentials (Hille, 1992). Thus these Na^+ channels can be in at least three states:

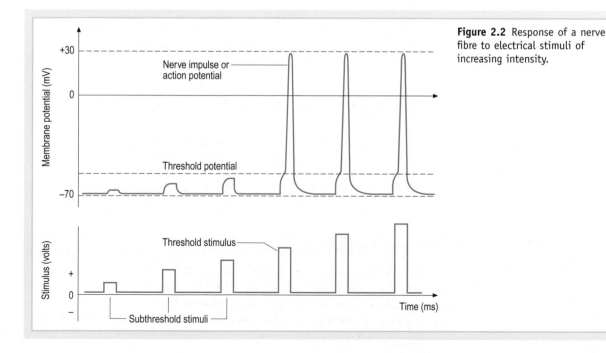

Figure 2.2 Response of a nerve fibre to electrical stimuli of increasing intensity.

Figure 2.3 Orthodromic and antidromic propagation of action potentials in response to electrical stimulation.

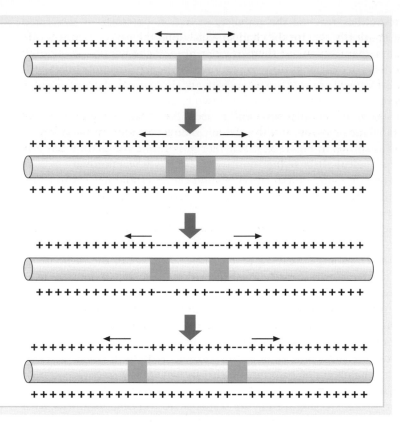

Figure 2.4 Stages of the action potential: (a) depolarization, (b) repolarization and (c) hyperpolarization.

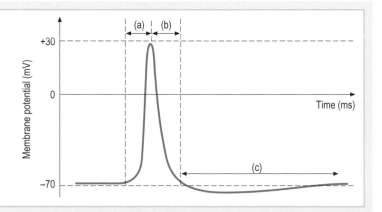

In reality, Na⁺ channels are constantly opening and closing due to random local voltage fluctuations, but this is inconsequential until a large number of channels are affected simultaneously.

- closed, but ready to open instantly
- open
- closed but unable to open instantly.

They go through these states in sequence in response to a voltage change beyond threshold, spending a very brief time open and a longer time – a millisecond or so – in a closed but inactivated state. These are absolute states for the channel which 'flips' almost instantaneously from one to the other: there is no half-open condition. The smooth rise and fall of the action potential, as in Figure 2.4, is due to many Na^+ channels opening and closing to cause an average voltage curve.

Although an action potential involves Na^+ ions moving into the cell and K^+ ions moving out, the change in concentration of these ions is extremely small. For example, it has been calculated that an outflow of only one hundred thousandth of the total K^+ in the cell can alter the membrane potential by 100 mV (Alberts et al., 1994). Similarly small quantities of Na^+ ions enter the cell. Ultimately the situation is restored by the Na^+/K^+ pump. Even without the activity of the pump, the impulse can occur many hundreds of times before the concentrations change enough to alter significantly the membrane potential. The ship analogy used above is appropriate; many small rushes of water could be allowed to enter the hull before the ship is in danger of sinking, even if the bilge pumps are not working.

The impulse will travel along the length of the fibre because the depolarization spreads in all directions. Since the voltage-dependent sodium gates are opened once the threshold is reached, the electrical charge spreading along the surface of the membrane causes the next area of the fibre to depolarize and so on. Once the impulse has passed, that particular part of the fibre membrane is refractory, i.e. it cannot be stimulated until it has repolarized. The first part of the action potential (Na^+ ions rushing in) is analogous to a line of dominoes set up so that when the end domino is pushed over it falls against the next which falls against the next and so on. A wave of falling dominoes thus travels along the prearranged line. Such a system has the characteristics of the initial part of the nerve impulse in that energy is stored in the upright position of the domino, like the store of energy in the membrane potential. Also the domino has to be disturbed sufficiently to bring its centre of gravity outside its base – beyond the threshold – from which point it accelerates downwards, tipping over the next domino as it goes. The falling domino has the same positive feedback properties – rapid acceleration to the limit of the system – as the reversal of membrane polarity due to the inrush of sodium ions. Of course, the nerve membrane potential is automatically reset but the domino line needs the attention of a dexterous human hand to reconstruct it.

The speed of propagation of the nerve impulse along the nerve fibre varies in different nerves. Generally, the larger the nerve fibre diameter the faster its conduction. Further, many nerve fibres are surrounded by an electrically insulating sheath, the myelin sheath, interrupted at intervals by the nodes of Ranvier which are exposed areas with no myelination and many voltage-gated ion channels. The electrical potential of the nerve impulse travels along the fibre but only triggers depolarization at the nodes of Ranvier. When one node is depolarized this triggers depolarization in the next node without the action

Figure 2.5 Saltatory conduction of the action potential in myelinated nerve fibres.

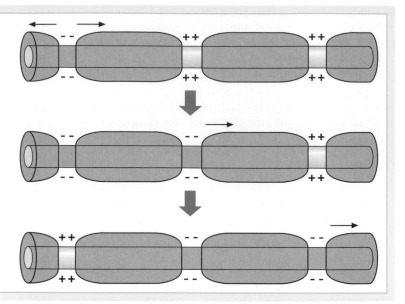

potential having to travel along the intervening myelinated region of the fibre. The change in the membrane potential when an action potential is produced at one node (about 100 mV) is large enough to trigger an action potential at the adjacent node. Thus the nerve impulse can be described as skipping from node to node (Figure 2.5) using less energy and travelling much faster. This is called saltatory conduction. Single nerve impulses can be recorded on the skin surface to investigate their conduction rates in peripheral nerve conduction studies.

The action potential will actually be spread over many nodes of Ranvier at any one time. The higher the conduction velocity the greater the length of fibre which is depolarized. At the extreme, for instance, an impulse travelling at 100 m.s^{-1} may occupy some 5 cm of axon length (Bray et al., 1986).

The transfer of information in the nervous system and the regulation of muscle contraction are 'coded' by the number and frequency of nerve impulses.

Summary

A nerve impulse is:

- an 'all-or-none' event
- triggered by a disturbance of the nerve fibre membrane electrical potential beyond threshold potential
- an electrochemical disturbance – a depolarization – which travels along the length of the nerve fibre
- identical in magnitude and velocity for any given nerve fibre
- able to travel more rapidly in a myelinated nerve fibre.

ACTIVATION OF MUSCLE FIBRES

Like nerves, muscle fibres also produce an electrical disturbance: this causes them to contract. Action potentials in motoneurons result in release of the neurotransmitter acetylcholine (ACh) at the nerve fibre ending, the neuromuscular junction. The ACh triggers depolarization of the muscle fibre membrane at the junction and a wave of depolarization spreads along the muscle fibre membrane. It is this wave of depolarization which causes the whole muscle fibre to contract. A single motor nerve innervates, i.e. synapses with, many muscle fibres and so will activate them as a group. A *motor unit* consists of a single motor nerve together with the muscle fibres it supplies, which can range from several hundred in a large muscle to only several in smaller muscles involved with precise movement and control. The central nervous system thus has control of motor units rather than individual muscle fibres. A fascinating feature of muscles is that they are extremely well designed to produce smooth, precise contractions regardless of the force required. For low force contractions, motor units with small numbers of muscle fibres are activated, and activated at a low frequency. For increased force production, motor nerves fire at higher frequencies and more motor units are activated. As the force requirements increase, motor units with larger numbers of muscle fibres are recruited. This is discussed further in chapters 4 and 5.

When many muscle fibres contract, the electrical signal produced is quite large, much larger than that of the motor nerve fibres activating them. This is simply because one motor nerve innervates many muscle fibres. The electrical activity of muscle can be measured at the body surface. Skeletal muscle activity can be detected using skin-mounted or needle electrodes and amplified, then displayed as an electromyograph or EMG. The size of the signals recorded depends on the number of active muscle fibres. There is, therefore, considerable variation in the size of the EMG signal, depending on the size of the muscle and the proportion of the muscle fibres activated.

Nerve fibre activity is much harder to detect and record because the electrical signal is so much smaller. The normal method of making non-invasive measurements is to use skin-mounted electrodes and record multiple events, e.g. the nerve response to repetitions of a single electrical stimulus, then average the measurements so as to reinforce the nerve activity signal while averaging-out the random variation in the electrical signal, which is called 'noise'.

Another example of this is the way in which information about the heart can be provided in the form of an ECG or electrocardiogram.

ELECTRICAL POTENTIALS OF OTHER CELLS AND TISSUES

Nerve and muscle cells are not unique in having a potential difference across their plasma membranes. All tissue cells have this characteristic. The difference is that nerve and muscle fibre membranes undergo large, transient changes in the membrane potential (action potentials) as part of their normal function, while other cells do not. The membrane potential is important in all cells as it acts as a source of energy for moving molecules across the membrane. This is important because the principal role of the membrane is to be a barrier to the ingress of most molecules. Nonetheless, there are many molecules which are needed by the cell and which must be able to enter without difficulty. The membrane potential is a source of energy for the process of secondary active transport, whereby molecules which would otherwise be unable to cross the membrane are moved across at specific transport sites using the electrical energy of the membrane potential.

Tissue potentials

A transcutaneous voltage normally exists in human skin. The stratum corneum is negatively charged with respect to the dermis, with an average potential difference of 23 mV (Foulds and Barker, 1983). One study reports that relatively hairless skin surfaces, such as the hands and feet, show a greater potential difference, but always negative to the dermis in all areas and with all subjects tested. Similar skin potentials occur in animals, and experiments on guinea pigs showed that incisional wounds are associated with a decrease in the measured potential difference (Barker et al., 1982). Similar changes have been observed in human subjects.

These differences have been argued as evidence that wound healing may be partly controlled by electrical signals and hence that electrical stimulation might influence wound healing. The argument is not fully convincing, particularly given the developing explanation of the possible contribution of another factor, the stimulation of the autonomic nervous system by cutaneous stimulation. The (limited) clinical findings are discussed in chapter 6.

Electrical charges generated by connective tissues

Strain generated potentials are found in bone and other connective tissues. These are charges resulting from, and proportional to, mechanical deformation of the tissue. The mechanism is not fully understood but is widely described as a piezoelectric effect (see chapter 9) though it involves greater complexities (Charman, 1990e). Bone growth and remodelling are known to be controlled by mechanical forces causing strain generated potentials, which in turn stimulate cells (osteoblasts or osteoclasts) and cause either bone growth or absorption. Similar mechanisms are believed to apply in the control of connective tissue remodelling in which the balance of collagen fibre synthesis and breakdown is controlled by strain generated potentials along the collagen fibrils.

Electrical gradients in embryonic development

In animals and plants that have been extensively studied, embryonic development is associated with potential gradients. These are generated by cellular activity and seem to have a growth-regulating function. Experiments with some simple animals have shown that artificially reversing the electrical polarity can reverse the direction of head-to-tail development. All embryos seem to have electrical polarity which develops soon after fertilization.

Electrical gradients in limb regeneration

Most adult animals including humans are entirely unable to regenerate the complex masses of tissues involved in the regrowth of limbs. A few, however, notably the salamander, have the ability to regrow a new limb after surgical amputation. This appears to be achieved by blastoma formation near the amputation site whose undifferentiated cells develop to form the new limb tissues. Innervation seems to be an essential component. A similar amphibian, such as a frog, that has no regenerative capacity shows a very much smaller change in potential across the wound.

There are claims of partial regeneration in non-regenerative animals produced by the application of artificial currents in various experiments; see Charman (1990d) for a review.

The importance of wound potentials in both healing and regeneration is uncertain, particularly in determining what is cause and what is effect. The importance has been shown in humans in the amputation of part of the terminal phalanx of a child's finger. Such a wound has been shown to heal and the end of the finger regenerate if kept moist (Illingworth and Barker, 1980). Several other small tissue potentials and gradients have been described, some in the nervous system but entirely separate from the impulses due to varying transmembrane potentials described above. For a review of this whole topic see Charman 1990(a–f) and 1991(a and b).

THE HEALING PROCESS

Throughout this book reference is made to the effects of various therapeutic modalities on the inflammatory, healing and repair processes, and pain symptoms of healing. It seems appropriate to give an outline of these changes at this point with some discussion of the mechanisms involved.

The tissue response to damage is often described in terms of mechanical injury to the skin and subsequent infection by bacteria. The series of changes that ensue are much the same whatever the tissue involved and however the injury is caused. Thus the visible changes of an accidental cut in the skin are very similar to the less visible changes following a muscle or ligament tear. The reason is, of course, that the response to any kind of damage is similar in all vascularized tissues; it is the response to some irritant. This could be the products of damaged cells or some introduced organism, say a bacterium, or a chemical or radiation irritant. It is usual and convenient to describe these changes as a sequence of stages which decidedly overlap and occupy varying lengths of time. Thus the process can be characterized in the four stages of initial injury, inflammation, proliferation and remodelling.

Initial injury

This results in damage to cells and small blood vessels. Cells die as a consequence of direct damage. This is followed by secondary cell death due to factors such as oxygen deficiency due to the damaged blood vessels, or chemicals released from other damaged cells. The extracellular structure of the tissues may also be damaged with tearing of fibres and disruption of the ground substance. If the damage is at the surface, bleeding is visible, otherwise the extravasated blood is trapped in the damaged tissue. Within a few minutes the released blood starts to clot, which serves to plug the leaking blood vessels, helps to immobilize the area and traps bacteria. Clotting is precipitated by the aggregation of platelets and the activation of a 'cascade' system of enzymes. These convert prothrombin to thrombin which causes the soluble plasma protein, fibrinogen, to become the insoluble fibrin. This complex process of blood clotting, which involves an extrinsic and intrinsic system, is an important trigger to the inflammation that follows. It causes, among many other important reactions, the production of bradykinin and initiation of the complement cascade, which is a system of interacting proteins in plasma associated with the activity of antibodies, especially in the presence of contaminants. The clots are dissolved after about 5 days by fibrinolysis.

Consider a slip with a kitchen knife resulting in a flesh wound. The initial laceration produces little damage or cell death. Far greater damage occurs secondarily when blood clotting, essential to prevent blood loss, causes local hypoxia and secondary cell death in the vicinity (see chapter 12).

Inflammation

This word, derived from a Latin word meaning to burn, is especially apt since, when the skin is involved, it becomes hot, red, swollen and painful (calor, rubor, tumour and dolor). These are the four cardinal signs of inflammation. To these it is appropriate to add a fifth – loss of function. Inflammation is basically the result of the microcirculation of the tissues reacting to injury.

Vascular changes

First, there is a very brief vasoconstriction of the non-injured vessels in response to irritation, followed by prolonged dilation. This dilation includes arterioles, venules and lymphatics in both active and dormant channels. The total blood flow to the region is, therefore, increased, although the rate of flow in individual channels may be diminished. This leads to both redness and increased temperature of the skin. White blood cells – polymorphonuclear leucocytes – move to the edge of the blood stream, lining up along the endothelial vessel wall, in a process called margination. They subsequently pass through the vessel wall into the adjacent tissue fluid. The endothelial cells forming the vessel walls partially separate at their junctions, leading to increased vascular permeability. This is due to direct damage which loosens the intercellular junctions in both capillaries and venules. The endothelial cells of venules are also able to contract – pulling away from one another – when affected by chemical mediators such as histamine. This has tremendously important consequences, because it allows much more plasma protein (albumin, globulin and fibrinogen) to leave the blood vessel and enter the tissue fluid. Because of this, the osmotic pressure between the blood and tissue fluid is altered so that fluid leaves the vessels and enters the tissue spaces. This is further encouraged by the increased capillary hydrostatic pressure due to arteriole dilation. The resulting increase of fluid in the tissues is called oedema and the fluid itself is called an exudate. This, then, is the cause of the swelling associated with inflammation. It seems to be beneficial in the presence of infection since it dilutes bacterial toxins and allows the passage of immunoglobulins (antibodies circulating in plasma) and complement (a system of plasma enzymes) which will promote the destruction of bacteria. By the same mechanism that leads to coagulation of blood, fibrinogen in the exudate is converted to a fibrin network. This both limits the spread of bacteria and makes them more susceptible to phagocytosis by white blood cells, as discussed later.

Activation and control

While the vasodilation and exudation are a standard universal response, the causative agents are complex and multiple. Initially, histamine, formed from the amino acid histidine, is released during many kinds of injury, much of it being from degranulated mast cells; these are wandering cells found in large numbers in connective tissue. Also at this stage, serotonin (5-hydroxytryptamine), probably from platelets, contributes together with local inactivation of adrenalin. Collectively, these allow early vasodilation to occur, which is maintained by the activation of kinins by enzymes triggered by some of the processes of blood clotting. (Kinins are a group of polypeptides, which includes bradykinin.) There are many other groups of substances which provoke features of the inflammatory reaction, particularly a group of fatty acids formed from arachidonic acid in or on the cell surface. These form a group called prostaglandins and another group called leukotrienes. Prostaglandins are affected by non-steroidal anti-inflammatory drugs and both groups by corticosteroids, which may account for the anti-inflammatory action of these drugs. Additionally, steroids may inhibit macrophage levels. Further mediators

Where no infection is present, the value of the laying down of fibrin is less evident, as it can lead to restriction of movement in the tissues and hence later functional impairment, which is sometimes permanent.

include enzymes from the complement pathway. These are also involved in histamine release and chemotaxis, specifically the attraction of neutrophils to the area. Among many other mediators are platelet activating factor, plasmin and cytokines. The complex sequential appearance of so many different substances to promote vasodilation seems complicated, but these are systems that control not only the initiation and completion of inflammatory change but also its nature and intensity.

Pain

The pressure applied to sensory nerve endings by exudate accounts for some of the pain associated with inflammation. This becomes very obvious if expansion of the tissues is restricted, leading to higher pressure. Pain is also provoked by all the chemical mediators that cause vasodilation, notably the kinins. Histamine may only provoke itching and the prostaglandins may act by potentiating the effect of other pain-provoking substances. Other chemicals liberated by cell injury may also cause pain.

Cellular response

Almost immediately after formation of the fluid exudate, polymorphonuclear leucocytes (neutrophils) start to pass through the vessel wall by inserting pseudopodia in the gaps between cells and 'flowing' through, a process called diapedesis and a continuation of the margination noted above. A little later, these neutrophilic granulocytes are joined by monocytes which, once in the damaged area, develop into macrophages. Both types are attracted to the area by chemotaxis due to many of the mediator factors noted above. The principal function of the polymorphonuclear leucocytes is phagocytosis of pathogenic bacteria. This process of engulfing and destroying bacteria and other unwanted particles invariably leads to the death of neutrophils. If very large numbers are involved due to the extent and virulence of the invading bacteria then pus is formed, which is usually extruded from the surface. Macrophage cells are not only phagocytic and much longer lived than neutrophils, they also release chemical factors needed for the proliferative and remodelling phases. Phagocytosis appears more effective when particles and bacteria are trapped in the fibrin mesh. Lysosomes release digestive enzymes which break down dead cells and bacteria.

The contribution of the higher levels of the nervous system can be seen from the fact that hypnosis can be used both to increase and decrease the vascular inflammatory response, although it does not directly affect cellular activity.

Influence of the nervous system

Although inflammation will proceed apparently normally in denervated tissues, the vascular responses, at least, are influenced by nerve fibre activity. At a very basic level the triple response occurs as a result of sensory and vasomotor nerve activity. At the site of the damage there is an initial red reaction which appears within a few seconds.

This is caused by capillary dilation due to direct pressure. It is followed by local mild swelling – a wheal – because of the increased permeability of capillaries and venules, and a more diffuse redness – a flare – caused by arteriolar dilation. It is due to an axon reflex in which sensory nerve stimulation results in impulses being relayed antidromically via a branch (axon) of the peripheral nerve to the arterioles. Stimulation of polymodal pain receptors also leads to the release of neuropeptides from the (pain signalling) C fibres which help to trigger inflammatory responses; substance P is probably the most important of these. Adrenalin, controlled by the sympathetic nervous system, can inhibit the vasodilation of inflammation. The effects of the higher centres of the nervous system on the perception of the pain of inflammation are well known and can both inhibit and exaggerate.

Summary

Initial injury:

- damage to cells
- damage to extracellular structures
- bleeding into or outside tissues
- blood clotting.

Inflammation – 'calor, rubor, tumour and dolor':

- vasodilation
- increased vessel permeability allowing plasma protein to leak into tissues which produces oedema to dilute toxins and promote destruction of bacteria
- local pain due to pressure of exudate and chemical mediators
- cellular activity
- polymorphs exhibit margination and diapedesis and phagocytosis
- macrophages appear later and are longer lasting than polymorphs. Macrophages are not only phagocytic but also release important chemical agents controlling later phases
- control of inflammation effected by complex sequential cascades of chemical activators including histamine, various kinins and prostaglandins
- leucocytes attracted by chemotaxis
- some influence from the nervous system.

Proliferation

This stage lasts about 3–4 weeks. It includes reconstructing the tissues, resurfacing if necessary and giving strength to the wound. It involves the activities of three kinds of cells: macrophages, fibroblasts and endothelial cells (to form new blood vessels, a process called angiogenesis). Acting in concert, these form new, highly vascular, wound-filling granulation tissue. It is called granulation tissue because of its grainy appearance when sectioned. Macrophages are essential for healing to occur. Not only do they digest and remove wound debris but they also migrate into the damaged area, releasing chemotactic agents which stimulate fibroblast activity and angiogenesis. These new blood vessels appear at first as buds of endothelial cells which grow into the damaged area, branching and eventually joining adjacent buds to form capillary loops when they canalize. As blood starts to flow through them, the oxygenation of the region increases and, at the same time, fibroblasts lay down new collagen fibres to provide a supporting framework. Thus new granulation tissue proceeds, growing in from the normal tissue edges, replacing the dead or dying injured tissues. The macrophages are notably able to tolerate low oxygen levels and thus tend to lead the process. Some of the fibroblasts become myofibroblasts which are able to contract and effect wound contraction by pulling the edges together. Dehydration (drying) also plays a role with skin wounds. The processes can, in certain circumstances, lead to contracture and considerable scarring of the affected tissues. Figure 2.6(b) illustrates the changing populations of the different cells during these phases.

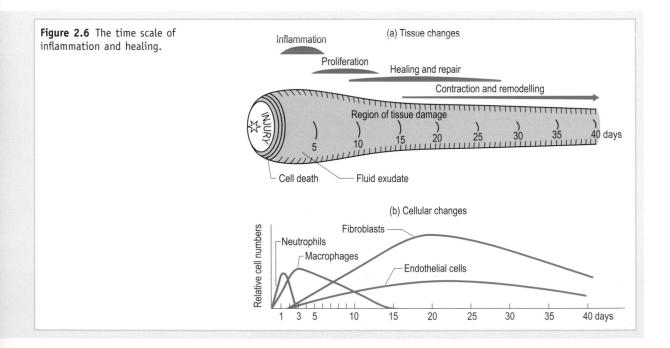

Figure 2.6 The time scale of inflammation and healing.

Remodelling

The repair process continues until the whole damaged area is replaced. At the same time the granulation tissue becomes more fibrous and less vascular, ultimately to become dense fibrous tissue (i.e. scar tissue). At 3 weeks the strength of the wound is only approximately 15% of that of the original tissue. The process of remodelling may continue for months, the structure of the new tissue altering slowly. The number of blood vessels reduces to that appropriate to maintain viability of the tissues. Arterioles, venules and lymphatic channels redevelop, and there is concurrent regeneration of small nerve fibres. The fibroblasts not only lay down new collagen fibres, but also the mucopolysaccharide (proteoglycan) matrix of typical connective tissue. Further, there is remodelling of the connective tissue with time. This phase can last for years, depending on the size of the connective tissue structure. At first the collagen fibres appear to be randomly oriented but subsequently they become rearranged in a way that best resists the stresses to which the tissue is normally subjected. Importantly, this last mechanism depends on appropriate stresses being applied by activity.

If the skin surface has been damaged, the epithelial cells are able to regenerate to cover the area with new skin, a process called epithelialization. A small wound can be covered in 48 hours. This forms a protective barrier which lessens the chances of infection and prevents fluid loss. However, no new hair follicles or sweat glands are formed. This is because some specialized cells are able to replicate while others are not. Most cells lose their ability to replicate when they become specialized (differentiate). Several more or less specialized cells are able to regenerate (i.e. replicate themselves to replace lost tissue) in humans; liver cells are particularly notable in this respect. The general repair of human tissue is, however, restricted by most differentiated cells not being able to replicate. A consequence is that dense fibrous tissue can replace the dead or damaged normal tissue, i.e. there is permanent scarring as a result of the injury.

Timing of the processes

The processes just described overlap to a considerable extent and the length of each phase is very variable depending on the severity of the original injury and whether injury continues over time. The initial bleeding usually lasts only a few minutes but cell death may continue over a few days. Vasodilation starts within an hour or so and continues over several days. Tissue oedema follows a similar pattern but often lasts rather longer. Phagocytosis starts within hours, reaches a peak about 3 or 4 days later, but continues over several days as the debris is cleared. The inflammatory phase lasts approximately 3–4 days. The development of granulation tissue can often be identified after a few days, merging into fibrous repair which may continue for

The application of stress to undamaged connective tissues is essential for them to retain their integrity and mechanical strength. Unstressed connective tissue will atrophy. Repetitive loading can produce tissue hypertrophy.

weeks or months. The time scales of these tissue and cellular changes are illustrated in Figure 2.6.

Summary

Proliferation, healing and repair:

- involves activity of macrophages and fibroblasts as well as angio-genesis to form granulation tissue
- also involves wound contraction.

Remodelling:

- more fibrous tissue formed and resorbed
- scar formation
- regeneration of vessels, nerves in the damaged tissue.

HEALING OF AVASCULAR TISSUES

Most tissues of the human body are vascularized. They have a good blood supply: an elaborate network of capillaries infiltrates the tissue, providing nutrients to the cells and removing waste products. Damage to vascular tissue has the characteristics described above and damage and repair follow the distinct phases described. Some connective tissues – most importantly articular cartilage and intervertebral discs – are avascular (and aneural) and the response to injury does not follow the same path. Because the tissues are avascular, blood clotting and the resulting hypoxia and secondary cell death are absent, as is the inflammatory response. An unfortunate consequence is that the third phase, repair, is also compromised. Tendon is not truly avascular but the blood supply is much lower than normal vascularized tissues and it repairs poorly and at a lower rate.

Generally speaking, the tissue cells function in, and are adapted to, an environment with restricted oxygen and nutrient supply so unless they are directly damaged, injury has little impact on their status. The downside is that because of the restricted supplies, their ability to carry out rapid and efficient repair is strictly limited.

Articular cartilage trauma and repair

Of all the avascular connective tissues, articular cartilage is least able to repair. When cartilage is lacerated superficially, i.e. when the damage does not extend to the underlying bone, very little necrosis occurs. Cell death is minimal as the cartilage cells (chondrocytes) are relatively insensitive to hypoxia and their oxygen and nutrient supply is relatively unchanged. Inflammation is absent as the tissue is avascular and the third phase, repair, is virtually non-existent. The lacerated region remains essentially unchanged. Chondrocytes are not triggered into repair mode as there are not the stimuli that are produced in injured vascularized tissues. Nor would chondrocytes be able to kick into high gear metabolically because of their restricted nutrient supply. A consequence is that damage remains and this can lead to a downhill spiral of events whereby the cartilage progressively degenerates.

Articular cartilage consists of a framework of collagen fibres embedded in a gel consisting principally of the mucopolysaccharide aggrecan and water. Aggrecan is needed to give the cartilage its compressive stiffness. If the collagen framework is disrupted, aggrecan can escape and the region becomes softer and mechanically weak. This means that, under compressive loading, the stress in adjacent regions will be increased. If the increase in stress is high enough to damage further the collagen fibre framework a vicious circle is set-up, whereby the tissue progressively degenerates.

Although superficially lacerated cartilage does not repair, damage which does not disrupt the cartilage surface at a microscopic level can repair effectively (Buckwalter, 2002). This is presumably because the collagen fibre damage is not extensive and aggrecan has not escaped, so the repair requirements are within the means of the chondrocytes.

With a deeper injury, extending to the vasculature of the subchondral bone, significant repair will occur. The normal response of necrosis, inflammation and repair is evoked. New bone is formed and calcification does not proceed beyond the cartilage–osseous end-plate boundary. A problem is that the cartilage is repaired with a plug of dense, fibrous collagen of a different type to the original and lacking in aggrecan. It is scar tissue rather than true cartilaginous tissue. The repaired cartilage is thus much weaker than the original as the stress distribution under load is quite irregular.

An interesting aspect of articular cartilage is that, because it is completely avascular, it is isolated from the immune system. The collagen in articular cartilage (type II collagen) is different to that of collagen fibres in vascular tissues such as skin and bone (type I collagen). A consequence is that the immune system does not 'know' type II collagen and if it is exposed, an immune reaction follows.

> The most abundant mucopolysaccharide in articular cartilage is aggrecan. Aggrecan attracts and binds water, resulting in a high internal osmotic pressure, which gives the cartilage its ability to withstand compressive loading.

> In rheumatoid arthritis, exposure and sensitization of the immune system to type II collagen leads to an ongoing attack on the microscopic fibrous framework of articular cartilage.

Intervertebral disc trauma and repair

Repair of damaged intervertebral discs is a relatively slow process as there is no inflammatory response. Nonetheless, they do have a limited repair capacity due to the vascularity of the vertebral end-plates and the soft tissue surrounding the disc. This provides a (strictly limited) supply of oxygen and nutrients. If the annulus fibrosus is punctured superficially then, providing that the damage does not extend to the nucleus pulposus, the structure will repair. If the damage extends to the nucleus, the annulus does not repair and major changes occur to the nucleus pulposus over time.

The end result is that the nucleus becomes more dense, fibrous and matted, both due to the accumulation of type I collagen and the depletion of aggrecan. Aggrecan depletion means that the nucleus pulposus also has reduced water binding and retention capability. The disc overall is thus more compressible, is intrinsically weaker (because greater compression focuses stress on the outer regions of the annulus fibrosus) and is hence more susceptible to further damage. A problem if the disc is re-injured is that it is not soft, jelly-like nuclear material which is squeezed through the damaged annulus but a tougher fibrous solid. If this impinges on and compresses nerves or the spinal cord, the effects are a good deal more severe and longer lasting than those of the original injury.

Tendon trauma and repair

Tendon is not truly avascular but the blood supply is much more restricted than in normal vascular tissues. Capillaries extend from muscle into the tendon at the musculo-tendinous junction. At the osteo-tendinous junction (the insertion) a much more limited supply is provided. The tissue surrounding the tendon is also well vascularized and so provides a source of oxygen and nutrients (Sharma and Maffulli, 2005).

When a tendon is torn, cellular injury is confined to a limited number of tendon cells (tenocytes) damaged directly by the trauma. The cells in tendons are widely dispersed in the much more extensive extracellular matrix of collagen fibres and it is the matrix which suffers the main injury. A systemic response is provoked but it is primarily the surrounding vascular tissue which responds and becomes inflamed. Tenocytes near the site of the damage respond slowly (because they can only operate within the limits set by their nutrient supply). In the torn, inflamed region much more dramatic events occur. Granulation tissue is produced and this gradually transforms into dense connective tissue as fibroblasts lay down a new extracellular matrix of collagen fibres joining the two torn ends. The joining region is bulbous and the collagen fibres are disorganized. With time, vascularization reduces and the tissue starts to resemble tendon. Over a period of months, the scar tissue remodels so that fibres are aligned along the axis of the tendon (Lin et al., 2004).

Tendon injury can provoke swelling and inflammation of the tendon sheath and surrounding tissues and this can produce the pain. The pain and inflammation follow the usual pattern and reflect the course of injury. The symptomatic changes which occur are rather unreliable indicators of the rate or extent of repair of the tendon itself as the mechanical strength may not be regained for several months, though the injury may be asymptomatic at a much earlier stage.

The development of a fibrous mass in the damaged nucleus is because the cells that are stimulated to produce aggrecan also produce collagen. When stimulated by injury, the cells produce not only type II but also type I collagen which forms the coarse fibres found in skin, tendon, ligament and scar tissue.

A complication with tendon repair is the formation of adhesions which can restrict tendon gliding and limit the range of movement (Woo et al., 2000).

Summary

- The ability of avascular tissue to heal is much more limited than vascular tissue.
- Of all tissues, articular cartilage has the least ability to repair.
- Intervertebral discs can repair if damage does not extend to the nucleus pulposus.
- Tendon is better able to repair because it is not truly avascular and surrounding vascular tissue assists the process.

THE APPLICATION OF ENERGY TO THE BODY FOR THERAPY

Physical energy can be applied to the body in various forms. The most obvious is mechanical energy, in the form of some appreciable mass, such as the hand, being pressed against the body surface. If this pressure varies at a suitable rate it is called a vibration (therapy 1, Table 2.1). If the frequency of vibration occurs between about 20 and 20 000 cycles per second, i.e. Hertz, it is detected as sound when it strikes the tympanic membrane of the ear. The tympanic membrane is not able to vibrate appreciably at frequencies above 20 000 Hz so sensory nerves cannot detect the vibration. For this reason, higher frequency oscillations are called ultrasound (therapy 2). This energy can be passed through the body tissues generating heat and causing other effects where it is absorbed.

Table 2.1 Forms of energy applied to the body

	Mechanical	Electrical	Radiation
Continuous	Pressure	Constant current	
Low frequency	Vibration	Low frequency currents	
Medium frequency	Sound	Medium frequency currents	
High frequency	Ultrasound	High frequency currents	Radiowaves Microwaves
Still higher frequencies	Heat	Electron oscillation	Infrared Visible Ultraviolet X-rays γ-rays
Therapies	1 Pressure and vibration 2 Ultrasound 3 Conduction heating 4 Cold therapy	5 Direct current 6 Muscle-stimulating currents and transcutaneous nerve stimulation 7 Shortwave diathermy	8 Microwave 9 Infrared 10 Visible light 11 Ultraviolet

If the atoms and molecules of the object placed against the skin are given more motion, i.e. the object is made hotter, this heat energy can be transferred to the skin and tissues. The tissues are thus heated by conduction (therapy 3). If the molecules of the object in contact have less motion than those of the tissues then heat is conducted from the tissues to the object, thus cooling the tissues (therapy 4).

If an electrical potential difference or voltage is applied to the skin surface this will cause ions in the tissues to move. The movement of charges is an electric current in the tissues (therapy 5). If these currents are varied, either in intensity or direction, at a suitable frequency, e.g. 50 Hz, it can disturb the ionic balance across nerve or muscle membranes, causing a nerve impulse or muscle contraction to occur (therapy 6). Both low frequency currents (up to 100 Hz or so) and medium frequency currents (in the range 1 kHz to 10 kHz) are used clinically for electrical stimulation of nerve and muscle. At still higher frequencies, in the megahertz range, nerve and muscle fibres cannot respond. The alternations are simply too rapid to cause fibre excitation. The French scientist, d'Arsonval, pioneered the study of the effects of alternating current (AC) on the human body. He reported (d'Arsonval, 1893, 1894) that a low frequency AC stimulus, at a level sufficient to cause muscle contraction, was very uncomfortable. At higher frequencies (1 kHz or more) the discomfort was diminished or eliminated while the force of the evoked muscle contraction was not.

d'Arsonval also demonstrated that at higher frequencies still (hundreds of kHz), high currents could be passed through the human body with no nerve or muscle excitation. He demonstrated this in a classic experiment where several volunteers joined hands to make a circle. A high frequency AC generator was included in the circle and, at a separate point, an electric light bulb. When the generator was activated the light bulb glowed brightly, indicating a high flow of current. The human participants felt no discomfort and no muscle contraction was evoked.

Thus high frequency current flow in the human body does not produce direct stimulation of nerve fibres. Rather the effect is one of heating because appreciable amounts of energy can be transferred to the tissue without nerve or muscle excitation. At high frequencies (typically 27 MHz in clinical applications) current flow is induced in tissue to produce heat and possibly other therapeutic effects (therapy 7). At these high frequencies it is not necessary to use electrodes in contact with the skin surface. Rather a current flow can be induced in the tissues by the electric field between two electrodes or by the magnetic field produced by alternating current flow in a coil of wire wrapped around some part of the body. This is discussed further in chapter 13.

When charges are made to accelerate, energy is given off in the form of electromagnetic radiation. This radiation can enter the tissues and cause effects when they are absorbed. When the electron movement is at frequencies of thousands of millions of Hz (GHz) it pro-

d'Arsonval's pioneering studies laid the groundwork for the clinical use of alternating current, both for nerve and muscle excitation and tissue heating.

Where electromagnetic radiation is of a single wavelength and the waves are in phase it is called 'laser' radiation.

duces microwave radiation (radar), which leads to heat when the radiation is absorbed in the tissues (therapy 8). At higher frequencies the radiation is called infrared and is absorbed at the skin surface but still causes heating (therapy 9). Still higher frequencies give radiation which stimulates the retina of the eye, i.e. it is visible (therapy 10). Frequencies immediately beyond the visible – ultraviolet (therapy 11) – cause marked biological changes when absorbed at the skin surface, e.g. sunburn.

Effects of an applied electrical potential

The effects on the body of an applied electrical potential or voltage depend on the amplitude and nature of the resulting current in the tissues. They can be rather simply summarized as having three basic effects, each of which may have various complex physiological and therapeutic consequences:

- Chemical changes occur in the tissues as a result of the application of unidirectional or direct current (DC). Such effects are described in chapter 6. If the current is sufficiently great, or of sufficiently long duration, tissue damage will occur.
- Excitable tissues, nerves and muscles, can be stimulated by currents that vary at a suitable rate. The change in current has to be quick enough to unbalance the ions around cell membranes, but not so quick that they do not allow time for the cell to respond. This may lead to many effects such as muscle contraction and altered pain perception. These currents are of various kinds and described in chapters 3 to 6.
- Significant heating can be generated in the body tissues if high frequency evenly alternating currents are applied because the rate of change is too high to allow time for excitable cells to respond and the chemical effects are insignificant due to the even alternation, so that relatively high current intensities can be applied. High currents cause significant heating in the tissues because they dissipate much more energy than low current intensities. Such currents, described as 'diathermy', are discussed in chapter 13. In addition to these three major effects, which may overlap, there are other less well-understood mechanisms. All are supported by some evidence and described more fully in the appropriate chapter.
- There are effects at a cellular level. Proliferation and increased migration of epithelial and connective tissue cells have been demonstrated due to the application of low-intensity current. DNA and protein synthesis may also be increased. This leads to accelerated wound healing, discussed in chapter 6. Enhanced fracture healing has been demonstrated using low intensity currents applied invasively as well as of using pulsed currents applied non-invasively (capacitatively or electromagnetically coupled). Such currents have also been applied successfully to treat connective tissue disorders.

The heating due to current flow depends on the square of the current intensity (Joule's Law:

$$H = I^2 Rt$$

where H = heat, I = current, R = resistance and t = time).

Principles Explained' by Low and Reed and 'Biophysical Bases of Electrotherapy' by Ward. Both of these books elaborate the basic science
concepts in more detail than here. Sometimes parts of the books are
explicitly referenced in margin notes. Even when not, the books may
be helpful when difficult ideas are encountered.

References

Alberts, B., Bray, D., Lewis, J. et al. (1994). Molecular Biology of the Cell, 3rd
    edn. New York: Garland Publishing Inc.

Barker, A., Jaffe, L., Vanable, J. (1982). The glabrous epidermis of cavies
    contains a powerful battery. Am J Physiol, **242**, 358–365.

Bray, J., Cragg, P., MacKnight A. et al. (1986). Lecture Notes on Human
    Physiology. London: Blackwell Scientific Publications.

Brown, W. (1998). The placebo effect. Sci Am, Jan, 68–73.

Buckwalter, J. (2002). Articular cartilage injuries. Clin Orthop Relat Res, **402**,
    21–37.

Charman, R. (1990a). Bioelectricity and electrotherapy – towards a new
    paradigm? Introduction. Physiotherapy, **76**, 502–503.

Charman, R. (1990b). Bioelectricity and electrotherapy – towards a new
    paradigm? Part 1: The electric cell. Physiotherapy, **76**, 503–508.

Charman, R. (1990c). Bioelectricity and electrotherapy – towards a new
    paradigm? Part 2: Cellular reception and emission of electromagnetic
    signals. Physiotherapy, **76**, 509–516.

Charman, R. (1990d). Bioelectricity and electrotherapy – towards a new
    paradigm? Part 3: Bioelectric potentials and tissue currents.
    Physiotherapy, **76**, 643–654.

Charman, R. (1990e). Bioelectricity and electrotherapy – towards a new
    paradigm? Part 4: Strain generated potentials in bone and connective
    tissue physiotherapy. Physiotherapy, **76**, 725–730.

Charman, R. (1990f). Bioelectricity and electrotherapy – towards a new
    paradigm? Part 5: Exogenous currents and fields – experimental and
    clinical application. Physiotherapy, **76**, 743–750.

Charman, R. (1991a). Bioelectricity and electrotherapy – towards a new
    paradigm? Part 6: Environmental current and fields – the natural
    background. Physiotherapy, **77**, 8–14.

Charman, R. (1991b). Bioelectricity and electrotherapy – towards a new
    paradigm? Part 7: Environmental current and fields – man-made.
    Physiotherapy, **77**, 129–140.

d'Arsonval, A. (1893). Influence de la fréquence sur les effets physiologiques
    des courants alternatifs. Comptes Rendus Acad Sci Paris, **116**, 630–633.

d'Arsonval, A. (1894). Action de l'électricité sur les êtres vivants. In Exposé
    des titres et traveaux scientifiques du Dr A. d'Arsonval, pp 37–77. Paris:
    Imprimerie de la cour d'appel.

Evans, D. (2003). Placebo: The Belief Effect. London: Harper Collins.

Finean, J., Coleman, R., Michell, R. (1978). Membranes and their Cellular
    Functions, 2nd edn. London: Blackwell Scientific Publications.

Foulds, I., Barker, A. (1983). Human skin battery potentials and their possible
    role in wound healing. Br J Dermatol, **109**, 515–522.

French, S. (1997). The Powerful Placebo in Physiotherapy: A Psychosocial
    Approach. Oxford: Butterworth-Heinemann.

Harrington, A. (ed.) (1997). The Placebo Effect. Cambridge, Massachusetts:
    Harvard University Press.

Hille, B. (1992). Ionic channels of excitable membranes. Sunderland, Massachusetts: Sinauer Associates Inc.

Illingworth, C., Barker, A. (1980). Measurement of electrical currents emerging during the regeneration of amputated fingertips in children. Clin Phys Physiol Measur, **1**, 87–89.

Kidd, G., Oldham, J., Stanley, J. (1988). Eutrophic electrotherapy and atrophied muscle: a pilot clinical trial. Clin Rehabil, **2**, 219–230.

Lin, T., Cardenas, L., Soslowsky, J. (2004). Biomechanics of tendon injury and repair. J Biomech, **37**, 865–877.

Sharma, P., Maffulli, N. (2005). Tendon injury and tendinopathy: healing and repair. J Bone Joint Surg, **87A**, 187–202.

Woo, S., Debski, R., Zeminski, J. et al. (2000). Injury and repair of tendons and ligaments. Ann Rev Biomed Eng, **2**, 83–118.

Electrical stimulation – currents and parameters

The discovery of electricity came piecemeal, having its origins with the discovery, around 400 BC or earlier, of the torpedo fish: a fish capable of generating an electric shock current of 100–150 V to stun its prey. It was used to treat a variety of ills and enjoyed limited but significant popularity for over 2000 years. Around 1750, batteries were invented. These provided a means of producing steady, direct current and were used by Galvani to demonstrate the effects of electric current on frog nerve and muscle. Some medical practitioners and other enthusiasts were quick to adopt the therapeutic use of electrical stimulation using batteries, then known as 'Voltaic cells'. Torpedo fish lost their popularity due to their higher maintenance cost and lesser general availability.

A problem with batteries and torpedo fish is that they produce painful jolts rather than a smooth, sustained physiological response. A turning point came in the 1800s, when the then newly discovered induction coil was used to generate current pulses by devices known as Faradic Stimulators, which were widely adopted by medical practitioners for patient treatment (Geddes, 1984). Faradic stimulators produce current pulses of brief duration, suitable for stimulating nerve, using electrodes in contact with the skin surface.

Around 1900 the alternator was invented: a device for producing sinusoidal alternating current (AC), which is still used, for example, to generate mains-supplied electricity. A French scientist, d'Arsonval pioneered the study of the physiological responses to AC electrical stimulation using the newly invented alternator and established that kHz frequency AC was best for producing comfortable, strong muscle contractions (d'Arsonval, 1894). In the 1950s Nemec (1959) promoted 'Interferential Therapy', a form of electrical stimulation, which is still popular, and which uses AC at a frequency around 4 kHz, produced electronically, for stimulation of nerve and muscle. In the mid-1970s, a Russian scientist, Kots, pioneered the use of 2.5 kHz AC for muscle strengthening and related uses and this led to the popularity of 'Russian' currents in clinical practice (Ward and Shkuratova, 2002).

Early (pre-1980s) electromedical equipment was purpose designed and easily identified. Thus a clinician might use an 'interferential', a

The modern day pulsed current stimulators used clinically are the descendents of Faradic stimulators. Most allow control of the pulse duration and frequency, which was not possible with Faradic stimulators. For comment on the history of the induction coil, see page 87 of the book 'Physical Principles Explained' on the CD which comes with this book.

'Russian current' or a 'Faradic' stimulator and could be reasonably confident of what kind of stimulus was being produced by the equipment. Modern electrical stimulators are microprocessor controlled. The heart of the stimulator (or, more correctly, the brain) is a microprocessor and the stimulus waveforms are generated by software. This means that a single machine can provide several different kinds of stimulus so it can function as any kind of stimulator with the stimulus type selected by the operator. It is therefore important that the operator knows the parameters of the available waveforms and their physiological effects. A potential further complication is that software allows many more options to users so if, for example, a wider pulse width or higher frequency can be selected, it is important that the clinician knows the effects of such choices. The advent of microprocessors and 'multi-stimulator' units has reinforced the view that electrical stimulators should be judged on the basis of the stimulus waveform parameters and the known or likely physiological effects, not on the name of the current.

The focus of chapter 3 is on the basic components of stimulation: how to use it and the currents and individual parameters. This chapter starts with an outline of the equipment used clinically and the electrode–skin interface, discusses the effects of changing different parameters, commonly available equipment and how currents are named.

Understanding the effects of the different parameters makes it possible for a user to assess the likely clinical usefulness plus the extent of any risks associated with a particular current. The next steps are to investigate the clinical effectiveness of a current and the treatment protocols used.

There are five questions which have to be answered in order for the clinician to make a rational choice between different stimulus types for treating a particular condition and achieving the desired outcome:

Some types of current cause less muscle fatigue, some more, depending on the parameters. Some currents are more likely to cause skin damage but with others it is highly improbable.

- can a particular current do what it is claimed to do and what are the clinical effects?
- are its effects different from other options?
- how credible are manufacturers' claims?
- how is it applied and altered for different outcomes?
- has it been properly tested and evaluated?

This chapter also describes the two different systems used to name currents. This, unfortunately, is a source of confusion for would-be users.

In summary, the focus of this chapter is on using electrical stimulation clinically and the parameters. To explain these, the first part describes how electrical stimulation is applied in practice and the effects of different parameters. This leads into a discussion of the different currents used clinically. The aim of this chapter is to provide a starting point for later chapters. Some of the ideas in this chapter are developed further in chapter 4, especially the underlying theory of the effects of pulsed and alternating currents. The clinical uses, effectiveness and other issues are the focus of chapter 5 (motor stimulation) and chapter 6 (sensory stimulation and pain control, iontophoresis and other uses).

USING ELECTRICAL STIMULATION CLINICALLY

Clinical applications of electrical stimulation require a power source, a stimulator, at least two electrodes and leads. This equipment can be miniature and located under the skin (a subcutaneous or indwelling stimulator), can be connected via leads on the skin surface (transcutaneous stimulation) or connected via leads which penetrate the skin (percutaneous stimulation). Examples of indwelling, or subcutaneous stimulators, include cardiac and gastric pacemakers and dorsal column stimulators. The stimulator and its power source, the leads and electrodes are all surgically located under the skin. Percutaneous stimulation is also located surgically. This is typically used for a shorter period, such as applying a direct current to a fracture site. The stimulator is kept externally but its output is applied via leads through the skin to implanted electrodes: one (the cathode) in the fracture site and the other (the anode) in more superficial tissues.

The focus of this chapter is on transcutaneous electrical stimulation. This does not require surgery for implanting as all equipment is used externally, is commonly available, and requires a broad knowledge of the effects of different parameters, as the existing options are many and varied.

Applying transcutaneous electrical stimulation

How electrical stimulation is applied will depend on the aims of treatment. Therapists need to know about the types of stimulators and electrodes and how to apply electrical stimulation to meet a range of different treatment aims. Applying stimulation transcutaneously means selecting a stimulator, electrodes and the connecting leads, understanding aspects of the electrode–skin interface and how to locate electrodes according to what is to be stimulated.

The integrity of the skin under the electrodes must be checked prior to placing them and applying current. If the skin is broken, current will selectively enter through that region as the resistance will be much lower at that point. This can cause considerable discomfort at the current intensities usually used clinically.

Assuming the skin is intact, then the electrode placement areas should be cleaned using an alcohol swab or soap and water and left slightly damp. This type of cleaning is primarily to remove any surface substances including oils that may increase the skin resistance. The next steps are to select the stimulator and the electrodes.

Stimulators

Stimulators can be mains or battery powered. The choice depends on the type of current and the number of options required. Some types of current cause too large a drain on batteries to be practical in a portable stimulator. Many clinically useful currents though, can be efficiently produced in battery-powered stimulator units. The number of hours for which a battery-powered stimulator can operate will depend on the type of current, the design of the circuitry, and the operating intensity.

The major advantage of a portable stimulator is that a user can carry it and apply current throughout the day or night, as needed. This is especially important if used for pain control, for joint or soft tissue mobilizing, and in some instances of strengthening muscle. Also, portable stimulators are often considerably cheaper than the mains-powered ones and safer if the maximum output intensity is suitably restricted.

Larger, mains-powered stimulators are effectively not portable as they are designed to be used while plugged in. Their main advantage is that they can be designed as a multistimulator and supply a large range of different types of currents at any required intensity with no limit on the treatment duration. Alternatively, they can be limited to the one type of current and this, typically, will be one that drains too much current to be practical in a battery-powered device.

While any mains-powered equipment is potentially not as safe as its battery-powered counterpart, the international safety standards for electromedical equipment ensure that the risk of shock from the mains supply is negligible. Stringent design and construction requirements ensure that compliant equipment is actually safer than many mains-powered domestic appliances. The danger with the equipment is that the available output intensity is often high enough to cause electrocution. It is for this reason that use should be restricted to appropriately qualified clinicians.

Stimulators can be constant voltage or constant current: they cannot be both at the same time. During stimulation the impedance (resistance to current flow) of the skin and electrodes may change, for example, during treatment the skin normally becomes slightly more hydrated under the electrodes and its electrical impedance decreases so current can flow more readily. Ohm's Law indicates that if the voltage is kept constant and the resistance drops then the current must increase. Conversely, if the current is to be kept constant, the voltage must decrease.

Whether a machine is a constant voltage or constant current machine depends on its design. For clinicians the focus is on the implications, summarized in Table 3.1.

Table 3.1 indicates the importance of the skin–electrode interface at the start and throughout a treatment in ensuring a constant flow of current through the skin. Over time the skin conductivity can

For example, the stimulus intensity required to produce a forceful contraction of the quadriceps could be fatal if applied trans-thoracically.

For more information on Ohm's Law, voltage and current see chapter 1 of the book 'Biophysical Bases of Electrotherapy' and chapter 4, page 35 of 'Physical Principles Explained' on the CD which comes with this book.

Table 3.1 Constant current and constant voltage stimulators

Event	Change in impedance	Effect if constant current	Effect if constant voltage
Electrodes drying on skin	Increase	None[1]	Reduced current, may no longer be enough
Electrodes pushed against skin	Decrease	None	Increased current, if sudden can feel like a small shock
Electrode lifting off skin	Increase	Increased current density	Drop in current, may no longer be enough
Increased sweating under electrode	Decrease	None	Increased current and current density

[1] Risk of localized increases in current density if drying is not uniform.

increase, i.e. the impedance can decrease, as the skin becomes better hydrated. If an electrode dries or contact with the skin decreases the conductivity will decrease, i.e. the impedance will increase. This table also indicates that users and therapists should be advised not to push on an electrode if current is flowing as, depending on the type of equipment, it can cause an increased current flow.

In terms of constancy of stimulation, constant current stimulators have the advantage as the current, the main stimulating component, remains constant irrespective of changes to the electrodes and skin. A single, major problem with constant current stimulators is that if there is any decrease in the area of electrode contacting the skin, the current density will increase and can cause discomfort and possibly skin damage (an electrical burn). Constant voltage stimulators offer less constancy of stimulation but are intrinsically safer as, if the contact area decreases, the current will decrease proportionally and the current density will not change. The decrease in impedance with sweating, a potential problem for constant voltage stimulators, is small and insignificant in practice and the resulting increase in current density is small. For safety reasons, constant voltage stimulators are preferred.

The risk of electrical burns from constant current stimulators is small, however, the possibility of skin damage and the potential legal consequences can mitigate against their use unless they have inbuilt detection and alarm systems to warn of excessive current density increases.

Safety recommendations

Before treatment, the output should be tested by the therapists on themselves. Electrical apparatus should be turned on and tested before connecting the patient to the circuit. At the end of the treatment, the output should be turned to zero and the patient disconnected. The machine should only be switched off after this. The reason is that on some older equipment there is a spike of output at switch-on and/or switch-off before the machine stabilizes and this might deliver a shock.

Summary

- The skin integrity should always be checked prior to electrical stimulation and protective measures implemented if necessary
- Battery-powered stimulators are:
  - not suitable for all current types
  - portable and often the cheaper, more convenient option
  - safer as the maximum output intensity is normally restricted
- Mains-powered stimulators can provide
  - a range of types of currents
  - unlimited treatment duration
  - output intensities sufficient to produce any desired effect
- Constant voltage stimulators are inherently safer than constant current devices
- Before treatment, the output should be tested by therapists on themselves.

ELECTRODES

The appropriate selection of electrodes for transcutaneous electrical stimulation is important. The type of electrode is the first of three issues to consider and the size, the second. The third concerns where on the body electrodes should be located.

Type of electrodes

Electrodes provide not just a means of applying current to the body, but also a means of distributing it. Electrode systems vary but there are two common elements:

- the electrode itself, which may be self-adhesive, metal foil or conductive rubber (carbon-impregnated silicone rubber). Metal foil electrodes were used traditionally but they have been largely superseded by self-adhesive and conductive rubber electrodes.
- the coupling medium which provides a conductive bridge between the electrode and the skin. This is an integral part of self-adhesive electrodes. With conductive rubber electrodes an adhesive gel pad is often used. The coupling gel-pad, which is solid but soft and flexible, is both electrically conductive and adhesive. There is no need to strap the electrodes onto the skin to ensure conduction unless electrode-gel (a spreadable conductive jelly) has been used instead. With metal foil electrodes, the coupling medium may be an electrode-gel or a wetted pad of lint, cotton gauze or some form of sponge material which absorbs and retains water. Metal electrodes using spreadable gel or wetted pads must be held in contact by straps or bandages.

Ordinary tap water is a reasonable conductor because of its ion content but in some soft-water areas a little salt or bicarbonate of soda may need to be added to increase the conductivity.

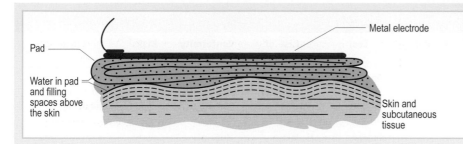

Figure 3.1 An example of how currents are applied to the tissues using a conductive couplant between the electrode and the skin.

Figure 3.1 illustrates the arrangement using the example of a metal electrode and a wet pad couplant. As noted above, the electrode may be self-adhesive or conductive rubber and the couplant may be a flexible adhesive gel-pad or spreadable gel. In each case, the aim is to ensure good electrical contact with the skin over the whole of the electrode area.

The choice of electrodes must be made on the basis of a cost/benefit analysis. Self-adhesive electrodes are simple to apply and require no strapping. They have an adhesive gel which is inseparable from the cloth/rubber backing so this means that the assembly is discarded in entirety. They can, however, be reused for the same patient. They must be stored in a sealed bag, as recommended by the manufacturer, and may require some rehydration after a few uses. Their advantage is convenience of use, as adhesion eliminates the need for strapping while ensuring good electrical contact over the whole of the electrode area. Their disadvantage is the cost. Metal electrodes applied with a wetted pad or sponge offer the lowest cost per treatment as they are reusable. The disadvantage is they have to be strapped or held on and they must be cleaned appropriately after every use. Reusable conductive rubber electrodes with gel or disposable adhesive gel pads offer a useful compromise. The gel is washed off or the gel pads are discarded after one use but the conductive rubber electrodes can be cleaned and reused.

The treatment period is a relevant factor. Reusable, self-adhesive electrodes or separate gel pads cost more to buy, but the convenience is much greater if the patient requires treatment over an extended period. With the metal electrode and sponge option, there is a known risk of transferring infection when the sponges used with metal electrodes are not properly cleaned (Lambert et al., 2000). This risk of cross-infection applies equally to the use of lint and cotton gauze and perhaps even to carbon rubber electrodes. In an era of increasingly antibiotic-resistant bacteria, the need to clean carefully and the risks and time and material costs of this process should be carefully considered by a therapist when selecting the type of electrodes to be used. Table 3.2 summarizes the important differences between electrode types.

Table 3.2 Summary of differences between electrodes

Type	Size	Reusability	Cost	Ease of application	Conformity to skin	Risks[6]	Cleaning
Self-adhesive	Range of shapes and sizes but some limitations	Yes, but limited to single patient	High	Very high	High	Low	See manufacturer's guidelines
Carbon rubber and gel[1]	Range of shapes and sizes but some limitations	Yes, after cleaning	Moderate to low	Moderate – limited by rigidity of electrode and slipperiness of gel	Moderate but must tape on	Low to moderate	Wash in soapy water, rinse, air dry
Carbon rubber and gel pads[1]	Range of shapes and sizes but some limitations	Yes, after cleaning but gel pad single use	Moderate as gel pads are single use	Moderate – limited by rigidity of electrode	Moderate	Low	Soak off and discard gel pad. Wash in soapy water, rinse, air dry
Metal[2] and sponge[3]	Any size required, can be cut to size and shape	Yes, after cleaning	Low	Moderate – needs firm covering to keep in place[5]	Moderate to high	Low to moderate	Wash electrode as above. Soak sponge in suitable cleaning solution, rinse thoroughly, air dry
Metal and lint[4]	Any size required, can be cut to size and shape	Yes, after cleaning	Low	Moderate but needs firm covering to keep in place	Moderate to high	Low to moderate	Wash electrode as above. Soak lint in suitable cleaning solution, rinse thoroughly, air dry
Purpose specific metal	e.g. vaginal and anal electrodes	Yes, after cleaning	Moderate	Moderate	Purpose designed	Low to moderate	Wash electrode as recommended by manufacturer

[1] electrically conducting gel designed for clinical use

[2] can be thin aluminium or lead, must be flexible to conform with skin curvatures

[3] damp first with either saline or water to enable conduction, depth should be at least 0.5 cm, more if area is irregular or near bony prominences

[4] lint or a similar material which can be folded and retains moisture, should be at least 1 cm thick to retain sufficient moisture for a 15 to 30 minute treatment

[5] alternative is to use a suction cup with inbuilt metal electrode and removable sponges, increases ease of use

[6] risks refer only to risks due to properties of the electrode; the type of current used changes the general level of risk

Size of electrodes

Electrode size is very important and has to be considered in conjunction with the types of electrodes available and where they are to be located. As a general principle, the larger the better. Larger electrodes result in more comfortable stimulation (Alon et al., 1994). When being used for sensory stimulation, for pain control, a greater level of stimulation is possible with larger electrodes. If using stimulation to produce a motor response, a stronger response is likely (Alon et al., 1994). These results have to be considered in relation to the size of the muscle or area being stimulated and the availability of the size needed in the different types of electrode.

Larger electrodes result in lower current densities. When current passes through the body the total current at each of the two electrodes will be equal but an important factor is that if the two electrodes are of unequal size, the current density (i.e. current per unit area) at each will be different. If being used to stimulate muscle, this means that most effects will occur close to the smaller electrode, which is usually called the 'active' electrode. The larger electrode is called the 'indifferent' or 'dispersive' electrode and is positioned so as to avoid direct stimulation of excitable tissue. Small electrodes have a higher current density than larger and are more likely to cause pain (Patterson and Lockwood, 1993). Another implication of using larger electrodes, relative to the size of a muscle being stimulated is that the current path must, of necessity, be larger. This means that more nerve fibres are likely to be stimulated as more will be in the path of the current. Similarly, if for pain control, a larger electrode will stimulate more cutaneous nerve fibres than a smaller electrode.

The effects of an applied current will be evident where the current density, the intensity of current per unit area ($mA\,cm^{-2}$) is highest. Because of current spreading (Figure 3.2), the current density is highest close to the electrodes and decreases rather dramatically with distance (the inverse square law is a rough but useful guide). In the example shown in Figure 3.2, the area shown at depth is about three times that of the electrode, so the current density is about one third. This means that the cutaneous sensory nerves which are close to the electrodes will be affected most readily and the more deeply placed motor nerves, less so.

As a consequence, when low current density stimulation is applied to the skin, the sensory nerves, which normally respond to touch, temperature and pressure, are the first to be stimulated. This causes a mild tapping or tingling sensation. As the current (and consequently the

To limit the effects to an area such as the motor point of a muscle, the active electrode can be a small metal disc covered with lint or other suitable material and attached to a handle. This is often called a button or probe electrode. In addition, purpose designed anal and vaginal metal electrodes are also available.

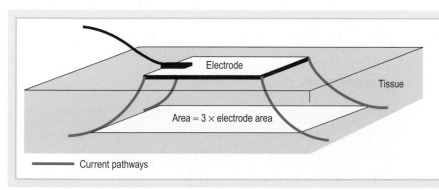

Electrode

Tissue

Area ≈ 3 × electrode area

Current pathways

Figure 3.2 Current spreading reduces the effective stimulation intensity which depends on the current per unit area, i.e. current density.

current density) is increased, greater sensory stimulation is produced and motor nerve fibres, located more deeply, are recruited, producing muscle contraction.

Further increases in the current produce rather large increases in the force of muscle contraction as recruitment increases rapidly, quite disproportionate to the increase in stimulus intensity. More motor units are recruited as action potentials occur in more of the small branches of nerves in the area where current is flowing. This results in both stronger and more widespread muscle contraction. Still further increases of current will eventually cause pain nerve fibres to be stimulated.

Location of electrodes

Notice that the phrase – 'to stimulate a muscle' – is a convenience. The current is stimulating the motor nerve which conveys nerve action potentials to stimulate the muscle fibres. The actual muscle fibres are not stimulated directly.

The third aspect to be considered is where to locate the electrodes on the skin. Clearly, the positioning of the electrodes is one determinant of the site of greatest current density and hence which nerves are affected. For example, in order to stimulate a normally innervated muscle effectively but painlessly the active electrode is applied to the motor point. This is a point on the skin surface at which maximum muscle contraction can be achieved. Motor points are usually close to the point where the motor nerve enters the muscle. Current applied at this point – often at the junction of the proximal third with the distal two-thirds of the muscle belly – will activate a large number of motor units as the innervating fibres are close together. Thus less current density will be needed than if the muscle belly were stimulated directly.

The specific locations for electrodes will depend on the treatment aims but there are guidelines to help a user make appropriate choices. If the aim is to stimulate an innervated muscle, it is important to ensure the nerve supplying that muscle is in the current path. That indicates two main options:

- over the nerve trunk or over the motor point of the muscle (Figure 3.3)
- at either end of the muscle so the nerve must be in the current path.

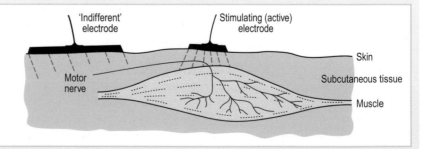

Figure 3.3 Stimulation over the motor point of a muscle using a 'unipolar' electrode setup.

The first option is to stimulate the nerve supply directly by deliberate placement and sizing of the electrodes. To concentrate the current to the one area requires using different sized electrodes. This means the current density will be higher under the electrode with a smaller surface area in contact with the skin than under the other, larger electrode. For example if the current flowing between the electrodes in Figure 3.3 is 10 mA and the area of the indifferent electrode is 25 cm^2 and that of the active electrode is 1 cm^2, then the current density under the indifferent electrode is $10/25 = 0.4$ mA cm^{-2}, while the current density under the active electrode is $10/1 = 10$ mA cm^{-2}. The current through each electrode is the same so the current density is inversely proportional to the electrode area. In the example used, the area of the active electrode is 1/25 that of the indifferent electrode so the current density is 25 times higher.

Unipolar electrode setup. The term 'unipolar' can be confusing. It does not imply stimulation using a single electrode (two must always be used). Rather it refers to one electrode being more 'active' than the other (see Figure 3.3). Unipolar electrode setups apply the concept of current density. The user places the smaller (active) electrode over the nerve supply. For example, if stimulating the quadriceps femoris, the smaller electrode could be placed directly over the femoral nerve as it transits under the inguinal ligament lateral to the femoral artery. The larger (dispersive or indifferent) electrode can then be placed where it is even less likely to stimulate anything, on the lower abdomen or back or on the lateral aspect of the contralateral leg.

Unipolar electrode setups are also used to stimulate a specific muscle or muscle belly. The electrode can be a smaller sized electrode of any type including a button or probe electrode. The indifferent electrode is usually applied away from the muscle being stimulated. Limitations of unipolar electrode setups include problems with stimulating a muscle when the nerve trunk cannot be accessed. Another problem might occur when a therapist wishes to stimulate a group of muscles at the same time. This is solved by using a bipolar electrode setup.

Bipolar electrode placements. A bipolar method of electrode placement uses two equal or nearly equal size electrodes placed at either end of the muscle belly or group to be stimulated (Figure 3.4). The size equivalence means equal current density under each electrode. Their location at either end of the belly or group means that the relevant motor nerves will inevitably be in the current pathway between the pair of electrodes and so can be stimulated.

The size of electrodes needed will depend on the size of the muscle or group to be stimulated. Generally speaking, small muscles should be treated using small electrodes and large muscles or groups, large electrodes.

If the aim is to stimulate a denervated muscle a bipolar placement is usually used. The reason is that a denervated muscle is much harder to stimulate than an innervated one. Motor nerves, like sensory nerve

Clinical guideline: look for a muscle motor point at the junction of the upper and middle third of the muscle belly.

Figure 3.4 Stimulation using a bipolar electrode setup.

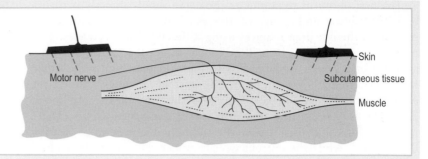

Skin

Subcutaneous tissue

Muscle

Motor nerve

fibres are highly excitable and so easily stimulated. When the motor nerve supply is damaged then the muscle fibres have to be stimulated directly. This means the current needs to flow directly through as many muscle fibres as possible so, generally speaking, large electrodes should be used. Greater electrical energy is needed and long duration current pulses are effective in achieving this end. With small muscles the therapist may use probes or purpose-designed caliper electrodes but again, long pulse durations would be used.

Another aim of using electrical stimulation might be to decrease a patient's perception of pain. This requires increasing the level of sensory input, ideally into the same dermatomes as the structures causing pain. This is best done by using a bipolar technique to reduce the chances of motor stimulation. Using relatively large electrodes for the area being treated ensures a reduced current density and a greater level of sensory input, as a larger number of superficial afferent sensory nerves will be directly beneath the electrodes, where the current density is highest.

Variations on bipolar and unipolar electrode placements exist. For example, one electrode can be replaced by two or more with a combined area equal to the one being replaced. Both setups can be modified in other ways to suit the particular aim of the therapist.

Water bath treatment. Water bath application of current typically involves a hand, forearm, leg or foot being immersed in water through which current is flowing. Either type of electrode placement can be used. Figure 3.5 shows a foot positioned between two equal-size electrodes for bipolar treatment. Bare metal or carbon rubber electrodes are placed within the water bath (no salt is used as it would facilitate current flow through the water, reducing it through the tissue). A smaller electrode can be placed adjacent to the area to be treated or nerve to be stimulated and the dispersive left in the water but to the side. Alternatively, a bipolar placement with both electrodes under the foot or hand can be used. The water provides a sufficiently conductive ionic medium that there is little risk of uneven applications of current to the hand, forearm, leg or foot being treated.

Summary

- Electrode placements may be 'unipolar' or 'bipolar'.

Unipolar:
- unequal current density. Current is concentrated under the smaller (can be button or probe) electrode
- use the smaller electrode over a motor point or stimulate over nerve trunk

Bipolar:
- equal current density under each electrode
- applied either end of a muscle belly or muscle group

Variations which depend on aim:
- can bifurcate one or both electrodes
- include using a water bath to treat a hand, forearm, leg or foot.

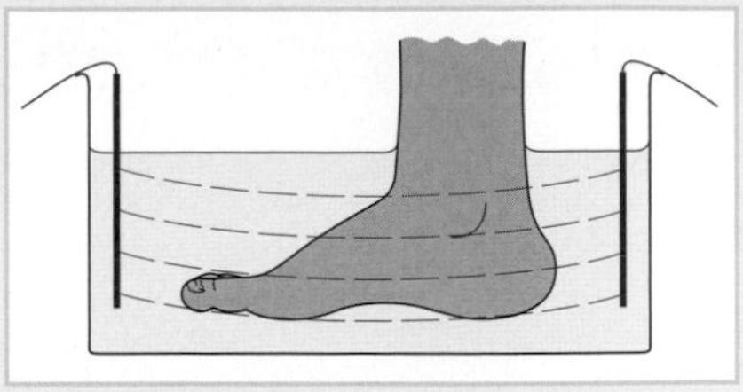

Figure 3.5 Water bath stimulation using a bipolar electrode setup.

The electrode–tissue interface

When electric current flows through tissue between a pair of electrodes, electrochemical effects can be produced. If the current flow is direct (DC), acid accumulates under one electrode and base under the other. The effect and its consequences are described in more detail later in this chapter. If the applied current is charge balanced (i.e. is alternating current, AC, so that equal amounts of charge flow backwards and forwards) there are no significant chemical changes; also if the total current, although unidirectional (DC), is very small (low-intensity and/or very short pulses) the chemical effects will be negligible.

A layer of ion-containing fluid is needed to pass current from the electrode to the tissues, normally skin. This is water or conducting gel. Gels used for this purpose are generally made primarily of water, ionic salts ($NaCl$ or KCl), a surfactant and fungicide and bactericide (McAdams et al., 1996). The gel or water provides a uniform conducting pathway between the electrode and the epidermis as it fills the pores and skin irregularities under the electrode. Otherwise, as the epidermal surface is very irregular a flat electrode pressed onto it would be in contact at only a few points, leading to a high current density at these points. Further, the epidermal surface has a high electrical resistance because it is largely dry keratin and because of the presence of oily sebum. This resistance is lowered by wetting the skin surface. It also reduces after an electrode and gel have been in contact with it as the water in the gel gradually diffuses through the skin and increases its conductivity (McAdams et al., 1996). Sometimes users may also warm the skin with a hot pack or infrared lamp prior to commencing treatment. The aim is to produce a local increase in sweat and a resultant increase in conductivity.

Warming the skin with a hot pack or infrared lamp prior to commencing treatment can produce a local increase in sweat and a resultant increased conductivity.

When the skin is not even, such as with large warts or scars, special care can be required. Applying current through them can mean uneven current distribution through the skin and insufficient conformity of the electrode to the skin. As with any other effective barriers to current flow through the skin this can produce areas of higher current flow than anticipated and may increase any risk of skin damage.

The integrity of the skin under the electrodes must be checked prior to placing them and applying current. If the skin is broken, current will selectively enter through that region as the resistance will be much lower at that point. This can cause considerable discomfort at the current intensities usually used clinically. The exception is when treating wounds. The difference with this type of treatment is the current intensity: much lower than is otherwise used. If the skin has a small area of damage, treatment can continue but the break must be covered by a non-conducting barrier such as a suitably sized waterproof dressing or lint or gauze with a petroleum jelly covering. Using this type of barrier is only justified if the treatment must be continued and there is no increased risk of infection or skin damage (Robertson and Ward, 2002). The option is to use a different electrode location, possible if aiming to provide sensory input but not always if stimulating a particular muscle.

Assuming the skin is intact, then the electrode placement areas should be cleaned using an alcohol swab or soap and water followed by careful drying so as to leave the skin moist but not wet. This type of cleaning is primarily to remove any surface substances including oils that may increase the skin resistance.

Skin

The amount of current flowing through tissue depends on the applied voltage and the resistance, according to Ohm's Law:

$$V = IR$$

where V is the applied voltage, R is the resistance and I is the resulting current flow. Current has to flow from one electrode through the couplant (water or gel) then skin and into the underlying tissues and must then flow through another layer of skin and couplant to the opposite electrode (see Figures 3.3 and 3.4). The resulting resistance is the sum of the resistances in each part of the current pathway (see chapter 4 for more details). This is because the parts are in series (meaning that the current must flow through each in turn).

In a typical treatment setup, the resistance of the electrodes and couplant are low as is the resistance of the subcutaneous tissue (which is highly hydrated). The skin resistance, however, is much higher. This is due to the high resistance of the stratum corneum.

Figure 3.6 shows some important features of skin, which comprises the dermis and epidermis. The epidermis is punctured by the skin appendages: the sweat gland ducts and hair follicles. Beneath the skin

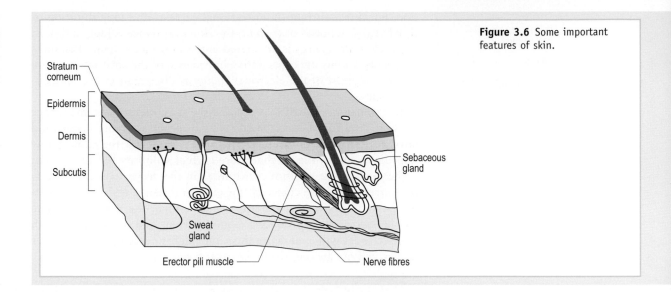

Figure 3.6 Some important features of skin.

is the subcutis, also referred to as the superficial fascia or simply sub-cutaneous tissue. In most areas of the body, the subcutis is predominantly adipose (fat storing) tissue. Blood vessels, lymph vessels and nerves infiltrate the subcutis and dermis but not the epidermis. The dermis and subcutis have low electrical resistance. It might be thought that the subcutis, which is often adipose tissue, would have a high resistance because fat is an insulator, but the resistance is low as conductive channels (blood and lymph vessels) infiltrate the tissue.

No blood or lymph vessels infiltrate the epidermis. It is avascular, meaning that the cells (keratinocytes) must derive their nutrients by diffusion from capillaries in the underlying dermis. The basal layer of the epidermis is metabolically very active, with the cells regularly undergoing mitosis. Keratinocytes, formed and pushed upwards from this layer, synthesize keratin, which is retained within the cell. In their life cycle, the keratinocytes move towards the skin surface, becoming less metabolically active as diffusion limits the rate of nutrient supply. Near the surface the cells die and shrivel, finally forming a scaly shell called the stratum corneum. The stratum corneum is thus a layer of shrivelled, dead, dehydrated keratinocytes. The dead keratinocytes are tiny packages of keratin. This has important implications when applying current transcutaneously.

Where two low-resistance regions are separated by a high-resistance region, i.e. a near insulator, a capacitor is formed and capacitive effects occur. Thus, where an electrode is separated from nerve and muscle in the underlying tissue by skin (more specifically the stratum corneum), there is a capacitor. The concept of these electrical pathways is illustrated in Figure 3.7.

A special thing about capacitors is that they impede the flow of current, but the extent of this impedance depends on the pulse dura-

For more information on capacitors and capacitative effects, see chapters 1 and 2 of the book 'Biophysical Bases of Electrotherapy' on the CD which comes with this book.

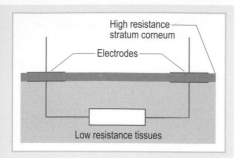

Figure 3.7 Electrical pathways of current applied to the tissues.

tion. For direct current (unidirectional current) and long duration or slowly varying pulses of current, the skin impedance is high and most of the electrical energy is dissipated in the stratum corneum. For short bursts of current, the capacitive impedance of the stratum corneum is low and most of the electrical energy is dissipated in the underlying tissues.

It is sometimes stated that because the skin offers a low impedance to short duration pulses, the current can penetrate more deeply and have greater effect on deeper structures. This is not the case. A low impedance simply means that more current will flow but the current is the same in the stratum corneum as in the deeper tissues and it is the current (or more correctly, the current density) which determines the biological effects. If the impedance is high, the stimulus voltage can be increased to produce a higher current and all tissue beneath the electrodes will experience the same, higher current, i.e. the deeper tissues will not be selectively disadvantaged.

Nerve fibres

Stimulation with short duration current pulses has long been recognized as more comfortable than with longer duration pulses. It is an interesting exercise to test this empirically using a clinical stimulator which can deliver, say, 50 μs, 200 μs, 1 ms and 5 ms pulses. If the intensity is adjusted to the motor threshold at each pulse duration, the subjective sensation of discomfort increases with increasing pulse duration. The reason is that different nerve fibre types respond differently to variations in pulse width.

The difference in behaviour of different nerve fibre types is seen in their strength–duration properties. A strength–duration (S-D) graph shows how much current or voltage is necessary to produce a particular response (pain, motor or sensory) when using pulses of different durations. Figure 3.8 illustrates the variation.

For very short duration pulses a very high current (or voltage) is necessary to get a response. Up to about 100 μs there is a steep drop in the amount of current required. From 100 μs to 1 ms the rate of drop is steady but less. When pulses are longer than 1 ms there is little change in the intensity of current required. The other noticeable feature of an S-D graph (which is relevant when deciding what type of current to use clinically) is the changing separation between sensory, motor and pain responses.

Figure 3.8 indicates that the first response will normally be a sensory one. This is because the nerves closest to the electrodes are the sensory nerves with receptors in the skin and subcutaneous tissues. This is where the current density is highest. Current density is an important factor with stimulation.

A second important factor is the nerve fibre diameter. The larger the diameter, the lower is the threshold for excitation. Sensory and motor fibres are similar: they are large diameter, myelinated, fast-

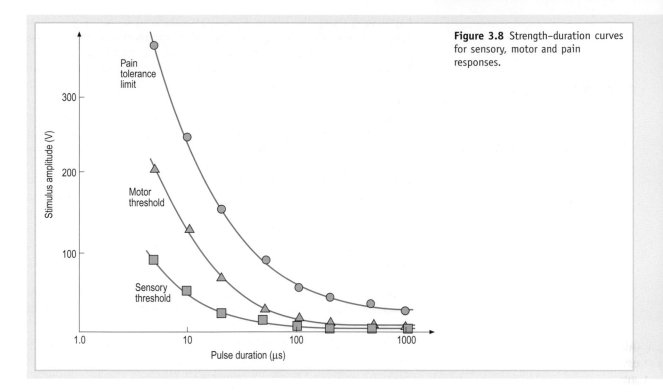

Figure 3.8 Strength–duration curves for sensory, motor and pain responses.

conducting fibres and are more readily stimulated than the smaller diameter pain fibres. Some motor nerves (A-α fibres or alpha-motoneurons) have larger diameters than the widest sensory fibres (A-β fibres) and on this basis should be excited before sensory nerves. In practice the sensory threshold is, more often than not, reached first because of the closer proximity of the sensory fibres to the electrodes. With some individuals, the motor threshold can be reached before the sensory threshold. These individuals have very little subcutaneous adipose tissue as assessed by measurements of skinfold thickness (Ward and Robertson, unpublished findings).

The sensation of pain is conveyed by A-δ and C fibres. A-δ are myelinated but are smaller diameter and slower conducting than sensory and motor fibres. They convey the sensation of prickling, stabbing pain. Their smaller diameter means that they are less excitable, i.e. have a higher threshold, so that pain is always above the sensory threshold even though most pain fibres are located superficially. C fibres have the smallest diameters. They are unmyelinated and have the slowest nerve conduction velocity. They convey the sensation of deep aching pain and have the highest activation thresholds.

Unlike the sensory and motor graphs shown in Figure 3.8, the pain graph is not a true indication of pain threshold but rather shows the maximum tolerable limit. Subjects are asked to turn the intensity up to a level beyond which they decide is 'too uncomfortable' (see, for

If you stand on a drawing pin, the sharp, stabbing sensation conveyed by A-δ fibres is quickly noticed. A deep, aching pain sensation is felt several seconds later because of the lower conduction velocity of the C fibres.

example Alon et al., 1983). Pain (particularly A-δ) fibres would be recruited far earlier than this threshold so the motor response could be painful but not intolerably so. The pain S-D graph indicates the maximum tolerable and this depends on the total amount of pain (A-δ and C) fibre activity. Although not indicative of actual pain thresholds, the pain S-D graph is a useful indicator of intensities which should not be exceeded in clinical practice. A lot of leeway is evident at short pulse durations, where the sensory and motor thresholds can be considerably exceeded without reaching the pain tolerance limit.

The S-D graph suggests a user who wants a sensory response (for pain control) and no motor response should use a shorter pulse than someone who wants to produce a muscle contraction, also called a motor response. A motor response with pulses of 300 to 600 μs is more likely to be comfortable than if a longer pulse, 1000 μs (1 ms) or more is used. With a longer pulse duration only a very small change in current intensity is required to change from a just perceived stimulus to a motor and then a pain response. Thus an S-D graph indicates how some of the parameters of a clinically used current might be used to produce different outcomes.

This explains why short pulse lengths are more easily able to stimulate deeply located fibres. As Figure 3.8 shows, with short pulses the stimulus intensity can be increased well above the motor threshold without reaching the pain tolerance limit. Hence the intensity at depth is more likely to be high enough to stimulate deeply placed low-threshold nerves, such as motor nerves. With longer duration pulses, stimulus intensities not much above the motor threshold are likely to be painful. Thus to stimulate high-threshold unmyelinated pain fibres (C fibres) in the skin it is appropriate to use longer pulses of a few milliseconds.

> This effect of pulse duration occurs with both single pulses and alternating pulses of appropriate frequency, i.e. a 4000 Hz medium-frequency alternating current is a series of 0.125 ms pulses (half cycles) and behaves in a similar way to separate single pulses of this duration.

EFFECTS OF DIFFERENT PARAMETERS

Current is defined as the rate of flow of charge, i.e. the amount of charge moved per second. The current can be unidirectional, steady and continuous (direct current, DC), a whole series of separate unidirectional pulses (pulsed DC), or a continuous set of alternating pulses (alternating current) which may be symmetrical or asymmetrical. The parameters are the variables that make each type of current different.

The main response of the body to clinical electrical stimulation is via the peripheral nervous system. Thus understanding action potentials and something of how a nerve responds to current makes it possible to understand about choosing currents and setting parameters. Some machines are supplied with preset currents and parameters. Others offer more options. To be an effective user, a clinician needs to understand how changing a parameter might affect the outcome for a patient.

The previous discussion of S-D graphs indicated the roles of pulse duration and intensity in excitation of different types of nerve. There are other effects that some current parameters have that can also be used clinically, as the following discussion indicates.

Polarity

Polarity, in the context of electric current, means charge imbalance. Current flow, the movement of charge, can be unidirectional or bidirectional. If unidirectional, the charges do not change direction and the current flow has (positive or negative) polarity. Unidirectional flow is a key feature of direct current (DC), such as that supplied by a battery which has a positive terminal and a negative terminal, i.e. positive and negative poles. When direct current flows through tissue, negative ions (anions) move from the negatively charged electrode (the cathode) to the positively charged electrode (the anode), while positive ions (cations) move in the opposite direction. Thus, if direct current is applied to the body via skin-mounted electrodes, there will be a build up of ions under the electrodes. Under the cathode (negative electrode) an excess of positive ions will accumulate. Under the anode (positive electrode) there will be a corresponding accumulation of negative ions. If the current is alternating (AC) there may be no accumulation of charge. The examples shown in Figure 3.9 illustrate the distinction between DC and AC.

The stimulus waveforms shown in Figure 3.9(a) and (b) would result in charge build up. The waveform shown in 3.9(c) would not as the positive phases are the same size as the negative phases, so the resulting charge movements would cancel.

The stimulus waveforms used clinically are often more complex than those shown in Figure 3.9 and it is important to know whether the current is balanced or imbalanced. For example, pulsed current could have a waveform resembling one of those shown in Figure 3.10. In each case the current flow is biphasic.

The amount of charge moving in each direction can be equal (balanced) or unequal (unbalanced). The waveform shown in Figure 3.10(a) is unbalanced: there is a greater net current flow in the positive than in the negative direction. The waveform shown in Figure 3.10(b) is balanced.

> For more information on DC, AC and charge movement, see chapters 1 and 2 of the book 'Biophysical Bases of Electrotherapy' on the CD which comes with this book.

Electrolytic effects of different waveforms

When DC (interrupted or continuous) or unbalanced biphasic pulses are applied via skin-mounted electrodes, electrolytic effects will occur. This is because of the build-up of ions under each electrode. The result is a change in the pH of the couplant between the electrodes and the skin surface. The area under the cathode will become more alkaline and that under the anode more acidic. A sufficient ionic build-up will

Figure 3.12 The variation in muscle force production with short-duration pulsed current in the frequency range 2 Hz to 50 Hz.

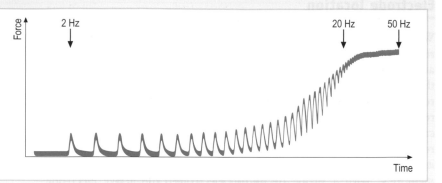

difficult to distinguish the effects of individual stimuli. The twitch responses fuse and the contraction becomes stronger still. With most human muscles, at a stimulus frequency of about 20 Hz, only small ripples are seen in the force record. This is described as partial tetany. Between 20 and 50 Hz, the ripples disappear, the contractile force reaches a plateau and the contraction is described as tetanic.

Figure 3.12 illustrates the effect of a progressive increase in stimulus frequency on the evoked muscle response. Here the frequency has been ramped from 2 Hz to 50 Hz. At about 20 Hz, the response is almost tetanic. Above this frequency complete tetany occurs. Note that the tetanic force is about four times greater than the twitch force.

In Figure 3.12, the fusion frequency is about 30 Hz. The fusion frequency varies between muscles and depends on the muscle fibre types present. In terms of twitch times, two groups of fibres are distinguished: fast and slow twitch. The soleus muscle contain mostly (about 80%) slow twitch fibres. The twitch contraction time is long and consequently the fusion frequency is low. At the opposite extreme, orbicularis oculi, an eye movement muscle, contains about 85% fast twitch fibres and the fusion frequency is high. Fusion frequencies can vary from less than 20 Hz to close to 80 Hz. Many human skeletal muscles have roughly equal proportions of slow and fast twitch fibres. For example, biceps and triceps brachii are comprised of about 60% fast twitch fibres, while the figure for quadriceps is close to 50%.

The use of higher stimulus frequencies (50 Hz or more) for greater force production is questionable. Changing the frequency from, say, 40 Hz to 80 Hz will produce a marginal increase in force but the rate of fatigue will double.

Frequencies of around 30–40 Hz cause smooth contractions of muscle and are commonly used clinically unless a higher torque is required in which case the frequency is increased to 50 Hz or more. Frequencies below 30 Hz are not normally used for muscle contraction because of the lower resulting force and the twitching or fluttering nature of the contraction.

In voluntary contractions, motor nerve firing rates rarely exceed 40 Hz (McComas, 1996). In a sustained, weak voluntary contraction, firing rates of 8–12 Hz are typical. Lower firing rates are found with repetitive weak contractions. For a steady, sustained forceful contraction, an upper limit to the firing rate seems to be about 30 Hz in human skeletal muscle. These are firing frequencies which result in a partially fused contraction. This raises the question of how smooth, controlled voluntary movements are possible when low forces are involved and the nerve firing rates are very low. Figure 3.12 indicates that twitching or fluttering will occur when the firing rates are below the fusion frequency. However, the voluntary activity of different motor units is asynchronous. Although individual motor units may be firing at low frequency and producing a fluttering, partly fused contraction in individual muscle fibres, there is no synchronization between different motor units. At the level of the whole muscle, the total force is the sum of the contributions of all active motor units so the ripples in force output from each motor unit are smoothed, i.e. lost in the total. By contrast, when muscles are activated electrically, all of the activated fibres are synchronously activated so smooth contractions are only possible when the induced firing frequencies are greater than, or equal to, the fusion frequency.

Shape of pulses

For the most efficient stimulation of nerve fibres, a rectangular stimulus (see Figure 3.9b) is optimal. A vertical leading edge means an almost instantaneous increase in current to the maximum level. This increases the likelihood of an action potential occurring. All that is required is sufficient charge movement due to the pulse. If the current increases more slowly, the nerve fibre can accommodate to the current flow. The threshold potential increases and generation of an action potential is less likely (Spielholz and Nolan, 1995). Figure 3.13 illustrates the effect.

This means that nerve stimulation is ideally done using a rectangular pulse, capitalizing on the lack of time for the nerve fibre to accommodate. However, if the pulse is of sufficiently short duration, the rise time is not an issue: it will be short enough to avoid any measurable accommodation. For example, rectangular and triangular pulses of 250 μs or less are functionally equivalent as the difference in slope does not affect the chance of an action potential: accommodation is negligible with either pulse. For pulses of several ms duration, accommodation can be clinically important and will mean either that no action potential will result or that a higher current intensity will be needed.

Pulse duration

A pulse duration is measured in μs or ms for most clinical purposes. An electrical pulse needs to produce a certain minimal amount of charge movement to cause an action potential. Thus, if short dura-

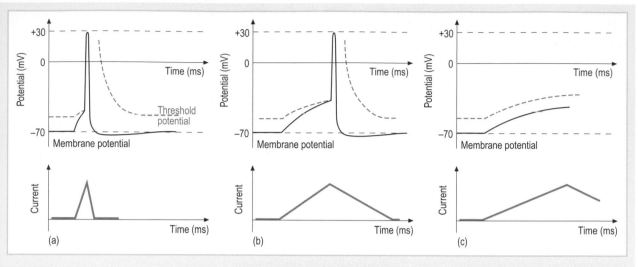

Figure 3.13 The effect of pulse rise time on the nerve fibre threshold potential.

Rather longer pulses of duration 10 ms or more can provoke two nerve action potentials, one when the current rises and the other when it falls. The reason for this is explained later.

tion pulses are used, the current will need to be high. Longer duration pulses can be effective at lower peak currents but can be uncomfortable and increase the risk of skin damage. These ideas are based upon the strength–duration (S-D) behaviour of nerve fibres described previously (see Figure 3.8). One type of clinically used current (High Voltage Pulsed Current) is based on the knowledge that with a very short pulse duration a high voltage or current is required to produce an action potential. This highlights how useful the S-D graph is for predicting aspects of the uses for a particular current if you have sufficient details of its parameters.

If a pulse delivers a greater amount of charge than is needed to trigger an action potential it will still only have that effect on a nerve fibre. No matter what current amplitude is applied, the same nerve action potential is triggered. Increased sensory effects or stronger muscle contractions are due to a larger number of fibres being stimulated. Similarly if the pulse has a longer duration no further effects occur, as implied by the S-D curve in Figure 3.8. Thus the same current triggers an action potential at 1, 10 and 30 ms pulse duration. It is the initial half-ms or so of the pulse which produces the charge movement needed to initiate an action potential.

Time between pulses

The time between pulses can also affect the outcome. If instead of a series of individual pulses, trains or bursts of pulses are used the effect can also be different. If the time between pulses is greater than the refractory period, the nerve will fire at the same frequency as the stimulus pulses. If the time between pulses is within the relative refractory period, the nerve firing rate will be less than the pulse frequency unless high stimulation intensities are used. This effect and the clinical uses and implications are discussed in detail in chapters 4 and 5.

Amplitude

The amplitude is the size of the stimulus applied. It is measured either as the stimulus voltage or current. Stimulus voltages used clinically are typically in the range 10 V to 100 V or more. Stimulus currents are typically in the range 10 mA to 100 mA for clinical treatments. The amplitude is usually set according to the patient's level of comfort and to the aims of a treatment.

Microampere (µA) level currents are used under some treatment conditions but such stimulation is subthreshold as far as the generation of action potentials is concerned if applied transcutaneously.

Duty cycle

Time is a very important variable with electrical stimulation. The way of describing the proportion of time for which current is actually flowing or a stimulus burst is actually being applied is by specifying the duty cycle. Examples are shown in Figure 3.14.

Duty cycle can apply at different levels as the word 'cycle' can refer to the level of on-off times for either bursts or trains of individual pulses. For example, if bursts of pulses are applied with 5 s 'on' followed by 10 s 'off', the burst duty cycle is 33%.

In Figure 3.14(a) the bursts are 10 ms 'on' and 15 ms 'off' and so the burst duty cycle is 40%. At the level of individual pulses, the percentage of time the current flows before the next pulse is the (pulse) duty cycle. If the pulse duration is 200 µs with a frequency of 50 Hz, one complete cycle is 1/50 s or 20 ms so the duty cycle is 1%. In Figure 3.14(b) the pulse duration is 1 ms and one complete cycle is 20 ms so the duty cycle is 5%.

As the above examples indicate, duty cycle describes the proportion of time for which current flows during the different cycles that

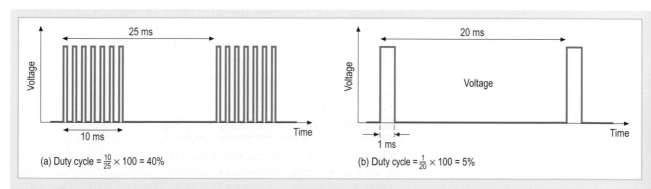

(a) Duty cycle $= \frac{10}{25} \times 100 = 40\%$

(b) Duty cycle $= \frac{1}{20} \times 100 = 5\%$

Figure 3.14 Duty cycle with formula for (a) bursts and (b) continuous pulses or pulses within a burst.

Propagation failure is a term used to describe failure of the action potential to spread through the muscle fibre's t-tubule system.

comprise a treatment session. The main relevance of duty cycle is that it is one of the factors determining the extent of electrolytic effects and, in the case of burst duty cycle, it is a factor determining the rate of fatigue.

Fatigue can occur at different levels of the neuromuscular system. In this instance we are not considering central fatigue, which occurs in the central nervous system, only peripheral fatigue. Peripheral fatigue involves the neuromuscular system and can have effects at different levels in that system. Fatigue due to neurotransmitter depletion or propagation failure will occur if the action potential frequency is much in excess of 50 Hz. This is sometimes called 'high frequency fatigue' (Jones, 1996). Its onset is rapid (a matter of seconds), as is recovery. Similarly, muscle fibres can fatigue due to the metabolic changes occurring within the muscle fibre as a result of heightened activity. When, for example, quadriceps is being stimulated, the area experiencing the highest current density, immediately under the electrodes, demonstrates fatigue first. To maintain the same level of force, adjacent or deeper motor units must be recruited, meaning that the therapist will need to increase the intensity to increase the current density and recruit sufficient deeper motor units. This has an important implication for many clinical uses of electrical stimulation (Vanderthommen et al., 2002) as the pain tolerance limit may restrict sustained force production.

Modulations

The phenomenon of habituation is sometimes (incorrectly) referred to as accommodation or adaptation, which are quite different processes (Spielholz and Nolan, 1995).

Modulations are systematic variations in a particular parameter: frequency, amplitude or duration. With therapeutic currents modulations are used to reduce the rate of habituation (Spielholz and Nolan, 1995). Habituation is the decrease in response to a repeated stimulus and is responsible for the decrease in perception of a sensory stimulus. Thus, if electrical stimulation is applied at an intensity just above the sensory threshold, the initial tingling sensation will fade and disappear in seconds or tens of seconds. Habituation is thought to be important when electrical stimulation is used for pain control.

Figure 3.15 illustrates the three ways of modulating a stimulus waveform.

Frequency and amplitude modulation are the two commonly employed means of modulating pulsed current. Their clinical usefulness is discussed in chapters 5 and 6.

Ramping, peak on-times, surging

When a clinical stimulator is used to elicit a muscle contraction, the current is normally ramped, i.e. gradually increased and decreased, rather than changed abruptly. This is to avoid a 'startle' reaction as

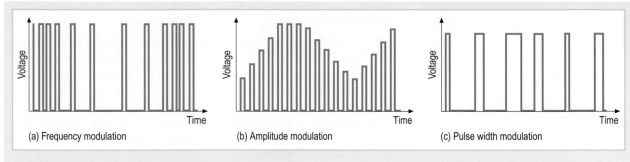

Figure 3.15 Different ways of modulating a pulsed stimulus.

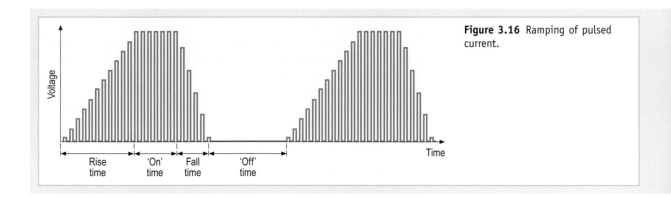

Figure 3.16 Ramping of pulsed current.

the peak intensity will normally be well above the sensory threshold. Ramping (or surging) is the systematic increase or decrease in the intensity of a train of pulses (Figure 3.16) or bursts of pulses. 'Ramping up' means the amplitude of successive pulses or bursts is systematically increased. To avoid a startle reaction, the ramp up time should be at least 0.5 s. The time at peak intensity can usually be set by the user. It is followed either by ramping down or by an immediate cessation of current. The ramp down time is unimportant as far as the startle reaction is concerned. Ramping is also used when the aim is to mimic a voluntary contraction where the muscle force increases progressively to maximum, is sustained, then decreases progressively to zero. In this case the ramp up and down times might be several seconds and the peak intensity time could be as little as a fraction of a second or several seconds, depending on the desired clinical outcome.

Ramping is particularly important when there is an issue of tolerance of surface electrical stimulation.

Summary

- *Polarity* refers to charge imbalance. Current flow may be unidirectional (fixed polarity) or bidirectional (alternating polarity). Unidirectional current flow affects the choice of electrode location and alters the skin pH under the electrodes. If the pH change is excessive it may produce irritation or chemical burns.
- *Frequency* is the number of pulses (or bursts) per second (Hz). Stimulus frequency affects the clinical response, e.g. twitching or tetanic muscle contraction.
- *Shape* of pulses. If the rise time is longer than a few hundred μs, accommodation will occur, i.e. the action potential threshold is increased.
- *Pulse duration* affects the current amplitude necessary to elicit an action potential. It also determines the amount of discrimination between sensory, motor and painful stimulation.
- *Time between pulses*. This is important as pulses falling within the relative refractory period will not produce action potentials unless the stimulus intensity is sufficiently high.
- *Amplitude* is important as it describes the current *intensity* and hence determines the total number of nerve fibres activated.
- *Duty cycle* is the relative time for which current is flowing. It is expressed as a percentage of the time in each cycle for which current flows.
- *Modulations* of pulses may take the form of frequency modulation, amplitude modulation or pulse width modulation.
- *Ramping or surging* of the stimulus is commonly used either to avoid a startle reaction or to produce a muscle contraction that mimics a voluntary contraction.

DIFFERENT TYPES OF CURRENTS

Each type of current has a defining set of parameters. There are three main types of currents defined clinically: direct, pulsed and alternating. The first section discusses each of these and what differentiates them. They are described by the American Physical Therapy Association (APTA, 2000). We call this system the 'descriptive system' as it describes the current by providing parameter details. The second section discusses a number of currents usually referred to by name and describes for each which one of the three types of currents they are. This system is referred to as the 'named current system'. The final part explains how users can manage the complexities of having to use two quite different ways of labelling currents. It also explains why both systems continue to be used despite many users having problems interchanging between them.

The advantage of having a number of different types of currents available is a larger set of possible uses. As discussed previously in this chapter, different parameters have different effects and changing a parameter can increase or decrease a particular effect. Some changes will be minor and unimportant but some can be clinically important. Occasionally, two or more parameters are changed at a time. The disadvantage is the confusions with the naming of currents and different opinions on the details for some.

The descriptive system

Three types of current are distinguished for clinical purposes: direct, alternating and pulsed. Direct at its most basic level is continuous. Alternating is, as described previously, current that passes in one direction and then in the other. The clinical addition is pulsed current. This type of current can flow in the one direction only or in both. The main distinguishing feature is the gap between successive pulses. As this outline suggests, pulsed current has a number of variations. The main features of all three types of currents are described below. Pulsed and alternating are also described in considerably more detail in chapter 4. The reason is, they are used more clinically and understanding their uses and options is more complicated than is the case with direct current.

Direct current

As explained previously, direct current (DC) is current which flows in one direction only (see Figure 3.9a and b). From a general scientific perspective, any current which satisfies this criterion is classed as DC. Clinically, a more restrictive definition is used, namely that the current flows in one direction only and that the current flow is sustained for at least one second. Direct current (using the restricted definition) is used clinically for iontophoresis which is the pushing of therapeutically beneficial ions through the skin barrier.

Potential variations to direct current include interruption or ramping of the current intensity. Thus pulsed DC could be rectangular, triangular or sawtooth in shape. For iontophoresis, sustained, unvarying current (see Figure 3.9a) is used as any interruption or diminishing of the current is counterproductive.

From the point of view of nerve excitation, DC (as defined clinically) can be thought of as an 'infinite duration' pulse. As S-D curves indicate (see Figure 3.8), if the pulse duration is increased above about 100 ms, the duration becomes unimportant. Thus a 500 ms (half second) pulse would have the same effect as a 5 or 50 s pulse. Threshold is reached at the same stimulation intensity (i.e. the rheobase) regardless of pulse duration after 100 ms. More importantly, if the threshold intensity is exceeded, the nerve will fire once then begin

Direct current with a duration less than 1 second is, in APTA terminology, called pulsed current or more specifically monophasic pulsed current.

accommodating and either immediately, or rapidly, cease firing. Although current durations of 1 s or so seem short to us, at the level of the nerve fibre it is effectively an 'infinitely long' pulse. For this reason DC is clinically unimportant other than for iontophoresis where moving charged molecules through the skin barrier is the aim rather than nerve excitation and wound healing, where the physiological mechanisms have not been established (iontophoresis and wound healing are discussed in chapter 6).

Alternating current

Alternating current (AC) comprises a continuous series of alternating pulses. Their main uses are to cause contraction of innervated muscle and to provide sensory stimulation for pain control.

The distinguishing feature of alternating current is the fact the pulses are joined and continuous. There is no interpulse interval. The shape of a pulse may be sinusoidal, triangular or rectangular.

Figure 3.17 shows three examples of AC: (a) shows continuous sinusoidal AC; (b) and (c) are modulated. AC used clinically has a frequency in the range from 1 kHz to 10 kHz. This means that one complete AC cycle has a duration between 100 µs (at 10 kHz) and 1 ms (at 1 kHz). Since each complete cycle consists of two phases, one positive and one negative, the phase (or pulse) durations are in the range 50 µs to 500 µs. The current flow is balanced, i.e. the amount of charge in each phase is identical.

The relationship between frequency, f, and period, T (the time for one complete cycle), is:

$$f = \frac{1}{T}$$

so a frequency of 1 kHz (10^3 Hz) corresponds to a period of 10^{-3} s or 1 ms.

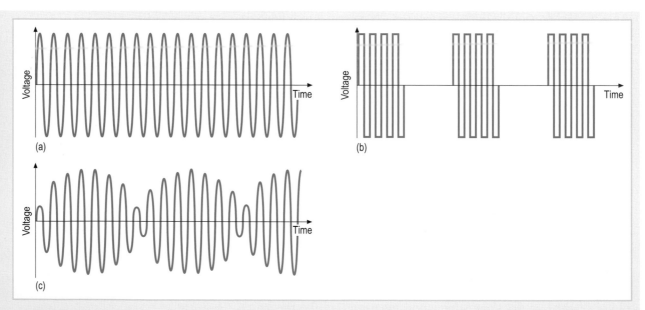

Figure 3.17 (a) Continuous sinusoidal AC, (b) rectangular AC, burst modulated, (c) sinusoidal AC, sinusoidal amplitude modulated.

The frequency of alternating current is within the range traditionally called 'medium frequency'. Medium frequencies cover the range from 1 kHz to 100 kHz. Frequencies above 10 kHz are not normally used as nerve fibres become less excitable at higher AC frequencies. The oscillations are simply too rapid for the nerve fibre to respond. Thus, at, say, 100 kHz the intensity required to depolarize a nerve fibre would cause tissue burns immediately beneath the electrodes.

AC used clinically is normally modulated either as rectangular (Figure 3.17b) or sinusoidal (Figure 3.17c) bursts. The burst frequency is normally in the 'biological' range, 1 Hz to 120 Hz. It has been claimed that if the burst frequency is, say, 50 Hz then nerve fibres will fire at the same low frequency, i.e. once with each burst. This is not true. The physiological response to a burst of current is quite different to single pulses as nerve fibres can fire repeatedly within a burst if the burst duration is sufficiently long. This point is elaborated in chapter 4.

The low frequency bursts of current may be ramped, generally over a period of seconds or tens of seconds. Figure 3.18 illustrates this. Each shaded bar in Figure 3.18(a) is a burst of AC and the bursts might have a frequency of, say, 40 Hz. Within each burst (two are shown in Figure 3.18b) the AC frequency will normally be between 1 kHz and 10 kHz.

Four important characteristics of the stimulus waveform shown in Figure 3.18 are:

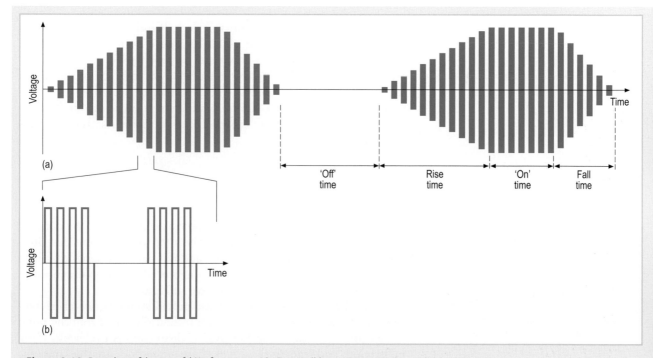

Figure 3.18 Ramping of bursts of kHz frequency AC. Bursts (b) are represented as solid bars in (a).

- the *AC frequency* of pulses in each burst (also called the carrier frequency). This determines the pulse width. For example if the AC frequency is 4 kHz, 1 cycle has a duration of 1/4000 s or 250 μs so each pulse or half-cycle has a duration of 125 μs. This affects the discrimination between sensory, motor and pain responses (see Figure 3.8)

- the *burst frequency*. If the time between the start of each burst in Figure 3.18b is 25 ms or 1/40th of a second the burst frequency is 40 Hz. The burst frequency affects the nature of the physiological response. Thus, with motor stimulation, the burst frequency affects whether the elicited contraction is twitch or tetanic and how forceful (see Figure 3.12). It also determines the rate of fatigue (see chapter 4).

- *ramping* of the burst intensity. Ramping is used to avoid a sudden change in the elicited response, in particular to avoid a 'startle' reaction and can also be used to mimic more closely voluntary muscle contractions.

- *on–off duty cycle*. To obtain a muscle contraction current may be on for, say, 6 s and then off for 12 s before another 6 s of stimulation commences. The duty cycle is the percentage of time in a cycle for which stimulation is applied:

$$\text{duty cycle } (\%) = \frac{\text{‘on-time’}}{(\text{‘on-’} + \text{‘off-time’})} \times 100$$

so with a 6 s on time and 12 s off, the duty cycle is 6/18 of 100% = 33%.

Calculation of the on–off duty cycle in Figure 3.18 is complicated by the rise and fall times. It could be argued that the current is on during ramp-up and ramp-down and so they should be included as 'on-time'. Strictly speaking this is true. However, much of the stimulation will be subthreshold so the physiological response will be a small during most of the ramp-up and ramp-down periods. From a clinical perspective it makes more sense to count the rise and fall times as 'off-time'.

Pulsed current

Pulsed current is a third type of current used clinically. The defining feature, which distinguishes it from the alternating current described above, is that each pulse is separate and not part of a series of joined pulses. All pulses are separated by an appreciable inter-pulse interval. Examples of pulsed current are shown in Figure 3.19.

Figure 3.19a shows a monophasic pulsed stimulus, which technically is DC, while (b), (c) and (d) are technically AC. From the point of view of nerve excitation the AC/DC distinction is irrelevant. If the pulse width and leading (positive) phase amplitudes are the same, the nerve response to the four stimuli will be virtually indistinguishable.

Note that for illustrative purposes, the horizontal blue lines in Figures 3.19a to c are drawn touching the horizontal axis. This represents zero volts, not 'small but slightly positive'. The corresponding line in (d) represents small but negative.

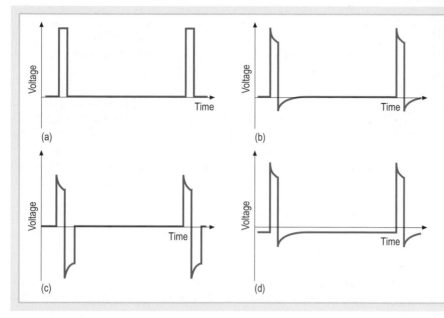

Figure 3.19 Pulsed current (a) monophasic, (b) biphasic asymmetrical (unbalanced), (c) biphasic symmetrical (balanced), (d) biphasic asymmetrical (balanced).

The pulses can be balanced or unbalanced. As indicated previously, unbalanced pulses result in a net flow of current in one direction and there will be resulting electrolytic effects. This could pose a hazard when current is applied for long periods, such as when self-administered for pain control for hours per day. However, for short duration pulses (less than 1 ms) applied at a low frequency (less than 120 Hz) for 10 or 20 minutes the electrolytic effects are unlikely to pose a hazard. Nonetheless, since there is no apparent advantage in using an unbalanced stimulus for nerve excitation, a balanced waveform is preferred. Most clinical stimulators provide biphasic asymmetrical (balanced) stimulus pulses (Figure 3.19d). Others offer a choice of symmetrical or asymmetrical pulses.

As noted earlier (see Figure 3.15), frequency, amplitude or duration of pulsed currents can be modulated. Also as with alternating current (see Figure 3.18), ramping can be used to vary the physiological response. The difference with bursts of pulsed current is that the combination of interpulse and interburst intervals can mean a very low duty cycle. Figure 3.20 illustrates ramping of pulsed current.

Assuming a pulse frequency of 50 Hz and a pulse duration of 300 μs, the time for which current flows in a second is $50 \times 300\,\mu s = 15000\,\mu s = 15\,ms$ or $0.015\,s$. The duty cycle for this pulsed current is then $= ([.015/1.0] \times 100) = 1.5\%$. That indicates how little current actually flows and why pulsed currents can be successfully used in battery-powered portable stimulators.

The usefulness of having the option of symmetrical or asymmetrical balanced pulses has yet to be established. There appears to be no evidence of any clinically significant differences in their effects.

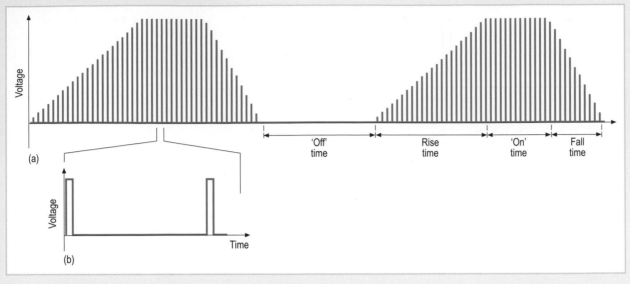

Figure 3.20 Ramping of pulsed current. Pulses (b) appear as vertical lines in (a) because of their short duration.

Summary

Three types of described currents are distinguished clinically:

- direct current which is
  - continuous
  - monophasic
- alternating current which is
  - biphasic
  - continuing, i.e. no interpulse interval
  - sinusoidal, triangular or rectangular in shape
- pulsed current which is
  - monophasic or biphasic
  - separated by interpulse intervals
  - rectangular, triangular and other.

The named current system

The second way of describing clinical currents is by name. Above, three types of current were described along with their differences. That method is a more recent development actively promoted by some groups to facilitate understanding and to promote consistency between users of clinical electrical stimulation (APTA, 2000). This is, however, not the way many people describe or discuss clinically used currents. The second is the 'named current system', so called because each type of current has an understood set of parameters. This system and the most commonly used named currents are described below.

The naming of some currents has a historical basis. For example, galvanic and faradic currents are named for early investigators of the biological effects of electric current. 'Russian current' is named with the nationality of the scientist, Kots, who first promoted it (Ward and Shkuratova, 2002). Other names relate more to characteristics of the current such as interferential and high voltage pulsed current. Some of the most commonly known named currents are listed alongside.

A problem with the named current system is that the stimulus parameters are not rigidly defined. For example, the name 'faradic current' originated on equipment, now no longer available, which produced pulsed current with certain specific characteristics by electromechanical means (Geddes, 1984). The equipment has been replaced by electronic stimulators which produce currents similar to the original but which often allow the operator greater control over the stimulus parameters. The term 'faradic type' current is often used – however, if the parameters are changed, at what point does the stimulus cease to be 'faradic'? The descriptive system avoids this confusion by focusing on the parameters and physiological effects of the stimulus.

Named currents and their effects and implications for clinical users are now discussed.

A list of named currents	
● faradic	● galvanic
● Russian	● interrupted
● interferential	galvanic
● diadynamic	● TENS
● high voltage	● microcurrent
pulsed (HVPS)	

Faradic current

Faradic current is a low frequency pulsed current similar to that shown in Figure 3.19d. The pulses originally produced were asymmetrical biphasic with a frequency of between 30 and 70 Hz and a pulse duration of 1 ms or less but usually greater than 300 µs. These parameters are within the usual range used for stimulating innervated muscle. For that reason, many manufacturers label the current intended for stimulating innervated muscle as 'faradic'.

Figure 3.21 illustrates the difference between the original faradic current and the monophasic version of its modern day incarnation. Biphasic pulses with a similar phase duration and frequency are also called 'faradic current'.

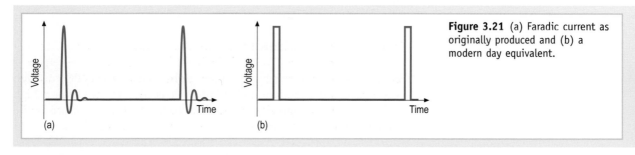

Figure 3.21 (a) Faradic current as originally produced and (b) a modern day equivalent.

(a)   (b)

Some pulsed stimulators offer a choice of pulse widths and frequencies, which was not a possibility when the term 'faradic current' was coined and widely understood and used. This, combined with the range of possible interpretations of what 'faradic current' really is, suggests that if the name is to be retained, specific waveform characteristics using the descriptive system should be agreed upon.

Galvanic current

'Galvanic current' is another name for continuous direct current (DC). It is not used for nerve stimulation but rather for iontophoresis, i.e. for driving therapeutically beneficial ions through the skin barrier. Because of this there is no point in interrupting or pulsing the current flow as this would only increase the required treatment time. Nor would reversing the current flow be appropriate (to avoid electrolytic effects), as this would drive the therapeutically beneficial ions back across the skin.

In terms of the descriptive system, galvanic current is defined as current which flows for 1 s or more.

TENS

TENS is the popularized name for electrical stimulation produced by a portable stimulator and used to treat pain. However, TENS stands for Trancutaneous Electrical Nerve Stimulation and so, by definition, covers the complete range of transcutaneously applied currents used for nerve excitation. Nonetheless, the term TENS is often used with a more restrictive intent, namely to describe the kind of pulses produced by portable stimulators used to treat pain.

Pain control TENS units typically produce a continuous train of pulsed current at frequencies in the range 1 to 120 Hz, some as high as 200 Hz (see chapter 6).

The pulses are normally rectangular, or close to rectangular, in shape (see Figure 3.19), biphasic and the pulse duration is normally 50–200 µs. Sensory stimulation is usually applied at a 'strong but comfortable' level. The aim is selectively to excite A-β (sensory) nerve fibres and produce an analgesic effect by 'gating' signals conveyed by pain (A-δ and C) fibres (see chapter 6).

> Strictly speaking, faradic, Russian, interferential, high voltage pulsed current, etc. are all 'TENS'.

High voltage pulsed current

As the name suggests, high voltage pulsed current (HVPC) or high voltage pulsed stimulation (HVPS) as it is also known, has a high voltage output, originally up to 500 volts. A special feature is the shape of the pulse, a twin spike as shown in Figure 3.22.

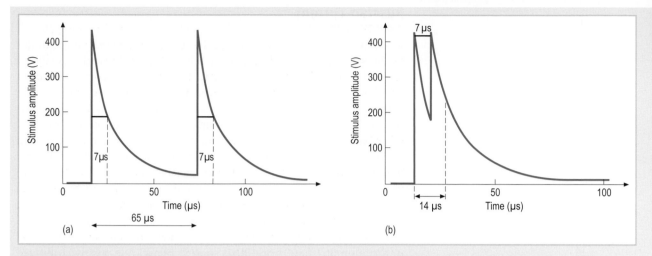

Figure 3.22 The two common forms of high voltage pulsed current: (a) wider separation of pulses and (b) closer separation.

The frequency of the double pulse combination can be varied, usually from 1 to 100 Hz. Two spike options are commonly used. The first is a short duration twin pulse with a small interpulse interval (Figure 3.22a). The pulses have an almost instantaneous rise time and are of very brief duration (the intensity drops to half of maximum in about 7 μs). The pulse separation is about 65 μs. The second (Figure 3.22b) uses the same 7 μs pulses but the time between the start of each pulse is reduced to about 7 μs so the twin spikes overlap.

The overlapping twin spikes (Figure 3.22b) reinforce and the effective pulse duration is about 14 μs. This results in a stronger motor response with the overlapping waveform.

With such short duration pulses, very high voltages are needed (hence the name) to provide high enough current to stimulate nerve fibres (see Figure 3.8). Peak currents of 2–2.5 A may be generated during the few microseconds of peak voltage (Alon, 1987), but the average current is very low, at around 1.2–1.5 mA.

The potential clinical uses of this type of current can be predicted by reviewing S-D graphs (see Figure 3.8). The marked separation of the graphs at short pulse durations indicates that this type of current is likely to be very comfortable. The pain threshold for very short duration pulses (HVPS) is much higher than for longer pulses (i.e. >200 μs) and the separation between thresholds means the difference in intensity required to get a pain response is much greater at shorter pulse durations. This indicates this type of current is well suited to pain-free sensory stimulation and should provide a very comfortable way of producing muscle contractions.

The peak voltage is set by safety considerations. Above 300 V, skin breakdown is possible. Skin conductivity increases dramatically and burns can result. The need for twin pulses with HVPC may be simply because a double pulse of 300 V would not cause skin damage, while a single 600 V pulse would.

Russian current

Russian current is 2.5 kHz alternating current delivered in rectangular bursts with a burst frequency of 50 Hz and a burst duty cycle of 50% (Figure 3.23). The name derives from work conducted by a Russian scientist, Kots, who reported significant strength gains in trainee athletes as a result of electrical stimulation using 2.5 kHz sinusoidal AC with trains of 10 ms bursts, applied 10 s on and 50 s off (Ward and Shkuratova, 2002). Kots' findings had a major impact on sports science and other parts of clinical practice in the late 1970s and in the 1980s. As a result, 2.5 kHz alternating current with a burst frequency of 50 Hz became known as Russian current. The pulse shape originally used was sinusoidal but at kHz frequencies it makes little difference whether the shape is sinusoidal, rectangular or triangular.

At a frequency of 2.5 kHz, one sinusoidal oscillation has a period or duration of 1/2500 s or 400 μs so each phase (one positive followed by one negative) has a duration of 200 μs. This is similar to the pulse widths produced by conventional TENS stimulators. The difference is that with conventional TENS, the pulses are separated by a very large interpulse interval while with Russian currents there is no interpulse interval: positive pulses are immediately followed by negative pulses. The short pulse duration (see Figure 3.8) allows for efficient, pain-free motor stimulation.

As noted earlier, technological change has meant that it is easy to produce electronic stimulators with stimulus parameters adjustable over a wide range. A device claimed to be a 'Russian current' stimulator may offer burst on/off times other than 10 s on and 50 s off for 10 minutes. The on-time may be adjustable from 1 s to 20 s (of 10 ms, 50 Hz bursts) and the off-time from 1 to 50 s. The treatment time can also be varied. If the stimulus parameters are changed, at what point does the stimulus cease to be 'Russian current'?

Along with knowing a current is a Russian current a would-be user also needs to know if any parameters offered by the manufacturers are different to those of 'true' Russian currents.

Figure 3.23 Russian current: 2.5 kHz sinusoidal AC delivered in 10 ms bursts with a 50% duty cycle.

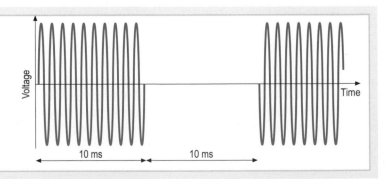

Interferential current

The word 'interferential', suggests some sort of interference and this is the basis for the name of this current. Interferential currents (IFC) are two kHz frequency alternating currents applied in a continuous train (see Figure 3.17a). The currents have a slightly different frequency (for example, one might be 4000 Hz, the other 4050 Hz). Two pairs of electrodes are positioned so that the currents intersect deep within the tissue volume (Figure 3.24b).

A claimed advantage of interferential currents is depth efficiency of stimulation. It is argued that in the region of intersection, the reinforcement of the currents will result in a greater total stimulus intensity so maximum stimulation is produced at depth (Figure 3.24b) rather than superficially as occurs with normal bipolar stimulation (Figure 3.24a). Whether this is true is questionable as current spreading reduces the intensity at depth so even if two currents are superimposed, the total intensity could (and probably would) still be less than immediately under the electrodes.

Modern interferential stimulators offer a selection of AC frequencies in the range 1 to 10 kHz and may use either sine wave or square-wave pulses. The original interferential stimulators used sinusoidal AC at a frequency of 4 kHz. As noted earlier, at kHz frequencies it makes little difference whether the shape is sinusoidal, rectangular or triangular.

Interferential stimulators also offer the option of 'premodulated interferential current' where the two slightly different frequency currents are combined within the stimulator and a current is applied using a single pair of electrodes (Figure 3.24a). The term 'premodulated interferential' illustrates the problem with the named current system. If the current is premodulated and no longer interferes and reinforces at depth in the tissues then it should not be described as 'interferential'. The interferential label is, however, argued to be justified as the current is still the same kHz frequency AC.

'Premodulated interferential' is a contradiction in terms. If the current is premodulated and applied using a single pair of electrodes, there are no two currents to interfere within tissue so the current cannot be 'premodulated' and 'interferential' at the same time.

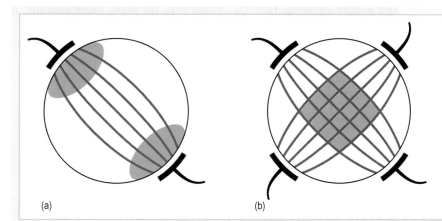

(a)

(b)

Figure 3.24 (a) Conventional bipolar and (b) quadripolar application of currents showing the (claimed) regions of maximum stimulation.

Robertson, V., Ward, A. (2002). Vastus medialis electrical stimulation to improve lower extremity function following a lateral patellar retinacular release. J Orthop Sports Phys Ther, **32**, 437–445.

Spielholz, N., Nolan, M. (1995). Conventional TENS and the phenomena of accommodation, adaptation, habituation and electrode polarization. J Clin Electrophysiol, **7**, 16–19.

Vanderthommen, M., Depresseux, J., Dauchat, L. et al. (2002). Blood flow variation in human muscle during electrically stimulated exercise bouts. Arch Phys Med Rehabil, **83**, 936–941.

Ward, A. (2004) Biophysical bases of electrotherapy. Mount Waverley: Excell Biomedical Publications. (on the CD accompanying this text).

Ward, A., Shkuratova, N. (2002). Russian currents: the early experimental evidence. Phys Ther, **82**, 1019–1030.

Effects of electrical stimulation

Electrical stimulation affects a range of tissues but most directly nerve and muscle. The previous chapter focused on aspects of how to use electrical stimulation. It also outlined the effects of different parameters and the different current types and their uses. This chapter looks in more detail at the stimulus waveforms used clinically and attempts to assess their likely effectiveness in terms of known physiological effects.

There are three sections: first, how voluntary and electrically produced contractions differ; second, the effects of different parameters of alternating and pulsed currents; and third, the clinical implications of stimulus parameters. The first section starts with a discussion of the different muscle fibre types and the implications of their properties and nerve supply. This is followed by discussions of torque production and fatigue and of how contractions produced electrically differ from voluntary contractions. The second section discusses in detail the effects of different parameters of alternating current and how using it differs from using a pulsed current for muscle stimulation. The third section covers the practical implications of stimulation using different current types. This chapter builds on chapter 3 and discusses in more detail the effects of different stimulus parameters.

VOLUNTARY VERSUS ELECTRICALLY INDUCED CONTRACTIONS

Although they can appear superficially similar, the nature of a muscle contraction induced by transcutaneous electrical stimulation is quite different to that produced voluntarily. The differences have important implications for users of electrical stimulation. One important difference is the muscle fibre types which are preferentially activated.

Muscle fibre types

Muscle fibres within a whole muscle are not homogeneous, i.e. they do not all have the same properties. One important distinction is in

Three different schemes are used to categorize muscle fibres: histological, biochemical and mechanical. We will make most use of the mechanical categorization.

Fast-fatigable fibres, while inefficient, have an obvious survival advantage. The ability to escape a predator or capture prey is enhanced by these energy-inefficient muscle fibres.

With fast and powerful rather than progressive contractions, the size principle may not apply (McComas, 1996).

the twitch response. When a single action potential reaches the neuromuscular junction, the resulting muscle fibre response is a single twitch. Some muscle fibres are 'fast twitch', having a duration of 50 ms or so. Others are 'slow twitch' with a duration of 90 ms or more. Note that the twitch duration (whether fast or slow) is much longer than the action potential which initiates the contraction. The duration of an action potential spike is typically 1 ms or so. In general, fast twitch fibres produce high peak forces of short duration while slow twitch fibres produce a much lower peak force with a longer duration. The fibres also differ in terms of their fatigability. Slow twitch fibres are fatigue-resistant. Two kinds of fast twitch fibres are identified: 'fast-fatigable' and 'fast-fatigue-resistant'. Fast-fatigable fibres produce the highest peak force while fast-fatigue-resistant fibres produce somewhat lower force.

It should also be noted that the muscle fibre type is not fixed. Fast twitch fibres can convert to slow and vice versa. Muscle fibre type changes are an integral part of normal growth, development and adaptation.

Fatigue-resistance depends on cellular metabolism. Slow twitch fibres have high numbers of mitochondria, a good blood supply (are close to capillaries) and rely on aerobic glycolysis for energy production. The metabolic mechanisms of energy production are suited to endurance: sustained or repetitive contractions. Fast-fatigable fibres have far fewer mitochondria but high levels of glycolytic enzymes in the cytoplasm. They are designed to produce very high peak forces for a very short time (from a fraction of a second to a few seconds). They rely on anaerobic metabolism for peak energy production: an oxygen supply from the bloodstream is not an immediate requirement. A problem with anaerobic glycolysis is that it is inefficient: only two molecules of adenosine triphosphate (ATP) are produced per molecule of glucose catabolized. Glucose levels are thus depleted very rapidly. Aerobic catabolism is much more efficient: almost twenty times as many molecules of ATP are produced from each glucose molecule under aerobic conditions.

In a steady or repetitive voluntary contraction it is the slow, highly fatigue-resistant motor units which are recruited first. For contractile forces up to about 20% of maximum, slow motor units dominate. Above this level, the contribution of fast-resistant units increases. Fast-fatigable units are the last to be recruited. The process of recruitment is thus metabolically efficient with the energy-inefficient (fast) fibres recruited last and only if needed.

Recruitment order

If the fibres within a nerve trunk are dissected and measured, it is found that motor nerves differ in diameter according to the muscle fibre types which they innervate. Slow, fatigue-resistant muscle fibres are innervated by smaller diameter nerve fibres. Fast-fatigue muscle fibres have larger diameter motor nerves controlling them. The observed order of muscle fibre recruitment (fatigue-resistant before fast-fatigue) is because small diameter motor nerves are activated before larger diameter ones, at least in slow or repetitive movements. This observation led Henneman et al. (1965) to propose the 'size principle', which states that the order of recruitment in a normal voluntary contraction is from small to large nerve fibre diameters.

When nerve fibres are activated by transcutaneous electrical stimulation, the order of nerve fibre recruitment does not follow the size principle but rather its opposite. Fibre diameter is a key factor as depolarization depends on the potential difference between two adjacent nodes of Ranvier (McNeal, 1976) and the spacing between adjacent nodes is proportional to the fibre diameter. Larger diameter fibres are bigger in all respects and have larger internodal distances, while smaller diameter fibres have smaller internodal distances. An increased diameter and proportionally increased internodal distance will result in a larger potential difference between two adjacent nodes when current passes through tissue. Consequently, the larger the fibre diameter, the more easily excited the fibre. It is for this reason that sensory and motor responses, involving relatively large diameter fibres, are generally evoked at lower stimulation intensities than the pain response associated with stimulation of smaller diameter fibres. It is for the same reason that, other things being equal, fast-fatigable motor units will be recruited at lower stimulation intensities than slow, fatigue-resistant motor units.

Fibre diameter is not the only factor determining recruitment. Proximity to the electrodes is also important. The proximity of fibres to the electrodes is a factor because current spreads through the underlying tissue volume (see Figure 3.2), so the effective stimulation intensity decreases with distance from the electrodes. This means that there will be a 'zone of effectiveness' under each electrode where stimulation is maximum. Outside this region, recruitment will diminish as a lesser proportion of the fibres will be excited. At a sufficient distance from the electrodes, no stimulation will occur as the local stimulation intensity will be subthreshold.

The recruitment order with transcutaneous electrical stimulation thus depends on both the distance of the nerve fibre from the stimulating electrode and the nerve fibre diameter. The larger the fibre diameter and the closer the fibre is to the electrode, the greater the excitability.

Fatigue

Any form of sustained or repetitive muscle contraction will result in fatigue, which is defined as the progressive decrease in the ability of a muscle to generate force as a result of ongoing motor activity. The complication is that muscle force generation is the end product of the sequence or chain of events illustrated in summary form in Figure 4.1

Figure 4.1 The chain of events in voluntary production of muscle force.

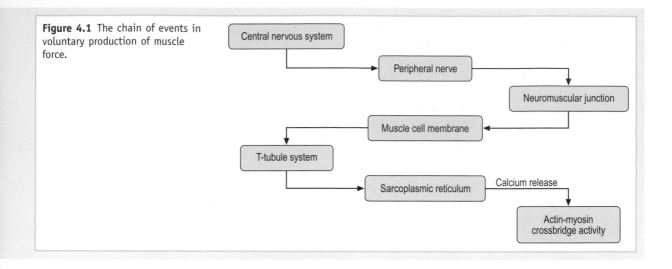

and each step in the sequence has the potential to contribute to fatigue.

For normal, voluntary contractions, the chain of events involves central nervous system activity resulting in firing of fibres and their peripheral nerves, the α-motor neurons. The signals are transmitted to the neuromuscular junction where the neurotransmitter acetylcholine (ACh) is released. Binding of sufficient ACh to the motor end plate results in an action potential being produced and propagated over the muscle fibre membrane. A wave of excitation spreads across the membrane and is transmitted into the interior of the muscle fibre via the transverse tubules (T-tubules). Depolarization of the T-tubule membrane results in release of calcium ions from the stored reserves in the sarcoplasmic reticulum. Calcium ions released from the sarcoplasmic reticulum bind to troponin molecules and this binding activates actin-myosin crossbridge cycling with ATP used as the energy source. This is the basis of muscle fibre contraction.

Central versus peripheral fatigue

Fatigue can have its origins at any of the steps involved in muscle contraction (see Figure 4.1) and can be a result of either a decrease in the neural activation of muscle fibres or a decrease in the muscle fibre response to repeated stimulation. These decrements can be usefully categorized as central in origin or peripheral. Central fatigue is when the average motor nerve firing frequency decreases, either because of a lesser central nervous system (CNS) drive or because of reduced transmission of CNS drive to the motor neurons. Peripheral fatigue occurs at or beyond the neuromuscular junction.

With electrical stimulation, peripheral nerves are stimulated directly so any fatigue observed must be of peripheral rather than central origin. Electrically induced peripheral fatigue can involve a variety of mechanisms, including an impaired ability to evoke an action potential at the site of stimulation. Other effects are implicit in Figure 4.1.

There is the possibility of impaired transmission at the neuromuscular junction. In a normal voluntary contraction where the firing frequency is low, the amount of ACh released per action potential is far in excess of that required to depolarize the muscle fibre membrane. However, with higher frequency stimulation the limited stores of ACh in the motor axon terminal can become depleted because the time constant for replenishing the ACh is relatively long, in the order of 5 s (Otsuka et al., 1962). With higher frequency stimulation (50 Hz or more), neurotransmitter depletion can result in failure to initiate depolarization of the muscle fibre membrane.

The muscle fibre response to constant frequency stimulation can also diminish because of reduced spread of the action potential over the muscle fibre membrane. Jones et al. (1979) demonstrated that if skeletal muscle is fatigued rapidly by stimulation at 100 Hz for a few tens of seconds and then the stimulation frequency is decreased to 20 Hz, without any rest period, there is a sudden partial recovery of force output. This recoverable loss of force is given the name 'high frequency fatigue'. The effect is thought to be due to changes in the inter-fibre and T-tubule cation (K^+ and Na^+) concentrations. Like neurotransmitter depletion, high frequency fatigue is unlikely to occur with voluntary contractions but is likely at frequencies typically used in transcutaneous stimulation (50 Hz or higher).

Fatigue can also occur within the muscle fibre, as a result of metabolic changes and changes in ion concentrations. Factors include inadequate supply of oxygen, glucose depletion and accumulation of metabolic byproducts including hydrogen ions within the muscle fibre. Variation in the concentrations of free and bound calcium ions (Ca^{2+}) in the cytoplasm can also play a part. The relative contribution of these factors to electrically induced muscle fatigue is not completely understood and analysis is complicated because the relative contributions depend on the particular stimulus parameters used.

Whether fatigue induced by electrical stimulation is detrimental to muscle strengthening is arguable. One argument is that a fatigued fibre has dropped-out so there is no benefit to be gained by further stimulation, hence fatigue is to be avoided. The counter-argument is that strengthening will only occur if the muscle fibre is worked to its fatigue limit. The answer seems to be that fatigue results in strengthening but only if it is the muscle fibre which fatigues. Fatigue can result from neurotransmitter depletion or propagation failure, in which case the muscle fibre is not activated and is not strengthened. If fatigue occurs within the muscle fibre, cellular processes are triggered which result in strengthening.

Neurotransmitter depletion does not occur in a normal, voluntary contraction where the firing frequencies of individual motor units are either relatively low or in the form of brief duration bursts. It is much more important in transcutaneous stimulation (Mizrahi, 1997; Clamann, 1981) where a limited number of motor units are firing at a relatively high frequency.

Nerve fibre types, firing rates and force production

In graded voluntary contractions, fatigue-resistant muscle fibres are preferentially recruited for low contractile forces. Increased muscle force is achieved partly by increasing the firing frequency of the activated motor units and partly by recruiting more motor units.

Fatigue-resistant motor units are small: the innervating fibres have a small diameter and the number of muscle fibres per motor unit is small. So recruitment of fatigue-resistant fibres produces low increments in muscle force which can be finely graded to produce a smooth, continuous increase. Greatest force is achieved by the additional recruitment of fast twitch, fast-fatigue motor units. Fast-fatigue motor units are large: the innervating fibres have a large diameter and the number of muscle fibres per motor unit is high. Thus recruitment of fast-fatigue fibres produces very large increases in muscle force but the force increase cannot be sustained. Figure 4.2 shows the relationship.

Normal physiological recruitment of motor units is thus an efficient process. Energy efficient, fatigue-resistant motor units are recruited first and fast twitch, fast-fatigue fibres are kept in reserve as a means to produce shorter duration, unsustainably high forces.

As noted previously, with electrical stimulation, recruitment depends on the proximity of nerve fibres to the electrodes and the nerve fibre diameter. This means that in an electrically induced contraction, there will be a disproportionate recruitment of large-diameter fast-fatigue fibres and consequently a rapid rate of fatigue. The problem is compounded by the fact that the fusion frequency of

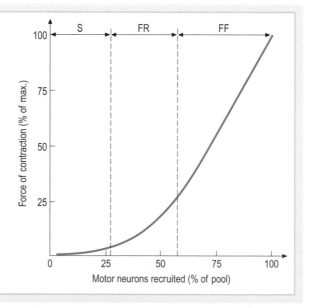

Figure 4.2 The pattern of recruitment in a smooth, graded voluntary muscle contraction. Fibres are recruited in the order slow (S), fast-fatigue-resistant (FR) then fast-fatigue (FF).

fast-fatigue fibres is high so the stimulation frequency must be high if a smooth, tetanic contraction is to be produced.

Force production and fatigue

It might be thought that if higher force is produced by higher intensity electrical stimulation, the rate of fatigue would be higher. It is certainly true that with voluntary contractions, the higher the force produced, the greater the rate of fatigue. This is not the case with electrically induced contractions. Higher intensity electrical stimulation recruits more of the smaller diameter nerve fibres innervating fatigue-resistant muscle fibres as well as recruiting more deeply located larger diameter fibres. The net effect is little change in the fatigue rate at higher stimulation intensities.

Summary

The main factors affecting the response to electrical stimulation are:

- the muscle fibre type, i.e. whether
  - slow twitch, fatigue-resistant
  - fast twitch, fatigue-resistant
  - fast twitch, fatigable
- the recruitment order, which is very different to that of a voluntary contraction:
  - large diameter motor nerve fibres are activated before smaller diameter
  - the distance of the motor nerve fibre from the electrodes is also important
- peripheral fatigue can occur in different ways. It:
  - is more pronounced if there is a higher frequency of activation than voluntary, as is usually the case
  - can be therapeutically beneficial if fatigue occurs within the muscle fibre
  - will be counterproductive if it results in the muscle fibre not being activated.

TYPE OF CURRENT AND IMPLICATIONS OF DIFFERENT PARAMETERS

The type of current used can have a major effect on the outcome as discussion of the effects of different parameters indicated in chapter 3. The focus here is particularly on pulsed as compared to alternating current and how this can change the outcome, especially when requiring muscle contractions. The effect of varying the stimulus parameters is described. An implicit issue, the advantages and disadvantages of alternating versus pulsed current, is also addressed.

Pulsed current (PC)

Pulsed current used clinically normally uses pulses of 1 ms duration or less, delivered at frequencies up to 100 Hz or so. Whether the pulses are monophasic or biphasic, balanced or unbalanced is not particularly relevant at these pulse widths and frequencies. If the stimulus is above threshold, one action potential (nerve impulse) will be produced by each current pulse. Thus a 40 Hz pulsed current stimulus will result in a nerve fibre firing frequency of 40 Hz. In theory, if the stimulus frequency were higher, pulses could be applied within the relative refractory period and not produce a response but, in practice, most nerve fibres are stimulated at intensities well above threshold with transcutaneous stimulation, so refractoriness is not an issue.

Fatigue

Fatigue is an important issue with transcutaneous stimulation when a motor response is required. As noted earlier in this chapter, muscle fatigue can be the result of the muscle fibre working hard and producing a sustained high force or can result from neurotransmitter depletion or propagation failure, in which case the muscle fibre is not activated and does no work. Activation failure is more likely to be therapeutically disadvantageous than beneficial. To minimize activation failure, the lowest pulse frequencies should be used. For most skeletal muscles stimulated at 15 Hz, fluttering will be evident. Depending on the muscle, by 20 Hz or more, the contraction will become smooth and continuous. Stimulation at the fusion frequency will provide a good compromise between peak force production and non-strengthening (activation failure) fatigue. In this way, the muscle fibre can be strengthened, by doing work with minimal activation dropout.

The approach often advocated is to use higher frequencies (typically 50 Hz) for motor stimulation and is based on the fact that 50 Hz stimulation will produce a contraction which is close to maximal in most human skeletal muscles. This ignores the fact that most skeletal muscles have a much lower fusion frequency and that fibre dropout due to activation failure will occur rapidly at 50 Hz. Direct nerve stimulation at 50 Hz for a period of as little as 0.2 s has been shown (Otsuka et al., 1962) to produce a marked drop in ACh release at the neuromuscular junction. To minimize activation failure, the fusion frequency should be determined experimentally by simple observation and subjective reporting of the response to frequencies in the range 15–50 Hz. The observed fusion frequency can then be used as the stimulus frequency.

Practical point

For a motor response, use the lowest pulse frequency which will produce a smooth, non-twitching contraction. The stimulus frequency should be gradually increased from, say, 15 Hz until a frequency is reached where the observed contraction is continuous.

A frequency of 50 Hz is often advocated for motor stimulation and 80 Hz stimulation for a maximally forceful contraction. This is based on the fact that 50 Hz stimulation will produce a forceful contraction and 80 Hz stimulation a slightly more forceful one. While it is true that greater peak forces will be produced at higher than fusion frequencies, the clinical significance is called into question by the likelihood of activation failure occurring very rapidly. Consequently, while current practice is to use higher frequencies for strengthening innervated muscle, more research is needed to identify the point at which increased force production is compromised by a failure to activate muscle fibres.

Discomfort

A problem with pulsed current is that it can be uncomfortable. The discomfort is primarily produced by activation of A-δ nerve fibres which are small and myelinated. They convey the sensation of prickling-stabbing pain. C-fibres are smaller and unmyelinated. They convey deep, aching pain. With electrical stimulation, it is doubtful that C fibres are activated directly. The pain tolerance limit is set by A-δ nerve fibre activity, i.e. prickling-stabbing discomfort. This is because A-δ fibres, although of small diameter, have a larger diameter than C-fibres and the greater the diameter, the greater the ease of excitation.

Pulsed currents with a shorter pulse duration are less uncomfortable. As illustrated in Figure 3.8, at shorter pulse durations, discrimination between sensory, motor and painful stimulation is maximum. Nonetheless, as the intensity is increased to produce a stronger motor response, the stimulation becomes more uncomfortable and the maximum muscle force which can be produced is limited by the pain tolerance of the individual. Skinfold thickness is also an important factor. The higher the skinfold thickness, the lower the maximum force which can be produced. This is because many A-δ fibres are located superficially, in and above the adipose tissue, while motor nerves are located beneath the adipose tissue. Those at greater distance are less likely to be stimulated as current density drops with distance from the electrodes.

The pain tolerance limit may be due to direct electrical stimulation of A-δ fibres or to the pain associated with the forcefulness of contraction resulting in the perception that if the muscle contracted any harder, physical damage would occur.

Summary: pulsed current

- Nerve fibres will fire at the chosen pulse frequency, which is often higher than physiological.
- The fatigue rate can be reduced by using stimulus frequencies less than 50 Hz.
- Stimulation at the fusion frequency will provide a good compromise between peak force production and non-strengthening (activation failure) fatigue.
- Discomfort is due to stimulation of A-δ nerve fibres.

Alternating current (AC)

The two main versions of AC used clinically, Russian current and interferential current (IFT), were outlined in chapter 3. The focus in this section is on AC used clinically, with an emphasis on the sensory and motor responses and how the effects differ from those produced by low frequency (100 Hz or less) pulsed current. Clinical uses of AC and pulsed currents are described more extensively in chapters 5 and 6.

A distinguishing feature of alternating current is the fact the pulses are joined and continuous. There is no interpulse interval and each pulse is, by definition, biphasic. The shape of a pulse is usually sinusoidal (see Figure 3.17c) or rectangular (see Figure 3.17b) and the AC frequencies used clinically are normally in the range 1–10 kHz.

AC may be applied as a continuous train (Figure 3.17a) or an interrupted (Figure 3.17b) or amplitude modulated (Figure 3.17c) train of pulses. The trains of pulses are called bursts.

Discomfort

Anecdotally, kHz frequency alternating current is reported to be more comfortable than pulsed current stimulation. A study by Shanahan (2004), which compared pulsed and alternating current for relief of cold-induced pain, found that AC was perceived as more comfortable by the majority of participants. The study compared symmetrical biphasic pulsed current applied at a frequency of 100 Hz (phase duration 100 μs) with 'premodulated interferential' (see Figure 3.17c) which had a modulation frequency (also called a beat frequency) of 100 Hz and an AC frequency of 5 kHz (thus a phase duration of 100 μs).

Ward et al. (2004) compared the relative discomfort of sinusoidal AC with frequencies in the range 500 Hz to 20 kHz; 50 Hz bursts were applied using different duty cycles ranging from a minimum (one sine wave cycle) to 100% (continuous AC). Subjects were asked to report if the stimulus felt more uncomfortable than others. Figure 4.3 shows the variation in the number of reports of discomfort with AC frequency. The results show that frequencies of 1 kHz and above are relatively comfortable and, of the frequencies tested, 4 kHz is the best in terms of producing least discomfort. It is interesting to note that interferential currents normally have an AC frequency of 4 or 5 kHz and so might be expected to be well tolerated by recipients.

Figure 4.4 shows the variation in the number of reports of discomfort plotted against duty cycle. Duty cycles of 50% or less are associated with low discomfort and a duty cycle of 20% appears to be optimal. The relative discomfort of continuous AC (100% duty cycle) is clearly evident.

A study which compared the relative discomfort of 'true' and 'premodulated' interferential current (Ozcan et al., 2004) also found that continuous AC was less well tolerated than AC applied in bursts with a 50% duty cycle. In this study 90% of negative reports concerned continuous AC.

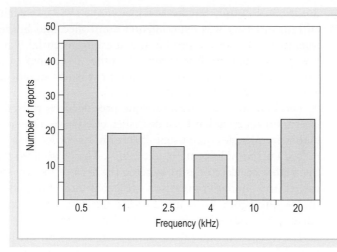

Figure 4.3 The variation in perceived discomfort with AC frequency.

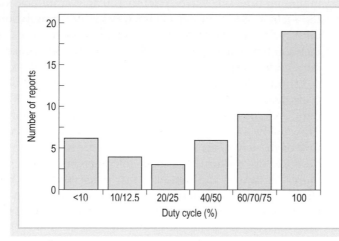

Figure 4.4 The variation in perceived discomfort with duty cycle.

A 20% duty cycle at 50 Hz is an AC burst duration of 4 ms. The burst duration is likely to be more important than the duty cycle as such.

Torque production

Both pulsed current and AC can be used for motor stimulation. AC stimulation is less uncomfortable (see above) and this raises the question of whether lesser discomfort allows, or is associated with, greater torque production. A comparison was made of the quadriceps torque generated by three types of currents: Russian current (2.5 kHz, 50 Hz burst frequency, 50% duty cycle); a quadripolar interferential current application (4 kHz and 4.050 kHz currents producing an amplitude modulated 50 beats per second and pulses with a phase duration of 125 µs) and pulsed current with a frequency of 50 Hz and a phase duration of 200 μs (Snyder-Mackler et al., 1989). In each instance the current intensity was experimenter controlled and limited by subject tolerance. The torque produced using interferential was significantly lower than that produced using the other two types of currents. The torque produced using Russian current was not significantly different to that produced by pulsed current.

The limited difference in torque produced by pulsed and 2.5 kHz alternating current has been described elsewhere. One such study used higher frequencies than usual: 90 Hz bursts for Russian and 90 Hz for pulsed current (Holcomb et al., 2000). They also used the quadriceps but with four electrodes to increase the area of muscle stimulated. An earlier and similar comparison identified more marked differences in the torque produced using 2.5 kHz alternating current than pulsed current (Grimby and Wigerstad-Lossing, 1989).

The torque produced by sinusoidal AC with frequencies in the range 500 Hz to 20 kHz has been measured (Ward et al., 2004); 50 Hz bursts were applied using different duty cycles ranging from a minimum (one sine wave cycle) to 100% (continuous AC). Although the focus was on current parameters for AC stimulation, the lowest duty cycle used was a single sine wave: in other words, a single symmetrical biphasic pulse. Figure 4.5 shows the variation in torque with duty cycle, averaged over frequencies of 1, 2.5 and 4 kHz. As Figure 4.5 shows, there is a smooth increase in torque with decreasing duty cycle over the range 100 to 10%. Maximum torque is produced at a duty cycle of about 10% which corresponds to a burst duration of 2 ms. Below 10% there is a small, insignificant decrease. An implication of these findings is that Russian currents, with a 50% duty cycle produce less torque at the pain tolerance limit than single biphasic pulses. A further implication is that when bursts of AC are used to elicit a forceful contraction, the duty cycle should be small, i.e. the bursts should be of short duration, optimally about 2 ms.

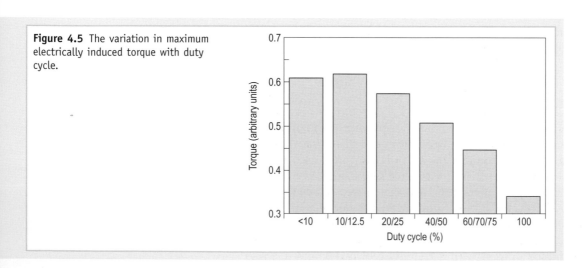

Figure 4.5 The variation in maximum electrically induced torque with duty cycle.

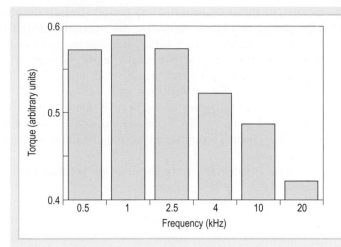

Figure 4.6 The variation in maximum electrically induced torque with AC frequency.

Figure 4.6 shows the variation in torque production with AC frequency, averaged across all duty cycles. Maximum torque is produced at a frequency of 1 kHz. At 500 Hz and 2.5 kHz the average torque is only slightly lower but the differences were found to be statistically significant. Above 2.5 kHz there is a marked decrease in torque with increasing frequency. An implication is that the 2.5 kHz AC frequency of Russian currents is well suited for maximum muscle torque production, though 1 kHz would be better. A further implication is that interferential current frequencies (4 or 5 kHz) are not the best for torque production, but are best from the point of view of minimizing discomfort (see Figure 4.3).

Nerve fibre firing rates

AC used for transcutaneous electrical nerve stimulation is normally in the frequency range 1–10 kHz. AC frequencies less than 1 kHz are too painful (see above) and at frequencies above 10 kHz, nerve fibre sensitivity decreases (Ward and Robertson, 2001). Above about 10 kHz, the current alternations are so rapid that the nerve fibre hardly has time to respond before the stimulus reverses direction. Consequently, high current intensities are needed to depolarize the nerve. High current intensities result in significant heat production and there is a risk of burns immediately under the electrodes where the current density is highest. These electrical burns, if relatively mild, can take the form of tiny white spots or blisters centred on the skin appendages, specifically the exits of the hair follicles and sebaceous glands. The risk of skin damage puts an upper limit on the AC frequencies that can be used clinically.

At AC frequencies in the range 1–10 kHz, the nerve fibre cannot respond by firing at the same frequency. The maximum firing rate is dictated by the absolute refractory period. Thus, if the absolute refractory period is 1 ms or 1/1000 s, the maximum firing rate is 1000 times per second (1 kHz). Firing frequencies approaching this limit have been observed experimentally using laboratory animals and directly stimulating a nerve trunk while monitoring the activity of individual nerve fibres (Bowman and McNeal, 1986). For example, stimulating at a frequency of 4 kHz at an intensity of two times threshold resulted in nerve fibre firing rates of 800 Hz (one fifth of the AC frequency). In this example, nerve impulses are triggered with every fifth AC pulse.

At kHz frequencies, nerve impulses are produced by *summation of subthreshold depolarizations*. Summation was first proposed by Gildemeister (1944) as an explanation for his observations that the subjective sensation, and whether there was any sensation, associated with bursts of kHz frequency AC depended strongly on the burst duration, i.e. the number of cycles in the burst, and also on the AC frequency. The AC frequency is important because successive pulses of an AC stimulus push the nerve fibre closer to threshold with each pulse in a burst. Membrane threshold is reached when successive pulses result in sufficient depolarization to produce an action potential. The Gildemeister effect, as it became known, requires that the pulses occur sufficiently rapidly that the membrane does not have time to recover between them. Depolarization due to summation thus occurs more readily at higher kHz frequencies.

AC used clinically is normally applied in bursts and the AC burst frequency is normally in the 'biological' range, 1 to 100 Hz or more. It has been claimed that if the burst frequency is, say, 50 Hz then nerve fibres will fire at the same low frequency, i.e. once with each burst. This is not true. The physiological response to a burst of current is quite different to the response to a single pulse as nerve fibres can fire repeatedly within a burst if the burst duration is sufficiently long and the stimulus intensity is sufficiently high.

Thus 50 Hz bursts of AC might be 10 ms long (10 ms on and 10 ms off) and the pulses have a frequency of 4 kHz. This means that each burst consists of $10/1000 \times 4000 = 40$ sine wave pulses. If every fifth pulse results in an action potential (nerve impulse), there are eight action potentials per burst so, although the burst frequency is 50 Hz, the fibre firing frequency is $50 \times 8 = 400$ Hz. Consequently, we would expect fatigue effects to be pronounced. On the other hand, if the duty cycle, and consequently the burst duration, was reduced there would be fewer action potentials per burst and the fatigue effects would be less.

An interesting predicted consequence of summation is that if the burst duration is increased, the thresholds for sensory, motor and pain responses should decrease. This is because longer burst durations would allow a greater time for the effects of successive pulses to summate. Two studies were identified which reported threshold measurements using premodulated interferential current (see Figure 4.7c) at an AC frequency of 4 kHz and modulation frequencies in the range

The Gildemeister effect was demonstrated quantitatively by Schwarz and Volkmer (1965) who measured the change in membrane potential of isolated nerve fibres as a result of successive pulses in a burst of kHz frequency AC.

0 (continuous) to 100 Hz (Boonsinsukh et al., 1987; Palmer et al., 1999). Both studies found that the thresholds decreased with decreasing modulation frequency, i.e. increasing burst (beat) duration. This is in contrast to pulsed current stimulation where an increase in threshold is observed with decreasing pulse frequency (Howson, 1978; Palmer et al., 1999).

Summary: alternating current

- The pulses are joined and continuous.
- Stimulation is less uncomfortable than with pulsed current.
- For minimum discomfort the parameters should be:
  - 4 kHz frequency
  - 4 ms burst duration.
- Torque production is slightly larger than with pulsed current.
- For maximal torque the parameters should be:
  - 1 kHz frequency
  - 2 ms burst duration.
- 2.5 kHz is a good compromise between comfort and force production (used with a 2–4 ms burst duration).
- Fibre firing rates are higher than the operator-set (burst) frequency if stimulation is above threshold because of summation of sub-threshhold depolarizations.

Russian current

As discussed in chapter 3, Russian current has a frequency (sometimes called the carrier frequency) of 2.5 kHz and a burst frequency of 50 Hz. This means that each burst is of 10 ms duration and the duty cycle is 50%. The main clinical uses of Russian current are for obtaining a motor response, specifically for muscle contraction and strengthening.

Russian current is applied in trains of bursts with a '10/50/10' treatment application. The bursts of current are applied for 10 s followed by a 50 s rest period and the stimulation is repeated for 10 minutes of treatment. Kots' original finding was that the '10/50/10' treatment regimen was needed to avoid muscular fatigue, which, he thought, would diminish the muscle strengthening effect. Kots found that if the rest period was reduced from 50 s or the 10 s of stimulation extended, fatigue (as evidenced by force decline) developed at some stage through the 10-minute treatment period (Ward and Shkuratova, 2002).

Kots reported large strength gains as a result of stimulation using the '10/50/10' regimen. He also noted that increasing a muscle's force-generating capability can be achieved by two means. One means is by

Kots' assumption that fatigue induced by electrical stimulation would diminish strengthening appears to be validated by the subsequent finding that the fatigue observed is likely to be due to propagation failure and neurotransmitter depletion, not actual muscle fibre fatigue.

It should be noted that many studies of muscle strengthening have reported appreciable strength gains ahead of any increase in muscle bulk (McComas, 1996), thus indicating central nervous system effects ahead of muscle fibre strengthening.

central nervous system adaptation, whereby a greater maximum voluntary contraction is produced by central nervous system 'learning' and adaptation to the pattern of excitation. In this case, the force gains are achieved by greater and more effective recruitment of muscle fibres. The second means is by building the physical bulk of the muscle to produce a greater force output for the same neural input. In this case, the muscle fibres grow in size and muscle volume increases. Kots found increases in limb circumference (and thus, by inference, muscle bulk) paralleling the increase in muscle force and concluded that the force gains were predominantly of peripheral origin.

Recent studies (Ward and Robertson, 1998; Ward et al., 2004) add support for the choice of a 2.5 kHz AC frequency for production of a maximum electrically induced torque. Although torque production is greater at 1 kHz, the difference is small and 2.5 kHz is less uncomfortable.

The 50% duty cycle of Russian currents is clearly not optimal, either from the perspective of comfort or torque production. Minimum discomfort appears to be achieved using a 20% duty cycle (see Figure 4.4) and maximum torque results when a 10% duty cycle is used (see Figure 4.5). A better choice of duty cycle would appear to be in the range 10 to 20%.

Interferential current

Two types of interferential current (IFT) were described in chapter 3: 'true' or quadripolar IFT and premodulated IFT. Quadripolar IFT uses two circuits to enable the crossing of two different currents within the tissues and premodulated (bipolar) IFT uses one circuit which produces current claimed as having similar parameters to the expected outcome of current mixing in tissues.

A claimed advantage of true interferential currents is depth efficiency of stimulation. It is argued that in the region of intersection, the reinforcement of the currents will result in a greater total stimulus intensity so maximum stimulation is produced at depth (see Figure 3.24b) rather than superficially as occurs with normal bipolar stimulation (see Figure 3.24a). Whether this is true is questionable as current spreading reduces the intensity at depth so, even if two currents are superimposed, the total intensity could (and probably would) still be greatest immediately under the electrodes. What is more likely to be true is that greater stimulation is produced at depth with true, i.e. quadripolar, interferential currents than with bipolar (premodulated) stimulation.

When the currents intersect within tissue they 'interfere' or superimpose. The total current at any point is the sum of the two currents. Figure 4.7 shows the effect. Current (a) might have a frequency, f, of 4000 Hz. Current (b) might be 4050 Hz. The resulting current would have a frequency of 4025 Hz and, more importantly, would be modulated in intensity at a frequency (δ) of 50 Hz in this example. This

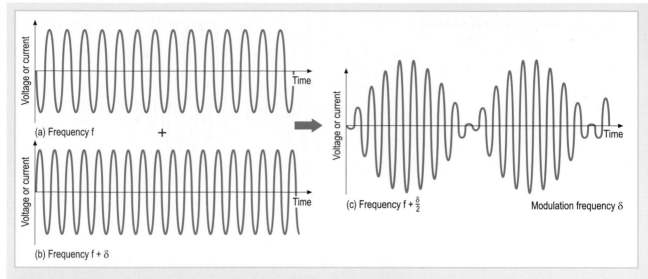

Figure 4.7 Interference of two currents of equal amplitude but unequal frequency.

frequency is called the *beat frequency*: it is equal to the difference in frequency between the two currents. Within tissue the current would be in the form of sinusoidal bursts of current with a burst (or beat) frequency of 50 Hz. In order to make a clear distinction, the AC frequency (4025 Hz in this example) is referred to as the *carrier frequency*.

'True' interferential current

It is claimed that when interferential currents intersect in tissue, the currents interfere (add) and the resulting stimulus intensity is burst modulated as shown in Figure 4.7c. This is a misleading oversimplification. If the currents in Figures 4.7a and (b) ran parallel, and were of equal intensity, then they would interfere and the resulting stimulus intensity would be as shown in Figure 4.7c, but two factors complicate the issue. When the currents are applied at right-angles (see Figure 3.24b) then:

- the two currents will, in general, not be of equal intensity even though the current intensities at the electrodes may be equal
- the resulting stimulus intensity depends on the direction so the stimulus applied to a nerve fibre will depend on its orientation.

In regions closer to an electrode, the current intensity will be higher because the current spreading effect (see Figure 3.2) will be less. When the two currents are not the same size, an interference effect will still be produced, but the resulting waveform will not drop to zero midway between the maxima. Figure 4.8 shows the effect of adding two currents of slightly different frequency when one current is twice as big

Figure 4.8 Interference of two sinusoidal currents of different frequency and different intensity.

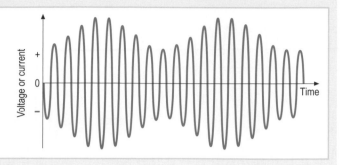

as the other. An interference effect is still produced but the depth of modulation of the waveform is less.

As noted in chapter 3 (see Figures 3.3 and 3.4), for maximum stimulation efficiency, current should flow parallel to the nerve fibres when there is a single current flow through tissue. When there are two intersecting currents of equal amplitude, maximum stimulation occurs along lines midway between the current paths. The reason is that the net current flow is the vector sum of the two currents. Consider first the situation where two current pathways are at right angles and the current intensities are equal. Nerve fibres aligned parallel to one of the current pathways will experience an unmodulated AC stimulus as shown in Figure 4.7(a) or (b). Fibres aligned along lines midway between the current paths will experience a modulated stimulus (Figure 4.7c) of higher intensity. Those fibres aligned in other directions will experience a partially modulated stimulus, similar to Figure 4.8, with a depth of modulation that depends on the fibre orientation.

Figure 4.9 shows the net current flow in different directions for the simple configuration in Figure 3.24b. The length of the black arrows is proportional to the current intensity. In the horizontal and vertical directions, the net current is maximum and the modulation is 100%. In directions at 45°, there is no modulation and the intensity is some 30% lower.

The pattern of stimulation is clearly more complex with interferential currents than with current applied using a single pair of electrodes. We can, however, draw some important conclusions:

- nerve fibres aligned in directions which bisect the angle between the current pathways (horizontally and vertically in Figure 4.9) will experience the greatest stimulation intensity and the stimulus will be a modulated AC signal
- fibres aligned parallel to the direction of the individual current flows will experience a lower, but still relatively high, stimulation intensity. The stimulating current will not be modulated
- fibres oriented at some other angle or positioned closer to one electrode will experience a stimulus which is partially modulated (see Figure 4.8). This would be the most common scenario

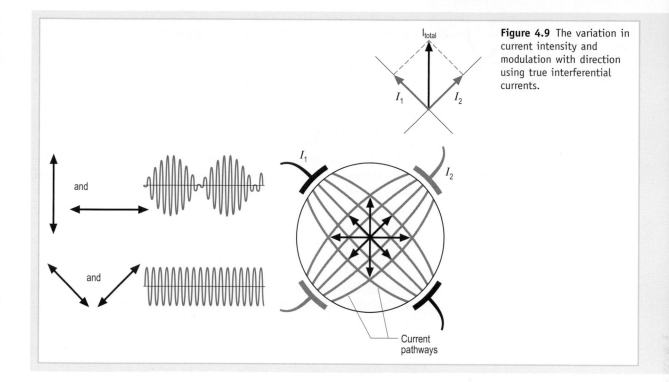

Figure 4.9 The variation in current intensity and modulation with direction using true interferential currents.

Current pathways

- nerve fibre firing rates will be much higher than with stimulation using single pulses applied at low frequency. Fibres aligned parallel to the direction of the individual current flows will fire at a rate determined by how far above threshold the local stimulation intensity is
- fibres aligned in directions which bisect the angle between the current pathways will fire in high frequency bursts. The bursts of activity will be at the beat frequency and the number of action potentials per burst will depend on how far above threshold the local stimulation intensity is.

A widespread misconception about interferential currents is that the pattern of stimulation is in the shape of a clover-leaf (a four-leafed clover, Figure 4.10) rather than the rounded-diamond shape shown in Figure 3.24b. The misconception seems to have originated from the idea that nerve fibres are insensitive to an unmodulated AC stimulus, i.e. that modulation at low ('biological') frequencies is necessary to produce a physiological response. Were this true, then fibres aligned parallel to the current paths would not be excited while those aligned along lines bisecting the angle between the current paths would be excited maximally. The pattern of stimulation would have four lobes, each lobe pointing to a corner of the rounded diamond shape.

In fact, the clover-leaf pattern shows the areas of maximum interference, not maximum stimulation. It indicates the direction in which

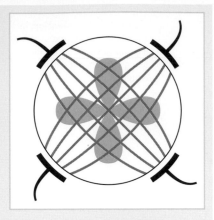

Figure 4.10 The 'clover-leaf' misrepresentation of the pattern of stimulation with 'true' interferential currents.

the stimulus intensity is greatest. It does not, in any way, represent the area of maximum stimulation. A pattern like this describes any small region of the tissue volume through which the currents are flowing. Within each small region, a clover-leaf pattern can be drawn, showing the directions of maximum interference: in other words, the directions in which nerve fibres must be aligned to experience maximum stimulation. A misleading implication of the pattern is that no stimulation is produced if the nerve fibres are aligned along either of the current paths.

Based on the above, it is reasonable to conclude that with clinical applications of 'true' interferential currents, nerve fibres stimulated above threshold will fire at high frequencies. Some will be subject to a relatively unvarying stimulus intensity and fire at a constant high frequency. Others will experience a smoothly modulated stimulus intensity (see Figure 4.9) and would be expected to fire at varying rates depending on the instant by instant variation in stimulus intensity. How this translates to clinical effectiveness is only partly known. Some implications for motor stimulation are apparent: fibre dropout as a result of neurotransmitter depletion or propagation failure or nerve fibre dropout at the stimulation site must result. The implications for sensory stimulation are not clear.

The decrease in discomfort with increasing frequency to about 4 kHz suggests that large diameter nerve fibres are better able to summate, meaning that recruitment of large diameter sensory and motor fibres is more efficient and there is less recruitment of smaller diameter (A-δ) pain fibres.

'Premodulated interferential' current

Premodulated current has the advantage that it is easier to apply, as only two electrodes are needed. A potential disadvantage is that there is no reinforcing at depth so maximum stimulation is produced immediately beneath the electrodes (see Figure 3.24a). This does not seem to be a problem in practice. Ozcan et al. (2004) compared true and premodulated stimulation of quadriceps using 4 kHz AC and a beat frequency of 50 Hz and found that premodulated (with a 50% duty cycle) produced more torque and was less uncomfortable than 'true' interferential. This is consistent with the findings of Ward et al. (2004), that continuous AC, which has an effective duty cycle of 100% is considerably more uncomfortable than burst modulated AC with a 50% duty cycle (see Figure 4.4) and also produces less torque (see Figure 4.6).

As noted previously, with 'true' interferential, some nerve fibres will experience continuous, unmodulated AC (see Figure 4.9), most will experience a partially modulated stimulus (see Figure 4.8) and some a fully modulated stimulus, depending on their orientation and location in the tissue. With premodulated interferential, all nerve fibres will be subject to a defined and predictable fully-modulated stimulus. The modulations may be sinusoidal beats or rectangular bursts. If a sinusoidal modulation is used the nerve firing rates will fluctuate, varying continuously in response to the modulation envelope. If rectangular bursts are used, fibres will alternate between high frequency firing during the burst and no firing during the inter-burst interval.

Frequency modulation

Interferential stimulators provide the option of rhythmically varying the beat or modulation frequency over a user-selectable range. For example a *frequency sweep*, sometimes called a *frequency swing*, of 80 to 100 Hz is normally recommended for pain control. The argument is that varying the beat frequency helps to avoid adaptation to the stimulus which would result in a progressive decrease in the physiological response. If the nerve firing frequency was equal to the beat frequency, this argument might have some validity, but the average nerve firing frequency will be very high and the same whether the beat frequency is 80 Hz or 100 Hz, so it is doubtful that the argument has any merit. The only study identified which casts light on the question compared changes in threshold after 3 minutes of repetitive stimulation using 4 kHz premodulated interferential with (a) a beat frequency of 100 Hz, (b) a beat frequency of 0 Hz, i.e. continuous stimulation and (c) a 50–100 Hz sweep of the beat frequency (Martin and Palmer, 1995). Thresholds changed, but there was no discernible difference between the three conditions. The evidence to date thus offers no support for the notion that a frequency sweep (frequency modulation) is of any advantage.

Vector rotation

Another feature of some interferential stimulators is 'vector rotation' or 'scanning'. This is achieved by rhythmically increasing and decreasing the amount of current applied between one pair of electrodes, while simultaneously decreasing and increasing the other, generally over a period of several seconds or tens of seconds. So when one current goes up, the other goes down and vice versa. This is often described as 'rotating' the clover-leaf pattern of stimulation (see Figure 4.10). As explained above, the pattern of stimulation does not have the shape of a clover leaf. Increasing the current between one pair of electrodes will stimulate more fibres lying parallel to the current path and if the other current is reduced, fewer of the fibres running parallel to it will be stimulated. Thus 'vector rotation' will change the pattern of stimulation in a tissue volume but the effect is best visualized as stimulation which progressively fluctuates between maximum along the path between one pair of electrodes and maximum between the other pair of electrodes.

There seems to be no reported evidence that 'vector rotation' is of clinical benefit, though it may be that the surging in intensity in different directions allows for some recovery between periods of high activity.

Suction cups

An important feature of commercial interferential stimulators is a vacuum unit which allows electrodes to be attached with suction cups. Metal electrodes within the cups are in contact with wetted sponges which conduct current from the electrodes to the skin. The ease of placement and securing of the electrodes is of great practical value. There is no need for strapping or use of conductive gel. If water from the local supply is not sufficiently conductive, a small amount of salt (about 1 flat teaspoonful per litre) can be added before the sponges are moistened. Some manufacturers advise against the use of salt as it can accelerate corrosion of any moistened metal in the suction unit but, if the unit is of quality, i.e. stainless steel and the amount of added salt does not exceed the recommended level, no adverse effects should occur. Suction cup electrodes are commonly used with interferential stimulators, perhaps because of the need to position four electrodes simultaneously. They are not normally used for other forms of stimulation but this is perhaps for historical reasons. Suction cup electrodes are quick and easy to position and could be used for any stimulus type, quadripolar or bipolar.

A potential risk with suction cup application is the vacuum produced. The vacuum must be great enough to hold the cup in contact with the skin but must not be high enough to cause tissue damage. The pressure in the suction cup can, if low enough, result in burst blood vessels and generalized reddening and bruising of the area immediately under the cups so it is important that suction units allow for sufficient operator control of the vacuum.

Pain control

Both interferential current and pulsed current (TENS) are used for pain relief. There is an appreciable body of evidence that pulsed current, as delivered by low-cost, small, portable TENS units, is effective for pain control (see chapter 6). Clinically, interferential current stimulation is often the modality of choice, but there is not a corresponding body of evidence that it is effective and, if it is, whether it has any advantage over a pulsed current.

The neurophysiological basis of pain, pain modulation and the effects of electrical stimulation are discussed in chapter 6. Although the basic mechanisms of pain signal processing are understood, as are the fundamental effects of electrical stimulation, from what is known it is not possible to predict whether interferential current will have different effects to pulsed current (Noble et al., 2000, 2001). With motor stimulation, the effects of varying the electrical stimulus parameters have been well studied. Thus, for example, we can predict when neurotransmitter depletion or propagation failure will be a consideration, whether the contraction will be twitching or tetanic and how rapidly fatigue will occur. We can also predict how the effects of AC and pulsed current will differ. There is not the same body of knowledge for sensory stimulation. Whether neurotransmitter deple-

Despite having been used clinically for over 50 years, it is only recently that the usefulness of interferential current has been called into question in the literature (Martin, 1996; Alon, 1999; Shanahan, 2004).

tion occurs when sensory fibres are stimulated at high frequency does not appear to have been studied. Nor have the effects of stimulus frequency on pain signal transmission or interpretation.

There are, however, some empirical studies which have attempted to establish the relative effectiveness of interferential and pulsed current for pain relief using healthy subjects experiencing pain induced by some standardized means (Johnson and Tabasam, 1999, 2003; Alves-Guerreiro et al., 2001; Cheing and Hui-Chan, 2004). Three of these four studies found that both TENS and IFT were effective in increasing the pain threshold, the exception being Alvez-Guerreiro et al. (2001) who induced pain by mechanical pressure applied to the palm of the hand. The three studies which did find an effect of both TENS and IFT found no significant difference between the two stimulus types. Of these three studies, one (Johnson and Tabasam, 1999) found a marked difference which approached statistical significance.

Johnson and Tabasam (1999) used a cold induced pain model to compare the effects of TENS and premodulated interferential currents. Subjects immersed their hands in ice-cold water and the time to the subjective report of the onset of deep, aching pain was measured. TENS elevated the pain threshold by an average of 35% while with IFT the increase was 24%. The low P value obtained ($P = 0.09$) suggests the likelihood of a type II statistical error (a conclusion that there is no difference when the difference is actually real but the sample size is too small to demonstrate the effect). A study by Shanahan (2004) repeated Johnson and Tabasam's study but included a training/familiarization component and found that TENS had a greater effect, and that the difference was statistically significant.

Although the evidence is strictly limited, it suggests that interferential current stimulation is less effective than pulsed current (TENS) for pain relief. There is clearly a need for further research on this topic.

One difference between clinical and laboratory uses of interferential and pulsed current is the electrode area in contact with the skin. Especially if 'true' interferential, the electrode area is usually considerably larger than if a TENS machine and a single channel is used. The effect, however, of stimulating a larger cutaneous area rather than one, say, 50% less, is not known.

Summary

Types of alternating current:

- Russian current
  - 2.5 kHz AC frequency
  - burst frequency 50 Hz
  - 50% burst duty cycle
  - applied with a '10/50/10' treatment protocol
- Interferential current
  - 1 to 10 kHz (carrier) frequency but normally 4 kHz
  - modulation (beat) frequency: operator-selectable frequency or frequency sweep
  - true (quadripolar) or premodulated (biopolar)

- true interferential uses two constant amplitude currents applied so as to 'interfere' in tissue. The stimulus experienced by a nerve fibre may be continuous or modulated depending on its location and orientation
- premodulated interferential current uses bursts with duty cycle of 50% or more
- there is some evidence that interferential current is less effective than TENS for pain relief.

CURRENT FLOW IN TISSUE

Pulsed current

An important point to note about pulsed current electrical stimulators is that most produce stimulus pulses with a controlled voltage, even though the readout may be in mA.

Most pulsed current stimulators produce a waveform resembling Figure 4.11a which shows a stimulus voltage varying with time in a rectangular manner. The resulting current flow through tissue will not vary in the same way but rather like Figure 4.11b. This is because current depends on the impedance of the tissue volume and the impedance increases with time during the pulse, so decreasing the current.

The reason that there is a negative spike, a negative flow of current in Figure 4.11b is that the first barrier to current flow is the skin. The electrical properties of skin and how it acts as a barrier to transcutaneous current were briefly introduced in chapter 3. The stratum corneum is an insulator so the skin acts as a capacitor and charge is blocked and builds-up on the skin surface. At the end of the pulse, the stratum corneum discharges. Charge which had accumulated on the skin surface flows back again, i.e. in the reverse direction so there is a brief negative (reverse) flow of current. Whether the stimulus shape is rectangular (Figure 4.11a) or drooping (Figure 4.11b) is not particularly important, the current flow in tissue in either case will be as in Figure 4.11b, i.e. drooping and with a subsequent reverse flow of current at the end of the pulse. The amount of droop depends on

For more information on skin and current flow see chapter 3 of the book 'Biophysical Bases of Electrotherapy' and chapter 4, page 60 of 'Physical Principles Explained' on the CD which comes with this book.

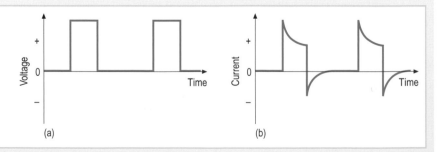

Figure 4.11 (a) A rectangular pulsed voltage stimulus applied to the skin and (b) the resulting current flow.

the electrical properties of the skin and underlying tissue and the pulse duration. With pulses of 100 μs or so, the amount of droop is small. It is not the pulse shape which dictates the nerve fibre response but the amount of charge flowing through tissue, which is determined by the pulse duration and amplitude and indicated by the area under the current versus time graph (Figure 4.11b). So whether the current pulse has a shape like that shown in Figure 4.11a or 4.11b is largely irrelevant as far as nerve fibre excitation is concerned.

With longer duration pulses (1 ms or more) the current drops to virtually zero before the pulse is over (Figure 4.12b). A current spike is produced at the beginning and end of the pulse. If the pulse duration is increased, the same spiked current pulses will be produced but the separation between them will increase. The physiological response will be virtually the same. This is why the strength–duration curve (see Figure 5.2) always has a plateau (the rheobase) at longer pulse durations. Any increase in the pulse width, above a certain limit, will produce no further decrease in the threshold stimulus intensity because the area under the spike, and therefore the charge delivered, does not increase.

Alternating current

AC with a rectangular voltage waveform will produce a current waveform which droops (Figure 4.13b) but at the frequencies used clinically, 1 to 10 kHz, the droop is relatively small and the physiological consequences are insignificant.

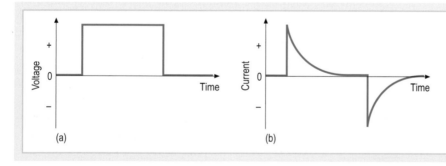

(a) (b)

Figure 4.12 (a) A long duration (> 1 ms) pulsed voltage stimulus applied to the skin and (b) the resulting current flow.

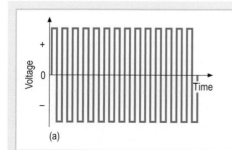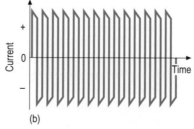

(a) (b)

Figure 4.13 (a) A rectangular, kHz frequency AC stimulus applied to the skin and (b) the resulting current flow.

AC with a sinusoidal waveform is unaffected by the skin acting as a capacitor. The stimulus voltage is sinusoidal and so is the resulting current. The skin impedance limits the amount of current flow so that at lower frequencies the impedance is higher and the current flow is less but the current waveform is still sinusoidal.

Skin breaks

Electrical stimulation through broken skin should be avoided unless using an appropriate method and type of current as for wound healing (see chapter 6). The reasons are twofold. First, because if the skin is damaged the skin impedance is compromised. Damaged areas will have a lower electrical impedance than those surrounding so the current density will be higher. The high current could produce further tissue damage. Second, a superficially damaged area will be hypersensitized so pain receptors will be more readily excited by the current flow. The combination of hypersensitivity and higher stimulating current density will have adverse effects. For this reason, stimulation over broken skin is either avoided or, if very small, a piece of impervious dry dressing or petroleum jelly is used to cover the break.

The risk of harm is increased markedly if AC is used rather than pulsed current because of the pulse duty cycle. For example, if true interferential current is applied at a current level of, say, 40 mA to produce a strong motor response, the stimulus voltage will be about 40 V and the power dissipated in tissue will be of the order of 1.6 W. Because the duty cycle is 100%, the average power is 1.6 W and, if the current is focused over a small area, the power density may pose a hazard. If pulsed current of duration 200 μs and frequency 50 Hz is used instead, the peak voltage to produce the same response would be about 60 V and the peak current about 60 mA, so the peak power will be of the order of 3.6 W, but the pulse duty cycle is only 1% so the average power will be 36 mW or about 1/40th of the power of the continuous AC.

As noted in chapter 3, the power dissipated, P, is given by the formula:

$$P = VI$$

where V is the stimulus voltage and I is the current.

Implants

Metal implants in tissue are not a contraindication for electrical stimulation. Rather there is a potential risk which must be assessed on a case-by-case basis by considering the lowest resistance pathways for current flow. For example, a metal pin inside a long bone would have little effect (provided the fracture has united) as cortical bone has a high electrical impedance so current flow would be mainly through the overlying soft tissues. A metal plate, secured to bone would provide an extremely low resistance current pathway so tissue adjacent and parallel to the plate would experience little current flow and minimal stimulation. The current density would be greatest in tissue immediately between the electrodes and the metal plate so the stimulation will be greatest in these regions.

In clinical practice, the therapist sets the stimulation intensity by assessing the physiological response. This includes the observed motor response (if any) and the subjective reports elicited from the patient. Since the current level is normally limited to avoid discomfort, the risk of any potentially adverse effects is minimal. If the patient does not have normal cutaneous sensation in the region then more care than usual is needed. The skin must be checked carefully under the electrodes to identify any possible or actual damage.

If an implant is an electronic device, current should never be allowed to flow through it. The risks are often incalculable and so current should not be passed through a body segment that contains an electronic device of any sort unless medical and manufacturers' clearances have been obtained.

Summary

Current in tissues:

- tissues change the pulse shape
- current passes through broken skin more easily
- damage is more likely with AC than pulsed current due to higher power
- not an issue with metal implants
- current must not pass through an implanted electronic device.

References

Alon, G. (1999). Principles of electrical stimulation. In: Nelson, R.M., Hayes, K.W., Currier, D.P. (eds). Clinical electrotherapy, 3rd edn. Connecticut: Appleton & Lange.

Alves-Guerreiro, J., Noble, J., Lowe, A., Walsh, D. (2001). The effect of three electrotherapeutic modalities upon peripheral nerve conduction and mechanical pain threshold. Clin Physiol, **21**, 704–711.

Boonsinsukh, P., Charmornnarumit, C., Chanpitayanukukij, R. (1987). Comparison of S-D curve in motor and sensory nerve. Paper presented at the 10th International Congress WCPT (Book 1), Sydney, Australia.

Bowman, B., McNeal, D. (1986). Response of single alpha motoneurons to high frequency pulse trains. Appl Neurophysiol, **49**, 121–138.

Cheing, G., Hui-Chan, C. (2004). Would the addition of TENS to exercise training produce better physical performance outcomes in people with knee osteoarthritis than either intervention alone. Clin Rehabil, **18**, 487–497.

Clamann, H. (1981). Discussion following Bigland-Ritchie B. EMG and fatigue of human voluntary and stimulated contractions in Porter, R., Whelan, J.

(eds). Human Muscle Fatigue: Physiological Mechanisms, pp.148–156. London: Pitman Medical.

Gildemeister, M. (1944). Untersuchungen über die wirkung der mittelfrequenzströme auf den menschen. Pflugers Arch gesamte physiol menchen tiere, **247**, 366–404.

Grimby, G., Wigerstad-Lossing, I. (1989). Comparison of high- and low-frequency muscle stimulators. Arch Phys Med Rehabil, **70,** 835–838.

Henneman, E., Somjen, G., Carpenter D. (1965). Functional significance of cell size in spinal motoneurons. J Neurophysiol, **28**, 581–598.

Holcomb, W., Golestani, S., Hill, S. (2000). A comparison of knee-extension torque production with biphasic versus russian current. J Sports Rehabil, **9**, 229–239.

Howson, D. (1978). Peripheral nerve excitability – implications for transcutaneous electrical stimulation. Phys Ther, **58**, 1467–1473.

Johnson, M., Tabasam, G. (1999). A double blind placebo controlled investigation into the analgesic effects of interferential currents (IFC) and transcutaneous electrical nerve stimulation (TENS) on cold-induced pain in health subjects. Physiother Theory Pract, **15**, 217–233.

Johnson, M., Tabasam, G. (2003). An investigation into the analgesic effects of interferential currents and transcutaneous electrical nerve stimulation on experimentally induced ischaemic pain in otherwise pain-free volunteers. Phys Ther, **83**, 208–223.

Jones, D., Bigland-Ritchie, B., Edwards, R. (1979). Excitation frequency and muscle fatigue: mechanical responses during voluntary and stimulated contractions. Exp Neurol, **64**, 401–413.

Martin, D. (1996). Interferential therapy. In: Kitchen, S., Bazin, S. (eds). Clayton's electrotherapy, 10th edn. London: WB Saunders.

Martin, D., Palmer, S. (1995). Sensory adaptation to interferential current is not affected by modulation of the stimulus. 14th World Congress of Physical Therapy. Washington, USA. Abstract PL-RR-0584-F.

McComas, A.J. (1996). Skeletal muscle form and function. Champaign: Human Kinetics.

McNeal, D. (1976). Analysis of a model for excitation of myelinated nerve. IEEE Trans Biomed Eng. BME-**23**, 329–337.

Mizrahi, J. (1997). Fatigue in muscles activated by functional electrical stimulation. Crit Rev Phys Rehab Med, **9**, 93–129.

Noble, J., Henderson, G., Cramp, A. et al. (2000). The effect of interferential therapy upon cutaneous blood flow in humans. Clin Physiol, **20**, 2–7.

Noble, J., Lowe, A., Walsh, D. (2001). Interferential therapy review part 2: experimental pain models and neurophysiological effects of electrical stimulation. Phys Ther Rev, **6**, 17–37.

Otsuka, M., Endo, M., Nonomura, Y. (1962). Presynaptic nature of neuromuscular depression. Japanese J Physiol, **12**, 573–584.

Ozcan, J., Ward, A., Robertson, V. (2004). A comparison of true and premodulated interferential currents. Arch Phys Med Rehabil, **85**, 409–415.

Palmer, S., Martin, D., Steedman, W., Ravey, J. (1999). Alteration of interferential current and transcutaneous electrical nerve stimulation frequency: effects on nerve excitation. Arch Phys Med Rehabil, **80**, 1065–1071.

Schwarz, F., Volkmer, H. (1965). Über die summation lokaler potentiale bei reizung motorischer nervenfasern mit elektrischen wechselimpulsen. Acta Biol Med German, **15**, 283–301.

Shanahan, C. (2004). A comparison of the analgesic effectiveness of IFT and TENS. Honours thesis, School of Physiotherapy, LaTrobe University, Australia.

Snyder-Mackler, L., Garrett, M., Roberts, M. (1989). A comparison of torque generating capabilities of three different electrical stimulating currents. J Orthop Sports Phys Ther, **10**, 297–301.

Ward, A., Robertson, V. (1998). The variation in torque production with frequency using medium frequency alternating current. Arch Phys Med Rehabil, **79**, 1399–1404.

Ward, A., Robertson, V. (2001). Variation in motor threshold with frequency using kHz frequency alternating current. Musc Nerve, **24**, 1303–1311.

Ward, A., Robertson, V., Ioannou, H. (2004). The effect of duty cycle and frequency on muscle torque production using kHz frequency alternating current. Med Eng Physics, **26**, 569–579.

Ward, A., Shkuratova, N. (2002). Russian currents: the early experimental evidence. Phys Ther, **82**,1019–1030.

Motor electrical stimulation

Since clinical electrical stimulation first became available researchers and clinicians have explored its possible uses. Modern technology allows more control over the stimulus parameters. The equipment has increasingly become miniaturized: it is more portable, cheaper and some of it implantable. This changes how electrical stimulation can be used and the range of conditions for which it might be used. For this reason alone, clinical users need to remain aware of current research that extends possible uses beyond those described in this chapter.

Four main categories of use of electric current exist in clinical practice. One of these categories is motor stimulation. This includes stimulation of both innervated and denervated muscle. The categories are not all mutually exclusive as stimulation for a motor response will, of course, also stimulate sensory receptors and have other effects. For this reason the categorization is made according to the main aim of treatment; if principally to obtain a motor response the use is considered in the motor and not the sensory category of uses.

This chapter discusses the relevant physiology and then the clinical and research evidence supporting motor electrical stimulation. Where relevant, the principles used to set stimulator parameters are outlined and the types of suitable current detailed. The chapter concludes with an outline of how motor stimulation is applied clinically and the risks and contraindications associated with its use. Given the range of possible uses the outline is necessarily general.

The main aim of this chapter is to present the range of uses of clinical motor stimulation so clinicians know how it is used and how to do it themselves in practice. The aim is also to promote understanding of present and possible future uses of motor stimulation. The principles governing the setting of parameters to achieve specific aims are provided to assist users. The descriptive system of identifying currents will be used throughout to ensure clarity. Named currents will be explicitly mentioned to indicate their main roles.

The other three categories of uses of electric current are the focus of chapter 6. They are sensory stimulation, iontophoresis and 'other'.

MOTOR STIMULATION

Motor stimulation means the production of a muscle contraction by the use of electrical stimulation. This can be stimulation via the motor nerves to obtain a muscle contraction or, if the muscle is denervated, direct stimulation of the muscle fibres.

This distinction between the stimulation of innervated and denervated muscle is very important as they are quite different. Nerve fibres are much more excitable and much more easily stimulated than muscle fibres.

However, the electrical stimulus parameters can be chosen preferentially to activate muscle fibres. This means the parameters for stimulating a denervated muscle will be quite different than if it were innervated. This also means that if the muscle is partly denervated then one set of stimulus parameters might only cause one part of the muscle to contract, either the innervated or the denervated part, depending on the parameters used.

Given this distinction, this chapter is divided into three sections: innervated muscle, functional electrical stimulation (FES) and denervated muscle. The innervated muscle section starts by describing the essential component of muscle contraction, the motor unit, and how it functions normally and in response to electrical stimulation. This leads to discussion of the range of clinical uses and issues of fatigue and changes in muscles following stimulation. Section two briefly discusses functional electrical stimulation, which may involve stimulation of innervated or denervated muscle to restore function. Section three describes the 'best' stimulus parameters for stimulating denervated muscle and how to test whether a peripheral nerve is damaged. The different types of damage that usually occur are also described.

The motor unit

A motor unit is defined as a single motor neuron and all the individual muscle fibres it innervates. The number of muscle fibres supplied by a single nerve fibre varies from very few where low force but precise control of movement is required up to one or two thousand for large postural muscles which must produce large forces.

An individual muscle is made up of many motor units which can be fast-fatigue or fatigue-resistant, giving the muscle its particular characteristics. All fibres in a particular motor unit are the same type but the proportion of different motor units, hence fibres, varies between muscles.

Slow twitch fibres are also described as *type I fibres*. They are red because they are highly vascular, and predominate in postural muscles such as soleus. They are slow to contract and relax. The motor neuron supplying them is of small diameter and innervates a relatively small number of muscle fibres. Slow twitch motor units are thus best suited

While we now know why early attempts to restore the dead with electrical stimulation were doomed to fail, we still have much to learn about clinical effects and the best uses of electrical stimulation.

Soleus, which is a major postural control muscle, has about 80% fatigue-resistant fibres. Gastrocnemius has a little under 50% (Johnson et al., 1973).

to produce low-level sustained contractions. The motor nerve typically fires at a continuous, low frequency. Slow twitch muscle fibres have many oxidative enzymes, have a good blood supply and fatigue slowly.

Fast twitch fibres are also described as *type II fibres*. These, which predominate in sternomastoid, are white, glycolytic fibres. They have a lower level of myoglobin and capillary content (Scott et al., 2001). The motor neuron supplying them is of larger diameter and supplies a larger number of muscle fibres. They are thus best equipped for brief, forceful contraction. They are divided into two subgroups. *Fast-fatigue-resistant* or *type IIA* have fewer oxidative enzymes than type I, but are relatively fatigue-resistant. They predominate in ordinary low force movement. *Fast-fatigable* or *type IIB* have the least oxidative enzymes and fatigue rapidly. They produce a large force for short periods and are only brought into play during forceful contraction.

Voluntary contraction of muscle

During voluntary contractions the firing of motor neurons is asynchronous and this produces a smooth muscle contraction. The force of a contraction is graded, in general, by an increase in (a) the number of motor units recruited (spatial summation) and (b) the frequency of nerve action potentials (temporal summation). As described in chapter 4 (see Figure 4.2), at low force levels, force increases are produced by recruiting more muscle fibres and the motor units recruited are fatigue-resistant. Only at high force levels are fast-fatigue fibres recruited. What Figure 4.2 does not show is the increase in nerve fibre firing frequencies which accompany increasingly forceful contractions.

The number of motor units recruited is most relevant in the low-force stages of contraction. Firing frequency is also used to increase muscle force and this becomes more important at high force levels. Figure 3.12 shows how muscle fibre force varies with stimulus frequency. The force of contraction changes quite markedly in the frequency range 5 to 20 Hz in this example.

Changes to muscle following electrical stimulation

Electrical stimulation initiates contractions of muscle, if innervated, by stimulating the nerve, and if denervated, by direct stimulation of the muscle fibres. To an innervated muscle, electrical stimulation appears as a usual initiator of a contraction. So, just as changing voluntary demands on a muscle initiate physiological changes in that muscle, changing the electrical parameters can also change the muscle in different ways. Electrical stimulation can mimic a range of conditions similar to those that are produced naturally. This suggests that

Low force, high repetition training will cause a reduction in the rate of fatiguing but typically little change in strength. High force, low repetition training will produce strength increases with a minimal change in endurance.

the effects on the muscle will be similar to those produced with specific voluntary patterns of contraction. Strengthening requires strong contractions and the number of daily repetitions does not need to be high. Endurance training requires many repetitions but the strength of contraction does not need to be high. Both forms of training will produce some degree of hypertrophy of muscle.

Muscle is essentially plastic and responds according to the particular demands made of it. This is the basis for establishing which parameters to choose to achieve a specific aim. The following section describes some of the effects on muscle when electrical stimulation is used.

Muscle fibre plasticity

The size of muscle fibres can change and the fibres can convert from one type to another (Scott et al., 2001). An increase in fibre size and consequently muscle bulk (hypertrophy) is a response to, particularly, a demand for regular repeated strong contractions. Decreases in fibre size and muscle bulk (atrophy), are associated with inactivity such as occurs following a tendon rupture.

Changes in skeletal muscle type occur in response to the frequency of stimulation. This has been demonstrated in cross-innervation experiments and studies using transcutaneous stimulation (Pette et al., 1973; Salmons and Sreter, 1976; Pette, 1994). The fibres innervating fatigue-resistant muscles such as soleus, fire at a low frequency (less than 10 Hz) for prolonged periods of time. Nerves innervating fast twitch fibres fire at higher frequencies but only in infrequent, short-duration bursts. Cross-innervation experiments have demonstrated conclusively that the muscle fibre adapts and changes in response to the changed neural activation pattern and thus that the muscle fibre type is controlled by neural activation. Continuous stimulation for up to 20 weeks of the fast twitch muscle fibres in rabbits and cats, with a frequency of 10 Hz, produces a significant increase in the twitch time (Salmons and Sreter, 1976). Less stimulation repeated across a number of days produced the same effects. Stimulation (300 μs pulses, 10 Hz frequency) of the muscles of rabbits for 28 days produced a 23% reduction in force over a 10-minute test period, compared to 75% at the start of the study (Hudlicka et al., 1977). In addition, changes consistent with altered fatigability also occurred in the capillary system and different metabolic markers of muscle activity.

Little is known about the time required for changes in the fatigue response in human muscle nor how best to exploit this property of plasticity. Strength changes following transcutaneous electrical stimulation are evident after as few as eight contractions per session, twice a week for 5 weeks (Soo et al., 1988). This degree of change, however, is probably also partly due to changes in the neurological system producing contractions more efficiently.

Few studies have investigated changes in the responses of slow twitch fibres to electrical stimulation (Gordon and Pattullo, 1993).

In a cross-innervation experiment, the nerve supply to a muscle made up of predominantly slow twitch fibres, such as soleus, is surgically cut and exchanged with the nerve trunk innervating a muscle with a much higher proportion of fast-fatigue fibres (such as gastrocnemius). What is observed is a progressive change in the twitch time, with the soleus becoming faster and gastrocnemius, slower.

Stimulation of denervated muscle leaves slow twitch fibres relatively unchanged if frequencies of 10–15 Hz are applied for 2 to 21 days, but the muscle response resembles that associated with fast twitch fibres if the stimulation frequency is 100 Hz (Gorza et al., 1988). This is consistent with the ideas that slow twitch fibres require a continuation of their normal pattern of activation (low frequency but often) otherwise they transform to fast twitch fibres and that activation at a high frequencies, which is typical of fast twitch fibres, does not prevent the slow to fast transformation.

Another factor contributing to the ineffectiveness of 100 Hz stimulation in preventing the slow to fast fibre transformation is activation failure (chapter 4) whereby the nerve fibre fires at high frequency but the contractile apparatus of the muscle fibre is not activated.

Strengthening and delayed onset muscle soreness

Strengthening following voluntary exercise has been shown to be associated with some damage at the microscopic level, involving tearing of actin/myosin contractile filaments in the muscle fibre. This damage is the cause of delayed onset muscle soreness (DOMS). The torque the muscle can produce is particularly affected both by active insufficiency and inhibited neural drive. Recovery is slow, taking hours or even days (Stokes et al., 1989; Jones, 1996). Nonetheless, if exercise is continued, the muscle strength can increase markedly (McComas, 1996). It is not known whether DOMS is necessary for strengthening but it is known that it accompanies most strengthening programmes. Intense electrical stimulation also presumably results in microscopic damage of activated fibres as anecdotally DOMS is reported after its use, especially if intense or after a period of little activity of the muscle.

Delayed onset muscle soreness would be more likely to occur with an electrically induced contraction than with a voluntary contraction of the same magnitude because a smaller proportion of the fibres would be activated and induced to work harder by the higher than physiological stimulation frequencies normally used (50 Hz or so).

Fatigue and fatigue-resistance

Muscle fatigue is a well-known consequence of voluntary contraction but it is complex, as discussed in chapter 4. Fatigue at submaximal voluntary contractions is minimized by preferential recruitment of fatigue-resistant fibres and by varying the activity of the particular motor units involved. This indicates that electrically stimulated muscle will undergo a more rapid rate of fatigue as a high proportion of fast-fatigue fibres will be recruited and there will be little or no change of the particular fibres recruited. The story is more complicated as the stimulating frequency also affects the rate of fatigue development and frequencies applied clinically do not normally correspond to those used physiologically to produce the same effect.

Two kinds of fatigue are identified with electrical stimulation: these are called 'low frequency' fatigue and 'high frequency' fatigue (see chapter 4). Low frequency fatigue follows the use of frequencies of approximately 20 Hz or lower. It is due to the failure of excitation-contraction coupling, i.e. the failure of depolarization of the muscle fibre membrane to result in force production (Matsunaga et al., 1999). The time-course of recovery is similar to the time-course of the fatigue. It is typically measured in minutes or tens of minutes, reflecting changes in metabolite concentration (including glucose, oxygen and carbon dioxide) in the muscle fibres. Fatigue from low frequency

High frequency fatigue is something which only occurs with electrical stimulation. It appears to be clinically undesirable as muscle fibres are not worked to the point of fatigue; rather the muscle fibres are no longer activated.

stimulation is like that produced by voluntary contractions. High frequency fatigue is also well documented (Jones, 1996). It is obvious at frequencies of 50 Hz and above and especially at higher frequencies (see chapter 4). Force recovery is relatively rapid (measured in seconds) and is thought to reflect re-establishment of ion concentrations in the T-tubule system and metabolite concentrations (particularly creatine phosphate) following fast-fatiguing activity. High frequency fatigue does not occur with normal, voluntary activities as the firing rates are either too low or, if high, are not sustained.

Fatigue is an important issue for users of electrical stimulation. High frequency fatigue should be avoided as it contributes nothing to strengthening, fatigue-resistance or fibre-type transformation (or its prevention). Thus stimulation frequencies of 50 Hz or more should be used only when the on-time is relatively short (a few seconds or less) and the off-time is at least as long as the duration of the on-time, to allow recovery. In practice for strengthening the off-time is usually at least one to three times longer than the on-time for this reason.

Extended periods of daily use, such as following a stroke or a spinal cord injury (see FES below), means consideration of fatigue is important when planning a treatment regimen. Treatment requires low frequency stimulation applied as often and for as long as possible. The daily duration of stimulation should be increased gradually and in response to how the treated muscles are affected. Low levels of electrical stimulation, for total stimulation of up to two hours a day, appear to maintain fatigue-resistance in muscles without reducing force (Gordon and Pattullo, 1993).

Blood flow increases

Besides direct effects on fatigability and strength, electrical stimulation has also been shown to produce long-term changes in vascularization at the capillary level. Low frequency stimulation of the triceps surae or tibialis anterior for 28 days (8 Hz, 3×20 minutes per day, 5 days per week) altered both limb blood flow and the associated microvascular filtration capacity (Brown et al., 1998). A later study using the same frequency and daily sessions routine (3×20 minutes daily, 5 days per week) and dynamically trained the plantarflexors at 70% of their peak torque or stimulated the muscles electrically (Brown et al., 2001). Electrical stimulation again produced structural changes with extended periods of application.

Low frequency stimulation for prolonged periods (and it is both the low frequency and the long periods which are needed) promotes fibre transformation from fast twitch, fast-fatigue to slow twitch, fatigue-resistant fibres. Slow, fatigue-resistant fibres rely on an adequate supply of oxygen for their function, so changed vascularization is an essential part of the transformation process.

There is a close link between vascularization and neural activity. Infiltration of nerve fibres into repairing tissue is a necessary precursor to capillary invasion and if the nerve supply to the area is damaged, normal vascularization and repair are markedly inhibited. Conversely, if nerve growth is stimulated, vascularization proceeds more rapidly (Grills et al., 1997). It would appear that increasing the activity of existing, active nerve fibres by electrical stimulation can also promote vascularization.

Trophic stimlation

Stimulation at particular frequencies to achieve a beneficial aim by changing the physiological response has been called 'trophic' or 'eutrophic' stimulation. These terms are most often used to describe the range of beneficial changes obtained when stimulation, usually with a frequency of less than 15 Hz, is applied to muscles for extended periods of time. One condition for which this has been used is non-recovering Bell's palsy (Farragher et al., 1987). The mean frequency of motor unit firing in selected facial muscles was used to choose the frequency (5–8 Hz) of 80 μs rectangular pulses applied to the facial nerve in bursts, 2 s on and 2 s off, for up to 8 h over several weeks. Considerable objective improvement was noted. There is, however, little evidence that the frequencies used need to be established by using EMG, as implied by Farragher et al. (1987). Rather, the benefits of what is called 'trophic stimulation' appear to be those of long-term, low-frequency stimulation of muscles.

The muscles may be innervated but the patient may have a central nervous system lesion such as spinal cord damage or their muscles may be partly or near totally denervated. As explained above, chronic low frequency stimulation can slow or even prevent atrophy and slow to fast fibre conversion and increase the amount of microvascularization (Brown et al., 2001).

The promotion of vascularization by low frequency electrical stimulation applied for long periods suggests a possible future treatment for some instances of intermittent claudication of the calf muscles (see chapter 6).

Summary

Electrical stimulation can be used to alter or maintain the properties of muscle fibres.

- Muscle is plastic, meaning that it will adapt its properties to respond best to the pattern of neural activation.
- Stimulation at low frequencies (<10 Hz) for sustained periods is best for stimulation of slow twitch, fatigue-resistant fibres. It can be used to prevent slow twitch fibres transforming to fast twitch; an undesirable process which is part of muscle atrophy. It can also be used to promote hypertrophy.
- Stimulation at high frequencies (>30 Hz) for brief periods is best for stimulation of fast twitch, fast-fatigue fibres. It can be used to increase muscle strength (peak force) by promoting hypertrophy of fast twitch fibres.

The experimental evidence thus indicates that the muscle fibre response to electrical stimulation can change in response to the stimulation parameters including the total duration of stimulation over weeks, the frequency applied, and the force demands. This is the basis of many clinical uses that are explained in the following sections of this chapter.

ELECTRICAL STIMULATION OF INNERVATED MUSCLE

The pattern of activation of fibres in the muscle cannot be the same with electrically induced and voluntary contractions. Electrical stimulation of muscle differs from voluntary contraction in three main ways. First, with electrical stimulation there is synchronous firing of all motor neurons stimulated. This means that to produce a non-twitching muscle response high stimulation frequencies (>20 Hz) must be used. Lower nerve firing frequencies are used physiologically as the firing of different motor units is asynchronous, so while individual motor units may be twitching, the muscle as a whole undergoes a smooth, non-twitching contraction. Second, electrical stimulation will not stimulate motor units in the same recruitment order as a voluntary contraction. Rather, the order is largely reversed because of the greater excitability of larger diameter motor neurons (see chapter 4). Third, sensory (A-β) nerves are inevitably stimulated, as are A-δ (pain) fibres. There is thus a substantial afferent component of electrical stimulation which is not produced in a voluntary contraction.

Electrical stimulation of a muscle via its motor nerve has both immediate and long-term effects. Muscle contraction and increases in force production as a result of CNS reprogramming are the immediate effects. Vascular changes, muscle strengthening and fibre type transformation can result from longer-term, chronic stimulation.

There is both neural plasticity and muscle fibre plasticity. Neural adaptation is rapid and strength gains reflect changes in the pattern and amount of neural activation. How this change occurs is unknown, but that it occurs, and occurs rapidly, has been convincingly demonstrated. Muscle fibre plastic changes are only noted with extensive periods of electrical stimulation. This contrasts with the effects of relative inactivity which promote rapid atrophy. There is a balance between the synthesis and breakdown of muscle proteins. The rate of this can be as much as 10% of skeletal muscle protein per day, occurring at a higher rate in type I slow twitch than in type II fibres. More anabolic than catabolic activity will lead to muscle hypertrophy with more muscle protein and collagenous tissue produced, while the reverse will cause atrophy. Similarly, the fibre type (and so the fatigue response) of the constituent muscle fibres will alter with long-term electrical stimulation.

Electrical stimulation of innervated muscle is used for the following:

The speed of muscle atrophy is highlighted in studies of astronauts' muscles following relatively short periods of weightlessness during space flight. After only one or two days, muscle atrophy and weakness are marked.

- strengthening normal muscle
- strengthening post-surgery and prevention of, or recovery from, disuse atrophy
- re-education of muscle control
- maintaining or increasing range of joint movement
- increasing muscle endurance
- changing muscle structure and function (trophic changes).

When voluntary active exercise of innervated muscle is restricted, electrical stimulation may be substituted. The usual parameters include a ramped (surged) series of short duration pulses at frequencies between 30 and 100 Hz. The choice of a high frequency ensures a smooth, tetanic contraction. The durations of the on- and off-times and the rate of ramping can be varied on most clinical stimulators. The choice of the 'on-time' and rate of ramping will vary according to the aims of treatment. If the on-time lasts for, say, 2 s and the interval between (off-time) for 4 s and appropriate ramping is used (1 s ramp up and down), then a physiological muscle contraction and possibly even joint motion will be mimicked. Some equipment also allows choice in the duration of the pulse selected. Altering the stimulus parameters enables the range of clinical uses of electrical stimulation for innervated muscle described below. Current types commonly used are pulsed (includes HVPS, TENS and faradic) and alternating (Russian or interferential).

The list in the margin includes a number of uses of electrical stimulation for innervated muscles that may have normal strength or be weak. The first of these is strengthening. Increases in the strength of a muscle of 10 to 25% following 15 treatments over 3 to 6 weeks are typical of normal young subjects (Balogun et al., 1993; Bircan et al., 2002). Similar results have been obtained with healthy subjects aged over 65 years (Pfeifer et al., 1997). Strength gains of about 25% occurred in the triceps surae of those given electrical stimulation and those performing voluntary exercise. This occurred over a 6-week period and the electrical stimulation was well tolerated by the subjects. Increases of approximately 10% in torque occurred in patients with knee osteoarthritis whose affected quadriceps muscles were strengthened (Talbot et al., 2003). Concurrent functional outcome measures included chair rise time, which decreased in those who received stimulation. Patients following a stroke also had increases in strength in stimulated quadriceps muscles (Newsam and Baker, 2004). Those in the untreated control group had increases of 31% in maximum voluntary isometric torque and those treated with stimulation, 77%. This was attributed to considerably greater motor recruitment in those who had stimulation, an increase from 35% to 53%, versus no change in those who did not.

Electrical stimulation can be used as the sole treatment (Bircan et al., 2002), superimposed over exercise (Strojnik, 1998) or as an adjunct to an exercise and a physical activity programme (Fitzgerald et al., 2003). Superimposing electrical stimulation or, better still, using

Uses of electrical motor stimulation

Innervated or partly innervated muscle: normal or weak

- strengthening
- increasing endurance
- mobilization – joint and soft tissues
- muscle re-education
- functional electrical stimulation (FES or FNS)
- stabilization and oedema control

Denervated muscle

- maintaining contractability.

Consistent reports indicate that maximum tolerable levels of torque should be used for muscle strengthening (Snyder-Mackler et al., 1994).

it as an adjunctive treatment overcomes a possible limitation of the method. Most strengthening is intended to improve function, and most functional activities involve complex movements. Electrical stimulation technology cannot yet accurately reproduce the complex interactions of groups of muscles, nor of the agonist and antagonist interactions that are needed to produce complex motor activities. Added to a programme that does include voluntarily produced activities, however, electrical stimulation can increase the overall success of that programme (Fitzgerald et al., 2003). Patients with chronic obstructive pulmonary disease receiving mechanical ventilation obtained greater strength gains and their ability to transfer from bed to chair improved faster with electrical stimulation than if they had voluntary exercise alone (Zanotti et al., 2003). Along with the range of programmes which include electrical stimulation, not surprisingly, there are considerable variations in the treatment protocols and parameters and in the methods of assessing change. Table 5.1 indicates guidelines for strengthening. The main features are the need for the muscle or group being strengthened to produce a high level of force (torque).

Principles of strengthening and selection of parameters

The main principles are that the electrical stimulation, as in an active strengthening programme, should:

- produce high force (torque) output of stimulated muscles. If a manually graded 5/5 muscle this will clearly be more than if graded 3/5. It is generally not possible with electrical stimulation to produce torques comparable to that of a maximum voluntary contraction (MVC). Maximum electrically induced torque is limited by pain tolerance and even in healthy individuals is typically 20–30% of an MVC, though there is much between-subject variation. The aim should be gradually to progress the torque production during the course of treatment to the highest possible level.

- use a maximum tolerable current amplitude (essentially the same point as above). This is usually neither desirable nor possible in the first treatment but tolerance usually builds quickly. Early in the treatment programme, the intensity limit is set by the discomfort of stimulation. As treatment progresses, tolerance of discomfort increases as the patient learns that discomfort does not equate to physical harm. With increased tolerance the limit becomes more dictated by the subjective sensation (as reported by many patients) that any greater stimulus intensity might cause tearing of muscle or tendon due to the force of contraction.

- usually involve a relatively low number of repetitions per day (e.g. 5 to 10 between 1 and 3 times). The force of contraction is more important than the number of repetitions per day, though it is also

If the current is poorly tolerated, change the type of current or the pulse duration or increase the size of the electrodes or move them. Also, see points in the section on increasing comfort.

Table 5.1 Summary of guidelines for setting parameters for motor stimulation

Objective	Torque	Number of repetitions	Intensity	Frequency	On-off cycle	Limiting factors
Strengthening	High (graded to tested muscle strength)	Low, ≈10 1–3/day[1]	High	50 Hz or higher[2]	1:3 to 1:5 'on-time' 5 s or less[3]	Comfort Muscle soreness (DOMS) especially during the first few days[4]
Mobilizing	Low to moderate torque at end of reduced ROM	200 to 1000+ per day	Moderate	The fusion frequency (determined by testing) or <50 Hz	1:1 or 1:2 'on-time' 3 to 8 s	Muscle soreness (DOMS)[4]
Increasing endurance	Moderate	High	Moderate[5]	Less than 15 Hz[6]	1:1 or 2:1 'on-time' 8 s or more	Muscle soreness (DOMS)[4] Sufficient number of contractions per day
Re-education	Low, sufficient to elicit the required action	To near fatigue	As low as needed for the response	The fusion frequency (determined by testing) or <50 Hz	1:2 or 1:4 'on-time' to suit muscle action	Local muscle fatigue
Oedema reduction	Low, sufficient to obtain contraction of the muscle group	10–30 minutes 1 to 10× or more per day	Low	50 Hz or less	1:1 'on-time' 2–5 s	Producing a sufficient number of contractions per day[7]
Stabilizing (e.g. shoulder subluxation post-CVA)	Low, sufficient to obtain adequate contraction of the muscle group	5–6 h per day or more	Low	The fusion frequency (determined by testing) or <50 Hz	1:1 'on-time' up to 10 s	Producing a sufficient number of contractions per day[7]

[1] more frequent repetitions will produce better effects but low repetition rates are adequate.
[2] if higher frequencies are used the 'on-time' must be low to avoid muscle fibre dropout (activation failure).
[3] 5 s 'on' is a recommended maximum at 50 Hz. At higher frequencies the maximum 'on-time' is proportionately reduced.
[4] Increase the torque and number of contractions per day carefully.
[5] moderate stimulation intensities are adequate but the higher the better. The stimulus frequency is more important.
[6] higher frequencies are sometimes used when endurance training is not the sole objective (see text).
[7] an aim of treatment is to increase the torque produced per contraction and number of daily contractions.

true that the greater the number of repetitions, the greater will be the effect.

- use a frequency high enough to produce tetany to ensure high force production, e.g. 50 Hz.
- have a strong contraction for 5 to 10 seconds, followed by an 'off-time' of 3 to 5 times the 'on-time'. This minimizes the extent of local muscle fatigue (duty cycle of 33 to 20%).

One study showed that the quadriceps could be strengthened using quite low amounts of electrical stimulation (Soo et al., 1988). Producing a torque equal to 50% of a maximum voluntary contraction, for eight contractions of 15 s duration twice a week for 5 weeks, led to a statistically significant increase in quadriceps torque. Thus surprisingly little electrical stimulation, a total of only 2 minutes stimulation in each of 10 sessions, produced an effect.

Although commonly used, pulses with a duration less than 100 µs (such as HVPS) are likely to be less effective than longer duration pulses for maximum force production.

Another outcome of using electrical stimulation is possibly some degree of cross-transfer effect. A study by Balogun et al. (1993) reported a 24% strength increase in the treated muscles and 10% in the untreated contralateral muscles after 6 weeks. Similarly, the strength in untreated legs contralateral to proximal femoral fractures improved without stimulation (Barber et al., 2002). Another possibility is that as the patients' level of mobility and their activity levels improved, this rather than a crossover effect from the electrical stimulation, could have benefited the untreated leg.

For a new programme, do not attempt to achieve the full dosage in the first treatment. Delayed onset muscle soreness (DOMS) can occur with electrical stimulation as with active exercise, probably more so with the considerably greater activity of a smaller number of fibres than in a voluntary contraction.

Stimulus parameters are based on the above principles. Two types of currents are commonly used:

pulsed

- balanced biphasic pulses with a rectangular leading edge, a duration less than 1 ms (200 to 600 µs) and adjustable frequency (e.g. faradic-type current).
- uniphasic pulses with a duration less than 100 µs and adjustable frequency (e.g. HVPS).

alternating

- carrier frequency of 1 to 4 kHz with rectangular, triangular or sinusoidal pulses with adjustable burst frequency (e.g. Russian current, premodulated interferential current if the bursts are rectangular rather than sinusoidally modulated).

Torque can be increased by making the following changes either together or singly:

pulsed

- increase the frequency from 50 to 65 Hz (only if the 'on-time' is short so that activation failure is avoided)
- increase the pulse duration to about 600 µs. Compared to 200 µs, the difference is small but significant.
- increase the amplitude to maximum tolerable.

alternating

- decrease the carrier frequency to 1 kHz. Compared to 2.5 kHz, the difference is small. Compared to 4 kHz, the difference is larger and clinically significant.
- increase the burst frequency from 50 to 65 Hz (only if the 'on-time' is short so that activation failure is avoided)
- decrease the burst duty cycle from the usual 50% to 10–20%, if equipment permits. The difference is large and clinically significant.
- increase the amplitude to maximum tolerable.

Note that changing the frequency from 50 to 65 Hz will have only a small effect on torque production, as evidenced in Figure 3.12.

Principles of reducing rate of fatigue and selection of parameters

There are two questions concerning fatigue which are important to the clinician: how to minimize fatigue during electrical stimulation and how to improve the fatigue-resistance of the stimulated muscle.

The questions have different but related answers. As described previously, maintaining fatigue-resistance means stimulating slow twitch muscle fibres at low frequencies for prolonged periods of time to prevent slow to fast fibre transformation. Similarly, stimulating fast fibres at low frequencies for prolonged periods can induce a transformation from fast twitch to slow twitch. In this way the fatigue-resistance of the muscle can be maintained or increased. Since the stimulus frequency is low (<15 Hz), a physiologically unnatural twitching response is produced. Although physiologically this is optimal for slowing the development of atrophy, this may not be the sole aim of treatment and it may be important to elicit a smooth, graded contraction resembling a voluntary contraction. For example an aim might be increasing joint stabilization or muscle re-education. For this reason higher frequencies (at or above the fusion frequency) are sometimes used clinically. Consequently, while the outcomes will generally be less effective at preventing muscle atrophy they will produce more normal forces on associated joints and structures. The user should question whether smooth, graded contractions are really needed for a particular treatment. The following addresses how to minimize fatigue during electrical stimulation, assuming that the contraction should be smooth (fused) so as to resemble a voluntary contraction.

Fatigue can be a problem with electrical stimulation. It can reduce the level of torque produced very quickly and, at the level of the contractile elements of the muscle fibre, can result in delayed onset muscle soreness from the tearing of actin/myosin filaments. A prudent approach is to start with perhaps 1 hour per day of low to moderate intensity stimulation and observe the patient's response, then increase up to the goal time (possibly 5 to 6 hours per day) as their tolerance increases. The main way of limiting fatigue is to change the time-based stimulation parameters, i.e. the on/off times and the on/off duty cycle. The other option is to reduce the pulse frequency. A combination of these changes can be used, as when stimulating the rotator cuff muscles for hours per day following a stroke.

For pulsed current, there is a novel way of effectively reducing the frequency. Based on observations of molluscs and later of New Zealand mantis-like insects called wetas, a phenomenon called 'catchlike tension' was identified (Hoyle and Field, 1983). The catchlike properties of weta muscle allow the insect to maintain particular postures for minutes to hours with minimum fatigue. Some stimulators offer a method of invoking an equivalent phenomenon in humans: the frequency of the first few pulses in an 'on-time' are at a higher frequency than the remainder. The commonly used pulse frequency is 80 Hz for the first few and 40 Hz for the remainder of each cycle. This appears to reduce the amount of energy necessary to maintain the force produced by the muscle (Binder-Macleod and Clamann, 1989; Binder-Macleod and Barker, 1991; Binder-Macleod and Russ, 1999). Alternatively a more complex modulated frequency can be used.

When a mollusc closes its shell there is a brief burst of nerve fibre firing which initiates the contraction. This is followed by very low frequency firing which maintains a high muscle force with little metabolic cost and correspondingly little fatigue.

Stimulus parameters are based on the above principles. Two types of currents are commonly used:

pulsed

- balanced biphasic pulse with a rectangular leading edge, duration less than 1 ms, adjustable frequency (e.g. faradic-type current)
- uniphasic pulse with duration less than 100 μs, adjustable frequency (e.g. HVPS)

alternating

- carrier frequency of 1 to 4 kHz with rectangular, triangular or sinusoidal pulses with adjustable burst frequency (e.g. Russian current, premodulated interferential current if the bursts are rectangular rather than sinusoidally modulated).

Fatigue can be further reduced by making the following changes either together or singly:

pulsed

- decrease the frequency to the lowest value practical (the fusion frequency, determined by observation) or use catchlike stimulation or some other type of frequency modulation
- increase the pulse duration to about 600 μs

alternating

- decrease the carrier frequency from 4 or 2.5 kHz to 1 kHz
- decrease the burst frequency to the lowest value practical (the fusion frequency, determined by observation)
- decrease the burst duty cycle from usual 50% to 10–20%, if equipment permits
- increase the 'off-time' (i.e. reduce the pulse train on/off duty cycle).

Principles of decreasing discomfort and selection of parameters

Less discomfort is likely to allow a greater acceptance of a higher level of current. This may be of central importance if the patient has an especially low tolerance of transcutaneous stimulation. There are ways of selecting parameters to reduce discomfort. They principally involve a reduction in activation of A-δ (pain signalling) nerve fibres.

The parameters of the different types of current or the method used to apply it should be changed in one or more of the following ways:

if *pulsed* current (e.g. faradic, TENS, HVPS), use:

- short pulse durations which produce less torque due to lesser activation of smaller diameter motoneurons but also produce less discomfort as there is less activation of small diameter A-δ fibres
- low amplitude which simply activates fewer nerve fibres

As noted previously, pulses of duration less than 100 μs (such as HVPS) are likely to be more fatiguing than longer duration pulses.

Note that decreasing the stimulus intensity (amplitude) of pulsed or alternating current does not affect the rate of fatigue, only the force of contraction.

HVPS, which uses very short duration twin pulses, is well suited to produce comfortable, though not maximally forceful, contractions.

- larger sized electrodes which will lower the current density under the electrodes and reduce stimulation of superficially located, small diameter pain fibres.

if *alternating* current (e.g. Russian, IFT) use:
- a higher carrier frequency (4 kHz or higher). Note, however, that the trade-off is a lower force production and more rapid fatigue
- a low amplitude to activate fewer nerve fibres
- a lower burst duty cycle than the usual 50%; reduce it to 10–20% if equipment permits
- larger sized electrodes (see above).

CLINICAL APPLICATIONS OF MOTOR STIMULATION

The electrical stimulus parameters required for torque production, fatigue reduction and discomfort minimization have been described above and are summarized in Table 5.1. This section describes some clinical uses of electrical stimulation and the application of the previously described principles.

Re-education of muscle control

Stimulation is extensively used therapeutically to re-educate and facilitate voluntary contraction of muscle. A re-education programme using electrical stimulation often precedes its use for muscle strengthening. The two reasons for using electrical stimulation for muscle re-education are often related; first, the muscle has insufficient or no voluntary control or, second, the muscle action is extremely weak or inhibited. The main aim is to facilitate and encourage movement. This implies the patient attempting to contract the muscle throughout the stimulation and changing the stimulation parameters to ones that produce less torque as the patient increases their contribution to each contraction. The number of contractions will typically be low, to encourage voluntary activity while limiting the extent of fatigue (see Table 5.1). As the patient regains more control, the extent of the electrical stimulation contribution should be decreased proportionately. Some examples of re-education studies using electrical stimulation are given below.

- Following a stroke when the patient has little voluntary control of a movement. One such randomized controlled design study investigated using electrical stimulation to improve wrist and hand function (Cauraugh et al., 2000). They randomly allocated seven patients to receive electrical stimulation and four to a control group. All 11 patients had had a stroke at least 12 months previously so function could be expected to have reached a plateau. The motor function of each patient's hemiplegic wrist was evaluated using five separate clinical and laboratory measures of motor function both before and after the trial. For the experimental group subjects the stimulator was one in which the output was triggered using electromyography such that when the preset level of motor activity was produced, the stimulation commenced. The results show clear functional gains and an enhanced ability to sustain wrist extension in this group.

- Where voluntary muscle contraction is inhibited by pain or injury. Anecdotally, stimulating the quadriceps, especially the vastus medialis, is commonly done after knee surgery, including arthroscopies, if the patient has problems starting to contract them again. Similarly stimulation is used with other muscles inhibited in the post-surgery period such as the calf following Achilles tendon surgery.

- When a person has knee osteoarthritis, electrical stimulation can assist with pain control and strengthening of the quadriceps femoris. It is associated with improvements in function, including sit to stand and use of stairs, in patients with radiological evidence of knee osteoarthritis (Talbot et al., 2003).

- Where muscle action is not readily under voluntary control without practice, e.g. stimulation of the pelvic floor muscles in the control of incontinence (Truijen et al., 2001). In this instance biofeedback can also be used when the person regains some voluntary control of the relevant muscles.

- When a new muscle action has to be learned, for example where a muscle or a motor nerve has been transplanted. Following the transfer of trapezius after a brachial plexus lesion (Ruhmann et al., 1998) patients re-learnt use working with a physiotherapist. How they re-learnt use is not explained but one method would have been to use electrical stimulation and gradually work with it. Another could have been by using biofeedback.

- In situations in which it is necessary to demonstrate to the patient that a particular muscle action or movement can occur normally, where hysterical paralysis is present, for example.

'Strengthening' post-surgery

Many recent reports of uses of electrical stimulation involve normal muscle postoperatively. Following orthopaedic surgery the surrounding muscles remain normal but are usually weak, either due to the surgery or to a combination of this and a pre-existing joint pathology. Following the repair of an anterior cruciate ligament of the knee, a randomized controlled trial found that the groups of patients treated with electrical stimulation had greater increases in strength and self-reported function after 12 and 16 weeks of rehabilitation than those not treated with it (Fitzgerald et al., 2003). Similarly, electrical stimulation has been shown to improve function faster following proximal femoral fractures (Barber et al., 2002) and total knee arthroplasties (Lewek et al., 2001; Avramidis et al., 2003). A series of cases showed that with bilateral knee arthroplasties, when both legs were exercised but only the weaker leg was stimulated, the initially weaker leg was (in 4/5 patients) stronger than the 'normal' at 6 months post-surgery (Stevens et al., 2004). This did not occur in those who had exercise only (3/3). The beneficial outcome is likely to be due to muscle re-education rather than muscle fibre strengthening.

There are three commonly used explanations for the greater rate of improvement using electrical stimulation:

- *The different recruitment pattern.* Fast twitch fibres, type II, are recruited at the same time as slow twitch fibres, type I, rather than after. This would cause a greater initial increase in peak, short-term strength than would occur if only voluntary muscle contractions were used.
- *The changes are due to neural mechanisms, at least initially.* Several factors suggest this: the speed with which the increase occurs – it can be demonstrated within a week – and the speed with which it can decline, as well as the lack of evidence of any changes in muscle volume. Several neural mechanisms have been described. Cortical activity has been shown to increase as a result of peripheral nerve stimulation and to continue for at least 30 minutes (Knash et al., 2003). Increased motor-evoked potentials in the muscles supplied by the stimulated nerve are indicative of more than just muscle activation, possibly also to an increased corticospinal excitability. The input from afferent nerves also possibly increases the excitability of the spinal motor neuron pools. This would help account for the cross-transfer effect described previously. In this case the effect can be described as re-education.
- *Contractions may cause pain or the patient may anticipate pain* and reduce the strength of any contraction and hence the effectiveness of a voluntary exercise programme. For example, following a joint replacement, a major joint reconstruction or in the presence of an incompletely united fracture, movement and muscle activity can cause pain. Using electrical stimulation can produce muscle contractions while possibly also reducing pain through a gating action, discussed in chapter 6. In particular, electrical stimulation can increase strength at quite low exercise intensities. This is another example of muscle re-education.

Stimulation parameters for muscle re-education

The claims made by manufacturers that their stimulators, of various kinds, are effective for muscle re-education are probably true. Thus the common current types, pulsed (i.e. includes HVPS, TENS, faradic) or alternating (premodulated IFT or Russian) are suitable. The stimulus intensity, and torque produced, can be low so the choice of the best or most effective means of stimulation should be made on the basis of patient tolerance and minimizing discomfort.

and low frequency would mean that the AC bursts would be too long and nerves would fire at multiples of the burst frequency. AC could be used if the apparatus allows selection of a low duty cycle, i.e. short burst duration.

Stimulation parameters for reducing the risks of skin damage

Skin damage is a possible risk when using electrical stimulation. With normal skin and appropriate methods of applying stimulation the risk is very low. This is not always the situation in clinical practice. The principles for minimizing any risks relate to the following factors:

- *charge balance*, i.e. if using direct current the flow of charges in one direction will, necessarily, be high. If the current is biphasic but has unbalanced pulses there will be a charge imbalance. Using a balanced pulsed current reduces the risks considerably. Similarly using AC stimulation means that there is, of course, no charge imbalance.
- the *current density*. This is the amount of charge flowing per unit area of skin per second; in other words the current per unit area. For example, an AC stimulus such as interferential has a much higher average current than a pulsed current (see chapter 3). More current flows through the skin and the level of risk of damage is higher. Using small electrodes also increases the risks as the current per unit area of the skin is commensurately higher.
- the *skin quality*, e.g. extent of hydration, if friable etc.

The parameters used must reflect consideration of these factors. Practical applications will depend on the reason for using electrical stimulation and hence the current and electrode options available to the user at that time. Ideally:

- pulsed current or AC with a small (<20%) duty cycle
- balanced pulses (this is implicit with AC)
- electrodes as large as practicable
- well hydrated skin and not adhesive electrodes if the skin is friable or at risk.

FUNCTIONAL ELECTRICAL STIMULATION (FES)

The terms neuromuscular electrical stimulation (NMES) and FES are sometimes used interchangeably. NMES is a more general term and includes any form of electrical stimulation to elicit a motor response. When NMES is used to produce a functional movement it is more commonly called FES.

Functional electrical stimulation (FES) uses electrical stimulation to produce a functional movement, or series of movements, that is not otherwise possible. Some users of electrical stimulation differentiate neuromuscular electrical stimulation (NMES) from FES. An example of NMES would be stimulation of the rotator cuff and abductor muscles of the shoulder following stroke to prevent or limit joint sub-luxation. The problem is, arguably this could also be called FES. This section avoids having to make such fine distinctions by labelling all functional uses as FES.

Most uses of FES follow problems caused by damage to the central nervous system. As long as the peripheral nervous system is intact, the muscles can be stimulated as previously. This means that after a stroke, for example, it is possible to stimulate muscles that the person can no longer voluntarily contract. In most cases when the central nervous system (CNS) is damaged, such as with cerebral palsy or following a stroke or spinal cord lesion, the peripheral nervous system remains intact.

FES can be used in the short term if recovery is expected or long term if recovery is unlikely. This distinction can affect the type of equipment used. Short-term uses or trials are most often with transcutaneous (i.e. surface) stimulation. Depending on the problem, if longer term, percutaneous or implanted stimulation systems may be preferable if the expected functional gain is a major one for the patient.

The range of uses made of FES is wide and rapidly increasing. Uses include cardiac and gut pacemakers (implanted forms of FES), implanted stimulators and those used transcutaneously to overcome some of the problems associated with spinal cord injuries and following a stroke. The diversity of uses means that providing specific parameter guidelines is not always possible but they can generally be anticipated using the research outlined in this chapter. Some current examples of using electrical stimulation to improve function are provided below.

Upper limb rehabilitation following stroke

Increasingly, the possible roles for electrical stimulation in the recovery of the upper limb function following stroke are being investigated. This section discusses the role in preventing shoulder pain and loss of function and improving hand function. Another role, not yet well understood, is in changing the adverse outcomes of reduced autonomic functioning, including oedema, which are common after stroke (Wang et al., 2004).

The subluxation that can result from a stroke affecting the upper limb can cause both a loss of function and pain in the arm, partly due to the primary damage to the central nervous system, but also to secondary problems following a protracted loss of return of function (Faghri et al., 1994). The range of different methods used to reduce pain and any secondary damage includes slings, corticosteroid injections, electrical stimulation (see case study) and EMG biofeedback. Both injections and electrical stimulation have been shown to be promising (Snels et al., 2002).

A comprehensive meta-analysis endorsed the role of electrical stimulation in preventing or reducing subluxation of the shoulder after stroke but was unable to provide optimal stimulation parameters (Ada and Foongchomcheay, 2002). The recommendations in Table 5.1 are based on existing case studies (Faghri et al., 1994; McKenzie, 1999)

26 recent hemiplegic patients having physiotherapy were randomly allocated to have or not have daily electrical stimulation of the rotator cuff and shoulder abductor muscles on their affected shoulder for 6 weeks. One outcome measure: the change in extent of X-ray demonstrated subluxation of the affected head of humerus in the glenoid fossa. The results were as follows: 6 mm baseline subluxation reduced to 3.5 mm in those receiving electrical stimulation and 4 mm subluxation baseline increased to over 9 mm if not having stimulation. In addition, pain was reduced and function increased in those having electrical stimulation (Faghri et al., 1994).

As noted in chapter 4, AC stimulation using a small duty cycle is more comfortable than pulsed current. If portable, low duty cycle AC stimulators were available they would likely be more effective than the present generation of pulsed current stimulators.

The use of stimulation to moderate spasticity is discussed further in chapter 6, along with other uses of sensory stimulation. Considerably more research is needed on this topic to establish which patients may benefit from this approach and to ascertain its cost effectiveness.

and our own clinical experience. The important feature is the number of hours per day for which contractions of the relevant muscles are required. This means users need gradually to increase the duration of stimulation while continuing to use short on- and off-times.

Typically, pulsed current is used. This allows the use of a portable stimulator to enable the necessary daily duration of stimulation. The pulses can be biphasic or, if very short duration, monophasic (HVPS). The stimulation can be applied either as surface electrical stimulation (Faghri et al., 1994; McKenzie, 1999; Ada and Foongchomcheay, 2002) or as intramuscular stimulation (Yu et al., 2004).

Electrical stimulation is also used to improve hand function following stroke. Stimulation of the wrist and finger flexors and extensors, used in conjunction with functional activities, can improve recovery (Alon et al., 2003; Gritsenko and Prochazka, 2004; Popovic et al., 2004).

Gait assistance for children with cerebral palsy

Transcutaneous and percutaneous stimulation have been used to improve the gait patterns of children with cerebral palsy (Carmick, 1993; Pierce et al., 2004). For example, Pierce et al. (2004) reported two cases of children with hemiplegic cerebral palsy with improved ankle kinematics and kinetics following the use of fine wire percutaneous electrical stimulation. By contrast, a study of 22 ambulant children with diplegic, hemiplegic or quadriplegic cerebral palsy all had stimulation for 8 weeks (changing over the weeks from 10 Hz to 30 Hz frequency and pulse width from 75 µs to 100 µs, duty cycle of 50 to 33% for up to 60 minutes daily) of their gluteus maximus on their most affected leg (van der Linden et al., 2003), but no significant changes were identified. Another study used stimulation of quadriceps, which was shown to be effective in a child with spastic diplegia (Daichman et al., 2003).

Perhaps the most interesting issue with using electrical stimulation to improve gait for children with cerebral palsy is that of what to stimulate. Should it be the extensors to reduce their tone or their antagonists to strengthen or regularize sensory input to the agonists. One study which used surface stimulation of the dorsiflexors at 40 Hz demonstrated marked improvements in gait including an increase in the heel-toe interval (Durham et al., 2004). Why this was so effective is unclear. Whether dorsiflexor stimulation altered the level of spasticity in the calf muscles or increased the strength of the dorsiflexors is unknown.

A comparison of the effects on gait of stimulation of gastrocnemius and of gastrocnemius and tibialis anterior showed both were effective (Comeaux et al., 1997). Similar benefits are obtained using percutaneous stimulation (Bertoti et al., 1997).

Upper limb treatment for cerebral palsy

Electrical stimulation can also improve upper limb function in children with cerebral palsy. Specifically, applied to wrist extensor muscles, electrical stimulation can also improve hand function (Carmick, 1997; Wright and Granat, 2000a). Similar functional gains were found in hand and wrist function in an adult with cerebral palsy treated with electrical stimulation (Wright and Granat, 2000b) and in children treated with sensory level rather than motor stimulation (Maenpaa et al., 2004). Aspects of this topic are discussed further in chapter 6.

Foot drop 'splinting'

A foot drop due to a CNS lesion can be treated using electrical stimulation of the dorsiflexors, triggered by a switch in the shoe or by a changed tilt of the leg (Stein et al., 2002). Most commonly, this type of stimulation is applied transcutaneously but can also be percutaneous or via an implanted stimulator. Implanting, when it is suitable, can overcome some of the problems of surface stimulation including locating the best points for stimulating the dorsiflexor muscles and stimulating sufficient volume of the muscles, especially the deeper parts (van der Aa et al., 2001; Wilder et al., 2002). While not a perfect solution and with all the risks attendant upon surgery, implanted stimulation can increase the distance walked in 6 minutes considerably and without the skin problems and discomfort that can affect some users of the surface method (van der Aa et al., 2001).

Stimulation cycling

Following a major spinal cord lesion, cycling using electrical stimulation provides a number of potential patient benefits. For example, one patient report described a sequential stimulation of gluteal, hamstring and quadriceps muscles. The goal was one hour of stimulation cycling per day, three times a week (McDonald et al., 2002). Six months after the introduction of stimulation cycling and aquatherapy, improvements were identified in sensory awareness and motor function in a range of muscles as well as a 90% reduction in the number of days taking antibiotics (McDonald et al., 2002).

Another reported benefit of spinal cord injured patients training using stimulation cycling three times weekly for a year is an increased insulin sensitivity, possibly the result of the increased muscle mass produced (Mohr et al., 2001) There is a reversal of muscle atrophy and an increased cardiovascular fitness (Faghri et al., 1994; Fitzwater, 2002) and an increased bone density (Stein et al., 2002). A consequence of the reduction in muscle atrophy can be fewer pressure sores as the bulk increases in response to stimulation (Levine et al., 1990; Rischbieth et al., 1998). Cycling, however, even if started soon after injury, cannot prevent the development of osteopenia, but merely reduce the subsequent extent (Eser et al., 2003).

After an incomplete spinal cord lesion, cycling has been shown to improve lower limb function and the extent of independent mobility (Donaldson et al., 2000). Cycling produces fatigue but there is no evidence that the stimulation should be changed as a consequence (Sinclair et al., 2004).

Electrically induced ambulation and rowing

Increasing cardiovascular fitness is another potential benefit to a patient with a spinal cord injury using ambulation by electrical stimulation. This method does not have the disadvantages of increased levels of upper extremity pain and injury associated with wheelchair propulsion activities or arm cranking exercise (Jacobs and Mahoney, 2002). Similarly, electrically assisted rowing offers a method for patients with a spinal cord injury to regain some fitness by repeated stimulation of the knee flexors and extensors (Wheeler et al., 2002). At present, the rowing technique produced differs considerably from that used by able-bodied rowers, a point that suggests possible scope for improvement in the technology (Halliday et al., 2004).

Gait and mobility retraining following spinal cord injury

Spinal cord injured patients can improve both their level of control and their speed of walking over ground on a treadmill following walking training in a safety harness (Field-Fote and Tepavac, 2002). An interesting outcome of such studies is the broader possible implications of FES for retraining as the results, in this example, indicated an improved intralimb coordination and hip control (incomplete spinal cord lesions below T10). FES can also be used to improve transfers as well as mobility in circumstances in which using a wheelchair is not practical. A survey of 12 such users with spinal cord injuries reported how having FES implants had improved their health generally as well as their ability to execute specific functional activities (Agarwal et al., 2003). It can also increase walking speed (Stein et al., 2002) and improve oxygen uptake and cardiovascular responses (Jacobs et al., 2003).

Bladder and bowel stimulation

One type of problem treated with electrical stimulation is an overactive bladder (Grill et al., 2001). When the problem is not effectively treated by one of the options such as biofeedback, sacral root or pudendal nerve stimulation can be effective. The advantage of pudendal nerve stimulation is that a stimulator is relatively easily placed near the nerve in both men and women (Grill et al., 2001). The results show normal voiding can occur using a mean stimulation duration of 8.6 hours per day. So far there appear to be fewer instances of lead migration or of pain following the implantation of the stimulator.

Little is known yet about the mechanisms of action, or the effectiveness, of using transcutaneous electrical stimulation to alter bowel functioning. A series of cases identified marked changes in bowel functioning in children with slow colonic transit constipation (Chase et al., 2005). While interesting, these findings are yet to be replicated.

Upper airways stimulation

Conditions including obstructive sleep apnoea, dysphagia, bilateral vocal fold paralysis and laryngeal dystonia have all been successfully treated with FES (Grill et al., 2001). Similarly, it has been used to stimulate abdominal muscles to control blood pressure and facilitate coughing in a patient with a C3/4 level spinal cord injury (Taylor et al., 2002). These uses are relatively new but they indicate the future potential scope of electrical stimulation.

Scoliosis

Adolescent idiopathic scoliosis has been treated by night-time applications of electrical stimulation to the muscles on the convexity of the curve. This means, arguably, it is a form of FES as it replaces the bracing necessary to try to limit the extent of curvature developed. Previously thought to be effective, more recent studies indicate that using electrical stimulation to treat scoliosis is less effective than bracing (El-Sayyad and Conine, 1994; Michaud, 2000; Bowen et al., 2001). Both bracing and electrical stimulation raise issues of compliance, suggesting that, at most, it may have a role when bracing is not acceptable to the patient.

Summary of FES

Existing uses of electrical stimulation are broad: some replace normal functions of the body, and some assist with an activity or have a retraining role. The range of uses is increasing, along with major developments in technology, especially in the past ten years.

ELECTRICAL STIMULATION OF DENERVATED MUSCLE

Electrical stimulation is used to stimulate denervated muscle as well as innervated. This necessitates quite different stimulation and treatment parameters as muscle is much more difficult to stimulate than is nerve. Also, there is considerable disagreement regarding the role of electrical stimulation in the treatment of denervated muscle. This section outlines the issues, starting with a discussion of the different types of damage to peripheral nerves. This is followed by an outline of the effects on muscle of the more serious types of nerve damage and the possible roles of electrical stimulation. One type of nerve lesion will be discussed separately, Bell's palsy, as stimulation is frequently sought for this condition.

Damage to peripheral nerves

Peripheral nerve injuries are categorized according to the degree of damage (Table 5.2). The range of possibilities is best understood in terms of the structure of a nerve. Figure 5.1 shows the complexity of a peripheral nerve which comprises a number of sensory, motor and autonomic nerve fibres held together by different layers of connective tissue.

Individual nerve fibres are separated from each other by surrounding connective tissue called the endoneurium. The endoneurium is enclosed within and bounded by another layer of connective tissue, the perineurium. The perineurium and its enclosed tissue is called a fascicle. Many fascicles are bound together by the epineurium and run the length of the peripheral nerve.

Damage can occur to the entire nerve, to part of a nerve, to axons within an endoneurial tube or to the connective tissues such as the epineurium. The implications for the patient thus range from complete denervation of muscles supplied by the affected nerve and loss of relevant sensory and autonomic function to some denervated or partially denervated muscles or even some sensory or autonomic changes only. The mechanisms of nerve damage include direct trauma

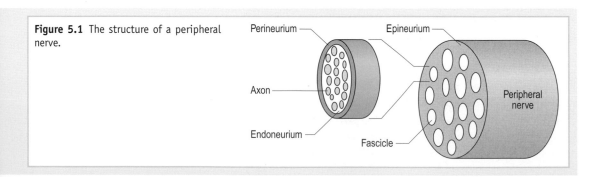

Figure 5.1 The structure of a peripheral nerve.

Table 5.2 Seddon's 3 categories of peripheral nerve injury

Category	Mechanism of injury	Description of damage	Clinical signs	Treatment	Prognosis
Neurapraxia (Sunderland I)	Prolonged compression, a sharp blow or traction, e.g. cyclist's palsy (Hankey & Gubbary, 1988)	Conduction block with local damage to myelin sheath	Loss of function below level of damage	Prevent damage while awaiting recovery	Spontaneous recovery in 6 to 8 weeks or less
Axonotmesis (Sunderland II)	Traction or a crush injury	Axon severed but endoneurial tube intact; degeneration of distal segment of nerve	Loss of all functions below level of damage (sensory, motor, autonomic)	Usually does not require intervention to nerve. Does require care of affected muscle and skin to ensure optimal outcome if regeneration successful	Regeneration is accurate with intact endoneurial tubes, rate depends on site of injury and rate of nerve regrowth ($\approx$1 to 2 mm per day)
Neurotmesis (Sunderland III–V)	Direct trauma, avulsion etc.	Loss of continuity of axon and all or some elements of endoneurial tubes, perineurium and epineurium; degeneration of distal segment of nerve	Loss of all functions below level of damage (sensory, motor, autonomic)	Surgical repair, primary or secondary, is required	Depends on the extent of injury and on the success of the surgery

and lacerations, compression, crushing, chemical irritation and stretching (Landers and Alternburger, 2003). The range of mechanisms of damage is consistent with many different consequences. Some or all of the peripheral nerve and its supporting connective tissue can be affected meaning the consequences also vary and it is important to know the type of lesion. Two systems are usually used to describe the different degrees of damage to a nerve. Seddon's system has three categories and Sunderland's has five (Sunderland, 1978; Omer et al., 1998).

Table 5.2 lists the three major types of damage: neurapraxia, axonotmesis and neurotmesis. Of these, this chapter primarily concerns the last two. The reason is that a neurapraxia is self-limiting as, assuming there is no other damage, the nerve will spontaneously recover. Some clinicians have incorrectly attributed successful outcomes to their treatment of Bell's palsy (a peripheral nerve lesion) with, for example, spinal manipulation. Most commonly Bell's palsy is a neurapraxia that will gradually resolve in 6 to 8 weeks or less following onset. This highlights the importance of correct diagnosis of the type of lesion to ensure appropriate treatment and accurate prognostication.

Effects of peripheral nerve damage

The loss of muscle bulk is due to microscopic level changes where individual muscle fibres become thinner due to loss of myofibrils. In addition, there is a reduction in the capillary network in the muscle. Increasingly the greater part of the remaining muscle is the supporting connective tissue, primarily collagen-based structures (Spielholz, 1999).

Nerve damage results in a loss of function, the extent of loss depending on the mechanism of injury. Muscle weakness or paralysis and changes in sensation occur immediately after the lesion (if due to trauma and not prolonged changes associated with other mechanisms such as toxic chemicals). Over the next 3 months affected muscles will atrophy, a process which stabilizes by 6 to 9 months (Spielholz, 1999). The muscle loses bulk and becomes thinner. At the same time the muscle fibres' sensitivity to acetylcholine increases and the muscle tends to twitch spontaneously, a response called 'fibrillation'. Fibrillation is usually visible and certainly evident on EMG testing. If the denervated muscle is re-innervated in sufficient time then some of these changes can be reversed.

At the tissue level, within 24 to 48 hours of a complete lesion of all or part of a peripheral nerve (axonotmesis or neurotmesis) the destruction of the distal myelin section of the nerve starts (Koeppen, 2004). This is irreversible and is called Wallerian degeneration. Proximal to the lesion, reversible changes will occur in the anterior horn cells together with Wallerian degeneration in the section of damaged nerve (Koeppen, 2004).

Direct Wallerian degeneration is the process of breakdown of Schwann cells and of macrophages digesting the debris, the axon and myelin distal to the site of damage (Landers and Alternburger, 2003). This stage takes time and in the first 3 to 7 days the section of the nerve distal to the lesion may still be electrically excitable. After 10 days Wallerian degeneration is usually complete and the complex changes necessary for re-innervation have started. Schwann cells start to proliferate distally as part of the process of nerve regeneration. As the damaged axons sprout they can be remyelinated by the Schwann cells (Koeppen, 2004). If, however, the Schwann cells remain denervated for more than a month, axonal regeneration tends to be limited (Gordon et al., 2003).

Early surgical repair to approximate the fascicles by suturing, nerve grafting or by using nerve conduits is very important to optimize the eventual outcome. Time and distance of site from denervated muscles are important. There is an increasing inability of motor neurons to continue axon growth as time passes. When axon growth does occur the patterns of innervation of an affected muscle are invariably different and incomplete which helps explain the functional impairment following a peripheral nerve lesion (Ijkema-Paassen et al., 2004).

Electroneurological testing

The tests commonly used to diagnose nerve damage and to differentiate the types of damage include the following:

- A sensory nerve is stimulated and the results are recorded either proximally (orthodromic) or distally (antidromic). The main recording measures are the:
  - amplitude of a sensory nerve action potential (SNAP)
  - sensory nerve conduction velocity.
- A motor nerve is stimulated and the following results are recorded, as appropriate:
  - compound motor action potential (CMAP) amplitude and duration
  - latency of response
  - conduction velocity
  - F-wave latency.
- Needle electromyography is used to determine the following:
  - signs of damage to a motor axon, e.g. abnormal spontaneous activity including fibrillations and positive waves in the motor units it supplies
  - motor unit action potentials (MUAPs) that have longer durations, higher amplitudes, a greater percentage of polyphasic potentials and a reduced pattern of recruitment (if more than 2 to 3 weeks since a lesion)
  - loss of nerve continuity
  - signs of regeneration or nerve sprouting.

Strength–duration testing

Another method of investigating the extent of nerve damage is by using strength–duration (S-D) testing (see chapter 3). This has long been used to test the extent of nerve damage and establish a possible prognosis. Motor S-D testing investigates the intensity of current required to obtain a threshold motor response using different pulse durations. This provides a clear measure of the responsiveness of any nerve stimulated, and in the absence of nerve, muscle tissue.

The type of current used is a rectangular, monophasic pulse, typically with a frequency of 1 or 2 Hz. A series of pulses each with durations of between 10 μs and 300 ms is used. The intensity is increased gradually until the motor threshold is reached. The intensity and pulse duration are recorded, then a new pulse duration is selected and the measurement is repeated. A graph (called the S-D curve) is then plotted of threshold intensity versus pulse duration. The responses of, usually, two muscles supplied by the nerve distal to the damaged area are examined, starting 7 to 10 days after the injury. The tests are repeated every 2 weeks or so (depending on site of injury and muscle

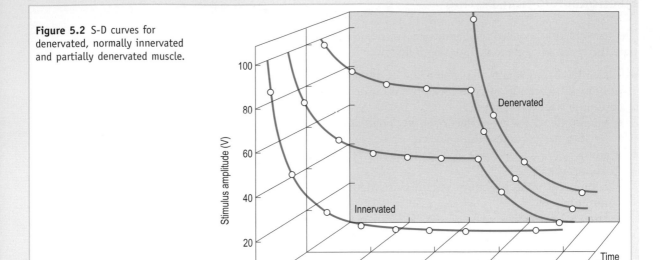

Figure 5.2 S-D curves for denervated, normally innervated and partially denervated muscle.

tested) to examine any systematic changes in response. Figure 5.2 shows a series of curves that can be obtained as a muscle is re-innervated and its level of responsiveness to short duration pulsed current increases.

A normal response is shown in a smooth curve. If completely denervated the curve is shifted upwards and to the right indicating that the muscle is less responsive to short pulses as the degree of innervation is either nil or close to nil. If the nerve recovers, this is typically first seen by a kink in the curve (see Figure 5.2) as some muscle fibres are supplied by nerves again. As the extent of re-innervation increases the curve gradually moves down and to the left and eventually the kink disappears.

S-D curves are evaluated both in terms of their shape and by using some of a range of different measures. The most common measures are called the rheobase and chronaxie. The rheobase is defined as the minimum intensity (V or mA) required to produce a threshold motor (or sensory or pain) response to an infinitely long pulse. In practice, the curve will have reached a plateau using a pulse of 100 ms duration so the rheobase is measured as the threshold stimulus amplitude at this duration. This measure, the rheobase, is then used to calculate the chronaxie. The chronaxie is defined as the pulse duration necessary to obtain a threshold response (motor, sensory or pain but most usually motor, as per the values in Table 5.3) using a pulse of twice rheobasic intensity. The chronaxie value obtained will depend on whether the threshold is measured in volts or mA (see Table 5.3).

Table 5.3 Normal values of rheobase and chronaxie

Outcome measure	Rheobase		Chronaxie	
	Innervated	Denervated	Innervated	Denervated
Threshold current	2–18 mA	higher	<1 ms	>10 ms
Threshold voltage	3–40 V	higher	<0.1 ms	>10 ms

In current clinical practice S-D curves are not commonly used and the electroneurological tests listed previously are preferred. The reasons include:

- issues of inter-tester reliability with serial S-D tests
- many therapists lack the knowledge and technical skills required accurately to perform S-D tests
- lack of diagnostic sensitivity as an S-D test cannot differentiate problems caused by nerve lesions from, for example, myopathies and motor endplate disorders.

Despite this, S-D curves obtained serially provide an easy and quick method of demonstrating change. They require easily available equipment and an experienced operator with a consistent technique can differentiate the following:

- a neurapraxia from the other two types of lesions
- change after a denervation, either deterioration or re-innervation.

Stimulating denervated muscle

Denervated muscle is different in many respects from innervated muscle. It will atrophy, motor units will degenerate, becoming thinner and weaker and converting from fatigue-resistant to fast twitch. This is accompanied by a decrease in vascularization which, in innervated muscle, is maintained by the trophic influences of nerve fibre activity. Neither voluntary nor reflex activity is possible from any denervated motor units. An aim of electrical stimulation is to reduce, prevent or possibly reverse the course of muscle atrophy. Electrical stimulation may also be beneficial for nerve regrowth and repair. Early electrical stimulation of denervated rat muscles has been shown to increase the rate of regeneration across the surgical gap (Gordon et al., 2003; Mendonca et al., 2003).

Without a functional nerve supply muscle can only be caused to contract by direct stimulation of the muscle fibres. There are therefore differences between stimulating muscle via its nerve and direct denervated muscle stimulation:

- muscle tissue is less excitable than nerve so that a greater electric charge is needed

The sluggish or worm-like response of denervated muscle occurs because, with each pulse, the muscle fibres close to the electrodes are activated sooner than those further away. Those further away experience lower stimulation intensities, which must be of longer duration to be effective, so depolarization is delayed.

For many years there has been confusion and controversy about the therapeutic use of electrical stimulation of denervated muscles. The rationale for this treatment is to maintain the muscle in as healthy a state as possible by electrically induced artificial exercise while awaiting reinnervation.

- slow 'worm-like' contractions result because of the slow spread of contraction through the muscle at a markedly diminished rate compared with innervated muscle
- slow-rising electrical pulses can stimulate muscle as it has less ability to accommodate than nerve.

Denervated muscle tissue may be stimulated by slow-rising triangular pulses, also called selective or accommodation pulses. Nerve fibres accommodate to slowly rising pulses (see chapter 3) so if a pulse has a sufficiently long rise time, nerve fibres will not respond. Unlike nerve, muscle accommodates only very slowly. Selective stimulation is possible by choosing a stimulus waveform which rises sufficiently slowly to allow accommodation of nerve fibres but which still rises rapidly enough to activate muscle fibres directly. To stimulate nerve, as previously discussed, a square wave pulse of less than 1 ms is best. To stimulate muscle fibre but not nerve, a triangular pulse with a rise time of 50 ms (100 ms pulse length) is used. To stimulate denervated muscle fibre only, a rise time of longer than 100 ms can be used; 300 or 500 ms triangular pulses are often selected.

The current has to be applied through the muscle tissue itself, because there is functionally no longer a motor point. The current is usually most successfully applied along the longitudinal axis of the muscle fibres, with the stimulating electrodes at each end of the muscle belly (a bipolar technique). The risks to the muscle of damage from using electrical stimulation have been well summarized (Spielholz, 1999). Any stimulation programme must carefully and gradually introduce stimulation as there is risk of further damage to a denervated muscle if excessive stimulation is used.

A recent study demonstrated considerable changes in the responsiveness of denervated muscle to regular electrical stimulation (Kern et al., 2002). Starting with pulses of 120 to 150 ms duration and a frequency of 1 Hz, over time the stimulated muscles equally effectively responded to shorter pulses, of 30 to 50 ms and a frequency of 16 to 25 Hz. For this a pulse amplitude of up to 250 mA was required (2 s on, 4 s off, 4 to 6 sets of 8 to 12 repetitions per set, once a day). The total time per day to stimulate adequately four major muscle groups, the quadriceps, hamstrings, gluteals and calf muscles is 1.5 to 2 hours. An unusual feature of this study was the use of biphasic pulsed current as most stimulation of denervated muscle is done using monophasic pulses. The benefit of using a biphasic pulse is that the risk of skin damage is markedly reduced with balanced pulses even if of long duration. The risk with monophasic pulses is of tissue damage with the build up of ions on the skin under the electrodes, especially if the stimulation is continued for hours per day, as in the Kern et al. (2002) study. There is, however, little functional difference between biphasic and monophasic pulses.

From a therapeutic point of view, regimens such as that described above are difficult to apply except to a few superficial muscles at a time. Such treatment tends to be limited to a small number of muscles and to those that patients can be taught to stimulate themselves. Self-treating patients must also have the time routinely to carry out the treatment which also needs a high degree of compliance and tolerance on the part of the patient to continue it over a long period of, perhaps, 1 or 2 years. If there is no chance of recovery, the value and cost of this type of programme has to be considered very carefully on an individual basis with each patient. When recovery is probable or highly likely, then this programme is more clearly of long-term benefit. However, as the previous discussion of FES indicated, there are probably still sufficient potential benefits to a patient's bone density and systemic functioning if large muscle groups are paralysed to at least consider using this type of treatment regularly, regardless of the prognosis.

Kern et al. (2002) found that even if there has been no treatment post denervation for many (15 to 20) years, stimulation can still be effective. They also point out that there is still a risk of overstraining and damaging muscle and note that endurance remains low, even with daily training.

Stimulation parameters for denervated muscle

The main principles are to introduce gradually electrical stimulation and increase the demands on a muscle or muscle group. The stimulation should be bipolar (electrode either end of the muscle) and each pulse must have a long duration. Rectangular pulses are relatively ineffective as the current flow in tissue resembles that shown in Figure 4.12. Because the stratum corneum is an insulator it acts as a capacitor which offers higher and higher resistance to current flow during applied constant voltage pulse. So if the stimulus voltage is rectangular and of long duration there will be a current spike at the start and end of each pulse but little in between (see Figure 4.12). The current spikes, being of short duration, will effectively stimulate any innervated muscle via the nerve supply and will also stimulate sensory and pain fibres.

By contrast, triangular long-duration pulses can selectively stimulate denervated muscle fibres. The reason is that nerve fibres accommodate to slowly rising pulses (see chapter 3) and so are less likely to respond to a triangular voltage stimulus when the rise time is 100 ms or more. Muscle fibres, however, do not accommodate (or accommodate only very slowly) so the current flow during the pulse pushes the membrane potential closer and closer to threshold and motor excitation is induced.

When a triangular stimulus voltage is applied transcutaneously, the current flow in tissue is close to constant during each pulse. The increasing voltage compensates for what would otherwise be a decreasing current flow.

In the beginning of treatment longer duration pulses (>100 ms) are used. As the (still denervated) muscle becomes more responsive to electrical stimulation shorter pulses with a gradually increasing frequency can be effective (Kern et al., 2002). This reduces the risk of skin damage with longer-term stimulation and any discomfort the person may feel during it (e.g. if an adjacent dermatome is still innervated). The stimulator should provide the following parameters (Hofer et al., 2002):

- up to 300 ms duration biphasic pulses
- triangular and other pulse shapes and ramping options

- a frequency range from 1 to ≈15 Hz (depending on and limited by the pulse duration)
- battery-powered operation, if needed, to allow safe unsupervised use between clinical assessments
- zero net DC output, meaning, no charge imbalance, to decrease any risk of skin damage (biphasic pulses ensure this).

Ideally, it should be a multichannel stimulator to enable multiple groups to be stimulated concurrently or alternately.

Bell's palsy

One of the most common causes of unilateral facial weakness is Bell's palsy, the other is stroke. A lower motor neuron lesion of the facial nerve (Bell's palsy) can seriously alter a patient's capacity to make facial movements. In turn, this can reduce their ability to control their saliva and can also cause lacrimation and difficulties with speech and eating. Of those affected approximately 20 to 30% do not recover near-normal function (Gilden, 2004).

The initial treatment of Bell's palsy usually involves the use of glucocorticoids to limit the extent of permanent damage to the nerve. Other medications, electrical stimulation and electrophysical agents are also used. A thorough review of the latter indicates the contributions of electrical stimulation and biofeedback especially with the more severe lesions (Quinn and Cramp, 2003). The extent to which facial muscles are affected can, however, vary. If only temporary damage to the nerve has occurred, a neurapraxia, it will respond to very short duration pulsed current applied distal to the site of damage to the nerve (300 μs or less) and recover in 6 to 8 weeks, irrespective of any stimulation or other treatment applied. More intractable cases may be completely denervated or they may have a mix of some innervated and some denervated motor units.

A study by Targan et al. (2000) confirms the extent to which electrical stimulation applied to a long-term case of Bell's palsy can produce changes. They used pulsed current (monophasic, 86 μs pulse duration, frequency of approximately 1.4 Hz), on for 6 s and off for 6 s (ramp up of 1 s, down of 0.5 s). The intensity was submotor so the patient could feel the stimulation but there was no motor response. Four facial muscles were stimulated initially in each of their 17 patients. The time was progressively increased from 30 minutes daily to 6 hours. Another four muscles were added and the time increased up to 60 minutes each. The results showed that the grade and appearance of movements decreased (House and Brackmann facial muscle grading system, grade 1 = normal to grade 6 = no movement). Fourteen of the 17 patients improved at least 2 grades.

These results are surprising in two respects: that a response was obtained after extended periods of denervation; and that this occurred using submotor intensities and very short duration pulses. While the explanations canvassed in the study do not address these issues, Targan et al. (2000) did suggest some explanations for the faster motor conduction: one is that re-innervation may occur either as a result of orthodromic stimulation of afferent trigeminal and facial nerve fibres, possibly promoting the generation of new terminal nerve fibres to the denervated motor units. This type of response has been described in experimental studies mainly involving rats. Typically the nerve is transected and the ends then re-opposed, sometimes with a fibrin glue added, and stimulation applied (e.g. English, 2005; Gordon et al., 2003). Stimulation is usually with a 20 Hz frequency for periods from 1 hour only to continuously for 2 weeks. The result is a faster repair if stimulation is applied.

Summary

The value of electrical stimulation for denervated muscle is generally limited unless the affected muscles are likely to be re-innervated or if the benefits of expected systemic effects justify the effort. However, while there is a suggestion that stimulation can increase or initiate re-innervation, the extent of usefulness remains unclear. Perhaps the most important change in recent years has been the introduction of biphasic pulses to stimulate denervated muscle.

Principles of stimulating denervated muscle

A realistic aim of stimulating denervated muscle is to maintain contractibility. It may also increase muscle strength and fatigue resistance so that if recovery occurs the muscle is in better condition. In achieving these ends, two practical considerations are important. First that the stimulation should involve minimum discomfort, i.e. minimum stimulation of pain (A-δ and C) fibres, assuming that some sensory awareness still exists if only in adjacent areas with an alternate nerve supply. Second, that there should be a minimal risk of skin damage. These principles can also be extrapolated to other uses of functional electrical stimulation (FES).

The actual method of applying electrical stimulation and the dosage used will depend upon the aims of treatment and can be derived by applying some relevant principles. The principles guide the selection of current parameters, the method of application and the specific treatment variables to be used in a particular instance.

Current parameters

For stimulation of denervated muscle, long duration pulsed current is needed. Alternating current is not used. The parameters that may need to be selected and set includes the following:

- polarity
- frequency
- shape of pulses
- pulse duration
- time between pulses
- amplitude
- duty cycle
- ramping, duration of ramp up, peak on-time, fall time and off-time of the stimulus pulse, i.e. the nature and rate of surging.

The type of current and stimulator used directs which specific parameters can be selected to meet a particular aim. The relevant parameters are described in this section (and chapter 3). Each parameter contributes to some aspect of the change electrical stimulation can produce in muscle.

METHODS OF APPLICATION OF ELECTRICAL STIMULATION AND DOSAGE

The method of application and dosage for most uses of electrical stimulation refers to the following:

- the electrode type, size, number and locations
- the number of contractions per session, sessions per day, and number of days and weeks using electrical stimulation (if relevant).

Stages of treatment with motor stimulation (transcutaneous)

Patient

Explanation: the reasons for using motor stimulation and why it is expected to be effective, the likely sensations during stimulation and the possible risks. Obtain the patient's consent to the treatment before proceeding. Often stimulation will be used without supervision. Ensure the patient fully comprehends how to use the equipment safely (provide written information as appropriate).

Preparation and testing the output of the stimulator

Turn the stimulator on and set the parameters required but ensure zero output. Connect the leads to the machine and the electrodes. The therapist should then use their hand or forearm (singular, i.e. one hand or forearm) to form a circuit between the electrodes and gradually increase the output noting what sensations they feel and at what intensity. (If using self-adhesive or pre-gelled electrodes, the therapist holds the pre-gelled ends of the leads 5 mm apart between two adjacent fingers or their index finger and thumb). If all is satisfactory, turn the output to zero and leave the stimulator on.

Test skin sensory awareness

Test the patient's ability to discriminate sharp and blunt sensation of the skin in the area where the electrodes will be placed. Use special testing tools, a pin or a toothpick with sharp and blunt ends. Note: a reduced awareness is not usually a contraindication but an indication that more care is needed with the level and type of current applied.

Setting

Ensure the patient is comfortable and the relevant muscles to be stimulated are accessible. If movement is expected, ensure it is possible. If weights or equipment are being used to resist movement set this up.

Electrodes

Clean the skin where the electrodes are to be placed with either 70% alcohol wipes or warm soapy water (pat dry). Select and apply either:

- single-person self-adhesive electrodes (reused only for that patient)
- multi-use carbon rubber electrodes each with a single-use gel pad or gel or with sponge
- electrode suction cups (used with sponges)
- multi-use metal electrodes and sponges or covers.

    See chapter 3 for more details.

Application

Electrodes – Attach the electrodes to the skin. If disposable, smooth them onto the skin and check that the entire surface area is adhering, including the corners. If not, use new electrodes and dispose of the old. If reusable (e.g. rubber or sponge), apply conducting gel (to carbon rubber electrodes) or water or saline (to sponge or lint) and bandage, tape or otherwise apply them to the skin ensuring a firm and even pressure.

Suction cups – If using suction cups, the level of suction should be the minimum needed to keep the sponge electrode in contact with the skin. High levels of suction can cause bruising, especially if the patient is taking anticoagulant medication.

Stimulator output – Gradually increase the output of the stimulator during the 'on-time' of the on/off cycle. Note: do not increase the intensity when the current is off: the possible sudden increase in intensity when the current is next on could cause a patient considerable discomfort. Modern electrical stimulators switch-off ramping when the stimulation intensity is adjusted. The stimulus ramps to maximum and holds. Only then can the intensity be increased. This avoids any startle reaction due to excessive stimulation during the on-time. Increase the intensity only within the patient's comfort range and note their responses and look for a motor response. If the motor response is not what is required, e.g. ulnar deviation when aiming to produce wrist extension, turn the stimulator to zero and reposition the electrodes so the current path is less likely to stimulate unwanted muscles or groups (the extensor carpi ulnaris muscle in this case).

Depending on the aim of the treatment, turn the intensity as high as required but always within the patient's level of tolerance.

Treatment

General guidelines (see text and Table 5.1 for specifics)

To increase strength: increase the intensity until a sufficient torque is produced (innervated or denervated muscle)
To mobilize: obtain full available range and limit torque to sufficient to pull into joint or muscle resistance
To increase endurance: use a high number of repetitions of moderate intensity
To limit fatigue: see text, this chapter
To increase comfort: see text, this chapter
To reduce risks of skin damage: see text, this chapter.

Termination

Stimulator – The intensity is slowly turned to zero output and the leads disconnected from the machine. The machine is then switched off and the electrodes carefully removed from the skin. If self-adhesive and they are to be reused (same patient only), they are stored in their original packaging and hydrated as advised by the manufacturer. (Usually in a plastic bag and some fresh water dripped on the non-skin surface of the electrode prior to resealing the bag.) If another type of reusable electrode it must be appropriately cleaned and stored.

Patient – Check the skin under the electrodes. It may be a little red and, depending on the type of current used, may itch a little (if monophasic or unbalanced biphasic pulses).

Electrodes – Clean multi-use electrodes, sponges, covers and probes then rinse each item thoroughly under running water and air dry on a drying rack:

- rubber electrodes/cups – clean in warm soapy water and rinse thoroughly (if using a single-use gel pad on each rubber electrode, soak off in warm water first)

- sponges/covers/probes – clean in a fresh disinfecting solution that contains chlorine, gluteraldehyde or alcohol according to the local protocol, or as advised by the manufacturer, and soak for at least 30 minutes. Rinse thoroughly before air drying as retained cleaning solution may cause skin burns. See chapter 7 for more discussion.

Record – Record the dosage parameters (including the date, duration of treatment, type of current, specific parameters, size, type and location of electrodes) and any patient responses, such as tolerance and level of torque produced.

Summary

1. Establish aims of treatment
2. Select appropriate current parameters and stimulator
3. Choose electrode type and plan size, number and location on skin
4. Explanation and warnings to patient
5. In electrode location – test ability to discriminate sharp from blunt sensations and then clean skin
6. Therapist test output via leads and electrodes
7. Apply electrodes, first checking the current intensity is at zero
8. Increase current intensity within patient tolerance and comfort
9. Monitor if required muscle action and relocate electrodes if not
10. At end of treatment turn current to zero and disconnect leads before turning off
11. Remove electrodes, check underlying skin and turn off the machine
12. Clean or dispose of electrodes
13. Record treatment details and consider treatment effectiveness.

Dosage

Dosage is very much a function of the aims of treatment. Guidelines regarding the number of repetitions per day for a range of aims are provided in Table 5.1, along with parameters to obtain a particular aim. In addition, the limiting factors for each aim are discussed.

Electrode size, number and location

Changing the electrode size, number and location will all affect the current path. They are therefore selected according to the aims of treatment; specifically, which muscles are to be stimulated and how strongly and if they are innervated. General principles are as follows:

- the size of electrodes and intensity govern the current density – use as low a current density as possible, i.e. electrodes as large as feasible given the size of the muscles or muscle group being stimulated

- Larger electrodes generally are more comfortable and, if relevant (e.g. using monophasic or unbalanced biphasic current), mean less risk of skin damage
- the number of electrodes is a minimum of two per channel but can be more if an electrode is bifurcated (e.g. with HVPS current). The most common use of bifurcated electrode systems is with HVPS current (see chapter 3) as it enables the location of a cathode over the motor point of each head of a multihead muscle or, each muscle in a group. Note the possible effect on current density of individual electrodes and that the combined area of cathodes (usually the divided electrode, see chapter 3 on polarity) should be approximately the same as that of the anode.

Current path

- For motor stimulation, the path should always be along the length of a muscle, not across it, to optimize the chance of stimulating motor nerve (if innervated) or muscle fibres (if denervated)
- The current path should not be trans-thoracic and possibly not through the anterolateral aspect of the neck or through the head. Passing current through the anterior muscles of the neck can make swallowing and speech difficult and so should be avoided when possible.

Progression of treatment

See individual sections in this chapter for progression of treatment. Specific parameters are provided to assist with optimizing treatment: specifically, to maximize comfort and to reduce the rate of fatigue development.

The reason for stimulating muscle dictates the number and frequency of sessions required to be effective. For example, for strengthening a normal quadriceps, three sessions per week is better than two (Parker et al., 2003). By contrast, daily sessions are recommended for mobilizing and stretching tight soft tissue (Robertson and Ward, 2002).

Dangers and contraindications

The safety of the equipment including the stimulators and leads should be checked and certified at least annually.

As with all electrical equipment it must be appropriately and regularly maintained by qualified electromedical technicians or engineers. In addition, users should always check individual leads and electrodes for integrity prior to testing the output of the stimulator on themselves before applying to the patient.

The user should always check the intensity is on zero prior to connecting the leads to electrodes on a patient. In addition, the intensity should only be increased while there is an output. This is evident from the muscle response, patient feedback or an output meter. Turn off the equipment only after it has been disconnected from the patient.

The main danger involving electrical stimulation applied transcutaneously is probably to the skin. However, skin breakdown is not common and electrical stimulation can generally be applied for a large number of hours with little risk, depending on the current type and density. With biphasic balanced pulses or alternating currents the risk is minimal unless applied at a high current density (i.e. small electrodes and/or high intensity). Therapists and home users must check the skin at electrode sites before and after each use. Also, electrodes must be carefully maintained. If disposable, they must not be used when the surface gel is too dry or altered by contamination by substances from the skin. If a reusable type of electrode such as a rubber or metal one, they must be intact and the contact medium (or sponges or lint pads) applied so an even contact with the skin occurs.

Pregnancy – There is little evidence of risk to the fetus or of initiating contractions of the uterus at clinical intensities. However, the risks are sufficiently important that passing a current through the uterus of a pregnant woman must be regarded as a contraindication. This advice errs very much on the side of caution as is clear from a review of the effect of TENS during pregnancy (Crothers, 2003). The summary of that review was that, although there was a lack of negative effects, there was no evidence that TENS was safe during pregnancy. This topic is further discussed in chapter 6 in the dangers and contraindications section as the main use of this treatment is to reduce low back pain during pregnancy.

Transthoracic or neck current – Passing a current through the thorax in any diameter must be regarded as a contraindication. (This does not preclude a coplanar application which is, by definition, not across a thoracic diameter). Current through the anterior neck region poses an unjustified risk. It should be avoided where possible because of the possible risk of unexpectedly strong contractions of muscles of the tongue and throat which could block respiration.

Indwelling stimulators – Current should not be passed through an indwelling stimulator or across the indwelling leads and electrodes (contraindication). The consequences can be serious if a stimulator, such as a pacemaker, malfunctions as occurred in two patients who had transcutaneous electrical stimulation (Chen et al., 1990). Assessing the risk can be difficult and must always be considered a contraindication unless recommended by the treating cardiologist or physician.

Tumours – Avoid treatment over known tumours as the level of risk of affecting malignant cell growth or metastasization is unknown. Also avoid locating electrodes or passing current through recently

Long-term transcutaneous electrical stimulation to the knee flexors and extensors has been shown safe in a sample of six patients with an indwelling cardioverter defribrillator (Crevenna et al., 2004). Note that in this instance the current path would not be through the implanted stimulator and that this should be done only on the advice of the treating cardiologist.

irradiated areas (the level of risk to skin following X- or γ-ray irradiation is unknown).

Damaged skin – Avoid passing current through a skin break (the risk is directly proportional to the intensity and inversely to the wound size). The markedly lower skin impedance will result in a high current flow through a small area with possible pain and further damage. If treating wounds a very low intensity is used. If current must be applied over a skin break, cover with a dressing which can remain dry or use an insulating jelly that will not adversely affect the wound.

Infection – Infection may be disseminated if large strong contractions occur in co-located muscle. The level of risk is unknown but it seems unlikely. The greater risk is of cross-infections by poor cleaning of equipment and by reusing infected electrodes on other patients (Lambert et al., 2000). This is easily avoided by either using single-use electrodes only or by implementing appropriate methods of cleaning electrodes.

Note that the following are not contraindications:

Indwelling metal – Metals have a much higher conductivity than subcutaneous tissue and fluids and will affect the current path and current density near the metal. However, current spreading (see Figure 3.2) will predominate and the effects of the metal will be small unless it is located immediately subcutaneously (e.g. tibial plate and screws) or penetrates through the skin (e.g. external fixation) and is in the current path.

Current through pelvis – There is no known risk to the bladder or genitalia from passing current through the pelvis using the electrode arrangement described: place the indifferent electrode (dispersive) on the unaffected hamstrings and the active electrode over the femoral nerve on the contralateral leg.

References

Ada, L., Foongchomcheay, A. (2002). Efficacy of electrical stimulation in preventing or reducing subluxation of the shoulder after stroke: A meta-analysis. Aust J Physiother, **48**, 257–267.

Agarwal, S., Triolo, R., Kobetic, R. et al. (2003). Long-term user perceptions of an implanted neuroprosthesis for exercise, standing, and transfers after spinal cord injury. J Rehabil Res Dev, **40**, 241–252.

Alon, G., Sunnerhagen, K., Geurts, A., Ohry, A. (2003). A home based, self-administered stimulation program to improve selected hand functions of chronic stroke. Neuro Rehabilitation, **18**, 215–225.

Avramidis, K., Strike, P., Taylor, P., Swain, I. (2003). Effectiveness of electric stimulation of the vastus medialis muscle in the rehabilitation of patients after total knee arthroplasty. Arch Phys Med Rehabil, **84**, 1850–1853.

Balogun, J., Onilari, O., Akeju, O., Marzouk, D. (1993). High voltage electrical stimulation in the augmentation of muscle strength: Effects of pulse frequency. Arch Phys Med Rehabil, **74**, 910–916.

Barber, M., Braid, V., Mitchell, S. et al. (2002). Electrical stimulation of quadriceps during rehabilitation following proximal femoral fracture. Internatl J Rehabil Res, **25**, 61–63.

Bertoti, D., Stander, M., Betz, R. et al. (1997). Percutaneous intramuscular functional electrical stimulation as an intervention choice for children with cerebral palsy. Pediatr Phys Ther, **9**, 123–127.

Binder-Macleod, S., Barker, C. (1991). Use of a catchlike property of human skeletal muscle to reduce fatigue. Muscle Nerve, **14**, 850–857.

Binder-Macleod, S., Clamann, H. (1989). Force output of cat motor units stimulated with trains of linearly varying frequency. J Neurophysiol, **61**, 208–217.

Binder-Macleod, S., Russ, D. (1999). Effects of activation frequency and force on low-frequency fatigue in human skeletal muscle. J Appl Physiol, **86**, 1337–1346.

Bircan, C., Senocak, O., Peker, O. et al. (2002). Efficacy of two forms of electrical stimulation in increasing quadriceps strength: a randomized controlled trial. Clin Rehabil, **16**, 194–199.

Bowen, J., Keeler, K., Pelegie, S. (2001). Adolescent idiopathic scoliosis managed by a nighttime bending brace. Orthopedics, **24**, 967–970.

Brown, M., Cole, M., Jeal, S., Anderson, S. (1998). Chronic low frequency stimulation of normal and ischaemic human skeletal muscles: vascular effects and muscle fatigue. Abstract from Scientific Meeting: Human Motor Performance, The Interaction between Science and Therapy: University of East London.

Brown, M. D., Jeal, S., Bryant, J., Gamble, J. (2001). Modifications of microvascular filtration capacity in human limbs by training and electrical stimulation. Acta Physiol Scand, **173**, 359–368.

Carmick, J. (1993). Clinical use of neuromuscular electrical stimulation for children with cerebral palsy, Part 1: Lower extremity. Phys Ther, **73**, 505–513; discussion 523–507.

Carmick, J. (1997). Use of neuromuscular electrical stimulation and a dorsal wrist splint to improve the hand function of a child with spastic hemiparesis. Phys Ther, **77**, 661–671.

Cauraugh, J., Light, K., Sangbum, K. et al. (2000). Chronic motor dysfunction after stroke. Stroke, **31**, 1360–1370.

Chase, J., Robertson, V., Southwell, B. et al. (2005). A pilot study using transcutaneous electrical stimulation (Interferential Current) to treat chronic treatment-resistant constipation and soiling in children. J Gastroenterol Hepatol, **20**, 1054–1061.

Chen, D., Philip, M., Philip, P., Monga, T. (1990). Cardiac pacemaker inhibition by transcutaneous electrical nerve stimulation. Arch Phys Med Rehabil, **71**, 27–30.

Comeaux, P., Patterson, N., Rubin, M., Meiner, R. (1997). Effect of neuromuscular electrical stimulation during gait in children with cerebral palsy. Pediatr Phys Ther, **9**, 103–109.

Crevenna, R., Wolzt, M., Fialka, V. et al. (2004). Long-term transcutaneous neuromuscular electrical stimulation in patients with bipolar sensing implantable cardioverter defibrillators: A pilot safety study. Artific Orgs, **28**, 99–102.

Crothers, E. (2003). Margie Polden Memorial Lecture: The use of transcutaneous electrical nerve stimulation during pregnancy: the evidence so far. J Assoc Chartered Physiother Women's Hlth, **92**, 4–14.

Daichman, J., Johnston, T., Evans, K., Tecklin, J. (2003). The effects of a neuromuscular electrical stimulation home program on impairments and functional skills of a child with spastic diplegic cerebral palsy: A case report. Pediatr Phys Ther, **15**, 153–158.

Donaldson, M., Perkins, T., Fitzwater, R. et al. (2000). FES cycling may promote recovery of leg function after incomplete spinal cord injury. Spinal Cord, **38**, 680–682.

Durham, S., Eve, L., Stevens, C., Ewins, D. (2004). Effect of functional electrical stimulation on asymmetries in gait of children with hemiplegic cerebral palsy. Physiotherapy, **90**, 82–90.

El-Sayyad, M., Conine, T. (1994). Effect of exercise, bracing and electrical surface stimulation on idiopathic scoliosis: a preliminary study. Internatl J Rehabil Res, **17**, 70–74.

English, A. (2005). Enhancing axon regeneration in peripheral nerves also increases functionally inappropriate reinnervation of target. J Comp Neurol, **490**, 427–441.

Eser, P., de Bruin, E., Telley, I. et al. (2003). Effect of electrical stimulation-induced cycling on bone mineral density in spinal cord-injured patients. Eur J Clin Invest, **33**, 412–419.

Faghri, P., Rodgers, M., Glaser, R. et al. (1994). The effects of functional electrical stimulation on shoulder subluxation, arm function recovery, and shoulder pain in hemiplegic stroke patients. Arch Phys Med Rehabil, **75**, 73–79.

Farragher, F., Kidd, G., Tallis, R. (1987). Eutrophic electrical stimulation for Bell's palsy. Clin Rehabil, **1**, 256–271.

Field-Fote, E., Tepavac, D. (2002). Improved intralimb coordination in people with incomplete spinal cord injury following training with body weight support and electrical stimulation. Phys Ther, **82**, 707–715.

Fitzgerald, G., Piva, S., Irrgang, J. (2003). A modified neuromuscular electrical stimulation protocol for quadriceps strength training following anterior cruciate ligament reconstruction. J Orthop Sports Phys Ther, **33**, 492–501.

Fitzwater, R. (2002). A personal user's view of functional electrical stimulation cycling. Artific Orgs, **26**, 284–286.

Gilden, D. (2004). Bell's palsy. New Engl J Med, **351**, 1323–1331.

Gordon, T., Pattullo, M. (1993). Plasticity of muscle fiber and motor unit types. Exercise Sport Sci, **21**, 331–362.

Gordon, T., Sulaiman, O., Boyd, J. (2003). Experimental strategies to promote functional recovery after peripheral nerve injuries. J Periph Nerv Syst, **8**, 236–250.

Gorza, L., Gundersen, K., Lomo, T. et al. (1988). Slow-to-fast transformation of denervated soleus muscles by chronic high-frequency stimulation in the rat. J Physiol, **402**, 627–649.

Grill, W., Craggs, M., Foreman, R. et al. (2001). Emerging clinical applications of electrical stimulation: Opportunities for restoration of function. J Rehabil Res Devel, **38**, 641–653.

Grills, B., Schuijers, J., Ward, A. (1997). Topical application of nerve growth factor improves fracture healing in rats. J Orthop Res, **15**, 235–242.

Gritsenko, V., Prochazka, A. (2004). A functional electric stimulation-assisted exercise therapy system for hemiplegic hand function. Arch Phys Med Rehabil, **85**, 881–885.

Halliday, S., Zavatsky, A., Hase, K. (2004). Can functional electric stimulation-assisted rowing reproduce a race-winning rowing stroke? Arch Phys Med Rehabil, **85**, 1265–1272.

Hankey, G., Gubbary, S. (1988). Compressive mononeuropathy of the deep palmar branch of the ulnar nerve in cyclists. J Neurol Neurosurg Psychiatr, **51**, 1588–1590.

Hofer, C., Mayr, W., Stohr, H. et al. (2002). A stimulator for functional activation of dendervated muscles. Int Soc Artific Orgs, **26**, 276–279.

Hoyle, G., Field, L. (1983). Defense posture and leg-position learning in a primitive insect utilize catchlike tension. J Neurobiol, **14**, 285–298.

Hudlicka, O., Brown, M., Cotter, M. et al. (1977). The effect of long-term stimulation of fast muscles on their blood flow, metabolism and ability to withstand fatigue. Eur J Physiol, **369**, 141–149.

Ijkema-Paassen, J., Jansen, K., Gramsbergen, A., Meek, M. (2004). Transection of peripheral nerves, bridging strategies and effect evaluation. Biomaterials, **25**, 1583–1592.

Jacobs, P., Johnson, B., Mahoney, E. (2003). Physiologic responses to electrically assisted and frame-supported standing in persons with paraplegia. J Spinal Cord Med, **26**, 384–389.

Jacobs, P., Mahoney, E. (2002). Peak exercise capacity of electrically induced ambulation in persons with paraplegia. Med Sci Sports Exercise, **34**, 1551–1556.

Johnson, M., Polgar, J., Weightman, D., Appleton, D. (1973). Data on the distribution of fibre types in thirty-six human muscles. J Neurol Sci, **18**, 111–129.

Jones, D. (1996). High- and low-frequency fatigue revisited. Acta Physiol Scand, **156**, 265–270.

Kern, H., Hofer, C., Modlin, M. et al. (2002). Denervated muscles in humans: Limitations and problems of currently used functional electrical stimulation training protocols. Int Soc Artific Orgs, **26**, 216–218.

Knash, M., Kido, A., Gorassini, M. et al. (2003). Electrical stimulation of the human common peroneal nerve elicits lasting facilitation of cortical motor-evoked potentials. Exp Brain Res, **153**, 366–377.

Koeppen, A. (2004). Wallerian degeneration: history and clinical significance. J Neurol Sci, **220**, 115–117.

Lambert, I., Tebbs, S., Hill, D. et al. (2000). Interferential therapy machines as possible vehicles for cross-infection. J Hosp Infect, **44**, 59–64.

Landers, M., Alternburger, P. (2003). Peripheral nerve injury. Adv Physiother, **5**, 67–82.

Levine, S., Kett, R., Cederna, P., Brooks, S. (1990). Electric muscle stimulation for pressure sore prevention: Tissue shape variation. Arch Phys Med Rehabil, **71**, 210–215.

Lewek, M., Stevens, J., Snyder-Mackler, L. (2001). The use of electrical stimulation to increase quadriceps femoris muscle force in an elderly patient following a total knee arthroplasty. Phys Ther, **81**, 1565–1571.

Maenpaa, H., Jaakkola, R., Sandstrom, M. et al. (2004). Electrostimulation at sensory level improves function of the upper extremities in children with cerebral palsy: a pilot study. Dev Med Child Neurol, **46**, 84–90.

Matsunaga, T., Shimada, Y., Sato, K. (1999). Muscle fatigue from intermittent stimulation with low and high frequency electrical pulses. Arch Phys Med Rehabil, **80**, 48–53.

McComas, A. J. (1996). Skeletal muscle form and function. Champaign: Human Kinetics.

McDonald, J., Becker, D., Sadowsky, C. et al. (2002). Late recovery following spinal cord injury. J Neurosurg (Spine 2), **97**, 252–265.

McKenzie, M. (1999). Electrical stimulation in early stroke rehabilitation of the upper limb with inattention. Aust J Physiother, **45**, 223–227.

Mendonca, A., Barbieri, C., Mazzer, N. (2003). Directly applied low intensity direct electric current enhances peripheral nerve regeneration in rats. J Neurosci Methods, **129**, 183–190.

Michaud, L. (2000). Electrical stimulation in children. Physical Medicine and Rehabilitation: State of the art reviews, **14**, 347–362.

Mohr, T., Flemming, D., Hanberg, A. et al. (2001). Insulin action and long-term electrically induced training in individuals with spinal cord injuries. Med Sci Sports Exercise, **33**, 1247–1252.

Newsam, C., Baker, L. (2004). Effect of an electric stimulation facilitation program on quadriceps motor unit recruitment after stroke. Arch Phys Med Rehabil, **85**, 2040–2045.

Omer, G., Spinner, M., van Beek, A. (1998). Management of Peripheral Nerve Problems. Philadelphia: WB Saunders.

Pandyan, A., Granat, M. (1997). Effects of electrical stimulation on flexion contractures in the hemiplegic wrist. Clin Rehabil, **11**, 123–130.

Parker, M., Bennett, M., Hieb, M. et al. (2003). Strength response in human femoris muscle during 2 neuromuscular electrical stimulation programs. J Orthop Sports Phys Ther, **33**, 719–726.

Pette, D. (1994). Adaption of skeletal muscle to increased neuromuscular activity as induced by chronic low frequency stimulation. Scand J Rehabil Med, Suppl, **30**, 7–18.

Pette, D., Smith, M., Staudte, H., Vrbova, G. (1973). Effects of long-term electrical stimulation on some contractile and metabolic characteristics of fast rabbit muscles. Eur J Physiol, **338**, 257–272.

Pfeifer, A., Cranfield, T., Wagner, S., Craik, R. (1997). Muscle strength: A comparison of electrical stimulation and volitional isometric contractions in adults over 65 years. Physiother Can, **49**, 32–39.

Pierce, S., Laughton, C., Smith, B. et al. (2004). Direct effect of percutaneous electrical stimulation during gait in children with hemiplegic cerebral palsy. Arch Phys Med Rehabil, **85**, 339–343.

Popovic, M., Popovic, D., Schwirtlich, L., Sinkjaer, T. (2004). Functional electric therapy (FET): clinical trial in chronic hemiplegic subjects. Neuromodulation, **7**, 133–140.

Quinn, R., Cramp, F. (2003). The efficacy of electrotherapy for Bell's palsy: A systematic review. Phys Ther Rev, **8**, 151–164.

Rischbieth, H., Jelbart, M., Marshall, R. (1998). Neuromuscular electrical stimulation keeps a tetraplegic subject in his chair: A case study. Spinal Cord, **36**, 443–445.

Robertson, V., Ward, A. (2002). Vastus medialis electrical stimulation to improve lower extremity function following a lateral patellar retinacular release. J Orthop Sports Phys Ther, **32**, 437–445.

Ruhmann, O., Wirth, C., Gosse, F., Schmolke, S. (1998). Trapezius transfer after brachial plexus palsy. J Bone Joint Surg, **80-B**, 109–113.

Salmons, S., Sreter, F. (1976). Significance of impulse activity in the transformation of skeletal muscle type. Nature, **263** (Sept 2), 30–34.

Scott, O., Vrbova, G., Hyde, S., Dubowitz, V. (1985). Effects of chronic low frequency electrical stimulation on normal human tibialis anterior muscle. J Neurol Neurosurg Psychiatr, **48**, 774–781.

Scott, W., Stevens, J., Binder-Macleod, S. (2001). Human muscle fiber type classifications. Phys Ther, **81**, 1810–1816.

Sinclair, P., Fornusek, C., Davis, G. (2004). The effect of fatigue on the timing of electrical stimulation-evoked muscle contractions in people with spinal cord injury. Neuromodulation, **7**, 214–222.

Snels, I., Dekker, J., van der Lee, J. et al. (2002). Treating patients with hemiplegic shoulder pain. Am J Phys Med Rehabil, **81**, 150–160.

Snyder-Mackler, L., Delitto, A., Stralka, S., Bailey, S. (1994). Use of electrical stimulation to enhance recovery of quadriceps femoris muscle force production in patients following anterior cruciate ligament construction. Phys Ther, **74**, 901–907.

Soo, C., Currier, D., Threlkeld, A. (1988). Augmenting voluntary torque of healthy muscle by optimization of electrical stimulation. Phys Ther, **68**, 333–337.

Spielholz, N. (1999). Electrical stimulation of denervated muscle. In R. Nelson, K. Hayes, D. P. Currier (eds), Clinical Electrotherapy, 3 edn, pp. 411–446. Stamford: Appleton & Lange.

Stein, R., Chong, S., James, K. et al. (2002). Electrical stimulation for therapy and mobility after spinal cord injury. Prog Brain Res, **137**, 27–34.

Stevens, J., Mizner, R., Snyder-Mackler, L. (2004). Neuromuscular electrical stimulation for quadriceps muscle strengthening after bilateral total knee arthroplasty: a case series. J Orthop Sports Phys Ther, **34**, 21–29.

Stokes, M., Edwards, R., Cooper, R. (1989). Effect of low frequency fatigue on human muscle strength and fatigability during subsequent stimulated activity. Eur J Appl Physiol, **59**, 278–283.

Strojnik, V. (1998). The effects of superimposed electrical stimulation of the quadriceps muscles on performance in different motor tasks. J Sports Med Phys Fitness, **38**, 194–200.

Sunderland, S. (1978). Nerves and nerve injuries. New York: Churchill Livingstone.

Talbot, L., Gaines, J., Ling, S., Metter, E. (2003). A home-based protocol of electrical muscle stimulation for quadriceps muscle strength in older adults with osteoarthritis of the knee. J Rheumatol, **30**, 1571–1578.

Targan, R., Alon, G., Kay, S. (2000). Effect of long-term electrical stimulation on motor recovery and improvement of clinical residuals in patients with unresolved facial nerve palsy. Otolaryngol – Head and Neck Surg, **122**, 246–252.

Taylor, P., Tromans, A., Harris, K., Swain, I. (2002). Electrical stimulation of abdominal muscles for control of blood pressure and augmentation of cough in a C3/4 level tetraplegic. Spinal Cord, **40**, 34–36.

Truijen, G., Wyndaele, J., Weyler, J. (2001). Conservative treatment of stress urinary incontinence in women: who will benefit? Int Urogynecol J, **12**, 386–390.

van der Aa, H., Bulstra, G., Verloop, A. et al. (2001). Application of a dual channel peroneal nerve stimulator in a patient with a 'central' drop foot. Acta Neurochir, **79**, Suppl, 105–107.

van der Linden, M., Hazlewood, M., Aitchison, A. et al. (2003). Electrical stimulation of gluteus maximus in children with cerebral palsy: effects on gait characteristics and muscle strength. Dev Med Child Neurol, **45**, 385–390.

Wang, J., Chen, S., Lan, C. et al. (2004). Neuromuscular electric stimulation enhances endothelial vascular control and hemodynamic function in paretic upper extremities of patients with stroke. Arch Phys Med Rehabil, **85**, 1112–1116.

Wheeler, G., Andrews, B., Lederer, R. et al. (2002). Functional electric stimulation-assisted rowing: Increasing cardiovascular fitness through functional electric stimulation rowing training in persons with spinal cord injury. Arch Phys Med Rehabil, **83**, 1093–1099.

Wilder, R., Wind, T., Jones, E. et al. (2002). Functional electrical stimulation for a dropped foot. J Long-Term Effects Med Implants, **12**, 149–159.

Wright, P., Granat, M. (2000a). Therapeutic effects of functional electrical stimulation of the upper limb of eight children with cerebral palsy. Dev Med Child Neurol, **42**, 724–727.

Wright, P., Granat, M. (2000b). Improvement in hand function and wrist range of motion following electrical stimulation of wrist extensor muscles in an adult with cerebral palsy. Clin Rehabil, **14**, 244–246.

Yu, D., Chae, J., Walker, M. et al. (2004). Intramuscular neuromuscular electric stimulation for poststroke shoulder pain: a multicentre randomized clinical trial. Arch Phys Med Rehabil, **85**, 695–704.

Zanotti, E., Felicetti, G., Maini, M., Fracchia, C. (2003). Peripheral muscle strength training in bed-bound patients with COPD receiving mechanical ventilation. Chest, **124**, 292–296.

Sensory stimulation and other uses

This chapter discusses three of the four categories of clinical uses of electric current. The first category (motor stimulation) was discussed in chapter 5. Here we consider, sensory stimulation, iontophoresis and 'other' uses.

Sensory stimulation is the first category discussed in this chapter. It is a general term that covers using electrical stimulation to produce changes in the central nervous system to reduce pain and to change the effects of conditions such as spasticity. This section starts with a discussion of the general principles of afferent nerve stimulation and the types of associated changes in central excitability and their implications. This is followed by a discussion of pain, what it is, the different types, how electrical stimulation is used to treat it and an evaluation of its effectiveness. How electrical stimulation has been used to treat spasticity is briefly discussed. Iontophoresis is the next category of use of electric current. Iontophoresis is not electrical stimulation but rather the use of electric current (DC) to facilitate the passage of therapeutically useful molecules through the skin (see also chapter 9, sonophoresis). The final category discussed includes a range of clinical uses of electric current: using it to increase blood flow, for its effects on the autonomic nervous system, to promote wound and fracture healing and to reduce oedema.

As in chapter 5 this chapter also outlines, where possible, the principles used to set stimulator parameters, the types of suitable current and the relevant risks and contraindications to its being used. The main aim of this chapter is to relate the theory of using electric current to clinical uses and to provide the principles for deciding a suitable treatment regimen and for modifying it. The descriptive system of identifying currents is used throughout to ensure clarity. Mention is also made of specific named currents to indicate what they are and how they are used.

> Note the distinction between electrical stimulation and use of electric current. Iontophoresis is not a form of electrical stimulation.

SENSORY STIMULATION

Sensory stimulation means applying electrical stimulation with the intention of increasing the afferent nerve input. This is quite different from the uses discussed to this point as they relied on the effects of stimulating the efferent nerve supply. This discussion starts at the skin with stimulation of afferent nerves and moves centrally, the second part of the discussion being the effects of electrical stimulation on central activity, i.e. excitation.

Afferent nerve stimulation

Increasing the afferent input means effecting change at the spinal or supraspinal levels of the neurological system. There are two main indications for using sensory stimulation. The first is to alter pain perception. The second is to alter cortical activity, to improve motor function or to decrease spasticity or tone. Of these, considerably more is known about the effect of using stimulation to alter pain perception. The emphasis in this section is pain, the types of pain and how electrical stimulation is used and its effectiveness. This is followed by a brief section on the use of electrical stimulation for reducing spasticity.

CENTRAL EXCITABILITY

Sensory stimulation is used to alter the level of central excitability to facilitate recovery. Until recently little was known about the effectiveness of this use except for empirical evidence that surface electrical stimulation can decrease spasticity.

The introduction of more refined methods of assessing cortical activity in living people is increasing our knowledge of what happens at the central level when stimulation is applied to the skin.

Peripheral stimulation above the motor threshold increases the level of excitability of the relevant area of the motor cortex for a period of over 2 hours (McKay et al., 2002). The effects of a single session possibly last less than 24 hours but, if repeated, appear to last for more than 2 days after the last stimulation session. If combined with concurrent brain stimulation there is possibly a functional benefit because of the increased corticospinal excitability (Uy et al., 2003). This effect appears to be purely a cortical response and not due to any spinal input (Ridding et al., 2000).

Following a stroke there is some evidence that applying sub-sensory threshold level stimulation to the affected hand or foot is associated with improved function of that limb (Peurala et al., 2002). Considerably more evidence is needed to confirm the consistency of this outcome and to determine its clinical utility. However, this type of finding demonstrates potential future uses of electrical stimulation and the need for more research in the area.

PAIN

Almost everyone understands the concept 'pain' and has had experience of it. Pain has sensory and emotional dimensions and is associated with both actual and potential tissue damage (Walsh, 1997). Despite knowing this, pain is difficult to define as it is a complex and multifaceted response to noxious stimuli or to potential or actual tissue damage. Part of the complexity is due to the range of possible modifications to input that might be perceived as pain from the different parts of the body. These modifications can occur during or after a painful event or series of events.

Some of this complexity is indicated by the following:

- the response to injury is variable between individuals and over time
- apparently innocuous stimuli can cause pain
- the location of pain is not necessarily that of any physical damage
- the nature and location of pain can change with time.

The different methods of treating or alleviating pain include the following:

- ingesting, injecting or implanting medications, i.e. chemicals known to reduce pain
- surgery
- applications of electrophysical agents such as electrical stimulation, heat or cold, MHz frequency ultrasound, mechanical vibration therapy
- meditation, hypnotherapy and psychology based strategies including cognitive-behavioural therapy and behavioural therapy (Martin and Palmer, 2005)
- acupuncture and acupressure
- massage, manipulation and mobilization (Mior, 2001)
- exercise and movement (Hides and Richardson, 2002)
- rest or immobilization of the affected area.

Each method of treatment has some (often limited) evidence of effectiveness. Each also has limitations. Among the conditions for which surgery is possibly the optimal treatment are the following: cervical root avulsion, Pancoast's syndrome, or cancer-related visceral pain (Meyerson, 2001). Nowadays though, there are many more options with fewer attendant risks. The different categories of medication can cause a range of side-effects, some minor and some serious. Some can also be addictive and their effectiveness may reduce with duration of use. Different electrophysical agents are effective for some types and sources of pain but not others, or primarily affect the inflammation and not the pain. Meditation and hypnotherapy each have a long history of use and for some provide an ideal solution, as do the other options listed (Martin and Palmer, 2005).

This chapter focuses on just one method of treating pain: electrical stimulation, although mechanical vibration is also briefly considered. Electrical stimulation is a widely used alternative to medications for pain control. The rationale for this treatment was provided by the gate control theory of pain proposed in the mid-1960s by Melzack

Different methods of treating pain are available and effective. The complexity of pain and the breadth of treatment options are reflected in the range of excellent books on the topic (e.g. Walsh, 1997; Wall and Melzack, 1999; Hides and Richardson, 2002; Strong et al., 2002).

and Wall (Melzack and Wall, 1965). Essentially, the stimulation is aimed at modifying the peripheral input to change the level of excitability of the central components of the neurological system. Changing the sensory input alters pain perception. It cannot change the actual or perceived causes of the pain, merely its perception and experience.

Stimulation can be applied to the skin or via an implanted stimulator at the spinal, peripheral nerve or brain level. Examples of spinally implanted devices also include intrathecal pumps and, for shorter duration uses, epidural intraspinal pumps. Peripheral implants include those used to treat complex regional pain syndrome type 1, the condition known previously as reflex sympathetic dystrophy (Forouzanfar et al., 2003). Another implanted option is a deep brain stimulator (Simpson, 1999b). These will not be considered here but they are based on the same principle: a contrived input can alter the central state in the neurological system and change pain perception.

The following section briefly outlines the physiological aspects of pain, the types of pain and then how pain may be altered and controlled. This is followed by a discussion of the evidence for clinical effectiveness of transcutaneous sensory stimulation to control pain and a discussion of the parameters and dosage aspects of this approach.

Physiological responses to pain

Pain receptors (nociceptors) exist in the skin and a range of body tissues including joint structures, bone, muscles, viscera and meninges (Galea, 2002). The two types of cutaneous nociceptors are the A-δ receptors, which respond to strong mechanical stimulation and convey sharp or pricking pain, and the C-fibres which convey the sensation of deep, aching pain. Unlike the A-δ fibres the C-fibres are unmyelinated and are polymodal, meaning that they are responsive not only to strong mechanical stimuli but also to noxious heat and cooling and to irritant chemicals (Galea, 2002). C-fibres with their free nerve endings are found in all innervated body tissue except the central nervous system and have a transmission speed of approximately $1\,\mathrm{m\,s^{-1}}$ (The A-δ conduction velocity is 5 to $30\,\mathrm{m\,s^{-1}}$).

The faster A-δ fibres convey 'fast' pain. Fast pain helps the body avoid tissue damage as it provokes an immediate flexor withdrawal reflex and produces a rapid well-localized conscious awareness. By contrast the slower polymodal C-fibres produce 'slow' pain which is less well localized and fibre activation does not produce reflex activity. They are sensitive to the chemicals released from damage to tissue and inflammatory changes as well as several cellular metabolites such as ATP, ADP and lactic acid. The presence of these substances has the effect of causing tenderness (allodynia) and an exaggerated response to painful stimuli not only at the site of injury but in surrounding tissues.

A cost–benefit analysis of implanted stimulators showed their use can produce considerable savings in a range of medical procedures and visits (Mekhail et al., 2004).

Tissue damage causes the release of chemicals such as hydrogen ions (protons), histamine, serotonin, acetylcholine, bradykinin, kallidin and prostaglandins E and F.

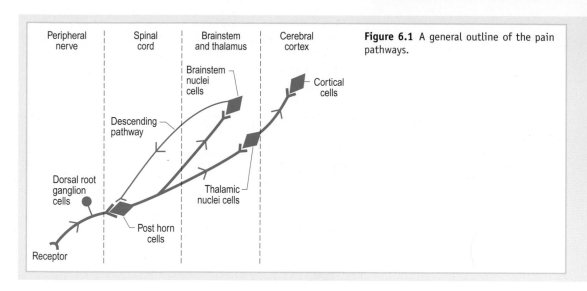

Figure 6.1 A general outline of the pain pathways.

If stimulated sufficiently intensely the evoked response is actually greater than might be expected (Li et al., 1999). The effect can be a long lasting central sensitization or a shorter-term up-regulation of the level of response to suprathreshold stimuli, as can occur following tissue damage. The mechanisms are complex but this form of neuronal plasticity is associated with many of the complex pain states. In addition, central sensitization can also occur in the absence of continuing peripheral nociceptor input (Wright, 2002). This is due to an increased level of excitability at the spinal cord level.

The other response to pain of relevance to this chapter is the release of chemical mediators that affect pain perception by altering the sensitivity of nociceptive pathways. The hypothalamus causes the pituitary gland to release a hormone, β-endorphin, which is a natural opiate. This strongly inhibits pain. Other chemicals released at different levels in response to pain include the production by the midbrain of noradrenalin, which inhibits spinothalamic tract activity in the dorsal horn; the release of serotonin by the raphe nuclei, which inhibits the wide dynamic range (WDR) neurons in the laminae; and the production of enkephalin, an inhibitory neurotransmitter, in the glomeruli in lamina 2 (Galea, 2002).

Pain pathways

All sensations are modulated by the central nervous system before they reach conscious level (Figure 6.1). The modulation can occur in each of the four stages between the stimulus and perception:

- peripheral nervous system
- spinal cord
- brainstem and thalamus
- cerebral cortex.

Figure 6.2 The principal nocioceptor connections and pathways.

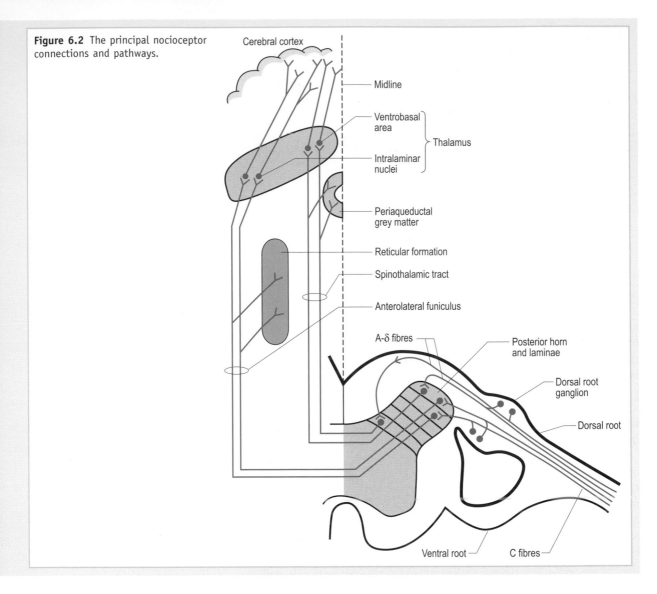

The cell bodies of the pain signalling A-δ and C fibres are in the dorsal root ganglion and their central connections enter the spinal cord via the dorsal root (except for some 30% of the C fibres which return to the peripheral nerve and enter the cord via the ventral root). Here they synapse with central nociceptive transmission cells. Lamina I contains mainly nociceptive-specific cells that respond only to nociceptors but also includes some wide dynamic range (WDR) neurons. WDR neurons (chiefly in lamina V) are so-named as they receive input from nociceptors and large-diameter A-β fibres. From here, information is transmitted via the spinothalamic tract directly to the thalamus or via the spinoreticular tract. The next stage is the transmission to the somatosensory cerebral cortex and other regions of the brain (Figure 6.2).

Modulating pain

The gate control theory of pain was first proposed by Melzack and Wall (1965) and has been expanded and modified since. It can be summarized as follows: pain perception is regulated by a 'gate' which may be opened or closed by means of other inputs from peripheral nerves or from the central nervous system, thus increasing or decreasing the pain perceived. Some low-threshold mechanoreceptors (A-β fibres) from the skin and elsewhere pass, without synapsing, up the posterior columns of the spinal cord. There they synapse with WDR neurons of the posterior horn which convey signals from nociceptor A-δ and C fibres. The WDR neuron integrates and modulates the pain fibre activity. In other words the WDR neuron firing rate depends on the nocioceptor activity and also on the activity of A-β fibres. A high A-β firing rate inhibits the response to nocioceptor activity.

While the focus of the gate control theory is inhibition of pain, it also explains the up-regulation or central sensitization that occurs following injury and nociceptive input (Hanai, 2000; Wright, 2002).

Electrical stimulation

The input of the mechanoreceptors reduces the excitability of the nociceptor responsive (WDR) cells to pain-generated stimuli; thus producing a presynaptic or segmental inhibition. This means that using electrical pulses to stimulate the A-β mechanoreceptor fibres can reduce pain perception. A-β fibres are large-diameter myelinated nerves which can be stimulated at lower current intensities than A-δ or C fibres. They have a similar diameter to A-α fibres. Effective stimulation therefore requires only relatively low intensity pulses to modulate or 'gate' nociceptive input. The conventional wisdom is that relatively high pulse frequencies (80–120 Hz) should be used, but there is no hard evidence. One study which examined the effect of frequency on relief of cold-induced pain found that lower frequencies (around 40 Hz) were more effective (Johnson et al., 1989).

Activation of the A-δ pain fibres may also provoke impulses in the midbrain that then travel back down the spinal cord to inhibit nociceptor neurons at the original level: a descending pain suppression system (Walsh, 1997; Galea, 2002; Wright, 2002). The A-δ nociceptors in the spinothalamic tract give off collateral branches to the periaqueductal grey matter in the midbrain. Descending neurons from this region pass to various subregions of the rostral ventral medulla and thence to the spinal dorsal horn generating encephalin in the substantia gelatinosa. Encephalin is a neurotransmitter which acts to inhibit transmission of C fibre activity. In the substantia gelatinosa (lamina II) there are interneurons which can produce encephalin to inhibit the C system cells in this region. An implication is thus that the deliberate stimulation of A-δ pain fibres will have an analgesic effect by inhibiting transmission of C fibre signals to the CNS. Another implication of this central response is that short-term sensory

Pins and needles

An interesting phenomenon where neural gating plays a part is the 'pins and needles' effect from sitting cross-legged (leg dysaesthesia). Both nerve compression and compression of blood vessels contribute. When a nerve is compressed, it may cease to conduct impulses through the compressed region. Larger diameter fibres are more easily compressed than small so sensory (A-β fibre) input is lost, resulting in numbness. Motor activity, requiring A-α motoneurons, largely ceases, resulting in a marked loss of strength and inability to weight-bear. The 'pins and needles' sensation is due to uninhibited A-δ fibre activity. A-δ fibres are relatively small and so less susceptible to transmission failure by compression. Slow firing of A-δ fibres elicits a 'pins and needles' sensation which is accentuated by the absence of A-β inhibitory activity.

stimulation can also modulate the activity of the motor system (Mima et al., 2004). Specifically, corticospinal excitability is transiently reduced.

Morphine acts on the C fibre system and hence controls tissue damage pain but not other types of pain. This occurs because morphine imitates naturally occurring groups of inhibitory neurotransmitters, encephalin, β-endorphin and dynorphin. In the substantia gelatinosa (lamina II) there are interneurons which can produce encephalin to inhibit the C system cells in this region. Collateral branches of A-δ fibres in the posterior horn connect with these interneurons and stimulate them. Thus stimulation of the A-δ fibres by electrical pulses is believed to act to damp down C fibre system-type pain. This is possibly also how acupuncture works as A-δ nerve fibres are stimulated by a pinprick in the same neural segment (dermatome, myotome or sclerotome). Evidence of this effect comes from studies of its reversal with naloxone, an opioid antagonist (Johnson, 1998). Also, there is some evidence from a study with rats to suggest that repeated administrations of high or low rate TENS causes increased tolerance of μ- and δ-opioids respectively (Chandran and Sluka, 2003). This is consistent with opioid users generally not responding to TENS.

Another aspect of applying electrical stimulation to consider is the extent to which any pain reduction during or following is a placebo effect. Studies evaluating electrical stimulation which use an active, a sham and a control method usually report a better outcome in the active TENS group. However, the sham group usually benefits more than the control but less than the active group suggesting that the specific parameters have more than a placebo effect (e.g. Marchand et al., 1993). Why is not clear, although there is a clear effect of stimulation that is typically greater than sham stimulation. The placebo effect is complex and incompletely understood (Kradin, 2004; Spiegel, 2004; Finniss and Benedetti, 2005; Fricchione and Stefano, 2005).

Mechanical vibration

Mechanical vibration is also used to reduce or modify pain. It is applied to the skin over or near the pain. While not the topic of this chapter, it is mentioned as the effect is also explained using the gate control theory. Additional sensory input in the A-β fibres can modulate pain and one source of such input is vibration. One evaluation of sham, 20 Hz and 100 Hz vibration on temporomandibular pain found that 100 Hz vibration (amplitude of 200 μm) consistently reduced the pain (Roy et al., 2003). Depending on the durability, tested only for 12 minutes in this study, this method of pain modulation is possibly very useful. It is easy to apply and safe: vibrators can be built into a chair, a seat cover or be a separate handheld unit.

Summary

The mechanisms of pain modulation by electrical stimulation described so far are summarized in Figure 6.1 and below:

- pain gate theory explains many of the effects of electrical stimulation and mechanical vibration
- the pain gate effect (gating) on both A-δ (fast) and C (slow) pain fibres in the posterior horn is due to stimulation of mechanoreceptors (A-β) fibres. Theoretically this is best achieved by applying high-frequency, low-intensity electric pulses, variously called high rate TENS, conventional TENS, hi-TENS or traditional TENS
- there is a morphine-type effect on the C fibre system. This is due to encephalin produced by interneurons in the posterior horn, which have been stimulated by A-δ pain receptor fibres. These

A-δ fibres are effectively stimulated by low frequency, high-intensity electrical pulses, which are called low rate TENS, ALTENS (acupuncture like TENS), lo-TENS or acupuncture TENS.

- there is a morphine-type (encephalin) effect on the C fibre system as in the point above but via centres in the midbrain and involving serotonin as a neurotransmitter; also activated by A-δ stimulation by low-frequency, high-intensity stimuli
- optimum frequencies for 'high' and 'low' frequency TENS have yet to be established.

Types of pain

Pain can be categorized in different ways including by immediacy and duration: acute and chronic. Pain can also be categorized in terms of its origin: somatogenic, neurogenic or psychogenic. Neither category is mutually exclusive as, for example, pain can be neurogenic and acute or chronic. There are also other categorizations, such as in terms of the causal mechanism or pathology (e.g. cancer pain). They will not be considered here as the physiological and chemical aspects and the mechanisms are no different from other types of pain, although the outcomes may be (Turk, 2002). The diversity of approaches to treatment is even evident in the categorization of centres for treating pain; modality based, syndrome oriented or comprehensive centres (Main and Spanswick, 2000).

Immediacy or duration of pain

Acute pain – If tissue damage is negligible, acute pain is transient, ceasing after a few seconds or so. Continuing acute pain is closely associated with tissue damage. The developing inflammatory changes and exudation in the first hours can cause increasing pain. This tends to limit movement or stress on the injured tissue, which, at this stage, can benefit healing.

Chronic pain – Chronic pain is defined by its persistence for at least 3 to 6 months beyond the initial cause and after healing is presumed to have happened (Dworkin, 2002). Changes occur in the spinal cord: an increased level of excitability and a central hypersensitivity that results in a lowered pain threshold. When this is present, stimulation of A-β afferents can cause pain, a secondary hyperalgesia (Devor and Seltzer, 1999). Pain that is associated with degenerative disease is also termed chronic.

Site or type of origin of pain

Somatogenic pain – Somatogenic pain is musculoskeletal or visceral pain and it can be well localized or diffuse, felt at the affected site or

Pain originating in deep structures is often perceived as originating in some other (superficial) site. This type of pain is called referred pain. Referred visceral pain is explained by the convergence of nociceptors from both the skin and the viscera onto the same dorsal horn cell.

referred. Surface pain is usually highly localized; deep pain from tendons, muscles and joints tends to be more diffuse. Pain originating in the parietal membrane – pleura, pericardium, peritoneum – is often sharp and well localized. These structures have more A-δ innervation. By contrast, pain arising in the viscera themselves, associated with the autonomic system, is usually not well localized, although often severe (e.g. spasm of the ureter due to a kidney stone).

Clinicians need to be able to distinguish visceral pain from cutaneous or deeper sources in the same dermatome. The nociceptive afferents for the heart, for example, enter the spinal cord at the C3–T5 level, explaining why cardiac pain can be felt in the left shoulder and upper arm. However, patients will often not recognize some types and patterns of upper arm pain as having a cardiac rather than a local origin; or diffuse calf pain as having an origin in central compression of the spinal cord or intermittent compression of a lumbar nerve root and not in the muscle. Understanding the mechanisms and implications of referred pain is clearly important in identifying the correct source of pain. It can also help to explain how stimulation, electrical or other, can affect visceral pain (Hanegan, 1992).

Neurogenic pain – Neurogenic pain such as post-herpetic neuralgia, complex regional pain syndrome type II pain (previously called causalgia) or central post-stroke pain is qualitatively different from other somatogenic pain. It is usually reported as a burning, throbbing or shooting sensation and it can be continuous or stimulus evoked (Dworkin, 2002). The common feature is the original cause; damage to some part of the neurological system. Damaged sensory neurons become hyperexcitable and tend to sensitize undamaged neurons. The result is the particular types of pain called neurogenic.

Psychogenic pain – Pain is markedly influenced by psychological factors such that a separate category of psychogenic pain is sometimes used.

Summary of pain categories

- Somatogenic pain
  - acute pain, associated with tissue damage
  - chronic pain persisting after tissue healing
  - referred pain, provoked in deeper or distant structures but recognized superficially or locally
- Neurogenic pain, qualitatively different from somatogenic, due to damaged neurological component
- Psychogenic pain, influenced by higher centres.

PAIN CONTROL WITH ELECTRICAL STIMULATION

One of the main indications for using electrical stimulation for pain control is when medication is not possible or desirable. Such situations include when the patient is to have nil orally, has allergies or a current or previous addiction to analgesics or when the side-effects of analgesics or of non-steroidal anti-inflammatories present a risk or a contraindication to their use. In some instances neurosurgical techniques are unable to stop or reduce the pain sufficiently. Anaesthetic blocks may not be able to be repeated as frequently as needed, as can occur following an amputation or nerve root damage. This is not to say that electrical stimulation is always effective, but it does offer an effective option in some situations, one that has no side-effects and is relatively safe, cheap and easy to use. The equipment commonly used is portable and easily available.

Repeated surveys show sensory stimulation for pain control is one of the most frequently and widely used electrophysical agents (Pope et al., 1995; Robertson and Spurritt, 1998). Different kinds of stimulators (e.g. interferential, HVPS, TENS) are all advocated by their manufacturers as being effective for pain control. While it is probably true that all are effective, there is still the question of whether some kinds of stimulators are more effective than others.

The explanation of gating and of how applying electrical stimulation can alter pain perception indicates that the effects of different stimulation parameters will vary, so different kinds of stimulator would be expected to vary in their effectiveness.

Ironically, the availability and low cost of pain control stimulators may not auger well if inexperienced users are not well informed about using the equipment. There is a risk that it may become unfairly undervalued in the future.

TENS machines

When electrical stimulation is used to treat pain it is usually from a small battery-operated transcutaneous electrical nerve stimulator. Colloquially the machine is called a TENS machine. Currents labelled 'TENS' and with the parameters shown in Table 6.1 are also available on some mains-powered clinical multistimulators.

The difference in frequency between 'high rate TENS' (80–120 Hz) and 'brief intense TENS' (125–150 Hz) is negligible from a physiological point of view and is probably a reflection of an attempt by the manufacturers to differentiate their products. Similarly, the difference in pulse duration between 'low rate TENS' (>300 μs) and 'brief intense TENS' (200–250 μs) is physiologically insignificant. The more general distinctions between high and low frequency and short or long pulse duration are the important distinguishing factors.

The usual pulse duration used for sensory stimulation is about 50 μs but may be higher. Longer pulse durations are better able to stimulate A-δ fibres. This is an objective of 'low-rate acupuncture-like' stimulation and 'brief intense TENS'.

For pain control via sensory stimulation, high frequencies are used (80–150 Hz), but there is little evidence that such high frequencies are

Table 6.1 Parameter sets typically used for pain control

Parameters	High rate TENS (conventional TENS)	Low rate TENS (acupuncture TENS)	Brief intense TENS
Frequency	High 80–120 Hz	Low 2–5 Hz	High 125–250 Hz
Pulse duration	Short ≈50 µs	Long >300 µs	Long 200–250 µs
Amplitude[1]	Strong tingling but below motor threshold	At or above motor threshold	Highest tolerable
Use	Extended period of time	45 minutes or so – limited by possible muscle fatigue	15 minutes or less

[1] The amplitude is set by the patient's response thresholds and a subjective assessment of pain relief.

appropriate. As noted previously, there is some evidence that lower frequencies might be more effective (Johnson et al., 1989). Pulse frequencies available on commercially available stimulators typically range from 1 to about 200 Hz so the operator is able to make an appropriate choice.

Clinical stimulators

A very low intensity direct current, sometimes called microcurrent because of its low intensity, is also used for pain control. The equipment usually comprises two self-adhesive electrodes that are a DC storage system which gradually discharges over a 24 to 48 hour period once the electrodes are connected to the skin and a circuit is formed. There appears to be no credible evidence of its effectiveness.

Other types of currents besides pulsed current are also used for pain control and these are normally provided by mains-powered clinical stimulators. The most common is an alternating current with a frequency of from 4 to 10 kHz; an interferential current provided by an IFT stimulator or a multistimulator. Although portable interferential machines exist, because of the high current, they typically either have limited settings or a very short battery life. IFT was described in detail in chapters 3 and 4. Currents such as high voltage pulsed current (HVPS) can also be used. All will produce an increased input from A-β fibres to the central nervous system.

There appear to be no reported clinical studies comparing the analgesic effects of different types of current. There also appear to be no published laboratory-based comparisons of HVPS with IFT or TENS. Only four studies directly compared the pain-relieving effects of IFT and TENS (Johnson and Tabasam, 1999, 2003; Alves-Guerreiro et al., 2001; Cheing and Hui-Chan, 2004). Three of these studies reported both IFT and TENS provide significantly greater analgesia than sham stimulation or control groups (the exception being Alves-Guerreiro et al., 2001). However, no significant difference in the analgesic effectiveness of IFT and TENS was identified in any study. A problem may have been the experimental design and the resulting statistical power. Other factors which may have contributed are the methods of inducing pain and the stimulus frequency used. Each of these differed between the reported studies.

The Johnson and Tabasam (1999) study clearly shows a greater analgesic effect with TENS, which peaked at the end of the stimulation period, but the difference was not statistically significant ($P = 0.09$). However, the number of subjects per group was seven. If the same mean and standard deviations are used to calculate P values for larger groups, a group size of 10 would have demonstrated significance ($P < 0.05$). This suggests inadequate statistical power rather than a lack of real difference between IFT and TENS. A later study, using a more tightly controlled experimental design with larger subject numbers (10) found a similar difference (i.e. TENS more effective than interferential) and the difference was statistically significant ($P = 0.015$, Shanahan et al., 2006). The limited evidence thus suggests that TENS is more effective than IFT for pain control. This stresses the need for clinical studies comparing the effectiveness of different currents. It also stresses the need to evaluate critically manufacturers' claims for their products. While interferential current may be correctly promoted as effective for pain control, this does not actually imply 'more effective than TENS' or even 'equally effective'. The evidence so far indicates that the opposite may be true.

> When a P value as low as 0.09 is obtained it suggests that, if the null hypothesis is retained, the risk of a Type II error is high. The P value suggests inadequate statistical power rather than a lack of real difference.

REAL AND EXPERIMENTAL PAIN

An issue with studies of the effectiveness of sensory stimulation on pain is its testing on induced and not 'real' pain. How much difference that might make to the measured effectiveness of electrical stimulation is not known. A further complication is that a range of models of induced pain is used, including cold-induced pain, ischaemic pain, heat-induced pain and mechanical (pressure) pain (McManus et al., 2006). A standardized method of pain induction permits the controlled evaluation and comparison of the effects of parameters and of different types of stimulators, but the penalty is that the effectiveness reflects the method of pain induction and may not be true of clinical pain which has different origins.

The issue of pain and what affects it is multifaceted. One factor that does affect it is gender, with males having higher thresholds for pressure pain than females (Rollman and Lautenbacher, 2001). With humans the contributions of contextual differences between a laboratory and clinical situation probably have considerable relevance in the modulation of pain by higher brain centres. Given this, the focus in the next section is on 'real' pain, clinical pain, and not on pain induced in humans in an experimental context. This is not to say that laboratory studies are not of use. They clearly are, but the results of some may not be generalizable with certainty to the clinical context.

The following section includes a range of studies. It is not an exhaustive review of literature on each reported use of electrical stimulation to treat pain. Readers are advised to read current systematic reviews and research publications. What the section does present is an overview of some of the uses known to be effective. Some areas of frequent use where there is less convincing evidence yet available are not included, such as the use of stimulation during labour or to treat the pain of haemophiliac joints after frequent bleeds or of post-herpetic neuralgia or caused by a malignancy.

CLINICAL STUDIES AND EXPERIMENTAL TRIALS

Evaluating the effectiveness of sensory stimulation can be difficult. Many studies do not accurately report their stimulation parameters. In addition, there is considerable diversity in reported parameters, making comparisons and evaluations difficult. Also pain control via electrical stimulation can be achieved using different types of stimulators which compounds the issue of the parameters used. The following section reports a selection of the better conducted studies which suggest when sensory stimulation might be effective.

Low back and neck pain

It should be stressed that a lack of evidence of effectiveness is not the same as evidence of ineffectiveness. A lack of evidence simply means that we do not know one way or the other.

A Cochrane Review into the effectiveness of TENS for chronic low back pain concluded that there was no evidence to support its use (Milne et al., 2004). A major problem identified by the reviewers was a lack of details concerning how, where and for how long it was used, and the parameters. A Philadelphia Panel review on low back pain reached a similar conclusion: there was a lack of evidence of the efficacy of TENS (Philadelphia Panel, 2001b). With neck pain, existing evidence is insufficient to indicate effectiveness. There are also insufficient data on other electrical currents such as interferential (Philadelphia Panel, 2001c).

A pilot trial showed patients with low back pain who had multiple sclerosis tended to benefit from TENS, both low and high rate TENS, more than placebo TENS (Al-Smadi et al., 2003).

Among the studies published since is one which compared the effectiveness of TENS, acupuncture-like TENS (ALTENS) and placebo on reducing chronic low back pain. It showed the following: compared to placebo, ALTENS was seven times more effective, and TENS 1.6 times (Fargas-Babjak, 2001). Both TENS and ALTENS were six times more effective at improving patients' functional status and return to work than placebo. An earlier study compared the effects of using TENS, placebo TENS or nothing (on a 6-month waiting list group) on 42 patients with low back pain of diverse origins, somatogenic, neurogenic or due to a specific pathology such as rheumatoid arthritis or osteoarthritis or scoliosis (Marchand et al., 1993). In the short term there was a marked drop in pain (42%) and in intensity (43%) in those treated with TENS. Those who had placebo treatment also benefited, 18% had a reduction in pain and 17% a reduction in pain intensity. This is clear evidence that there is both a stimulus-specific response and a perhaps equally important placebo response associated with using electrical stimulators.

Primary dysmenorrhoea

A Cochrane Review of the effect of TENS and acupuncture on primary dysmenorrhoea found that high rate TENS was effective but that more research was required to indicate if low rate TENS is also (Proctor et al., 2004). One study compared the effect of TENS to reduce primary dysmenorrhea to oral naproxen (500 mg) (Milsom et al., 1994). Both significantly reduced the pain scores but with an interesting difference: the response to TENS took 30 to 60 minutes and that to naproxen, 19 to 120 minutes; and changes in the pressure and frequency of contractions of the uterus changed only in response to the medication.

Knee and shoulder pain

Electrical stimulation has two associated roles in treating knee and shoulder pain of different types: pain control and muscle strengthening (see chapter 5). With knee pain, a review of earlier studies concluded that in general, TENS produces more pain relief than placebo TENS (Aubin and Marks, 1995). This was despite considerable variation in the TENS parameters and electrode locations used. A more recent comparison of two different stimulators on patients with atraumatic patellofemoral pain reported significant functional improvements (Callaghan and Oldham, 2004). However, both types of stimulators were used on the quadriceps muscle to reduce patellofemoral pain rather than just as sensory stimulators. An earlier case study demonstrated a similar finding when knee pain following a failed lateral patellar retinacular release started improving only after being treated with motor level electrical stimulation (Robertson and Ward, 2002). This suggests that stimulation has a possible dual contribution: in improving function by strengthening muscle and hence reducing pain or, primarily to reduce pain.

There is some suggestion that sensory stimulation and exercise might produce a better functional outcome in osteoarthritic knees (grade 2 or above) than either TENS or exercise alone (Cheing and Hui-Chan, 2004). Patients were treated five times weekly for 4 weeks and while the differences between the TENS + exercise and the TENS or exercise alone groups were not statistically significant the results suggest positive benefits of using both together.

Another treatment for knee pain is by non-steroidal anti-inflammatory drugs, in some cases easier to use than electrical stimulation. However, there are risks of using this type of medication and not all can take it successfully. The relative effectiveness of TENS and diclofenac sodium was compared (Lone et al., 2003). The results show that TENS is more effective at improving function and reducing pain in those with mild to moderate pain than diclofenac sodium alone or placebo medication or placebo TENS. Considerably more work is needed on the comparative advantages and disadvantages of anti-inflammatory medications and TENS.

TENS is unlikely to alter the inflammatory state itself. A study of the effects of TENS on the inflamed joints of rats found that both high- and low-frequency TENS were effective in reducing hyperalgesia but not the inflammatory response nor limb guarding (Sluka et al., 1998). The effects of low-frequency TENS lasted 12 h and those of high-frequency TENS more than twice as long.

The Philadelphia Panel (2001a) recommended the use of TENS for knee osteoarthritis. There was insufficient evidence to make recommendations on its use for some other types of knee pain or for other types of electrical stimulation. However, some of the more recent studies discussed here offer direction for using electrical stimulation for different types of knee pain.

With shoulder pain, there is little evidence of the effectiveness of TENS following most problems except for stroke. The effects seem both to be those due to the sensory input and to muscle strengthening (see chapter 5). Given a considerable percentage of those who have a stroke develop shoulder pain, this is an important treatment option that is easily used and has few possible adverse effects.

Chronic pain

Pain that continues for a long time, months, even years can be effectively treated with TENS. One study investigated patients who had TENS treatment for at least 6 months (Fishbain et al., 1996). Of these, 66% reported a higher level of activity since using TENS. For those for whom an increased activity was not possible, 86% reported that what TENS did was to enable them better to manage their pain at their current level of activity.

There is little evidence yet that particular sets of parameters are better for treating chronic pain. For example, no significant differences were identified in a study of patients with pain of at least 6 months duration (Koke et al., 2004). They used either low intensity TENS (80 Hz, 80 µs), high intensity (80 Hz, 250 µs) or a control TENS set by patients according to personal preference. Without a placebo group it is not possible to be sure how much the current contributed to the outcome and how much was the use of the stimulator itself. Similarly, the main findings of another study on the topic highlighted the diversity of parameters selected when users were able to self-set the equipment (Johnson et al., 1991a).

Intractable angina

Implanted stimulation has been particularly successful for patients with intractable angina (de Jongste et al., 1994). The aim is to produce sensory changes in the area where the patient usually feels the pain of angina. Implanted spinal cord stimulation has also been successfully used with patients with a pacemaker, precautions having been taken to avoid inter-device interference (Rushton, 2002). Stimulation in this instance improved their exercise capacity as well as reducing their pain and ischaemic episodes.

During painful procedures and postoperatively

A meta-analysis of 21 studies found that using TENS to treat postoperative pain can significantly reduce consumption of analgesics

(Bjordal et al., 2003). The studies reviewed investigated pain after procedures in 1350 patients, including arthroplasties of hips and knees, cholecystectomies, thoracotomies and abdominal surgery. No adverse events or side-effects were reported except a reduction in nausea in some patients taking opioid-based analgesics. To be effective TENS had to be administered in the region of the wound at a strong intensity, described as subnoxious. At lower intensities it was not effective.

The possible role of TENS in reducing pain during a painful procedure was investigated during shoulder manipulations done under local anaesthetic in 60 subjects (Morgan et al., 1995). This reputedly moderately painful procedure resulted in less pain in those treated with TENS (50% less in high rate TENS and 38% less in low rate TENS) compared to the controls.

Conclusions regarding TENS

- TENS is generally more effective than placebo TENS.
- TENS and placebo TENS are more effective than no TENS for many conditions.
- Convincing evidence exists of the effectiveness of TENS for treating conditions including the following:
  - different types of musculoskeletal pain
  - primary dysmenorrhoea
  - intractable angina
  - pain during painful procedures and postoperatively.
- TENS is equally or more effective than non-steroidal anti-inflammatories for treating some conditions and has no known side-effects.
- Considerably more research is required on the extent to which the effects of different parameters affect the outcome and when, and on patient selection.

Parameters and current types

The focus is on pulsed current as this is the most commonly used and reported current for sensory stimulation for pain control. The equipment is typically battery operated and is cheap and portable. Alternating currents, specifically IFT, are available in a portable stimulator form but, as the average current is much higher than with pulsed current stimulation, the time before the battery needs recharging is short. Also, as noted previously, the evidence available, though limited, suggests that IFT is less effective than pulsed current.

The direct current equipment mentioned previously is portable, single use and relatively cheap, but as there is very little evidence of effectiveness, it will not be discussed further.

Pulsed current

Three sets of parameters of pulsed current are commonly used (see Table 6.1). Their names are as follows: high rate TENS (also hi-rate or conventional TENS); low rate TENS (also acupuncture-like TENS,

AL-TENS), and brief intense TENS. High rate TENS optimally stimulates A-β fibres, not because of its higher frequency but because the pulse width is small (see Table 6.1). The short pulse duration results in preferential recruitment of the largest diameter nerve fibres (see Figure 3.8). At the intensities normally used (just below the motor threshold) it does not have the disadvantage of causing local muscle fatigue. Pain relief has a rapid onset and the stimulation can be used for extended periods of time in a day and for a longer period (months or years).

Low rate TENS is assumed by some to optimize the production of encephalins and endorphins. This is supported by existing evidence from laboratory and animal studies (Sluka and Walsh, 2003). Brief intense TENS has a rapid induction and is used for more intense pain, such as prior to or following a painful local procedure. Both low rate TENS and brief intense TENS use similar pulse durations (much greater than high rate TENS) and they would therefore activate A-δ fibres to produce both inhibition of (ascending) transmission of C fibre signals and activation of descending pathways resulting in encephalin and endorphin release. Low rate TENS and brief intense TENS thus have a physiological rationale but little supporting clinical evidence as yet.

> It may be that the stimulus intensities needed to produce sufficient endorphin and encephalin release to have a clinically significant effect are too uncomfortable to be practical.

Equipment

Depending on the equipment, high and low rate TENS can be used with any or combinations of the following modes:

- constant or modulated frequency
- constant or modulated pulse duration
- constant or modulated pulse amplitude
- burst mode delivery.

Most portable sensory stimulators provide one or more modulation options and a burst mode option. The burst mode option might allow selection of, say, a burst of $10 \times 200\,\mu s$ pulses applied 2 bursts per second. A study of long-term users showed that those able to choose between burst and continuous modes of stimulation tended to prefer continuous (56%) (Johnson et al., 1991b). Also, approximately 70% used TENS at an intensity more than 10 mA above their sensory threshold.

Duration of effect

The reported duration of effect due to TENS varies considerably. This could possibly reflect the range of conditions for which it is used. The usual expectation is from zero or a few minutes to over an hour. Some very interesting findings of 107 long-term TENS users showed that nearly half (47%) had their pain reduced by more than half as a result of this treatment (Johnson et al., 1991b). The onset was instantaneous for 30% and in less than half an hour for 75% of the 107 patients. Pain relief lasted less than 30 minutes after termination for over 50% of patients.

The other dimension of duration is the overall period for which stimulation offers pain relief. A study of 376 long-term users (over 6 months) showed 69% had used TENS for up to 12 months and 27% for longer (Fishbain et al., 1996). This is contrary to accepted wisdom that suggests TENS has only a limited period of effectiveness. These findings suggest the need for many more longitudinal studies of users. The study also investigated those who had stopped using TENS and found it was because their condition had improved (40%) or they needed more help with the equipment and using it (40%).

Habituation to electrical stimulation

Habituation occurs when electrical stimulating pulses continue to evoke action potentials but the response of the central nervous system reduces (Spielholz and Nolan, 1995). The CNS gets used to and ignores the sustained activity. For this reason most TENS machines provide a varying type of current, usually a modulated frequency, to reduce the likelihood of habituation. The theory is that if the pulse frequency is varied, say from 80–120 Hz this should result in less habituation than would occur with a constant 100 Hz stimulus. A study which compared fixed frequency IFT with sweep frequency stimulation found no difference between the two (Martin and Palmer, 1995).

The limited existing evidence suggests that modulating the frequency (i.e. providing 'frequency sweep' options on clinical stimulators) does not reduce habituation and does not extend the period for which a current can be used effectively. The usefulness of providing a frequency sweep option on clinical stimulators is thus questionable.

> It is important to make a distinction between habituation and accommodation. Accommodation occurs if a stimulus is applied at a low rate (e.g. a triangular pulse with a rise time of 10 ms). When the change in membrane threshold is sufficiently slow, an action potential does not occur and the nerve is said to have 'accommodated' (see Figure 3.13).

Principles of application

With sensory stimulation aimed at reducing pain the effect must be carefully evaluated. A lack of treatment effectiveness may be due to the inappropriate selection of electrical stimulus type or to factors such as the location of the electrodes or the parameters selected.

The principles of application are as follows:

- establish if the patient has an appropriate condition to treat with electrical stimulation and no relevant contraindications
- use expected optimal current parameters and electrode location (see below)
- evaluate the effect of initial treatment on pain
- if effective, decide a dosage and continue the procedures

- if not effective, re-evaluate and either change electrodes (location, size and possibly type) or parameters (intensity, frequency, pulse duration or type of modulation or a combination of these)
- if still not effective reconsider if electrical stimulation is an appropriate or optimal treatment.

Parameters

The parameters include those of the current used as well as the duration and frequency of use. Each of the selected parameters will affect which type of current is appropriate: alternating or pulsed (see chapter 3). The list of current parameters that may need to be selected and set includes the following:

- polarity
- frequency
- shape of pulses
- pulse duration
- amplitude
- modulations
- ramping, duration of peak on time, duration and rate of surging.

The type of current and stimulator used directs which specific parameters must be selected to meet a particular aim. The relevant parameters are shown in Table 6.2 and described in this chapter (and chapter 3) along with appropriate currents for the different aims (see principles). Note that these are guidelines only. Each parameter contributes to some aspect of the changes electrical stimulation can produce. Issues associated with the duration and frequency of applications are discussed in under the heading 'dosage'.

First select the type of parameters: high rate, low rate or brief intense TENS (see Table 6.1). If the pain is severe, maximize the sensory input (see Table 6.2). If for longer-term use, select conventional but use it, for example, with a burst setting during episodes of more acute pain. Alternatively, if for a short duration, use low rate or brief intense TENS. While the evidence concerning when high rate and when low rate should be chosen is incomplete, they have different implications for the duration of use and this and the intensity of pain should guide selection. Users should remember

Table 6.2 Selection of parameters depending on pain severity

Parameter	Severe pain	Less severe pain
Pulse width	Wide	Narrow
Frequency	High	High or low
Mode	Burst	Continuous ('Normal')
Intensity	High	Probably lower

though that the personal preferences of the patient must guide the final selection.

Stages of treatment with stimulation for pain control

Patient

Explanation: the reasons for using sensory stimulation and why it is expected to be effective, the likely sensations during stimulation and the possible risks. Obtain the patient's consent to the treatment before proceeding. If stimulation is to be used without supervision, ensure they fully comprehend how to use the equipment safely (provide written information as appropriate).

Preparation and testing the output of the stimulator

Turn the stimulator on and set the parameters required but ensure zero output. Connect the leads to the machine and the electrodes. The therapist should then use their hand or forearm (singular, i.e. one hand or forearm) to form a circuit between the electrodes and gradually increase the output noting what sensations they feel and at what intensity. (If using self-adhesive or pre-gelled electrodes, the therapist holds the pre-gelled ends of the leads 5 mm apart between two adjacent fingers or their index finger and thumb.) If all is satisfactory, turn the output to zero and leave the stimulator on.

Test skin sensory awareness

Test for ability to discriminate sharp and blunt sensation of skin in area under where electrodes will be placed. Use special testing tools, a pin or a toothpick with sharp and blunt ends. Note: a reduced awareness is not usually a contraindication but an indication that more care is needed in the level and type of current applied. Also note that the absence of afferent input means there is no point using sensory stimulation.

The patient

Ensure the patient is comfortable and there are no contraindications to using electrical stimulation.

Electrodes

Clean the skin where the electrodes are to be placed with either 70% alcohol wipes or warm soapy water (pat dry). Select and apply either:

- single-person self-adhesive electrodes (reused only for that patient)
- multi-use carbon rubber electrodes each with a single-use gel pad or gel

- electrode suction cups (used with sponges)
- multi-use metal electrodes and sponges or covers

  See chapter 3 for more details.

Selection will depend on why sensory stimulation is being used:

- if for home use then self-adhesive electrodes are optimal
- if a trial of a stimulator of any type, then multi-use or single-use may be appropriate
- if a single-use to reduce pain prior to an assessment or after a treatment then any option may be appropriate.

Application

Select electrode location and then the type, size and method of application.

Electrode location – The accepted hierarchy of electrode location is based on and explained by gate control theory. The aim of sensory stimulation is to increase the input to the same spinal levels as the nociceptive input. This means that ideally the electrodes should be located as near as possible to the painful area; on either side or immediately proximal to that area if the skin is broken to input into the same dermatomes, myotomes or sclerotomes as the pain; remembering that few structures are completely innervated by the one spinal level. Use the following as a guide, the higher on the list the generally more likely to be a successful location:

- one electrode on either side of the painful area or wound (note, not over broken skin)
- two electrodes proximal to the painful area but close to it and in same dermatomes, myotomes, sclerotomes or over the nerve or nerve trunk supplying the area
- one electrode proximal to the painful area (same dermatomes, myotomes, sclerotomes or over the nerve or nerve trunk supplying the area) and one very proximal (at the spinal level)
- two paraspinal electrodes at the ipsilateral area of the spine relevant to the painful area
- one electrode in the contralateral afferent input area and one at the same spinal level.

An alternative approach to electrode placement involves the use of acupuncture points. The comparative effectiveness of this approach is not clear, nor is the method of effect except to the extent that afferent spinal input may not have to be as specific as is sometimes thought with the multilevel sensory supply to most areas.

Having selected an appropriate location, the user should be prepared subsequently to move the electrodes if pain is not altered using

TENS. What is effective for a specific user in terms of electrode location and parameters will vary considerably between patients as shown in a study of 107 long-term users (Johnson et al., 1991b). They tended to place electrodes over or near to the site of the pain and most preferred a frequency between 1 and 60 Hz. The preferred frequency and mode in a set of 13 patients with chronic pain bore no relationship to the site of pain or to its cause (Johnson et al., 1991a).

Electrodes should not be placed over an anaesthetic area as, by definition, there is no or very little afferent input so stimulation cannot be effective. In this instance the electrodes should be moved to the next location in the hierarchy described above.

Electrode size and number. Large electrodes, relative to the size of the part are preferable.

Pain control relates to the extent of relevant sensory input. A larger area of stimulation means more afferent input. It also means a lower current density and less chance of motor stimulation if this is not required and a lower risk of skin damage. Skin damage can be an issue when using sensory stimulation for long periods for days on end.

The number of electrodes is not important except that more surface area stimulated means more afferent input. Generally only two electrodes per channel are used for sensory stimulation.

Electrode attachment – If disposable, smooth electrodes onto the skin and check their entire surface area is adhering, including the corners. If not, use new electrodes and dispose of the old. If reusable (e.g. carbon rubber), apply conducting gel (rubber) or water or saline (e.g. if with sponge or lint) and bandage, tape or otherwise apply them to the skin ensuring a firm and even pressure.

Suction cups – If using suction cups with sponge, the level of suction should be the minimum needed to keep the sponge electrode in contact with the skin. High levels of suction can cause considerable bruising, especially if the patient is taking anticoagulant medication.

Stimulator output – If on/off cycling is being used, gradually increase the output of the stimulator during the 'on-time' of the on/off cycle. Note: do not increase the intensity when the current is off: the possible sudden increase in intensity when the current is next on could cause a patient considerable discomfort. Increase the intensity only within the patient's comfort and until they report a strong tingling in the vicinity of the electrodes.

Turn the intensity as high as seems to be needed to decrease the person's awareness of the pain but it must always remain within their level of tolerance.

Treatment

See text and Tables 6.1 and 6.2 for details.

Termination

Stimulator – The intensity is slowly turned to zero output and the leads disconnected from the machine. The machine is then switched off and the electrodes carefully removed from the skin. If self-adhesive and they are to be reused (same patient only), they are stored in their original packaging and hydrated as advised by the manufacturer. (Usually in a plastic bag and some fresh water dripped on the non-skin surface of the electrode prior to resealing the bag.) If another type of reusable electrode it must be appropriately cleaned and stored.

Patient – Check the skin under the electrodes. It may be a little red and, depending on the type of current used, may itch a little (if monophasic or unbalanced biphasic).

Electrodes – Clean multi-use electrodes, sponges, covers and probes then rinse each item thoroughly under running water and air dry on a drying rack:

- rubber electrodes/cups – clean in warm soapy water and rinse thoroughly (if using a single-use gel pad on each rubber electrode, soak off in warm water first)
- sponges/covers/probes – clean in a fresh disinfecting solution that contains chlorine, glutaraldehyde or alcohol according to the local protocol, or as advised by the manufacturer, and soak for at least 30 minutes. Rinse thoroughly before air drying as retained cleaning solution may cause skin burns. See chapter 7 for more discussion.

Record – Record the dosage parameters (including date, duration of treatment, type of current, specific parameters, size type and location of electrodes) and any patient response, such as tolerance and level of sensation produced.

Summary

1. Establish the aims of treatment.
2. Select appropriate current parameters and the stimulator.
3. Choose the electrode type and plan the size, number and location on skin.
4. Give an explanation and any warnings to the patient.
5. Clean the skin in the electrode locations.
6. Therapist tests the output via leads and electrodes.
7. Apply electrodes, first checking that the current intensity is at zero.
8. Increase the current intensity within patient tolerance and comfort.

9. Monitor if reducing or altering the pain and relocate electrodes if not.
10. At the end of treatment turn the current to zero and disconnect leads before turning off.
11. Remove the electrodes, check underlying skin.
12. Clean or dispose of electrodes.
13. Record the treatment details and consider treatment effectiveness.

Dosage

Dosage depends on the clinical presentation: the type of pain, severity and effectiveness of TENS. A rule of thumb is to produce sufficient tingling that the pain perception is reduced. In practice this means turning up the intensity until the patient is aware of the tingling and less bothered by their pain.

Intensity is one parameter of dosage. The other main ones are the duration and frequency of applications. Both are affected by the characteristics of the pain being treated and by the response to electrical stimulation. A general guideline is: use TENS while it is reducing pain or during pain-inducing activities for up to one hour and repeat as necessary throughout the day. Do it for as many days as necessary, recognizing that habituation will occur in most patients over time. TENS has been shown to be of use in some patients for over a year (Johnson et al., 1991b; Fishbain et al., 1996).

Dangers and contraindications

The dangers and contraindications associated with electrical stimulation were described in chapter 5 and will not be repeated here. The main points made in chapter 5 are summarized below.

- All electromedical equipment must be appropriately tested at regular intervals. Some tests are carried out by the therapist, some must be performed by qualified electromedical technicians or engineers (see chapter 7).
- The main danger involving electrical stimulation applied transcutaneously is probably to the skin. Therapists and home users must check the skin at electrode sites before and after each use.
- Electrodes must be carefully maintained.
- Damaged skin: avoid passing current through a skin break.
- Infection: cross-infection is a risk which can be avoided by either using single-use electrodes only or by implementing appropriate methods of cleaning electrodes (see chapter 7).
- Contraindications:
  - a current path through the uterus of a pregnant woman
  - transthoracic current flow or through the anterior neck region

- current should not be passed through an indwelling electronic device such as a pump or a stimulator or across its leads and electrodes
- treatment over known tumours or passing current through recently irradiated areas (levels of risk unknown).

Although current flow through the pregnant uterus is contraindicated, this advice errs very much on the side of caution as is clear from a review of the effect of TENS during pregnancy (Crothers, 2003). Also, TENS has been used to treat low back pain in pregnant women with no adverse outcomes reported (Walsh, 1997). While the current will spread when using a coplanar method of application (e.g. all electrodes on posterior spinal area), the intensity at depth will be very low and there is no evidence that it is sufficient to stimulate uterine contractions. Similarly, TENS has been used to treat primary dysmenorrhoea. A comparison of the effect of TENS and oral naproxen monitored pressure in the uterus throughout (Milsom et al., 1994). Little change occurred in the intrauterine pressure or frequency of uterine contractions per half hour in those treated with TENS, while those receiving naproxen had significant reductions in both. The current path used in that study is unclear, but it seems unlikely that electrical stimulation offers an effective way of inducing labour.

Twenty pregnant subjects admitted to hospital post their due date were tested for the effects of electrical stimulation on uterine contractions (Dunn et al., 1989). Two hours of stimulation (30 Hz frequency) to acupuncture points on the same leg (spleen 6 on lower leg and liver 3, on the foot) caused uterine contractions. The current path was clearly peripheral but the response in those stimulated was significantly more high-intensity uterine contractions than in the placebo group (sham stimulation). Despite this, none proceeded to labour and the authors indicated considerably more and stronger contractions would have been necessary. No replications of this procedure or any similar studies have been identified. In summary though, the body of evidence on electrical stimulation and pregnancy clearly suggests no harm is likely but, if it were to occur, its import is such that pregnancy is better considered a contraindication in the absence of further relevant research.

SPASTICITY

Spasticity typically develops following an upper motor neuron lesion such as a spinal cord injury, a traumatic brain injury, some types of spinal or cerebral tumours or a stroke. The increased stretch reflex is typically explained by a reduction in the supraspinal inhibition. Spasticity limits the quality and ease of movement of antagonists to the affected muscles. During the swing phase in gait, for example, it can make foot clearance and hip swing difficult or even impossible. In a case study of a patient following an incomplete cervical spinal lesion, stimulation was applied over the L3,4 dermatomes on the affected limb. Qualitatively the range of hip and knee flexion and ankle dorsiflexion increased during stimulation, at an intensity below the motor threshold, while the patient was treadmill walking (Bajd et al., 2002).

Stimulation with a frequency of 100 Hz using biphasic pulses of 200 μs duration and an intensity below visible motor response was applied over the cutaneous distribution of the sural nerve on the affected limb for 20 minutes (Potisk et al., 1995). There was a reduction in the level of resistive ankle torque, which persisted for 30 to 45 minutes after stimulation (Potisk et al., 1995; Dewald et al., 1996). While not a functional study, the results demonstrate the effect of afferent stimulation. Sensory stimulation over an area proximal to the affected lower limbs, paravertebrally in the thoracolumbar region, has also been shown to reduce spasticity (Wang et al., 1998).

The spasticity associated with cerebral palsy is also treated with electrical stimulation, as discussed in chapter 5. A recent review of this treatment provides some supporting evidence (Kerr et al., 2004). The paper also makes the usual observations about the lack of high quality research on which to base treatments.

The ongoing questions relate to how to apply stimulation most effectively. When is it preferable to obtain a motor response and when is sensory stimulation preferable? The use of electrical stimulation for treating spasticity is still in the early stages of development but shows considerable promise under circumstances not yet fully described.

Yet another form of stimulation was used in the past to treat spasticity: deep brain stimulation. It is little used at present for this purpose (Simpson, 1999a).

IONTOPHORESIS

The third category of clinical use of electric current is iontophoresis. This is not a form of electrical stimulation but is included here because it is a use of electric current for therapeutic benefit. Iontophoresis is a method of treatment which uses current flow between two electrodes to push ions through the skin barrier. Clinically this means using direct current to move a drug or therapeutically active ion through the skin. The compound being used is placed under an electrode, the choice depending on its charge. The aim is to drive in active ions locally rather than having to inject them or have them taken systemically.

Historical uses of iontophoresis include the use of tap water or an aluminium compound to treat hyperhidrosis of the hands or feet. Iontophoresis has been used to accelerate wound healing using iodine, zinc or copper compounds (Sloan and Soltani, 1986). The problems with this were the need to use a comparatively high current (which presents a risk of chemical burns) as well as a limit on the number of times it could be applied given the likely development of sclerotic changes in the skin under the electrodes. Some commonly used compounds which are delivered using iontophoresis and which have a

Compounds applied using iontophoresis include:

- dexamethosone
- lidocaine
- hyaluronidase
- salicylic acid
- acetic acid/acetates.

lesser risk of skin damage are those listed alongside. Dexamethosone is used for its anti-inflammatory effects, lidocaine as a local anaesthetic, hyaluronidase to facilitate the breakdown of bruising or bleeding into the tissues, salicylic acid to reduce inflammation and pain and acetic acid to break down calcifications.

Iontophoresis is the single major use of direct current. Each electrode is either a cathode (negative) or an anode (positive). Which of these is called the 'active electrode' depends on which therapeutically active compound is being used and if its ions are positively or negatively charged. If positive, then the solution containing these ions is placed under the anode. Conversely, compounds with a negative charge are placed under the cathode. In both instances the aim is to repel the like charge, facilitating its entry through the skin more than would occur if massage were used. The current flow under the electrodes consists of positive ions moving towards the negative electrode and negative ions moving towards the positive electrode.

The mechanism by which iontophoresis works is that of current conduction generally. Ions pass through the skin barrier primarily via the hair follicles and sweat glands. This can only work if the drug or active compound is an ion (i.e. is positively or negatively charged). Most drugs are positively charged at low pH or negatively charged at high pH. This means that, in practice, the pH under the active electrode will need to be high or low to suit the drug being administered, i.e. to ensure that it is charged. Neutral (uncharged) molecules cannot be moved by iontophoresis. The choice of pH is a compromise between the risk of skin irritation or damage and the properties of the medication.

Other factors affecting the rate at which compounds pass through the skin include the following: hydration of the outer layer of the skin, the vascularization under the active electrode, the age of the patient (skin properties are affected by age), the location and the level of current used in the application (Leduc et al., 2003).

The factors listed above determine the rate at which compounds pass through the skin. Another, more important, factor is the amount of drug delivered. This depends on both the rate and the time. The greater the time for which the current is applied, the greater the dosage, i.e. amount = rate × time.

The equipment used for iontophoresis is increasingly a battery-operated portable unit which provides user selection of the (direct current) output. The electrodes can be any of the kinds described earlier as suitable for electrical stimulation (see Table 3.2). There are also purpose-designed electrodes (drug delivery systems) available for iontophoresis.

The current density with iontophoresis is an important consideration. The recommended maximum safe current density under the cathode is $0.5\,mA\,cm^{-2}$ and for the anode, $1.0\,mA\,cm^{-2}$ (Bélanger, 2002). In practice, most users use a cathode two to three times larger than the area of the anode.

Leduc's classic experiment

One of the best ways of explaining the importance of the charge on the electrodes (and the compound charge) is to refer to an often described experiment by Leduc. He had two rabbits arranged so that current passed through them in series. On one electrode on rabbit one he had strychnine sulphate and on the same sided electrode on the other rabbit, potassium cyanide (Sloan and Soltani, 1986). When current was on (40 to 50 mA), a rabbit with the anode over the strychnine and one with the cathode over the cyanide meant both died with signs of the relevant type of poisoning. If, however, the current flow was reversed (using new rabbits), neither died.

Skin hydration under the electrode normally increases with time. Thus the rate of drug movement through the skin may increase during the application. At the same time, the amount of drug remaining will decrease, which would tend to decrease the rate of delivery. A rough rule-of-thumb is that in practical situations, the rate of delivery will not change much during the application so the amount of drug delivered will be directly proportional to the treatment time.

Depth efficiency and clinical effectiveness

A practical problem with iontophoresis is that if the compounds administered are large molecules, they may not penetrate deeply but rather accumulate beneath the skin surface. When current flows between two electrodes, travelling through gel, the skin and then the underlying tissues, the flow of charges is constant. In the gel, the ions that move are the therapeutically active compounds and these are the ions that move through the drier layers of the skin. In and under the skin small ions (e.g. Na^+ and Cl^-) are in abundance and these will move more easily than the larger drug molecules. So current in the underlying, hydrated tissues is mostly by movement of small ions. Large drug molecular ions are more sluggish and are left behind. The result is an accumulation of the active compound immediately below the skin surface.

Drugs such as dexamethosone, lidocaine, hyaluronidase and salicylic acid are large molecules which accumulate under the skin surface. Their depth effectiveness depends on how rapidly they diffuse once under the skin. Acetate ions are small and so would be expected to penetrate further and diffuse more rapidly.

Clearly, there are two dimensions to the clinical effectiveness of iontophoresis: selecting appropriate compounds (taking into account their molecular size, charge and likely diffusion rate) and using it in appropriate areas. Unless the active treatment compounds are able to diffuse rapidly, or have effects at the very low concentrations which would be expected to result subcutaneously, they are unlikely to effect local changes. One study found that iontophoresis was not effective in treating calcific deposits in the shoulder (Leduc et al., 2003). The natural course of such deposits appears quite variable and this, however, may have obscured any effect due to the intervention.

Dangers and contraindications

The main danger from using iontophoresis is of chemical burns. One reason for using a purpose-designed drug delivery system is to reduce this risk by limiting the current density (sufficiently large electrode size and appropriate level of current). It is also important that the pH of the treating compound is appropriate and it is not applied over any areas of skin damage. Damage to skin means a considerably lower impedance and a selective flow of current where it has occurred. This can cause a major local increased ion concentration and hence risk of a chemical burn.

The usual contraindications (see section on pain control) also apply. Users should also note the importance when using direct current for iontophoresis of decreasing the intensity slowly and ensuring the circuit is not broken during a treatment.

Nerve fibres are relatively insensitive to steady direct current, but if the flow is changed suddenly, nerve fibre firing may result, producing pain and a startle reaction.

OTHER

The fourth category of clinical use of electric current is actually a miscellaneous collection. Some are clinically quite important, such as wound and fracture healing, but others may be less well known or used infrequently. This part of the chapter starts by considering some effects of electrical stimulation on the autonomic nervous system.

Effects on the autonomic nervous system

Little is known about the effects of stimulating autonomic nerves, even though they are an integral component of the nervous system and would be activated with transcutaneous electrical stimulation. Examples were given earlier of the vasomotor effects with the decrease in oedema associated with stimulation of the upper limb following a stroke. The oedema is clearly due to more than just a lack of muscle contractions, most probably to a reduced effectiveness of the vasomotor responses due to changes affecting the autonomic nervous system.

Sensory stimulation in rats shows the role of sensory nerve activity in modulating the peripheral vascular responses in healing (Merhi et al., 1998). If sensory nerves are damaged there is a reduction in the rate of wound healing. Electrical stimulation can compensate for the loss of neural activity. The parameters used were a pulse duration of 2 ms and a frequency of 5 Hz, which was more effective than 15 Hz. The extent to which sensory stimulation can affect other functions of the autonomic system needs more exploration.

One use of electrical stimulation is to alter bladder and bowel motility: this is clearly mediated by the autonomic system, although applied at a sub-motor level of intensity (Chase et al., 2005). The role of electrical stimulation of this part of the nervous system needs considerably more investigation to ascertain the limits of effects and the ideal parameters. Increases in blood flow occurred in patients with ischaemic leg pain if stimulation was applied at T12 (Ghajar and Miles, 1996). If applied between T8 and T10, vasoconstriction tended to occur. This differential response suggests a direct stimulation of the autonomic system.

Other evidence of the effect sensory stimulation can have on the autonomic system is the changes TENS can elicit in the sympathetic skin response (Olyaei et al., 2004). Low frequency TENS, 2 Hz with a pulse duration of 250 μs, was shown to have an inhibitory effect on the sympathetic nervous system: it increased the latency and skin temperature and decreased the amplitude of the response.

As indicated, there is relatively little systematic study of the possible clinical uses of electrical stimulation for stimulating the autonomic nervous system. This is an area requiring considerably more research.

In humans, transcutaneous electrical stimulation with a 4 Hz frequency and 250 μs pulse applied for 30 minutes to parts of the hand at an uncomfortably high intensity produced an increased hand temperature of 1.6°C at the end of the stimulation. This was higher than for the control (no stimulation) and high frequency (100 Hz) conditions (Scudds et al., 1995).

Blood flow increases

Electrical stimulation has been used to increase blood flow. Reddening of the skin may occur under the electrodes due to local irritation, especially with unbalanced pulses or direct current. The extent of change in local circulation with skin irritation is very small, an insignificant contribution to the whole limb supply. The increased flow in the area, has, however, been shown to be sufficient to contribute to wound healing, discussed in the following section.

A reliable and effective way of increasing blood flow to a limb by using electrical stimulation is to elicit muscle contractions. As with a voluntary initiated contraction, electrical stimulation will have the same effect and cause a temporary increase in muscle metabolism. There will be the associated consequences of increased oxygen uptake and carbon dioxide, lactic acid and other metabolite production, as well as raised local temperature and greater local blood flow. One study, with seven subjects, used venous plethysmography and showed a similar increase occurred 1 s after with both voluntary contractions (53% increase) and maximally tolerable electrical stimulation (57% increase). The notable difference was that the electrically induced increased blood flow continued for at least 15 s, whereas the drop following a voluntary contraction was much sooner (0% increase by 15 s) (Miller et al., 2000). This, and other studies suggest that the most reliable way of obtaining marked increases in blood flow is via large muscle contractions. This means that the level of stimulation must be above the motor threshold (Tracy et al., 1988; Cramp et al., 2002). Both tetanic (35 Hz) and 3 Hz frequencies producing contractions of lower limb muscles result in increased levels of blood flow in the stimulated limb (Janssen and Hopman, 2003).

Longer-term changes in the capillary system follow extended periods of electrical stimulation (see chapter 5). That is, extended low frequency stimulation produces structural changes in muscle (Brown et al., 2001). A study of 30 patients with stable ischaemic calf muscles were treated with either motor level stimulation (6 Hz, 250 μs pulses) or sensory stimulation only (90 Hz, 50 μs pulses) (Anderson et al., 2004). The motor level stimulation significantly increased the pain-free distance walked by patients without causing adverse changes in leucocyte levels or in vascular permeability, while no changes occurred with sensory level stimulation. This type of finding suggests a possible future, long-term treatment for some instances of ischaemic muscles.

Wound healing

Electrical currents applied to wounds have often been described as supplementing or altering the natural exogenous electrical activity of the body (see chapter 2). Studies using rabbits with surgically created wounds show a greater rate of increase in their regaining of tensile strength if treated with electrical stimulation. Similarly with surgically induced wounds in rats those treated with electrical stimulation, compared to controls, benefited at each stage of wound repair – inflammation, proliferation and remodelling. They were treated with the cathode over the wound for 3 days and the anode for the following 7, and a pulse duration of 300 μs for 30 minutes daily (Demir et al., 2004). In rats this effect has been shown to be due to the increased vascular response when transcutaneous electrical stimulation is applied. An increased microvascular flow occurs in rats with an intact sensory (afferent) nervous system. If a low frequency (5 Hz) long duration pulse (2 ms) is used it is argued that small unmyelinated sensory nerves are stimulated and they in turn stimulate the similarly sized sympathetic efferents (Khalil and Merhi, 2000).

Studies of humans have focused on chronic ulcers and pressure sores. The types of currents used are direct or a monophasic pulsed current (e.g. HVPS). For the first 2 to 3 days the cathode is placed directly over the wound. On subsequent days or when the bacterial count is reduced or zero, the anode is placed over the wound instead. If there is no change in the wound after approximately 3 days, the location of the two electrodes is again reversed (Watson, 1996).

The outcomes show that by using electrical stimulation for 2 hours per day, 5 days a week, the treated wounds can heal 1.5 to 2.5 times faster than untreated controls. One study reported decreases in the wound surface area of 44.3% (s.d. 8%) in chronic vascular leg ulcers treated with HVPS (100 μs, 100 Hz) versus changes of 16% (s.d. 8.9%) in the sham group (Houghton et al., 2003). The wounds were of at least 3 months duration and treated for 45 minutes three times a week for 4 weeks (12 treatments) and the extent of the improvement was both statistically and clinically significant.

This type of finding is relatively consistent across chronic wounds (Goldman et al., 2004). For 300 chronic wounds, if stimulated, healing of 90% occurred within 60 weeks, but for sham treated or conventionally treated wounds only 70% and 72% respectively healed in that time (Cukjati et al., 2001).

The use of microcurrent for wound healing is not generally any more successful than sham stimulation (electrodes placed but no current flows). Between them two studies investigated the effects of current densities of $0.92 \mu A\,cm^{-2}$ for 1 hour per day for 5 days (Byl et al., 1994) and $297 \mu A\,cm^{-2}$ for 2 hours a day for 14 days (Leffman et al., 1994) while both using an intensity of 100 μA. In neither case was the outcome better with stimulation than with sham stimulation.

Fracture healing

Electrical stimulation is used to promote fracture healing. Living bone is a complex, fluid-filled material with constant changes in the distribution of electrical charges on its surfaces with movements such as walking (Otter et al., 1998). A bony fracture also changes this distri-

The level of acceptance of electrical stimulation for wound healing is evident in the willingness of health insurance companies to pay for its use (Schaum, 2004).

bution of charges within the bone. For reasons not fully understood, applying electrical stimulation to the fracture site can expedite bony union by changing the usual complex interplay of electromechanical and biological processes in the bone (Lavine and Grodzinsky, 1987). This is called 'exogenous stimulation' to differentiate it from the endogenous, or naturally occurring currents within the bone.

Two types of currents are used: direct current, using implanted electrodes and alternating current, applied transcutaneously. One study used 4 kHz alternating current (IFT) on a series of 12 tibial shaft fractures, matched to 11 retrospective controls (Ganne, 1988). The 15 treatments resulted in 10 weeks to union for the electrically stimulated group and 17 weeks for the control group. An attempt to replicate this method did not obtain the same results (Fourie and Bowerbank, 1997). However, there were some differences in the methods used in the subsequent study, suggesting replications are still needed.

Considerable clinical and statistically significant success has been demonstrated with a higher frequency of alternating current, 60 kHz. For example, this was applied transcutaneously to 10 cases of non-union (at least 9 months since injury and no bony changes for 3 months) (Scott and King, 1994). Six were successful and four not, whereas 10 of the controls still had no signs of union when re-evaluated.

The role of electrical stimulation in treating both normal healing and delayed or non-union fracture healing merits more research. As with wound healing, guidelines indicating when a fracture may benefit from treatment with electrical stimulation need to be developed.

Reduction of oedema

Electrical stimulation is used to reduce oedema. Claims of how it works are based on at least two distinct mechanisms:

- a muscle pumping action, in which intermittent muscle contraction mechanically compresses adjacent soft-walled venous and lymphatic vessels to increase the flow of their contents. The consequent reduction of interstitial pressure is considered to be effective for all oedema, whatever the stage or cause. Healthy adults standing still for 30 minutes had an increase of 3.8% in their leg and ankle volume (Man et al., 2003). When electrical stimulation was applied to the anterior tibial and gastrocnemius muscles during the 30 minutes of standing, producing strong contractions in both, the volume increase was only 0.8%. This indicates a muscle pump effect produced by voluntary contractions.
- galvanotaxis provides another possible explanation for oedema reduction. This is the movement of charged molecules within the tissue in response to electrical stimulation. This theory is that the application of a monophasic current displaces the negatively

charged plasma proteins of the interstitial fluid of a traumatized region. The increased mobility of albumin in particular should accelerate the normal lymphatic capillary uptake, increasing the fluid return in the lymphatic system and reducing oedema. Evidence comes from animal studies which have applied monophasic pulsed currents (HVPS) immediately after trauma (i.e. while the oedema was developing). Macromolecular leakage from hamsters' cheeks was less when using cathodal HVPS than by anodal HVPS (Taylor et al., 1997). Not unexpectedly if galvanotaxis is the mechanism, using alternating current will not change the amount of leakage.

> There are issues of the relevance of animal study findings to humans. This is illustrated by a study which demonstrated a reduction in oedema but the extent varied between two different varieties of rats (Thornton et al., 1998).

Galvanotaxis may explain the more rapid reduction in the signs of delayed onset muscle soreness (DOMS) in one study using μA level current (Lambert et al., 2002). An electromembrane (negatively charged, discharge duration 48 h, total current 20 μA) reduced the subjective and objective signs of DOMS, including the level of serum creatine kinase. The reasons why are not understood.

Monophasic current is needed to produce a galvanotaxic effect and biphasic pulsed currents appear to hamper the rate of oedema reduction. The other points to consider are the timing of applications of current and the relevance to human clinical practice of these findings. Again, considerable laboratory and clinical research is required to establish the optimal timing and, beyond being a monophasic current, what parameters should be used.

Stimulus parameters for reducing oedema

As indicated above, there are two plausible mechanisms for oedema reduction using electric current: muscle pumping and galvanotaxis. For muscle pumping, electrical stimulation should:

- produce a low force (torque) output of stimulated muscles
- allow a relatively large number of repetitions per day
- use a low frequency, sufficient though to produce a tetanic response, i.e. just fused
- have short 'on/off-times' of 2 to 5 s.

Delayed onset muscle soreness (DOMS) can occur with electrical stimulation aimed at reducing oedema. This is why it is necessary to ensure that the torque is low (short pulse duration and low frequency) and the number of repetitions low until the person's response is evident. The parameters are based on the principles above. This means that two types of currents are appropriate (see Table 5.2):

- pulsed
  - balanced biphasic pulse with rectangular leading edge, duration less than 1 ms (100 μs to 600 μs), adjustable frequency (e.g. faradic-type current)

- uniphasic pulse with duration less than 100 μs, adjustable frequency (e.g. HVPS).
- alternating
  - carrier frequency of 2.5 or 4 kHz with rectangular, triangular or sinusoidal pulses with adjustable burst frequency (e.g. Russian current, interferential therapy).

As noted previously, if the mechanism of oedema reduction is galvanotaxis, the current should be monophasic or direct. Other parameters are yet to be established.

Diagnosis of damage to specific nerve fibre types

Nerve fibres respond to electrical stimulation according to their diameter. Radiculopathies and neuropathies tend selectively to impair fibres (Chado, 1995). Consequently, using sinusoidal pulses of 2 kHz, 250 Hz or 5 Hz means it is possible to diagnose differentially which fibre types are affected by identifying the current perception threshold for each frequency. A-β fibres respond to the 2 kHz frequency, A-δ to 250 Hz and C fibres to the 5 Hz. For example, the C fibres take more time to respond as they are unmyelinated and have a small diameter. This means they are unable to respond to 2 kHz frequency pulses but can to a slow rising 5 Hz pulse, whereas the A-β tend to accommodate to 5 Hz pulses (Chado, 1995). This type of test provides an early and a relatively simple method for detecting a diabetic neuropathy or for quantitatively assessing the extent of a sensory nerve block after a spinal anaesthetic (Liu et al., 1995).

Summary of effects of electrical stimulation

An alternative perspective on the effects of electrical stimulation is summarized below. Instead of a local approach, this provides a summary based on the broader neurological systems to clarify how electrical stimulation can be used.

- peripheral nervous system (intact)
  - elicit muscle contractions
  - alter muscle properties
  - increase local blood flow
  - decrease local oedema
  - maintain or increase tissue extensibility and joint range
  - improve motor skill performance
  - modulation of pain perception
- peripheral nervous system (damaged)
  - elicit muscle contractions
  - maintain contractility
  - maintain extensibility

- central nervous system (damaged)
  - maintain responsiveness of muscle, nerve and blood vessels (assuming intact peripheral nervous system)
  - improve cardiovascular fitness (intact peripheral nervous system)
  - reduce spasticity
- autonomic nervous system
  - not well understood but possibly maintain responsiveness of autonomic functioning such as vasomotor responses and regularize some bladder and bowel functioning.

In conclusion, there are many known uses of clinical electrical stimulation. Some are used frequently and widely and some are little used or known or understood. Some types of uses have not been well investigated (e.g. transcutaneous stimulation of the autonomic nervous system and galvanotaxis) and some are relatively well understood but can be time consuming for patients or therapists to use (e.g. stimulation to change muscle properties, to produce trophic changes). Another issue concerns understanding the implications of using different parameters and the options available to users.

THE FUTURE

Some possible future developments include the use of electrical stimulation to facilitate the regeneration of axons and to inhibit or increase the level of activity in a neuron. Stimulation might also be used more to increase the spontaneous regeneration at the spinal level by applying patterned sensory feedback (Grill et al., 2001). Considerably more research is needed to help us understand how best to use electrical stimulation and the optimal range of parameters for a condition. Although electrical stimulation has a long history of medical use we are, as it were, at the stage of running to the end of the pier while flapping wings – in the hope that one day we will take flight.

References

Al-Smadi, J., Warke, K., Wilson, I. et al. (2003). A pilot investigation of the hypoalgesis effects of transcutaneous electrical nerve stimulation upon low back pain in people with multiple sclerosis. Clin Rehabil, **17**, 742–749.

Anderson, S., Whatling, P., Hudlicka, O. et al. (2004). Chronic transcutaneous electrical stimulation of calf muscles improves functional capacity without inducing systemic inflammation in claudicants. Eur J Vasc Endovasc Surg, **27**, 201–209.

Aubin, M., Marks, R. (1995). The efficacy of short-term treatment with transcutaneous electrical nerve stimulation for osteo-arthritic knee pain. Physiotherapy, **81**, 669–675.

Alves-Guerreiro, J., Noble, J., Lowe, A., Walsh, D. (2001). The effect of three electrotherapeutic modalities upon peripheral nerve conduction and mechanical pain threshold. Clin Physiol, **21**, 704–711.

Bajd, T., Munih, M., Savrin, R., Benko, H., Cikaljo, I. (2002). Dermatome electrical stimulation as a therapeutic ambulatory aid for incomplete spinal cord injured patients. Artif Organs, **26**, 260–262.

Bélanger, A. (2002). Therapeutic physical agents. Baltimore: Lippincott Williams & Wilkins.

Bjordal, J., Johnson, M., Ljunggreen, A. (2003). Transcutaneous electrical nerve stimulation (TENS) can reduce postoperative analgesic consumption. A meta-analysis with assessment of optimal treatment parameters for postoperative pain. Eur J Pain, **7**, 181–188.

Brown, M., Jeal, S., Bryant, J., Gamble, J. (2001). Modifications of microvascular filtration capacity in human limbs by training and electrical stimulation. Acta Physiol Scand, **173**, 359–368.

Byl, N., McKenzie, A., West, J. et al. (1994). Pulsed microamperage stimulation: A controlled study of healing of surgically induced wounds in Yucatan pigs. Phys Ther, **74**, 201–219.

Callaghan, M., Oldham, J. (2004). Electric muscle stimulation of the quadriceps in the treatment of patellofemoral pain. Arch Phys Med Rehabil, **85**, 956–962.

Chado, H. (1995). The current perception threshold evaluation of sensory nerve function in pain management. Pain Digest, **5**, 127–134.

Chandran, P., Sluka, K. (2003). Development of opioid tolerance with repeated transcutaneous electrical nerve stimulation administration. Pain, **102**, 195–201.

Chase, J., Robertson, V., Southwell, B. et al. (2005). A pilot study using transcutaneous electrical stimulation (Inteferential Current) to treat chronic treatment-resistant constipation and soiling in children. J Gastroenterol Hepatol, **20**, 1054–1061.

Cheing, G., Hui-Chan, C. (2004). Would the addition of TENS to exercise training produce better physical performance outcomes in people with knee osteoarthritis than either intervention alone. Clin Rehabil, **18**, 487–497.

Cramp, F., McCullough, G., Lowe, A., Walsh, D. (2002). Transcutaneous electric nerve stimulation: The effect of intensity on local and distal cutaneous blood flow and skin temperature in healthy subjects. Arch Phys Med Rehabil, **83**, 5–9.

Crothers, E. (2003). Margie Polden Memorial Lecture: The use of transcutaneous electrical nerve stimulation during pregnancy: the evidence so far. J Assoc Chartered Physiother Women's Hlth, **92**, 4–14.

Cukjati, D., Robnik-Sikonja, M., Rebersek, S. et al. (2001). Prognostic factors in the prediction of chronic wound healing by electrical stimulation. Med Biol Eng Comput, **39**, 542–550.

de Jongste, M., Nagelkerke, D., Hooyschuur, C. et al. (1994). Stimulation characteristics, complications, and efficacy of spinal cord stimulation systems in patients with refractory angina. PACE, **17** (Part 1), 1751–1760.

Demir, H., Balay, H., Kirnap, M. (2004). A comparative study of the effects of electrical stimulation and laser treatment on experimental wound healing in rats. J Rehabil Res Dev, **41**, 147–155.

Devor, M., Seltzer, Z. (1999). Pathophysiology of damaged nerves in relation to chronic pain. In P. Wall and R. Melzack (eds), Textbook of pain, 4th edn, pp. 129–164. Edinburgh: Churchill-Livingstone.

Dewald, J., Given, J., Rymer, W. (1996). Long-lasting reductions of spasticity induced by skin electrical stimulation. IEEE Trans Rehabil Eng, **4**, 231–242.

Dunn, P., Rogers, D., Halford, K. (1989). Transcutaneous electrical nerve stimulation at acupuncture points in the induction of uterine contractions. Obstet Gynaecol, **73**, 286–290.

Dworkin, D. (2002). An overview of neuropathic pain: syndromes, symptoms, signs, and several mechanisms. Clin J Pain, **18**, 343–349.

Fargas-Babjak, A. (2001). Acupuncture, transcutaneous electrical nerve stimulation, and laser therapy in chronic pain. Clin J Pain, **17**, S105–113.

Finniss, D., Benedetti, F. (2005). Mechanisms of the placebo response and their impact on clinical trials and clinical practice. Pain, **114**, 3–6.

Fishbain, D., Chabal, C., Abbot, A. et al. (1996). Transcutaneous electrical nerve stimulation (TENS) treatment outcome in long-term users. Clin J Pain, **12**, 201–214.

Forouzanfar, T., Weber, W., Kemler, M., van Kleef, M. (2003). What is a meaningful pain reduction in patients with complex regional pain syndrome type 1? Clin J Pain, **19**, 281–285.

Fourie, J., Bowerbank, P. (1997). Stimulation of bone healing in new fractures of the tibial shaft using interferential currents. Physiother Res Int, **2**(4), 255–268.

Fricchione, G., Stefano, G. (2005). Placebo neural systems: nitric oxide, morphine and the dopamine brain reward and motivation circuitries. Med Sci Monit, **11**, MS54–65.

Galea, M. (2002). Neuroanatomy of the nociceptive system. In G. D. Baxter (ed.), Pain: A Textbook for Therapists, pp. 13–41. Edinburgh: Harcourt Publishers Limited.

Ganne, J. (1988). Stimulation of bone healing with interferential therapy. Aust J Physiother, **34**, 9–20.

Ghajar, A., Miles, J. (1996). The differential effect of the level of spinal cord stimulation on patients with advanced peripheral vascular disease in the lower limbs. Br J Neurosurg, **12**, 402–408.

Goldman, R., Rosen, M., Brewley, B., Golden, M. (2004). Electrotherapy promotes healing and microcirculation of infrapopliteal ischemic wounds: A prospective pilot study. Adv Skin Wound Care, **17**, 284–294.

Grill, W., Craggs, M., Foreman, R. et al. (2001). Emerging clinical applications of electrical stimulation: Opportunities for restoration of function. J Rehabil Res Devel, **38**, 641–653.

Hanai, F. (2000). Effect of electrical stimulation of peripheral nerves on neuropathic pain. Spine, **25**, 1886–1892.

Hanegan, J. (1992). Principles of nociception. In Gersh, M. R. (ed.), Electrotherapy in Rehabilitation, pp. 26–48. Philadelphia: F. A. Davis.

Hides, J., Richardson, C. (2002). Exercise and pain. In J. Strong, A. Unruh, A. Wright and G. D. Baxter (eds), Pain: A Textbook for Therapists, pp. 245–266. Edinburgh: Harcourt Publishers Ltd.

Houghton, P., Kincaid, C., Lovell, M. et al. (2003). Effect of electrical stimulation and chronic leg ulcer size and appearance. Phys Ther, **83**, 17–28.

Janssen, T., Hopman, M. (2003). Blood flow response to electrically induced twitch and tetanic lower limb muscle contraction. Arch Phys Med Rehabil, **84**, 982–987.

Johnson, M. (1998). Acupuncture-like transcutaneous nerve stimulation (AL-TENS) in the management of pain. Phys Ther Rev, **3**, 73–93.

Johnson, M., Ashton, C., Bousfield, D., Thomson, J. (1989). Analgesic effects of different frequencies of transcutaneous electrical nerve stimulation on cold-induced pain in normal subjects. Pain, **39**, 231–236.

Johnson, M., Ashton, C., Thomson, J. (1991a). The consistency of pulse frequencies and pulse patterns of transcutaneous electrical nerve stimulation (TENS) used by chronic pain patients. Pain, **44**, 231–234.

Johnson, M., Ashton, C., Thomson, J. (1991b). An in-depth study of long-term uses of transcutaneous electrical stimulation (TENS). Implications for clinical use of TENS. Pain, **44**, 221–229.

Johnson, M., Tabasam, G. (1999). A double blind placebo controlled investigation into the analgesic effects of interferential currents (IFC) and transcutaneous electrical nerve stimulation (TENS) on cold-induced pain in health subjects. Physiother Theory Pract, **15**, 217–233.

Johnson, M., Tabasam, G. (2003). An investigation into the analgesic effects of interferential currents and transcutaneous electrical nerve stimulation on experimentally induced ischaemic pain in otherwise pain-free volunteers. Phys Ther, **83**, 208–223.

Kerr, C., McDowell, B., McDonough, S. (2004). Electrical stimulation in cerebral palsy: a review of effects on strength and motor function. Development Med Child Neurol, **46**, 205–213.

Khalil, Z., Merhi, M. (2000). Effects of aging on neurogenic vasodilator responses evoked by transcutaneous electrical nerve stimulation: relevance to wound healing. J Gerontol: Biol Sci, **55A**, B257–263.

Koke, A., Schouten, J., Lamerichs-Geelen, M. et al. (2004). Pain reducing effect of three types of transcutaneous electrical nerve stimulation in patients with chronic pain: a randomized crossover trial. Pain, **108**, 36–42.

Kradin, R. (2004). The placebo response: its putative role as a functional salutogenic mechanism of the central nervous system. Perspect Biol Med, **47**, 328–339.

Lambert, M., Marcus, P., Burgess, T., Noakes, T. (2002). Electro-membrane microcurrent therapy reduces signs and symptoms of muscle damage. Med Sci Sports Exerc, **34**, 602–607.

Lavine, L., Grodzinsky, A. (1987). Electrical stimulation of repair of bone. J Bone Joint Surg, **69A**, 626–630.

Leduc, B., Caya, J., Tremblay, S. et al. (2003). Treatment of calcifying tendinitis of the shoulder by acetic acid iontophoresis: A double-blind randomized controlled trial. Arch Phys Med Rehabil, **84**, 1523–1527.

Leffman, D., Arnall, D., Holmgren, P., Cornwall, M. (1994). Effect of microamperage stimulation on the rate of wound healing in rats: A histological study. Phys Ther, **74**, 195–200.

Li, J., Simone, D., Larson, A. (1999). Windup leads to characteristics of central sensitization. Pain, **79**, 75–82.

Liu, S., Kopacz, D., Carpenter, R. (1995). Quantitative asessment of differential sensory nerve block after lidocaine spinal anesthesia. Anesthesiology, **82**, 60–63.

Lone, A., Wafai, Z., Buth, B. et al. (2003). Analgesia efficacy of transcutaneous electrical nerve stimulation compared with diclofenac sodium in osteo-arthritis of the knee. Physiotherapy, **89**, 478–485.

Main, C., Spanswick, C. (2000). The origins and development of modern pain management programmes. In C. Main and C. Spanswick (eds), Pain Management, pp. 107–114. Edinburgh: Churchill Livingstone.

Man, I., Lepar, G., Morrissey, M., Cywinski, J. (2003). Effect of neuromuscular electrical stimulation on foot/ankle volume during standing. Med Sci Sports Exercise, **35**, 630–634.

Marchand, S., Charest, J., Li, J. et al. (1993). Is TENS purely a placebo effect? A controlled study on chronic low back pain. Pain, **54**, 99–106.

Martin, D., Palmer, S. (1995). Sensory adaptation to interferential current is not affected by modulation of the stimulus. 14th World Congress of Physical Therapy. Washington, USA. Abstract PL-RR-0584-F.

Martin, D., Palmer, S. (2005). Soft tissue pain and physical therapy. Anaesth Intensive Care Med, **6**, 23–25.

McKay, D., Brooker, R., Giacomin, P., Ridding, M., Miles, T. (2002). Time course of induction of increased human motor cortex excitability by nerve stimulation. NeuroReport, **13**(10), 1271–1273.

McManus, F., Ward, A., Robertson, V. (2006). The analgesic effects of interferential therapy on two experimental pain models: Cold and mechanically induced pain. *Physiotherapy*. (In press).

Mekhail, N., Aeschbach, A., Stanton-Hicks, M. (2004). Cost benefit analysis of neurostimulation for chronic pain. Clin J Pain, **20**, 462–468.

Melzack, R., Wall, P. (1965). Pain mechanisms: a new theory. Science, **150**, 971–979.

Merhi, M., Helme, R., Khalil, Z. (1998). Age-related changes in sympathetic modulation of sensory nerve activity in rat skin. Inflamm Res, **47**, 239–244.

Meyerson, B. (2001). Neurosurgical approaches to pain treatment. Acta Anaesthesiol Scand, **45**, 1108–1113.

Miller, B., Gruben, K., Morgan, B. (2000). Circulatory responses to voluntary and electrically induced muscle contractions in humans. Phys Ther, **80**, 53–60.

Milne, S., Welch, V., Brosseau, L. et al. (2004). Transcutaneous electrical nerve stimulation (TENS) for chronic low-back pain. The Cochrane Library, 3.

Milsom, I., Hedner, N., Mannheimer, C. (1994). A comparative study of the effect of high-intensity transcutaneous nerve stimulation and oral naproxen on intrauterine pressure and menstrual pain in patients with primary dysmenorrhea. Am J Obstet Gynecol, **170**, 123–129.

Mima, T., Oga, T., Rothwell, J., et al. (2004). Short-term high-frequency transcutaneous electrical nerve stimulation decreases human motor cortex excitability. Neurosci Lett, **355**, 85–88.

Mior, S. (2001). Manipulation and mobilisation in the treatment of chronic pain. Clin J Pain, **17**, S70–S76.

Morgan, B., Jones, A., Mulcahey, K. et al. (1995). Transcutaneous electric nerve stimulation (TENS) during distention shoulder arthrography: a controlled trial. Pain, **64**, 265–267.

Olyaei, G., Talebian, S., Hadian, M. et al. (2004). The effect of transcutaneous electrical nerve stimulation on sympathetic skin response. Electromyogr Clin Neurophysiol, **44**, 23–28.

Otter, M., McLeod, K., Rubin, C. (1998). Effects of electromagnetic fields in experimental fracture repair. Clin Orthop Rel Res, **355S**, S90–S104.

Peurala, S., Pitkanen, K., Sivenius, J., Tarkka, I. (2002). Cutaneous electrical stimulation may enhance sensorimotor recovery in chronic stroke. Clin Rehabil, **16**, 709–716.

Philadelphia Panel. (2001a). Philadelphia Panel evidence-based clinical practice guidelines on selected rehabilitation interventions for knee pain. Phys Ther, **81**, 1675–1700.

Philadelphia Panel. (2001b). Philadelphia Panel evidence-based clinical practice guidelines on selected rehabilitation interventions for low back pain. Phys Ther, **81**, 1641–1674.

Philadelphia Panel. (2001c). Philadelphia Panel evidence-based clinical practice guidelines on selected rehabilitation interventions for neck pain. Phys Ther, **81**, 1701–1717.

Pope, G., Mockett, S., Wright, J. (1995). A survey of electrotherapeutic modalities: ownership and use in the NHS in England. Physiotherapy, **81**, 82–91.

Potisk, K., Gregoric, M., Vodnovik, L. (1995). Effects of transcutaneous electrical nerve stimulation (TENS) on spasticity in patients with hemiplegia. Scand J Rehabil Med, **27**, 169–174.

Proctor, M., Smith, C., Farquhar, C., Stones, R. (2004). Transcutaneous electrical nerve stimulation and acupuncture for primary dysmenorrhea (Cochrane Review). The Cochrane Library, 3.

Ridding, M., Brouer, B., Miles, T. et al. (2000). Changes in mucle responses to stimulation of the motor cortex induced by peripheral nerve stimulation in human subjects. Exp Brain Res, **131**, 135–143.

Robertson, V., Spurritt, D. (1998). Electrophysical agents: Implications of EPA availability and use in undergraduate clinical placements. Physiotherapy, **84**, 335–344.

Robertson, V., Ward, A. (2002). Vastus medialis electrical stimulation to improve lower extremity function following a lateral patellar retinacular release. J Orthop Sports Phys Ther, **32**, 437–445.

Rollman, G., Lautenbacher, S. (2001). Sex differences in musculoskeletal pain. Clin J Pain, **17**, 20–24.

Rushton, D. (2002). Electrical stimulation in the treatment of pain. Disabil Rehabil, **24**, 407–415.

Schaum, K. (2004). Decision on national coverage of electromagnetic therapy for wounds. Adv Skin Wound Care, **17**, 316–317.

Scott, G., King, J. (1994). A prospective, double-blind trial of electrical capacitive coupling in the treatment of non-union of long bones. J Bone Joint Surg, **76A**, 820–825.

Scudds, R., Helewa, A., Scudds, R. (1995). The effects of transcutaneous electrical nerve stimulation on skin temperature in asymptomatic subjects. Phys Ther, **75**, 45–53.

Shanahan, C. (2004). A comparison of the analgesic effectiveness of IFT and TENS. Honours thesis, School of Physiotherapy, LaTrobe University, Australia.

Simpson, B. (1999a). Spinal cord and brain stimulation. In R. Melzack (ed.), Textbook of Pain, 4th edn, pp. 1253–1381. Edinburgh: Churchill-Livingstone.

Simpson, R. (1999b). Neurosurgical management of chronic pain and spasticity. Crit Rev Phys Rehabil Med, **11**, 207–227.

Sloan, J., Soltani, K. (1986). Iontophoresis in dermatology. J Am Acad Dermatol, **15**, 671–684.

Sluka, K., Bailey, K., Bogush, J. et al. (1998). Treatment with either high or low frequency TENS reduces the secondary hyperalgesia observed after injection of kaolin and carrageenan into the knee joint. Pain, **77**, 97–101.

Sluka, K., Walsh, D. (2003). Transcutaneous electrical nerve stimulation: basic science mechanisms and clinical effectiveness. J Pain, **4**, 109–121.

Spiegel, D. (2004). Placebos in practice. Br Med J, **329**, 927–928.

Spielholz, N., Nolan, M. (1995). Conventional TENS and the phenomena of accommodation, adaptation, habituation and electrode polarization. J Clin Electrophysiol, **7**, 16–19.

Strong, J., Unruh, A., Wright, A., Baxter, G. (eds). (2002). Pain: A Textbook for Therapists. Edinburgh: Harcourt Publishers Limited.

Taylor, K., Mendel, F., Fish, D. et al. (1997). Effect of high-voltage pulsed current and alternating current on macromolecular leakage in hamster cheek pouch microcirculation. Phys Ther, **77**, 1729–1740.

Thornton, R., Mendel, F., Fish, D. (1998). Effect of electrical stimulation on edema formation in different strains of rats. Phys Ther, **78**, 386–394.

Tracy, J., Currier, D., Threlkeld, A. (1988). Comparison of selected pulse frequencies from two different electrical stimulators on blood flow in healthy subjects. Phys Ther, **68**, 1526–1532.

Turk, D. (2002). Remember the distinction between malignant and benign pain? Well, forget it. Clin J Pain, **18**, 75–76.

Uy, J., Ridding, M., Hillier, S. et al. (2003). Does induction of plastic change in motor cortex improve leg function after stroke? Neurology, **61**, 982–984.

Wall, P., Melzack, R. (1999). Textbook of Pain, 4th edn. Edinburgh: Churchill-Livingstone.

Walsh, D. M. (1997). TENS Clinical Applications and Related Theory. New York: Churchill Livingstone.

Wang, R., Tsai, M., Chan, R. (1998). Effects of surface spinal cord stimulation on spasticity and quantitative assessment of muscle tone in hemiplegic patients. Am J Phys Med, **77**, 282–287.

Watson, T. (1996). Electrical stimulation for wound healing. Phys Ther Rev, **1**, 89–103.

Wright, A. (2002). Neurophysiology of pain and pain modulation. In J. Strong, A. Unruh, A. Wright and G. D. Baxter (eds), Pain: A Textbook for Therapists, pp. 43–64. Edinburgh: Harcourt Publishers Limited.

Risk management

Risk management means identifying and managing relevant risks. Identification is critically important as it is only possible to minimize risk by implementing particular safety practices if the risk is known. Knowing the actual or likely risks and comparing these to the possible benefits and the probability of a desired outcome is also an integral part of clinical practice. This is especially important when using electrophysical agents as all have the potential to produce harm as well as benefits. It is thus important that the clinician is:

- aware of the risks so that appropriate practices and protocols can be adopted
- aware of the means of minimizing the risks for any particular treatment modality
- able to make an informed judgement about using a particular modality by making a risk/benefit analysis.

This chapter is divided into three sections and is intended to provide a basis for identifying and managing the risks associated with using different types of electrophysical agents (EPAs). The first section provides an overview of the categories of risks in using different EPAs and discusses risk management. The second section discusses the risks of using mains-powered equipment in the medical context. Issues of electrical safety testing and routine checking and maintenance are also discussed as they are integral to safe practice and risk minimization. The third section discusses another type of risk, infection, and the ways of reducing cross-infection during treatment with EPAs.

This chapter is located in between those that deal with different types of EPAs. It follows those on electrical stimulation which introduce the need for care of equipment and safety in usage. It precedes the chapters on most of the other types of EPAs currently used clinically because of its relevance to all. The importance of risk management in modern clinical practice must not be underestimated.

RISKS WITH DIFFERENT EPAS

Before any treatment is applied it is necessary to screen for specific treatment risks. This involves four stages:

- assessing the patient's condition and current problems
- identifying appropriate treatment options
- estimating whether the known risk of a selected option is greater than its expected benefits

● evaluating, after treatment, whether the intervention was effective and that no harm ensued.

The first of these is beyond the scope of this book. Aspects of the second are dealt with in chapters on specific modalities which address the issue of when each might be clinically effective. Similarly the benefits of different methods of treatment are discussed in the relevant chapters along with the known contraindications and risks.

The third of these four stages requires establishing which treatment options are appropriate. Some options may be precluded because of impaired sensation which makes use of the intervention an unacceptable risk. Table 7.1 lists the routine, pre-treatment checks which, if relevant, should be carried out prior to any intervention. The table lists the following four tests:

● thermal – a test of a patient's ability accurately to discriminate skin temperature (see chapter 10)
● cold – application of cold pack or an ice cube for a short time to confirm a normal reaction to cold and whether there are any adverse reactions, e.g. cold urticaria (see chapter 12)
● sharp/blunt – use of a pin with sharp and blunt ends to identify whether the large peripheral afferent nerve supply is intact before applying some types of electric currents (see chapter 6)
● erythemal test – the test used to identify level of skin responsiveness to UV as well as a treatment dosage (see chapter 17).

A problem with the third stage of screening is our relatively limited knowledge of the levels of risk associated with many uses of EPAs. A contraindication means a particular interaction has a high probability of a negative outcome in the context being considered, or that the outcomes are more likely to be adverse or negative than positive. As

Table 7.1 Routine pre-treatment checks

Modality	Sensation testing	Lead integrity and connections	Therapist test/ ascertain output
Deep heat (shortwave, microwave, ultrasound)	Thermal[1]	Visual check	Ultrasound – yes
Superficial heat (infrared, hot packs, wax, etc.)	Thermal[2]	Infrared – visual check	Yes
Ultrasound (no heat, very low heat)	n/a	Yes	Yes
Cold	Ice reaction test[1]	n/a	Yes
Electrical stimulation – direct	Sharp/blunt[3]	Yes – visual and machine output	Yes
Electrical stimulation – alternating or pulsed	Sharp/blunt[3]	Yes – visual and machine output	Yes
Phototherapy (ultraviolet)	UV – erythemal level	Yes	No
Phototherapy (laser)	No	As appropriate	n/a

[1] Contraindicated if not passed
[2] Extra precautions to limit level of heating required if test shows sensation limited
[3] Extra precautions to limit current density may be advisable if sensation is reduced.

empirical testing is generally neither feasible nor desirable, many contraindications are identified on the basis of adverse events or user experience or extrapolated from what is known of the relevant biophysical properties and likely effects. However, for medico-legal reasons it is likely that considerably fewer adverse events are reported than actually happen. Also, not all extrapolations from laboratory research or first principles are justified, as noted in the following margin text-box. This means all guidelines are necessarily incomplete, probably too conservative, and should be revised as more evidence comes to light.

The estimated level of risk associated with using each category of EPA is shown in Table 7.2. These are guidelines only and are graded from 0 to 3: 0 = no known risk; 1 = a low level of risk or an unlikely risk but the user may choose to apply relevant precautions; 2 = a possible risk and precautions should be used to reduce the risk; 3 = risk is high and use of the modality is contraindicated. The actual level of risk can also never be completely known given the contribution of different methods of using an EPA as well as a range of patient and environmental factors. This is especially important when a fetus is involved given the implications of an adverse consequence. This was discussed at length in chapter 6 when considering when the use of electrical stimulation might be contraindicated. Conversely, many claimed risks are repeated in the absence of either empirical evidence or theoretical justifications to substantiate them. In summary, the actual level of risk for some modalities is lower than generally accepted. However, sometimes other reasons, such as the serious nature of a possible adverse event, mitigate against a simple assessment of risk as offered in Table 7.2.

For example, the risk of damage from a treatment with ultrasound over an ephiphysis in a conscious child with normal sensory awareness is highly improbable and is probably based on studies conducted on animals in non-clinical conditions (see discussion in chapter 9).

USING MAINS-POWERED EPA EQUIPMENT

Any piece of equipment plugged into the electricity mains supply poses the risk of electric shock. If an equipment fault occurs, there is a risk that the mains voltage (240V or 120V AC) could be applied to anyone making contact with it. This problem is not confined to electromedical equipment, it also applies to normal household appliances such as televisions, computers, microwave ovens, etc. For this reason, commercial products must meet internationally agreed safety standards which ensure that the risk of electric shock is minimized.

The risk is amplified in a clinical context if electromedical equipment makes deliberate electrical connection to the patient. So if, for example, electrodes are deliberately secured to the skin or an ultrasound head is applied to the skin surface, normal reflex responses which might offer protection against a shock current can be circumvented. The good electrical contact (low resistance) would also allow a high level of current to flow. When deliberate contact is made and there is the possibility of current flow, the apparatus is defined as having a 'patient circuit'. The international standards for

If an electrical stimulus is of sufficiently high intensity to produce a powerful muscle contraction and activate a sufficiently large number of pain (A-δ and C) fibres, it is described as a shock current or electric shock.

Table 7.2 Estimated level of risk (on a scale of 0 to 3) with each modality under certain conditions

	Pregnancy[1]	Indwelling stimulator, pump, electronic device	Local sensory loss	Local circulatory insufficiency	Dissemination e.g. tumour, infection[2]	Exacerbation of existing local pathologies[3]	Other – see relevant chapter for details
Deep heat (shortwave)	3 if in vicinity of uterus	3 if within 3 m of device	3	3	3	3	3 metal implants, over anaesthetic areas
Deep heat (microwave)	3 if in vicinity of uterus	3 if a direct application	3	3	3	3	3 microwave to eyes
Deep heat (ultrasound)	3 if in vicinity of uterus	3 if in vicinity of device	2	3	3	3	2 over lungs, gut, testes, anaesthetic areas
Superficial heat (infrared, hot packs, wax, etc.)	0	0	2	3	2	3	1 (see chapter 11)
Ultrasound (no or very low heat)	2 if in vicinity of uterus	3 if in vicinity of device	1	2	3	2	1 (see chapter 9)
Cold	0	0	2	3	0	3	1 (see chapter 12)
Electric current (direct current)	3 if uterus in current path	3	2	3	1	2	2 if skin older and friable
Electrical stimulation (alternating or pulsed current)	3 if uterus in current path	3	1	1	1	2	2 if skin older and friable
Phototherapy (laser)	3 if in vicinity of uterus	0	0	0	2 over tumours	3 if post-radiotherapy	3 eye damage – goggles required
Phototherapy (ultraviolet)	0	0	0	0	0	2 some acute skin conditions, photoallergy	3 post radiotherapy, recent skin grafts

Table is modified from Table 1 in Robertson et al. (2001). Guidelines for the clinical use of electrophysical agents. Melbourne: Australian Physiotherapy Association.

Grade of estimated level of risk are: 3 accepted or justifiable contraindication; 2 possible risk, precautions important; 1 low level or unlikely risk, precautions may be advisable; 0 no known risk.

[1] Actual level of risk possibly lower than indicated but accepted because of implications of an adverse event to a fetus

[2] Includes acute infections and tumours benign and non-benign. The actual risk is dependent upon the problem and its precise location (see chapter on specific modality)

[3] Includes dermatological problems as well as local inflammation, local radiotherapy within past 6 months, haemorrhagic conditions.

electromedical equipment having a patient circuit are more stringent than for domestic or other equipment. The standards ensure that the risk of an electric shock is negligible provided that the equipment is properly maintained.

Electrical safety can also be enhanced if the mains supply to the clinical treatment area is shock protected. A simple and relatively inexpensive protective device, an Earth Leakage Core Balanced (ELCB) relay can be installed in the fuse-box. If an equipment fault occurs which could, or actually does, result in a shock current, the mains supply is disconnected. The response time of ELCB relays is normally 5 ms or less.

There is a sound argument for installing ELCB protection in the home, particularly if there are small, inquisitive children living there.

The stringent safety standards applying to electromedical equipment, agreed upon by members of the International Electrotechnical Commission (IEC) ensure that equipment, when purchased, is electrically safe for clinical use. The main or parent standard for electromedical equipment is IEC 601. Conformity to IEC 601 does not, however, ensure that the equipment will continue to be safe. The clinician must perform routine checks, such as inspecting leads and connectors and testing the output of the apparatus (where appropriate) on an ongoing basis. Electromedical equipment should also be subjected to regular testing (at least once a year) by an agency qualified to test and certify that the equipment meets the international standards. In other words, the clinic must have a documented risk management programme which includes the safety of all of its electrically-powered equipment, especially electromedical equipment.

The CE mark is the European symbol of safety and compliance with agreed international standards. All electromedical products which are intended for sale in any EU country must be CE marked.

Summary

Risk minimization as far as electrical safety is concerned involves four aspects:

- only using equipment which is certified as complying with the international electromedical safety standards
- having the equipment tested and certified on a regular basis (at least once a year)
- using mains-powered electromedical equipment in an area which has ELCB protection
- performing routine checks and maintenance.

The first two points in the above summary require no further explanation. The third and fourth points require some further elaboration.

Electric shock due to mains-type current

If an electric current is passed through the whole body it tends to spread throughout the low-resistance subcutaneous tissues. It will be

Applying Ohm's Law the current through a 1000 Ω resistance due to 240 V would be 240 mA which is enough to cause ventricular fibrillation in the heart muscle and could well be fatal. With dry skin having a resistance of, say, 100 000 Ω the current would be 2.4 mA, causing tingling sensations.

recalled that the skin resistance is very much greater than that of the internal tissues. Normal skin resistance is many thousands of ohms (Ω), but wet skin can be as little as 1000 Ω. The internal tissues have resistances of only a few hundred Ω; for instance, the resistance between a hand and foot excluding the skin resistance is about 500 Ω (Ward, 2004). The current through the body – it is the current which is the critical factor – will depend directly on the voltage (240 V in the UK and Australia) and inversely on the resistance ($I = V/R$), where I = current, V = voltage and R = resistance. Thus very much larger currents will flow if the skin is wet, because wetting greatly lowers its resistance; this explains why serious domestic accidents involving electrocution often occur in the bathroom or laundry.

It must also be understood that the likelihood of electrocution depends on the path the current follows in the body. Thus if the current passes from, say, a hand touching the live wire through the body to earth via the feet standing on the ground, the current then passes through the heart, lungs and abdomen and may well cause cardiac fibrillation and/or the cessation of respiration and thus prove fatal. Touching both contacts of a lighting socket with one finger would be likely to cause a painful shock and severe burns to the fingertip but would be less likely to be fatal.

Immediate treatment of mains current shock

First, the circuit must be disconnected to stop the flow of current through the victim. This may be simply a matter of switching off and unplugging, but it is important to ensure that disconnection has been made before touching the victim otherwise the rescuer may form another path to earth and also receive a shock. Second, the carotid pulse and respiration should be checked. If absent the airway must be cleared, mouth-to-mouth resuscitation and external cardiac massage immediately started and assistance summoned. In all cases the victim should be medically examined as soon as possible – urgently if there has been any loss of consciousness. Musculoskeletal damage can also occur as a result of abrupt muscle contraction due to the electric shock as well as cutaneous burns, which are usually evident.

Safety features of mains-supplied electrical apparatus

For more information on electrical safety and shock protection see chapter 13 of the book 'Biophysical Bases of Electrotherapy' on the CD which comes with this book.

The safety of electrical apparatus connected to the mains is ensured in several ways. The metal casing of the apparatus is connected to the earth terminal of the three-pin plug and socket. Thus if the live wire were to touch the casing of the machine a large current would flow to earth causing the protective fuse to 'blow' and interrupting the circuit. A problem with this is that if an earth wire is not present, or if it is broken, and the casing becomes live, anyone touching the machine may provide a low-resistance pathway to earth and receive an electric shock. One way to avoid this risk is not to rely on intact earthing but to make the apparatus 'double insulated'. Small portable pieces of electrical equipment such as radios and hair-driers are often double-insulated and connected to the mains by only two terminals, live and neutral. In these the casing is made of some non-conducting plastic material and the electrical conducting parts are separately insulated. Any exposed metal, such as the cutters of electric razors, is again separately insulated. All mains equipment is protected in one of these ways.

ELCB protection

Electrical safety is enhanced if the mains supply incorporates a core balance relay. ELCB protection for a treatment area is not mandatory if all the equipment has the necessary electrical protection built-in, i.e. if the equipment complies with IEC 601 and related standards. However, not all equipment will be so designed. Normal domestic appliances such as a fridge, table-lamp or clock are not designed to meet the standards required of electromedical apparatus so if they are present the patient, electrically compromised by low resistance wiring, could be at risk of shock if he/she touches the appliance. This is the argument for ELCB protection of the treatment area as a whole. ELCB protection of the treatment area is thus considered to be 'best practice'.

When the treatment area has ELCB protection, it is classed under the IEC standards as a type BF treatment area. This is also called a 'body protected' treatment area meaning that the maximum current which can flow through the patient's body even under fault conditions is too low to pose a risk. In areas of hospitals where patient monitoring or treatment may involve a direct electrical connection to a vital organ, the safety requirements are more stringent than those of a class BF area. Such areas are designated type CF and are called 'cardiac protected' areas.

The patient circuit of electromedical equipment is also categorized according to its level of protection. Most clinical stimulators have class BF patient circuits. External cardiac pacemakers are required to have a type CF patient circuit.

Routine checks and maintenance

International safety standards can ensure that equipment delivered to the clinician is safe and reliable but they cannot guarantee ongoing safety. This is why it is necessary to schedule routine qualified testing and certification of the equipment's safety, at least annually. It is also why the clinician should perform simple routine checks of the apparatus before each usage. Some of the checks are machine-specific and are described later, in the relevant chapter. Others are more general and apply to any kind of mains-powered electromedical apparatus. The following list includes the more general checks and is taken from the guidelines proposed by Robertson et al. (2001) with permission.

- Inspect the supply cord and plug before plugging equipment into the power outlet. Check for any physical damage such as a cracked or split plug casing or damage to the outer sheath of the power cord. Look for loose screw connections, frayed wires, signs of over-heating and loose cord clamps. Ensure the earth wire is intact (green/yellow or all green). The use of transparent plugs (now mandatory in some countries) facilitates this.
- Fault tag any suspected faulty leads and equipment, disconnect from the power, and remove from use. Fault tags should be readily available and identifiable and have space for a description of the fault symptoms. Ensure faulty equipment is not reused until tested by appropriately qualified engineering staff.
- Double adaptors and extension cords should not be used. Both can lead to overloading of a lead or wall socket and extension cords are hazardous in a work environment, where the wires (particularly the earth wire) may be damaged by crushing. Power boards are acceptable but only if used with caution because of the risk of overloading either the board or wall socket. The important factor is the load placed on the wiring. If the total current is less than the maximum (usually 8 A), it does not matter how many power boards and electrical sockets are used.
- Inspect patient leads (or cables) and electrodes prior to use. Frequent flexing of leads can result in broken wires in the lead or at the machine or electrode connections and can disrupt the output. With ultrasound machines, inspect the cable to the applicator and the cable insulation. Check that the applicator appears waterproofed if a bath treatment is to be used. With shortwave diathermy equipment check accessories including leads, pads, space plates and coils. Damage can lead to arcing within an accessory or at the socket.
- Connecting patients to more than one item of electrical equipment at a time increases the electrical hazard as well as possibly creating additional risks because of interactive effects and is ill advised.
- Space needs to be left around machines for ventilation as most electrical equipment generates some heat during use. Should the equipment emit an unusual odour or be too hot to touch, switch off immediately, fault tag it, and do not reuse until checked and cleared.
- Loose switches, controls, dials or non-functioning indicator lights/meters require repairing before the equipment is safe to use.
- If, during use, any unexpected disturbance in the output or an uncontrolled surge/shock occurs, turn off equipment immediately. Fault tag it and have it checked before further use.
- If a wax bath is used its temperature should be checked regularly to prevent fire and the bath should have a metal lid. Have a fire extinguisher suitable for oil and electric fires present (e.g. CO_2) and a fire blanket.

Risk associated with an electrical stimulator output

Another risk is electric shock from an electrical stimulator delivering an excessively high output current. Electromedical safety standards can ensure that the risk of electrocution from the electricity mains supply is negligible but there is still a risk that the maximum stimulator output may be applied inadvertently and deliver an electric shock. Such a risk is unavoidable with a muscle stimulator which must be able to elicit a strong contraction of a muscle group such as quadriceps femoris. The same stimulus intensity, applied trans-thoracically, could induce ventricular fibrilllation and death. Thus if safety was to be completely assured, the stimulator output would need to be limited to the extent that it would be clinically ineffective. This stresses the importance of usage being restricted to appropriately qualified, skilled practitioners who are able to use potentially dangerous equipment in a safe manner. It also stresses the importance of testing the output (where appropriate), moving the wires (or sound head if ultrasound) or whatever to identify any possible intermittent faults and performing other routine safety checks before any electrical equipment is connected to the patient.

A separate risk is of the current generated by the therapeutic stimulator interfering with demand-type pacemakers. This is a possibility with any kind of electromedical equipment which has an effect at depth.

An important point to note is that ELCB protection and class BF patient circuits provide a high degree of protection against electric shock from the electricity mains supply but they cannot protect against an electric shock from the normal stimulus generated by the apparatus. There is no borderline separating a normal therapeutic current and a shock current, so it is not possible to avoid completely the risk of electric shock.

One method of protection which has been made possible by the introduction of microprocessor-controlled apparatus is fault detection. Microprocessor-controlled equipment can easily compare stimulus voltages and currents. So if a wire is broken or an electrode becomes partially detached the current will be low or zero even though the stimulus voltage is normal. The apparatus can be programmed to detect 'out of normal' currents and voltages and immediately cancel the output stimulus. This is an important feature but it is not a mandatory requirement of the IEC standards so only some electromedical apparatus includes such protection.

> As noted previously, although there are few reports of patient injury due to inadvertent application of high intensity stimulation, this may be due to under-reporting because of the medico-legal implications.

> Before purchasing or using an electrical stimulator, the clinician should establish whether the equipment includes fault detection.

A practical problem: aversion

If current is applied at high amplitude very abruptly, the sensation and pain caused are likely to frighten the patient. Sensory nerves are stimulated by lower intensities than the pain nerve endings, so that high currents are more painful. Some discomfort may well be an inevitable consequence of a treatment, but it should never provoke anxiety or

> The term 'shock' is often used confusingly; any sudden sensory stimulation may produce a startle reaction and be described as a 'shock' (psychological); this would include electric 'shock' which refers specifically to electrical injury.

fear. Subjects become accustomed or adapt to electrical stimulation so that high intensities are easily tolerated if the current is increased gradually over a few minutes. Also, the risks of clinically applied electrical stimulation with appropriately maintained equipment used by a suitably trained operator are very low. Despite this, there is quite widespread apprehension about contact of the body with electricity. This is doubtless partly a fear of the ill understood. However, it is also culturally engendered in many places to suggest fear. There are even allusions to it in literature; for example, in Shelley's *Epipyschidion*: 'Her touch was as electric poison.' These anxieties may, at first, cause the sensations due to electric currents to be perceived as painful. With familiarization, tolerance rises. When applying treatment such fears must be taken into account; the patient must be carefully reassured and treatment applied initially at low intensity which can be gradually increased.

It should be emphasized that the pain due to electrical stimulation is not associated with, or due to, any tissue damage (except as noted below), but is the result of sensory, including pain, nerve stimulation and is thus harmless. As these currents can cause a strong muscle contraction it is possible that an exceptionally vigorous artificially produced contraction might cause mechanical muscle or tendon damage. However, the evidence for such effects suggests that they are no more serious than those caused during voluntary exercise. Similarly, delayed onset muscle soreness can occur with both voluntary and electrically induced exercise (Hon et al., 1988).

INFECTION CONTROL WITH EPAS

This section provides a very brief overview of infection control that must be read in conjunction with the relevant national and local requirements and guidelines. The focus is on the transmission of disease agents including those that are bacterial, viral or fungal between patients by virtue of using electrophysical agents.

An underlying assumption is that each facility which uses electrophysical agents has appropriate guidelines for users and standard requirements such as hand washing and equipment cleaning between patients. Some general advice is offered in Table 7.3 but this is subject to local requirements for infection control, to the specific condition of the patient, and to the manufacturers' recommendations for equipment. If a patient is immunocompromised, for example, the level of care required will have to be higher. Similarly, if a patient has an antibiotic-resistant strain of bacteria, a higher level of precautions against the cross-transfer of infection may be required. Unless the patient's condition or explicit advice to the contrary exists, users are generally advised to adhere to manufacturers' guidelines for the care of equipment for infection control (Lambert et al., 2000).

The level of precaution required for infection control is best categorized by the level of risk as follows: non-critical, semi-critical or

Table 7.3 Reducing known risks of infection

Items	Usual level of risk	Method of cleaning	Comments
Ultrasound applicator	Non-critical, intact skin	Alcohol wipes or equivalent	Clean after each use
Water container for ultrasound or stimulation	Non-critical, intact skin	Alcohol wipes or equivalent	Clean after each use
Reusable electrodes – sponge – metal – suction cups – lint	Non-critical, intact skin	Soak or wash in appropriate disinfectant as advised by the manufacturer, rinse thoroughly, air dry	Clean after each use
Single use electrodes or probes or covers over probes or equipment – vaginal or rectal electrodes – intravaginal pressure gauges – electrodes used directly over a wound with disposable cover – laser covers	Semi-critical as skin not intact or mucosal membrane surface in contact	Single use, dispose of single use cover or electrode appropriately after use	Therapist must observe the following precautions: – wear disposable gloves – ensure no dispersal of bodily fluids – clean and disinfect all equipment used
Wax bath	Non-critical risk, no reported incidence of infection transmitted via wax baths	Dispose of used wax or reheat and cool and remove debris from underneath when solid	No known risk of cross-infection as bacteria cannot live in paraffin oil/wax
Reusable heat/cold packs – plastic cover	Non-critical risk, cover completely with a clean towel each use, can clean with an alcohol wipe or equivalent	Towels laundered after single use	
Reusable heat/cold packs – non plastic cover e.g. canvas	Non-critical risk, cover completely with a clean towel each use	Towels laundered after single use	
EMG or acupuncture needles	Critical risk, submucosal insertion	Skin cleaned with alcohol prior to insertion, sterile needle used and disposed of in appropriate container after single use	

Note
All these recommendations are guidelines only. Current national or local guidelines, as appropriate, should always be used for all cleaning of equipment and of skin prior to using equipment to ensure appropriate methods of infection control. Users are also advised to follow manufacturers' recommendations for cleaning specific items.

critical. Most uses of EPAs are classified as non-critical. This means any equipment used contacts only intact skin. For example, an ultrasound applicator, an electrode or a hot pack wrapped in a towel is usually applied over intact skin. The general guidelines are that in this instance all reusable equipment that contacts a patient's skin, such as probes, reusable sponges or lint electrodes should be cleaned in an appropriate solution before being rinsed thoroughly and air dried.

Thorough rinsing is important – allowing some disinfectant solutions to remain in or on an electrode, for example, may increase the risks of local burning or skin damage during a subsequent use.

The type of disinfecting solution varies from country to country but may include alcohol or chlorite-based solutions. Thorough washing of items prior to air drying after is essential. All reusable electrodes that cannot be appropriately cleaned (see manufacturers' guidelines) must only be reused on the same patient. In between uses they should be stored as recommended by the manufacturer.

If equipment is used on non-intact skin or over an intact but non-sterile mucosal surface the level of risk is semi-critical. Typical examples include applications of ultrasound, UV or laser to wounds or the application of electrical stimulation rectally or vaginally. The types of precautions include the use of gloves by the operator and covering the surface of probes, where possible, with disposable covers. Electrodes should be single use and disposable. If equipment does come into contact and cannot be protected by a cover then a higher level of cleaning is required than for non-critical uses.

When the skin will be penetrated and the instrument will either be in the bloodstream or a sterile body cavity the risk is critical. This means that the highest level of precautions against infection is required. The few treatments by electrophysical agents in this category generally employ needles: for diagnosis with electromyography or for treatment with acupuncture. Both are beyond the scope of this book. Suffice to say, the precautions required are more critical because of the higher level of risk.

Summary

The risk of infection to the patient must always be actively minimized by all users of electrophysical agents. The types of precautions required are usually classified according to the use of the equipment: if to intact skin, to broken skin or intact mucosal membrane or if to the subcutaneous level, into the bloodstream or a sterile body cavity. The relevant category dictates the level of precautions required. The user is obligated to be aware of current national guidelines and those of the facility in which they are using equipment with patients.

References

Hon, S., De Domenico, G., Strauss, G. (1988). The effect of different electromotor stimulation training intensities on strength improvement. Aust J Physiother, **34**, 151–64.

Lambert, I., Tebbs, S., Hill, D. et al. (2000). Interferential therapy machines as possible vehicles for cross-infection. J Hosp Infect, **44**, 59–64.

Robertson, V., Chipchase, L., Laakso, E. et al. (2001). Guidelines for the clinical use of electrophysical agents. Melbourne: Australian Physiotherapy Association.

Ward, A. (2004). Biophysical bases of electrotherapy. Mount Waverley: Excell Biomedical Publications (on the CD accompanying this text).

Biofeedback

Most systems in the body rely on negative feedback to maintain homeostasis. For example, blood pressure, body temperature, blood glucose levels and extracellular pH are regulated in this way. The key feature of negative feedback is that the system responds to a deviation in one direction by opposing and correcting the deviation. Thus if the temperature of the body rises the thermoregulatory system makes modifications designed to cool it, such as increasing skin blood flow and sweating, which promote heat loss.

The word 'feedback' was long ago defined as 'a method of controlling the system by re-inserting into it the results of its past performance' (Wiener, 1948). Feedback can be positive, where a change in one direction causes further change in the same direction, but positive feedback is generally the opposite to what is required for homeostasis. For this reason there are many negative feedback systems on the body and only a few positive feedback systems.

An example of a physiological positive feedback loop is seen with childbirth when uterine contractions generate pressure on the cervix which results in release of the hormone oxytocin. Oxytocin stimulates more powerful uterine contractions which, in turn, result in more oxytocin release and so on.

Figure 8.1 illustrates some features of thermoregulatory negative feedback – in this case the response to a decrease in room temperature. The drop in environmental temperature promotes a decrease in body temperature which is countered by activation of physiological responses which have an opposite effect. Note that in Figure 8.1 the plus and minus signs refer to the effect on body temperature, not positive and negative feedback. The important point is that in a negative feedback system the signs are the opposite. Conversely, a positive feedback system would have either two minuses or two pluses.

The focus in this chapter is biofeedback, which refers to the application of negative feedback to biological systems and specifically to the conscious control of some of those systems which are usually considered to be autonomically (automatically) regulated.

As an example, the temperature of the skin of the fingers is under sympathetic regulation, which is largely dependent on the local and

As might be surmised, all physiological positive feedback systems must have a failsafe cutout mechanism to interrupt the cycle at some stage.

Figure 8.1 An example of thermoregulatory negative feedback: the response to cold.

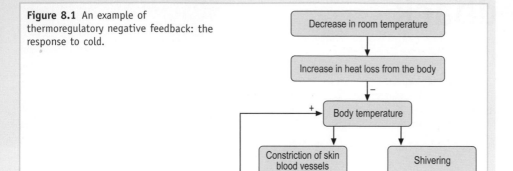

Figure 8.2 Skin temperature of the left and right middle fingers of a 58-year-old normal subject.

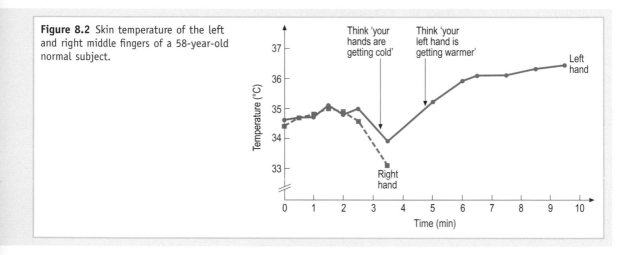

general environmental temperature, as described in chapter 10. If a sensitive skin thermometer is applied to the skin of the finger most people are able to make a small alteration of the skin temperature at will (Figure 8.2). This may take a little time and some practice but can be done providing the subject can see the thermometer reading and thus has immediate information of any change in skin temperature; this is the 'feedback'.

Many physiological changes of which people are normally unaware can be made visible or audible with suitable electronic instruments. This has enabled biofeedback control to be used for a whole range of activities, such as the control of blood pressure, heart rate, skin temperature, but principally for the contraction and relaxation of voluntary muscle using electromyographic signals. This effect can also be demonstrated in animals. Experiments have shown that the heart rate in rats and dogs can be controlled, in some cases, by operant conditioning.

The focus in this chapter is on the use of extrinsic biological signals to supplement feedback to the body concerned. In this instance equipment is used to provide an extrinsic feedback to supplement the normal intrinsic mechanisms of the body.

Extrinsic feedback is used deliberately in the clinical context to improve learning of a particular behaviour. Learning in this instance is like a 'black box'. The person may not be conscious of the actual process they use to recruit more motor units or to change the temperature of an area of their skin. Nor is that the aim. The aim is to have them 'learn' so that eventually they can make those same changes voluntarily, without having to use biofeedback equipment. The art of using biofeedback effectively lies in identifying which equipment might best be used to elicit which changes and using it to gradually shape the development of the new behaviour required. In this instance behaviour can mean relatively simple changes such as recruiting more motor units from a muscle or, considerably more complex changes such as improving a person's balance on a moving surface.

The chapter starts with a discussion of the different types of signals used clinically for biofeedback and how they are used. This is followed by a separate section that focuses on electromyography (EMG), probably the most commonly used form of biofeedback. Clinical examples that explore the range of uses and their effectiveness follow. Practical notes throughout will present information on how to use biofeedback clinically.

SIGNALS USED CLINICALLY FOR BIOFEEDBACK

The range of signals available for clinical use as extrinsic feedback to assist changes in behaviour is shown in Table 8.1.

As the table shows, these signals typically report electrical, pressure or temperature events or changes in position, angle or pressure. Some of these signals, such as the electrical output associated with muscle contractions, are very small and require a high level of amplification and signal processing. Others, such as changes in pressure in a bulb sphygmomanometer associated with grip strength, do not require additional or sophisticated equipment.

Some of the signals available for feedback are predominantly used clinically for diagnosis or for monitoring performance. All, however, can be used as feedback to facilitate change if provided in a suitable manner. Some signals, such as ECG, are rarely used, but others, such as EMG, are commonly used for biofeedback.

Table 8.1 Types and sources of signals used clinically for biofeedback and monitoring

Source	Signal type	Device	Uses include
Muscle	Electrical	Electromyogram (EMG)	Monitoring and to increase or decrease muscle activity
Brain	Electrical	Electroencephalogram (EEG)	Monitoring and to change the prevalence of some types of brain waves
Heart	Electrical	Electrocardiogram (ECG)	Monitoring and to change the heart rate
Blood pressure	Pressure	Sphygmomanometer	Monitoring and to change the reading
Local temperature	Temperature	Thermometer	Monitoring and to change local temperature, e.g. hand
Blood flow	Flow rate	Doppler flow meter	Monitoring and to change local blood flow volume, e.g. hands
Skin	Changes in conductivity	Galvanic skin response (GSR)	Monitoring and to change levels of anxiety and distress
Joint angle	Relative position of parts of a joint	Electrogoniometer	Measuring and to change range of movement used
Compression	Pressure dynamometer	Bulb sphygmomanometer,	Measuring or increasing grip strength, pelvic floor strength, muscle strength
Postural sway	Changes in pressure distribution (rate and magnitude)	Force platform connected to appropriate visual display	Monitoring and to improve balance

PRINCIPLES OF USING BIOFEEDBACK CLINICALLY

Providing feedback

If the aim is to increase active movement it might be appropriate to use EMG or an electrogoniometer. Which is chosen will depend on the specific outcome intended: EMG is more appropriate to affect the level of muscle activity and an electrogoniometer if increasing the actual range of movement is the objective.

There are two aspects to the provision of feedback. The first is that it should be appropriate for the change required. The second is that it should be easily recognized and used by the patient. Appropriate feedback can be a direct measure, e.g. changes in local blood flow measured using a Doppler flowmeter (see chapter 9), or an indirect measure, e.g. local skin temperature measured with a thermometer as an indicator of blood flow. The choice relates to the relevance of the options and the likelihood of the patient learning to control that measure. In the case of blood flow, an obvious starting point is with a thermometer; the cheaper, simpler and more portable method of providing feedback.

The feedback should be proportional to the response. Thus a strong muscle contraction should produce a strong signal. This suggests that visual signals such as a digital readout can be better than auditory feedback because it is easier to make direct comparisons within and between trials and a digital readout provides a more sensitive measure.

The equipment used to provide biofeedback must be sufficiently sensitive and specific. If not, the risk is changes in the signals may be too small or unreliable to assist the patient to learn what action on their part will change the output. An integral part of the success in using feedback is having the patient associate their actions or changes in their body with a change in the output signal. This is not always easy and may take considerable amounts of practice, as well as having appropriately sensitive and specific feedback. This also means that portable equipment that can be used at home, especially after the initial therapist-guided sessions, can be a considerable advantage.

The second aspect to consider when using biofeedback is how the feedback should be provided as it should be easily recognized and used by the patient. This means the method of feedback has to be appropriate to the patient and timely. The usual methods are visual or auditory. This means the person might need to see the output reading of a signal, as a number, a bar graph, or on a meter. If auditory, the signal might be adapted to increase in volume or pitch if there is an increased output and decrease if the signal drops. The equipment might provide details of the time or force produced during activity (Hartveld et al., 1996). Feedback can also be instrumental. Considerably more work is yet to be done on the development of a broader range of options to encourage appropriate actions or levels of relaxation in different people.

The other consideration when providing feedback is time. The contiguity of the signal and the patient receiving it as feedback are very important. If there is a delay of 5 minutes, for example, the patient may not associate the changes on the display with those they perceive in response to their effort. Unless the signal, like other biological signals, is almost instantaneous, there is a risk it will not be effective. Unless the patient can learn to connect or associate the initial actions with the feedback, change is unlikely. That is, delayed feedback is unlikely to be effective when trying to facilitate change.

Changes in the feedback signal may make a computer game available to the patient or make a DVD player or a train set work. In one example, the cursor was controlled by the EMG output associated with ankle movement in a patient following a stroke (Coleman and Harry, 2002). The extent (direction and magnitude) of change required in these instances can be preset by the therapist. This is particularly useful in gaining the interest and cooperation of children as well as many adults.

Summary

- Success with biofeedback is predicated on the development of an association between an externally provided signal and an outcome.
- The subject needs the following elements for success when using biofeedback:
  - feedback that is accessible to them
  - a willingness to practise
  - a desire to control the process.

User control

Biofeedback is controlled by the user. Once having learnt the ideas and how to use relevant equipment, the user does not usually need a therapist to provide ongoing feedback related to each performance of the selected task or activity. Instead, appropriately chosen biofeedback

Practical point – imagery

This must be appropriate to the context and aims. Consider social, geographical and cultural factors as well as usual triggers for that response. To increase blood flow, think of lying on an Australian or a Spanish beach. Sometimes warming both hands first in hot water and then focusing on maintaining the temperature in the one being monitored will help.

equipment can reliably indicate when performance is improving, not changing or deteriorating. Most therapies provide feedback and encouragement to help a patient gauge their progress: if a strengthening programme, the weight lifted; if an endurance programme, the distance walked or run or number of stairs climbed. (These are forms of feedback but not biofeedback.) Biofeedback is, though, also used to provide encouragement. Hence the need to ensure the user has a sufficient number of successes during early uses.

Selection of the starting position

This must be appropriate to the activity and one in which the person can most easily achieve an approximation of the goal – this is the first stage in shaping the eventual behaviour that is required. If relaxation is to be attempted then, to reduce general muscle activity, the body must be fully supported lying or half-lying with the EMG readout visible or audible, as required. If altering sequencing of muscle activity, select a position so that the particular movement can occur unhindered and be visible to the patient and there is little need for fixator or synergistic activity in other muscles. For example, if the activity of lower trapezius is to be increased in relation to upper trapezius, the person should be sitting comfortably on a stool, possibly facing a mirror and able to hear (or see) the feedback. After skin preparation and electrode placement ensure they know what is required. One strategy is to exaggerate the unwanted movement to show what is to be avoided. This could be shoulder abduction with the point of the shoulder leading. As they gain control of the required actions, change the starting position to standing, for example. Use biofeedback without a mirror, relying on intrinsic body awareness. Have them mimic a tennis stroke while minimizing activity of upper trapezius. As they manage this, repeat it with a very small weight in their hand. The progressions required to shape the behaviour depend on the aims of treatment and the rate at which the patient attains them. Therapist planning is important in this process, in shaping change and monitoring a patient's expectations and ensuring they continue to be reasonable.

Shaping behaviour

With biofeedback, the therapist selects a method of feedback that she/he believes will reliably provide evidence regarding a particular performance. In the beginning the tasks may only be an approximation of the actual goal. As the patient is able consistently to attain the preset goals the therapist will reset the threshold of performance required for success. With an EMG biofeedback unit this is usually simple. The threshold that the user is to beat or not to exceed is usually easily set. If the aim is to minimize muscle activity the threshold is set so that the user will consistently be able to keep their level of muscle activity below it. Depending on the equipment used this is usually indicated by a sound. When their level of activity is below the preset threshold the sound stops, starting again when or if the level of muscle activity increases. Conversely, some equipment permits the user to have the sound start once they have achieved the goal so that its stopping indicates too high a level of tension has again developed.

The same system of threshold setting is used when encouraging more muscle activity: the therapist initially sets the threshold so that a sound occurs once the user has a predetermined level of muscle activity.

Over time a therapist will change what is required as changes in behaviour occur. That is shaping, discussed above. This requires the therapist to select appropriate equipment, set suitable goals within the user's capacity, and make adjustments in response to changing behaviour.

Practical point – treatment sessions

Use short treatment sessions, 10 minutes or so, until some control is evident. Once some control is achieved, longer sessions may be used. Encourage home practice at least daily if an appropriate method of biofeedback is available. Practise in a range of situations, making it more difficult as control increases. If the aim is to reduce muscle activity, practise in situations or postures which previously consistently increased it. With more control intrinsic feedback should eventually replace extrinsic and the need for the biofeedback equipment.

Summary

- Use an appropriate method of biofeedback.
- Avoid fatigue and boredom – limit the duration of sessions and alter the tasks while ensuring success.
- Choose a suitable environment including starting position.
- Select an appropriate system for feedback
  - sensitivity and specificity of options
  - temporal contiguity.
- Teach user control.
- Shaping behaviour
  - ensure initial success
  - set upper and lower thresholds
  - change goals in response to changes in behaviour
  - gradually approximate required behaviour as goals are reached (shaping).

Electromyography (EMG) for biofeedback

Electromyography is the measurement of the electrical signals associated with muscle activity. The response of the fibres comprising a motor unit when they contract in response to an action potential is an electrical disturbance called the motor unit action potential (MUAP). During a normal muscle contraction many hundreds of motor units fire asynchronously, producing electrical potentials which can be detected either by needle electrodes in the muscle tissue or by surface electrodes.

An explanation of how EMG equipment works follows later in the chapter. The focus at this point is how to use EMG biofeedback

Practical note – increasing voluntary activity of a muscle group

First, explain the rationale for using the EMG biofeedback treatment to increase voluntary activity and emphasize its harmless and painless nature. Stress that it may take some time, perhaps many sessions, to achieve control.

Have the patient in a comfortable sitting position in a room at a comfortable constant temperature and where interruptions will not occur. Clean the skin over the relevant muscle group and locate the electrodes as closely as possible parallel to the direction of the fibres. Tape over the electrodes and leads to prevent artefacts (noise) caused by their movement on the skin.

Ask the patient to attempt to contract the muscles concerned. Assist by using techniques such as limb positioning, bilateral actions, patient's use of imagery, therapist instruction to increase the likelihood of the required outcome occurring. Focus on limiting the muscle action to the selected muscles. Have the patient watch the readout of the EMG during each contraction.

As the detected signal increases, focus on achieving a particular level and holding it for, perhaps, 2 s and then resting. Gradually shape the action until the patient can maintain the contraction for an appropriate period while limiting any extraneous muscle actions in the limb or region. Set frequent rest periods and have the patient attempt multiple EMG sessions during a day if possible.

Remember, a decreased EMG signal can be due to central fatigue (chapter 3). An increased EMG signal can be due to improved performance but can also be due to a different positioning of electrodes in a subsequent session (picking up more or different motor units than in previous sessions) or by crosstalk (increased activity of the antagonists may be detected and amplified, the larger signal quite erroneously suggesting a greater output from the muscles of interest).

The process continues with a decreasing reliance on extrinsic biofeedback and the introduction of more functional activities to retrain the muscle activity.

equipment clinically as this is probably the most commonly used method of biofeedback and it can be technically complex.

The action potentials occurring under or near the recording electrodes are amplified. These signals are very small, typically of the order of 1 mV or so. The output is usually displayed as a digitized number, or on a bar graph or analogue display, or as an auditory output. If sampling continues for the duration of the contraction it may be displayed on a computer screen as a graphed output over time or it may be heard as an output changing in volume and pitch as the strength of the signal changes. Whichever method and duration of display is used, a considerable level of amplification is necessary to make the signal available.

The EMG output bears only an approximate relationship to the magnitude of the muscle contraction causing it. The relationship is quite complicated because the MUAPs that occur will not all be equally detected and recorded. When surface electrodes are used, as for biofeedback, localization of the EMG signal is not precise. This also means it is really only useful for training involving reasonably superficial muscles and it is essential that users have an adequate knowledge of muscle anatomy. Another reason, explained later, is the need to arrange electrodes parallel to the line of fibres to optimize the pickup; this is especially important when few MUAPs are produced.

The amplified signal is the sum of all MUAPs near and between the active electrodes at a point in time. This means that the signal may come from adjacent muscles, even antagonists if EMG is used on a smaller part of the body such as over the wrist extensor muscles. Depending on the type of equipment, the active electrodes that pick up the signals may be close together or further apart. The further they are apart, the more MUAPs will be picked up and amplified so a stronger signal is obtained. A disadvantage of the wider spacing is a greater pickup of interference (noise and mains frequency signals induced in tissue). If closer together the volume of muscle tissue from which signals may be picked up will be smaller and more accurately represent the muscle(s) under the electrodes. The signal is smaller but there is less pickup of interference. These points are considered further later in this chapter.

The asynchronicity of firing, when numerical outputs are used for feedback, can result in considerable variation in the output. With audible biofeedback, the overall effect of stronger contractions if an audible output is used is more and louder clicks, merging into a roar and so is little affected. With numerical output the situation is different. Manufacturers of EMG biofeedback equipment either build in a fixed rate of sampling or the user can choose a period over which the signal is averaged. Averaging over a slightly longer period produces a more even output and is usually easier for a patient to work with than if a short period is used. If a short averaging period is used the signal can be very difficult to relate to a particular muscle action and trends, such as an increased output, become harder to identify.

USES OF BIOFEEDBACK

Biofeedback is used for one of two broad purposes:

- to increase activity or the level of output or
- to decrease activity or the level of output.

The following section presents a range of current clinical uses. This is not an exhaustive list but one that is intended to be broad and to show that the range of uses is limited only by the imagination of a therapist, the equipment available, and a patient's willingness to try an alternative method of treatment.

The descriptions of some uses are brief and focus on one or a small number of studies. Where possible systematic reviews or meta-analyses are described as a starting point for those interested in the particular use. Also, the descriptions of some studies raise issues that at times relate more to study design and at others to issues implicit in using the equipment. Where relevant, these issues are also discussed.

Stroke

Many published accounts of the use of EMG biofeedback have been for the treatment of stroke patients. The results of the meta-analyses below suggest some of the possible roles for EMG biofeedback following stroke and its level of effectiveness. It also suggests how clinicians might use it to improve outcomes following stroke.

Following a stroke, the focus is usually on retraining the voluntary activation of the wrist extensors, shoulder abductors and ankle dorsiflexors. The aim in this instance is to increase the output or number of MUAPs in response to the biofeedback output readings. EMG biofeedback can also be used to decrease the output of selected muscles, such as those with increased tone, like the wrist flexors and the calf. In this instance the aim is to decrease the number of MUAPs. Treatment usually commences with the patient in a comfortable position with the limb at rest and well supported. As their control over the level of MUAPs produced by muscle spasm increases, the aim is to keep the reading low while, perhaps, moving the contralateral limb or, changing the position of their body. Again, planning this type of shaping is integral to the likely success of this intervention as is patient motivation and willingness to use this method of treatment.

A review of 11 randomized controlled trials (RCTs) that investigated the contribution of EMG biofeedback to improving lower limb function post stroke suggests that it does have a clear benefit in gait retraining (Teasell et al., 2003). Most of these RCTs used EMG biofeedback to strengthen dorsiflexor muscles; others used different forms of feedback to equalize weight distribution over both limbs during sit-to-stand or to prevent knee hyperextension during walking. An earlier meta-analysis has also identified some effects of using EMG biofeedback post stroke to improve factors affecting mobility (Moreland et al., 1998). The results suggest that biofeedback is effective at increasing the strength of ankle dorsiflexors by an average of about 2.5 kg. The clinical significance of this extent of change is unknown. The same meta-analysis also found that EMG biofeedback is effective in improving the quality of gait post stroke but noted the need for many more trials to provide some more certainty of its effectiveness.

EMG biofeedback is also used to treat upper limb problems following stroke. A meta-analysis of 14 trials compared three systems of treatment: EMG biofeedback, conventional physical therapy and neurodevelopmental treatment (Hiraoka, 2001). The results suggest that of these EMG biofeedback is the most effective. This contrasts with the results of an earlier meta-analysis of six studies which compared EMG biofeedback and conventional physical therapy (Moreland and Thomson, 1994). The result was no clear difference but the authors did note the possibility of a type II statistical error.

Some of the difficulties inherent in evaluating the role of biofeedback for stroke patients are evident in a randomized controlled trial of placebo EMG and EMG biofeedback to wrist extensors to improve hand function (Armagan et al., 2003). Patients in both groups improved with treatment. The difference in functional improvement between those having real and those having sham EMG was not statistically significant. At the same time, the EMG surface potentials and the active range of wrist extension improved more for those patients treated with EMG biofeedback than those treated with sham EMG biofeedback. The issues are the natural course of change following stroke and the need for large subject numbers to avoid a type II statistical error.

The extent of weight bearing on each leg can also be monitored and used as biofeedback. Any type of pressure sensitive shoe insert can be used with appropriate signal processing circuitry. In turn the therapist needs to set the level of compression (body weight) necessary to stop a sound or to make a sound as the preset level (goal) is attained. Alternatively, this can be used to limit the amount of weight bearing on a lower limb – if a certain level is exceeded a noise can be preset to warn the patient to change how they are weight bearing.

Studies of the use of biofeedback, as indicated above, suggest it can be useful in improving some sequelae of a stroke. The differences in the capacity and needs of patients mean it can be difficult being prescriptive about the role of any particular type of biofeedback following a stroke. Reports of some of the other methods of biofeedback that might be of use following stroke are covered in other examples below, such as for improving balance and controlling movement. Again the issues are the aims of treatment and the patient's capacity and wish to use biofeedback.

Using biofeedback for a patient following a stroke is not always effective. Besides the therapist needing to ensure an appropriate

A quite different type of purpose-specific biofeedback used with stroke patients feeds back knee joint position. To improve control over knee extension during the stance phase of gait the position of the knee can be monitored and feedback provided. If the knee moves into hyperextension the monitor produces an audible signal. In one study the pitch of the signal increased with greater angles of hyperextension (Morris et al., 1991). Use of this device significantly enhanced the effect of treatment.

method and type of feedback is used, there are clearly other issues such as patient preference. If the person does not wish to use biofeedback or is unable to, perhaps because of the stroke, then methods of treatment that rely less on the patient's active participation are more likely to be effective than biofeedback with its reliance on the patients acting as their own therapist.

Spinal cord injury

The role of EMG biofeedback following spinal cord injury is not well established. Many investigations are explorations of the outcomes of particular interventions following a cord lesion rather than attempts to improve a patient's functional outcomes. For example, one study found that using EMG biofeedback, after improvement had plateaued, increased the electrical activity in triceps in subjects with quadriplegia at the C6 or higher level (Brucker, 1996). The important implication of this type of finding is not the improvement per se but that it can occur when other gains are no longer being obtained. The study also enables the exploration of the types of processes, like operant conditioning, that must underlie successful uses of biofeedback. As discussed above, the actual process or mechanism of learning is not the focus here and can be considered as a black box. In clinical uses of biofeedback, success is ascertained pragmatically, without the therapist or patient knowing or needing to know the process by which it was obtained.

Although the therapist does not need to know the process by which an intervention achieves its results, speculation as to the mechanism is useful as it can guide the exploration of future untested interventions.

A comparison between treatments involving physical exercise and electrical muscle stimulation with and without EMG feedback in spinal cord injury (Klose et al., 1993) showed no significant advantage of biofeedback. Patients had defects involving C5–7 and could produce at least some voluntary contractions. However, the study commented on the marked differences between individuals. Some patients particularly benefited with biofeedback, suggesting that particular subsets of spinal cord injury patients who might respond need to be identified.

Spasticity

Attempts have been made to reduce and control spasticity from a range of causes including head injury, multiple sclerosis, stroke and cerebral palsy. For example, EMG biofeedback has been used to retrain dorsiflexor function to improve the gait of cerebral palsy children (Toner et al., 1998). Three one-hour therapist-conducted EMG biofeedback sessions for 6 weeks and a daily home programme increased active and passive ranges of dorsiflexion and, in some subjects, the rate of foot tapping and the strength of the muscles. The effect on gait was not evaluated and there was an incomplete retention of all gains. This type of use of EMG provides a guide though as to how biofeedback can be used to produce change in the presence of spasticity.

Recovering and improving muscle function

Biofeedback is used to improve the outcomes of a range of problems affecting voluntary muscle contraction. These include the following: after a nerve injury, after a nerve or tendon transplant and to increase strength.

Following peripheral nerve injuries and once motor unit activity has been detected with an EMG, voluntary repetition can be encouraged. In clinical practice it is usually the therapist, rather than biofeedback that encourages progression beyond this stage by commenting on the change and offering verbal encouragement. The advantage of biofeedback is that it can be used independently by a person after instruction and frequently each day and at home. The changes indicated by the equipment can provide sufficient feedback to encourage an increase in activity and number of practice sessions.

Using biofeedback for long-standing facial muscle paresis can be effective (Ross et al., 1991). This study compared a group of patients who were taught exercises with a mirror (visual feedback) with a group taught with EMG biofeedback. There was no statistically significant difference between these groups. This is perhaps not surprising as both are forms of biofeedback – the mirror is simply low-tech. The implication is that EMG biofeedback offers an alternative method of treatment that may or may not be preferable in a particular instance: predicting which is preferable and when is not yet possible.

In cases of nerve transplant, biofeedback can be used to help the patient learn the new muscle action. This issue is discussed in more detail later, when the roles of EMG biofeedback and electrical stimulation are discussed together. Similarly, after trauma to a muscle or its attachments or after a tendon or muscle transplant it may not be possible for the patient to perform a particular voluntary movement. If some minimal voluntary movement is possible, there is evidence, identified above, that a biofeedback-type intervention can be of benefit. Where no voluntary movement is possible, a combination of electrical stimulation (see chapter 5) and biofeedback may be beneficial.

Muscle-strengthening and endurance training devices in clinical facilities and gymnasia have electronic displays which indicate the strength or power developed. These can also be viewed as biofeedback devices as the subject can exercise at a predetermined rate, for example at 50% of maximum, thus learning to maintain a particular training schedule. They can also use their previous measure as a target to be exceeded. The difference, namely that the signal (force) is a less direct biological signal, is small.

In the mirrors versus biofeedback comparison both methods require at least some motor units to be innervated. If the facial muscles were totally denervated, neither biofeedback nor exercises using visual feedback would have been effective.

Chronic musculoskeletal injuries

EMG can be used to treat musculoskeletal injuries produced by cumulative or repetitive trauma in situations ranging from process work to playing musical instruments. The importance of a cumulative trauma injury is that it implies the person has an ongoing need to repeat the movement or movements that are producing pain or a pain-producing musculoskeletal pathology. That is, avoidance of those movements is not necessarily easy.

The possible role of biofeedback in preventing recurrences of shoulder and neck pain in some industries was investigated in one study. The aim was to decrease the level of activity in specific muscles, including trapezius, during work (Palmerud et al., 1995). The six subjects in this study had fine-wire intramuscular electrodes inserted into supraspinatus, infraspinatus, anterior and middle deltoid and upper trapezius. They learnt, by watching their EMG outputs on a visual display unit, selectively to decrease muscle activity in trapezius without changing arm posture or their hand load.

EMG, relaxation training, a combination of both, and no treatment were compared in one study as ways of reducing what was described as 'muscle hyperactivity' (Spence et al., 1995). The results showed all three active methods were better than no treatment but that the relaxation training was most effective.

> EMG offers another treatment option for clinicians to reduce the level of overactivity of muscle that can develop following a chronic cumulative trauma.

Pain

Intractable rectal pain has been treated effectively with EMG biofeedback in some patients in which the cause was a paradoxical increase in puborectalis muscle activity (Gilliland et al., 1997). In this instance, an intra-rectal EMG electrode can provide feedback enabling patients to learn the sensations associated with effectively relaxing the muscle. Other methods of promoting relaxation are also often used in conjunction with EMG biofeedback such as visualization and a range of relaxation techniques. A finding of Gilliland et al. (1997) was that biofeedback was effective in some instances and, perhaps not surprising, that those patients tended to complete the treatment plan. Those for whom it was not effective tended not to complete the treatment. As discussed earlier, the effectiveness of biofeedback varies with the patient's willingness to use it and, presumably, the evidence they obtain regarding how effective it is.

Chronic pain can produce reductions in joint movement and associated muscle tightness. EMG biofeedback has been used to promote relaxation to enable stretching when patients have chronic musculoskeletal pain (Neblett et al., 2003). For example, a patient can be taught with feedback to maintain relaxation of their lumbar paraspinal muscles during stretching that was previously not possible.

A different type of study investigated 30 patients with patellofemoral pain syndrome (Dursun et al., 2001). The experimental group was given conventional exercise therapy and EMG biofeedback and the control group, the exercise therapy only. The results indicate that those who had EMG biofeedback developed a greater increase in the level of electrical activity in vastus medialis. While this is not the same as quadriceps force and there was no difference between the groups in functional status this does suggest that biofeedback can be a more effective treatment in some instances than conventional exercise therapies alone at restoring muscle activity in the presence of pain sufficient to reduce function.

Posture control

For postural control, monitors are worn to signal tilt away from the vertical. A typical scenario is that an inclination monitor is worn on the trunk and a head-position trainer is worn as a helmet. As the trunk or head moves from the vertical a receiver worn on the belt vibrates or makes a noise. Other types can indicate a change in a movement and have been used with patients with low back pain to limit trunk flexion in sitting. This type of biofeedback provides a more functional approach than, for example, a form of bracing or a corset. Normal movement is possible and there is no reduction in muscle activity.

Balance and mobility

Forceplates can provide feedback to patients about their balance and aspects of their mobility. The type of feedback provided to the patient ranges from simple sounds if a preset level of perturbation occurs to complex visual screen displays. In each instance a single or dual force plate provides ongoing feedback. This may be during activity, such as reaching out to touch an object, or it may be during single or double leg stance and aimed at minimizing the extent of postural sway movements.

Whether force plate biofeedback is more effective at a certain time post stroke or for a certain type of stroke or for other conditions remains open to question.

The contribution of force plate biofeedback and the methods usually used by physiotherapists to retrain balance were compared in a randomized controlled trial (Geiger et al., 2001). The results show that both treatments were equally effective. This indicates that force plate biofeedback can be less cost effective, i.e. the capital costs are higher but it does not markedly improve the clinical outcome.

Trunk muscle re-education

Pressure biofeedback is used as a way of facilitating trunk muscle re-education. Most particularly, this method is used to provide feedback when exercising the deep abdominal and posterior spinal muscles to treat or prevent low back pain (Richardson and Jull, 1995; Hodges et al., 1996). The patient is required to maintain a level of pressure in the unit for the duration of a contraction. At its simplest, this type of unit comprises an inflatable air-filled bag with one or more chambers with a sphygmomanometer like pressure gauge attached. The unit is placed between the patient and a hard surface and the patient is required to keep the unit compressed by contracting the deep abdominal muscles – if in prone, by increasing posterior pelvic tilt by 'drawing in' the relevant abdominal muscles without breath holding. This method is relatively cheap and has been shown to be effective at increasing strength of the relevant muscles and decreasing low back pain symptoms and the number of future episodes.

A pressure biofeedback unit can also be used to distinguish between people who have asymptomatic, resolved symptomatic and currently symptomatic low back pain (Cairns et al., 2000). Those with current or previous symptoms of low back pain are less likely to be able to produce and maintain a change in pressure than those with more normal deep abdominal musculature. Clinically this is not an especially useful test. There is also some evidence that the intra-tester reliability of a pressure biofeedback unit, at least in subjects without a history of low back pain, is only 0.59 (Storheim et al., 2002). This does not detract from the value of pressure biofeedback units as a way of teaching deep muscle stabilization, especially as this may otherwise be very difficult.

Another way of developing postural muscle control is by using feedback from a diagnostic ultrasound unit (Hides et al., 1995). The unit is used to provide an image of the relevant muscle group, be it transversus abduminus, multifidus or the pelvic floor (see chapter 9). As the person contracts the muscle real-time ultrasound permits them to 'see' their deep muscles changing size. With practice it becomes possible to increase control without always needing to see the ultrasound image. This method is increasingly used by physiotherapists (Frost and Clarke, 2004).

Respiratory control

Biofeedback has been used to assist in the process of weaning some patients from respirators. By increasing their ability to relax, biofeedback can reduce the neural parameters that drive respiration (Holliday and Veremakis, 1999). This study used audible feedback to indicate to the patient when the level of EMG activity of their third intercostal muscles rose above the initial resting level while they were rebreathing some CO_2.

Incontinence

Biofeedback has been used for retraining with both faecal and urinary incontinence. With faecal incontinence a pressure biofeedback device

On a related topic, constipation, the same findings were made of the use of both pressure and EMG biofeedback: the success rates are generally over 60% but more, methodologically acceptable studies are required (Heymen et al., 2003).

or EMG biofeedback can be used. The pressure biofeedback method requires the use of a rectal balloon. The balloon is used either to teach patients to identify a sensation of rectal stimulation and contract their external anal sphincter or to retrain differentially to rectal volumes (Norton, 2001). EMG biofeedback uses an intra-anal sensor or surface electrodes to teach effective use of the anal sphincter (Patankar, 1997; Norton, 2001). Existing studies using biofeedback to treat faecal incontinence have success rates of over 60% (Heymen et al., 2001; Norton, 2001). This needs, however, to be read in a context in which both a critical review (Heymen et al., 2001) and a systematic review (Norton, 2001) raise similar issues with existing research on this topic: many existing studies have methodological and other problems.

EMG biofeedback is also used to treat urinary incontinence of different types. Typically intravaginal electrodes are used. The results are positive for many and the benefits persist for a clinically significant proportion of those treated using biofeedback (Glavind, 1998; Jundt et al., 2002). Again, an alternative is to use a balloon type method of measuring pressure, a strategy especially designed for improving pelvic floor strength (Glavind, 1996). An analysis of which patients might benefit from which type of biofeedback or conservative treatment regimen considered many variables but was inconclusive (Truijen et al., 2001).

Another issue with the use of biofeedback is shown in many studies of its use for treating constipation and faecal and urinary incontinence. There is generally little difference in the outcomes in group studies between those who use whichever type of biofeedback and other types of home training (Heymen, 1999; Laycock et al., 2001; Norton et al., 2003). This suggests the need for more research to identify the condition and person specific characteristics that might guide clinicians in deciding which method of biofeedback, or which alternative type of treatment, is likely to be more successful in a specific context.

Stress-related conditions

This method of biofeedback, the galvanic skin response, is also the basis of a 'lie-detector'. Increased or decreased stress is reflected in the amount of sweating that occurs, which in turn determines the skin resistance.

One example of the use of biofeedback for relaxation is the use of a galvanic skin response sensor with computer input (Leahy et al., 1998). Depending on the patient's control, if relaxed they could play an outcome related game. If their level of relaxation decreased, their progress through a game was reversed until they again achieved a sufficient level of relaxation. The aim was to teach each patient a method of stress reduction sufficient to reduce their symptoms of irritable bowel syndrome. This approach has been used in other instances where the aim is to teach relaxation.

EMG biofeedback, especially using the cervical muscles or occipito-frontalis muscle has been used for the same purpose. Other conditions in which biofeedback might be used to promote a reduction in muscle tension include writer's cramp and blepharospasm (Marcer, 1986).

Hypertension

Blood pressure readings can be used as extrinsic feedback to reduce blood pressure. A randomized, double-blinded study was conducted with 30 men with mild unmedicated essential hypertension (systolic pressures in the range 140–200 mmHg and diastolic 90–115 mmHg) (Henderson et al., 1998). Laboratory instruction in the use of biofeedback was followed by home sessions using a purpose designed finger pressure cuff. The result was a clinically significant reduction in blood pressure after 4 weeks and an increased ability of the biofeedback trained group to lower systolic pressure on demand. Prior to the study approximately half of the subjects in each group could lower their blood pressure on demand. This raises questions of the role of biofeedback. It enabled more who had the training to reduce their blood pressure by clinically significant amounts than was otherwise possible. This suggests that for some people it is a particularly useful option and that others are less likely to benefit from its use.

Raynaud's disease

Biofeedback is used to treat idiopathic Raynaud's disease. As the primary symptom of Raynaud's disease is vasospastic attacks, the feedback used is thermal changes, an indirect measure of blood flow to an area. A summary of the alternate methods used to treat this disease concluded that thermal biofeedback can provide substantial relief for 80–90% of people with it (Sedlacek and Taub, 1996). They suggested that outcome takes 10 to 20 sessions over a 3–6 month period with subsequent follow-up. Some people, however, especially those with Raynaud's disease have difficulties in learning to control their skin temperature (Middaugh et al., 2001). Someone without the disease can usually learn temperature control (hand warming with thermal feedback) more easily than someone with Raynaud's disease. Factors affecting the likely success of a thermal biofeedback are the quality of the biofeedback training and the skills of the trainer as well as learning to apply the hand warming during an attack (Middaugh et al., 2001). Also, success in early sessions is important for a successful outcome.

Summary

- The general aim when using biofeedback is either to:
  - increase activity or output or to
  - decrease activity or output
- Biofeedback is used to improve aspects of the following conditions:
  - stroke
  - spinal cord injury
  - recovering and increasing muscle activity
  - chronic musculoskeletal injury
  - pain
  - posture control
  - balance and mobility
  - trunk muscle re-education
  - respiratory muscle control
  - stress-related conditions
  - hypertension
  - idiopathic Raynaud's disease.

MECHANISMS OF BIOFEEDBACK

Biofeedback is designed to work by initially making the patient aware of his or her own sensations when a dysfunction occurs, e.g. spasticity, or a change is to be made. The aim is that they can then consciously identify and actively prevent what is happening. Eventually the response should be automatic and not necessarily active or conscious on the part of the patient. That is, the response can be conditioned. In many patients, however, control is gradually lost when the immediate feedback is stopped. In order to maintain control the feedback must be withdrawn from some of the trials so that the patient gradually learns the response with progressively fewer feedback reinforcements; and then, methods to generalize the training to different contexts etc. must be introduced. The precise mechanisms by which biofeedback works are, as discussed earlier, treated as a black box in the context of this chapter. The focus here is using biofeedback clinically and readers are advised to search quite different literature for theories on how biofeedback works.

In all studies the successful outcomes occur in some, but not all, patients treated and the success that does occur is often modest. This happens in most therapeutic situations. As with many other methods of treatment, biofeedback is not a universally successful, powerful panacea for all problems. In fact, biofeedback is probably most effective when an integrated part of an appropriate treatment programme (Hanke, 1999).

As indicated throughout this chapter, clinicians are often not able to identify in advance the patients for whom biofeedback might be more effective than other treatment methods. Considerably more research is needed on this topic. Irrespective of the outcomes biofeedback is clearly effective in one domain: it sets out to teach patients control of their own body, be it a specific movement or the level of relaxation. In the long term this is probably in itself beneficial for many users, especially those with chronic problems that are difficult to treat.

BIOFEEDBACK EQUIPMENT

Figure 8.3 shows the feedback loop created when a subject uses biofeedback equipment. So far, the general principles, effects and uses have been discussed but the equipment has only been briefly described. Here some of the more important aspects of biofeedback equipment are discussed in more detail.

All biofeedback equipment has three essential components. The first is a transducer which might take the form of a pair of electrodes, a pressure transducer, a temperature transducer or whatever. The transducer detects a physiological variable such as blood flow, heart rate, EMG activity or skin temperature and produces a corresponding signal (often an electrical signal) which changes as the physiological variable changes. The second component is a signal processor. This may amplify, filter and/or average the signal and convert it to a useful form – one which can be displayed or communicated to the patient. The third component is the visual or audible display.

Some equipment is relatively simple. For example, the simplest form of temperature biofeedback requires only a glass thermometer which the patient can see. The liquid in the bulb of the thermometer (mercury or alcohol) acts as a transducer and expands in proportion to the temperature. This 'signal' is processed by a thin glass tube – the mercury or alcohol level in the tube is proportional to the expansion of the liquid. A visual display is created by labelling the tube so that the fluid height in the tube indicates the temperature. Digital thermometers use a thermistor as the transducer. When a voltage is applied to a thermistor, the amount of current flow depends on the

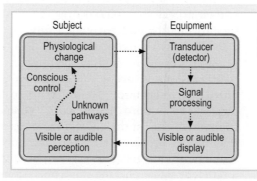

Figure 8.3 The feedback loop created when a subject or patient uses biofeedback apparatus.

temperature of the thermistor. The measured current flow is converted to a corresponding temperature value and shown on a digital display or simple analogue meter.

Other equipment is more complex in its nature and more demanding in terms of proper use. EMG equipment is the best example because of its widespread usage and complex features.

EMG equipment

There are differences between the quality of EMG equipment used for diagnostic purposes, research and biofeedback. EMG used for biofeedback equipment is usually considerably cheaper, less sensitive and with a different (more limited) range of options. Also, most biofeedback units use surface electrodes (surface EMG, SEMG). By contrast, EMG equipment designed for diagnosis and research uses a wider range of electrodes – from fine wire or needle electrodes to surface electrodes. A typical research use is kinesiology research to identify aspects of muscle timing and function (Cowan et al., 2000). Despite the differences, all EMG equipment has the features shown in Figure 8.3. The transducer may be surface mounted electrodes (biofeedback and some research use) or needle electrodes (electrodiagnosis or research). Both detect an electrical signal which is processed (amplified and filtered then averaged and smoothed). Finally the resulting signal is displayed and sometimes recorded.

Electrical noise

The EMG signal is very small, typically of the order of 1 mV or less, and a problem with its detection is that of electrical noise, i.e. unwanted (non-EMG) electrical signals. The most common form of electrical noise is from sources of electromagnetic radiation, such as radio and television transmitters, power lines, light bulbs and fluorescent lamps. Of these, the most problematic are those involving the electricity mains supply which uses alternating current at a frequency of 50 or 60 Hz (depending on the country). Mains frequency voltages induced in the human body in modern homes and workplaces are between 10 and 1000 times bigger than a typical EMG signal, so if two electrodes were placed over the muscle a clear mains frequency signal would be detected with a tiny superimposed EMG signal and a small radio/TV frequency signal. In short, the EMG signal would be swamped, i.e. masked by the noise.

Noise from the above sources can be eliminated (or at least minimized) by using three electrodes – two 'active' electrodes over the muscle and a third 'indifferent', 'ground' or 'reference' electrode somewhere else on the body: all connected to a differential amplifier (Figure 8.4). Because there is the same noise at each electrode, we have signal plus noise going into one input of the differential amplifier and a different signal plus the same noise going into the other input. The

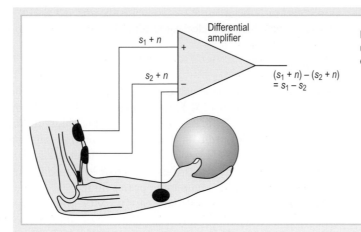

Figure 8.4 A differential amplifier is used to detect the EMG signal and eliminate unwanted noise.

differential amplifier subtracts the two and amplifies the difference so the noise is eliminated and the signal (s_1–s_2) only reflects the EMG – at least in theory.

The symbols '+' and '–' in Figure 8.4 do not represent polarity: they are not positive and negative inputs. Rather the symbolism indicates that whatever is applied to the '–' terminal will be subtracted from that applied at the '+' terminal. The amplifier is thus a difference or differential amplifier.

The differential amplifier might typically have a gain (amplification) of 50× so, for example, a 1 mV EMG signal becomes 50 mV and the noise is removed. The quality of a differential amplifier is principally determined by what is called its common mode rejection ratio (CMRR). If an identical signal is applied to the + and − inputs of the differential amplifier the output should be zero. In practice it is close to, but not exactly zero. The size of the output is used to calculate the CMRR. The smaller the output, the higher is the CMRR. Recent advances in electronics have made CMRR a less important issue. Most modern differential amplifiers have CMRRs which are so high that they are more than adequate for the job of EMG measurement.

The length of the wires between the electrodes and the differential amplifier is also important. It must be kept to a minimum as the wires act as aerials and pick-up electromagnetic signals which induce electrical noise. Although both wires would be expected to pick-up the same noise which would be eliminated by the differential amplifier, the longer the wires, the greater the likelihood of a difference in the signals. For this reason most clinical EMG apparatus has a small preamplifier (the differential amplifier), which is about the size of a postage stamp and separate from the main EMG unit so it can be mounted close to the measurement site on the body.

The output of the preamplifier is supplied to the main unit which further amplifies the signal by between 20× and 200× so the overall

Practical point

Electrical interference can pose a problem in clinical practice, especially with shortwave diathermy equipment (chapter 13) and, to a lesser extent, microwave apparatus (chapter 15). The problem is that although a differential amplifier subtracts the signals applied to each input, if the noise signal (n in Figure 8.4) is too large, the differential amplifier inputs will be saturated and the amplifier will subtract 'max' from 'max' to give an output of zero and no EMG signal will be detected. Shortwave diathermy administered in the clinic while EMG equipment is being used is likely to be a problem. It is possible that if the induced noise is too large, the EMG circuitry will be damaged and need replacement. Mobile phones operating near the equipment may also cause interference but not damage to the EMG circuitry.

amplification is between $50 \times 20 = 1000\times$ and $50 \times 200 = 10\,000\times$. The main unit also has electronic filters.

Filtering

EMG signals are in the range 0 to 500 Hz with most of the energy in the frequency range 50–150 Hz so frequencies above 500 Hz are deliberately filtered out. This removes any residual high frequency noise from, for example, radio, TV or microwave transmissions without compromising the EMG signal. The kind of filter used is called a 'low pass filter' because it allows the passage of low frequencies while filtering out those higher than some preset limit.

Most electrodiagnosis and research EMG apparatus also has a 50 Hz (or 60 Hz) 'notch' filter. An ideal notch filter removes signals of just one precise frequency from the total signal. Thus mains frequency noise can be selectively removed. In practice, notch filters are not ideal and signals with frequencies either side of the notch frequency are attenuated. Since the dominant energy of the EMG signal is in the 50–150 Hz range, it is not advisable to use a notch filter if fidelity of the EMG signal is required.

An additional source of electrical noise is movement – either movement at the electrode/skin interface or movement of the wires connecting the electrodes to the preamplifier. This introduces low frequency noise, mostly in the frequency range 0–20 Hz and called motion artefacts, into the signal. Motion artefacts can be minimized by secure mounting of the electrodes and the preamplifier, but some of this kind of noise is inevitable. For this reason, frequencies below 20 Hz are normally filtered out using a high pass filter, i.e. one which only allows the passage of signals with frequencies above the preset lower limit.

Another reason for filtering out frequencies below about 20 Hz is the inherent instability of the EMG signal at such low frequencies. This is because motor units fire in this frequency range and the firing rate is quasi-random.

Interpreting the EMG signal

The raw EMG signal (Figure 8.5c and d) is a pattern of overlapping spikes which appear almost as a blur in Figure 8.5, each spike being a motor unit action potential (MUAP). The chaotic pattern of the EMG signal is due to motor units being activated asynchronously and at different frequencies. Although an overall indication of muscle activity can be obtained by inspecting the raw EMG signal, a more useful quantitative assessment can be made from the integrated EMG signal (Figure 8.5a and b). The integrated EMG is obtained by rectifying the raw EMG signal (converting all the negative spikes to positive) then averaging the spike activity. The integrated EMG graph has three important features. First and fundamentally, it shows the time course of muscle activation. Second, it gives an indication of peak force production. Third, the area under the graph gives an indication of overall energy expenditure in a contraction. The integrated EMG is thus a less subjective measure of muscle activity.

In apparatus used for electrodiagnosis and research, the raw and integrated EMG signals are displayed and quantified. In EMG

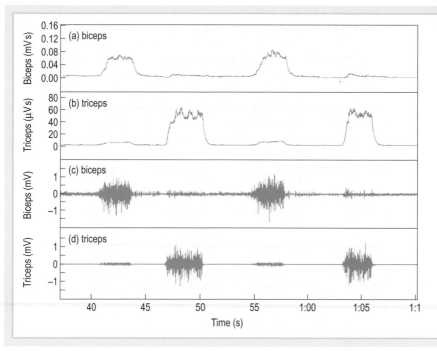

biofeedback apparatus the integrated EMG is also used, but more qualitatively. For biofeedback purposes, accurate quantification of the EMG signal is less important than showing its variation. Some biofeedback units do not use separate preamplifiers but rather rely more heavily on filtering to remove unwanted noise. This distorts the signal but the output is still a useful, though less quantitative, indication of muscle activity.

The integrated EMG signal may be used to drive a bar graph display so as to provide a qualitative visual indication of muscle activity at any instant or may be used to produce a sound with a pitch increasing with the amplitude of the EMG signal. Most biofeedback units allow the therapist to set a threshold, above or below which a sound is produced. Thus, for example, if the objective is to re-educate muscles which are not sufficiently active, the threshold can be set so that a sound is produced when a certain level of activity is produced. The patient has immediate feedback when this is achieved and is also informed if the level of activity falls below threshold. Some two-channel units allow comparison of the two signals with a sound produced when one signal exceeds (or exceeds some fraction of) the other by a therapist-preset amount. This is a useful feature when part of a muscle group must be retrained.

Signal variability is a major issue with surface EMG. This limits its usefulness in practical terms. Even with isometric contractions the signal can vary 20% or more in healthy subjects with nothing having apparently changed (Araujo et al., 2000). Extrinsic sources of variation such as placement, location and type of electrodes were controlled. This left intrinsic sources of variability such as the degree of skin and tissue hydration and changes in motor unit recruitment as possibilities. Other sources include muscle fatigue as it results in greater MUAPs to maintain the same force output and changes in ambient temperature, especially if the variations were sufficient to increase sweating. This extent of variability highlights the problems inherent in reporting changes between or within sessions as evidence of improvement or otherwise.

EMG electrodes

The size and spacing of EMG electrodes is important. If the electrodes are large and spaced far apart the signals captured are maximized. The downside is that there is also greater noise pickup and the risk that the electrical activity of nearby muscles will be recorded. This is described as 'crosstalk'. Note that in Figure 8.5, there appears to be simultaneous electrical activity of the antagonists with each contraction. This could be a real effect, with co-contraction to stabilize the joint, or could be just the detection of electrical activity by the electrodes overlying the opposite muscle, in which case it is crosstalk.

A simple test to distinguish co-contraction from crosstalk is to move the electrodes closer together. If the signals remain in the same proportion this indicates co-contraction. If there is crosstalk, it will be reduced by the closer electrode spacing.

Apparatus used for electrodiagnosis and research normally has separate electrodes and a choice of sizes. EMG biofeedback equipment often has the three electrodes mounted on a single sensor unit. Where a single sensor unit is used, the electrodes are relatively closely spaced. This is for two reasons:

- to allow measurement of the activity of small muscles and avoid crosstalk
- to reduce the problem of making good contact on curved or irregular surfaces.

Disposable sensor units, which have the three electrodes mounted on a flexible adhesive pad, have a practical advantage over rigid plastic units in terms of ensuring good electrode contact. Separate electrodes have the advantage that the therapist can choose the electrode spacing to suit the particular muscle, i.e. wider spacing for bulky muscles, closer for small muscles, particularly when other muscles are immediately adjacent. It is not possible to specify the volume of pickup with a particular electrode configuration, as there is no boundary to the region of detection, rather the signal becomes progressively smaller with distance. A rule-of-thumb which has been suggested is that with electrodes of area $0.5\,cm^2$ and spaced 2 cm apart the effective depth of pickup is about 2 cm (Morrish, 1999).

There are three possible arrangements for EMG electrodes applied transcutaneously:

- two separate active electrodes with a separate ground
- a bi-electrode with two active electrodes and a separate ground electrode

- a tri-electrode that has both active electrodes and the ground together.

For separate ground electrodes, read the manufacturer's guidelines, as the recommended placement varies from equidistant from both active electrodes to anywhere over a bony area being acceptable. Tri-electrodes and bi-electrodes are probably better in terms of amplifier properties but can be difficult to place in small areas, depending on their size.

As a guideline, use the idea that for a small area use small electrodes and small inter-electrode distance to increase the accuracy and reliability of measurement and to decrease crosstalk.

An important practical point is that the active electrodes should be aligned along the muscle belly (see Figure 8.4) so as to detect the potential difference produced as the wave of depolarization (the action potential) spreads along the muscle fibre membrane. If the electrodes are positioned transversely, i.e. across, rather than along, the muscle belly the signal detected will be weak and will only poorly reflect the muscle fibre activity.

Transcutaneous electrodes used for surface EMG (SEMG) are generally more reliable than intramuscular ones, such as fine wire. Unlike the wire, they do not tend to move or to produce local trauma (Soderberg and Knutson, 2000).

Skin preparation

It is best practice to wipe the skin with an alcohol swab prior to applying EMG electrodes. This removes dead cells and skin oils and reduces the electrical resistance of the skin. Traditionally, skin abrasion (using sandpaper or abrasive gel) and hair clipping were also used to reduce the resistance of the electrode/skin boundary. This is not necessary if a good quality, high impedance EMG preamplifier is used, so the practice is now largely obsolete.

EMG AND ELECTRICAL STIMULATION

New users can confuse biofeedback and electrical stimulation, although they are totally dissimilar. Biofeedback picks up body signals and produces information about them for the user. There is no current applied to the body. By contrast electrical stimulation does apply a current to body. The confusion in part arises because the roles of EMG biofeedback and electrical stimulation can overlap.

EMG biofeedback is used to facilitate the learning of voluntary changes in behaviour. Electrical stimulation can be used similarly. The difference is that electrical stimulation causes action potentials that, depending on the nerve, can produce a muscle contraction or physical sensation. If electrical stimulation is used, no initial voluntary contribution is required of the patient for the contraction to occur. By

Practical points – detecting the EMG signal

The quality of electrical contact with the skin surface is very important when using EMG. Poor contact means either a reduced signal or noisy artefacts. The amplifier amplifies the signal irrespective of whether it is from underlying muscle or the heart, or one produced by an electrode moving on the skin.

The active electrodes should always be aligned along the muscle belly.

The skin should always be cleaned with soapy water or an alcohol wipe.

Silver/silver chloride electrodes and purpose-made EMG or ECG gel (not ultrasound gel) provide the best option for surface (transcutaneous) electrodes. Fix the electrodes and leads firmly on the skin with tape to preclude movement over the skin, a major source of noise.

The depth of subcutaneous fat affects EMG readings when surface electrodes are used (Biedermann and Hemingway, 1996). An increased depth produces an underestimation of muscle activity. Normally this is not an issue, especially when using EMG as biofeedback. When, however, an EMG readout is used for other purposes, such as an evaluation of function secondary to chronic pain, this may be a problem.

contrast, some voluntary contribution is required for EMG biofeedback to be of use clinically.

The question of which to use, EMG biofeedback or electrical stimulation arises when working with a very weak muscle. This can occur when only a few motor units are innervated (following a Bell's palsy for example) and after other types of neurological injury when the person has a diminished capacity to elicit a contraction, perhaps because of the site of the lesion or because of alterations in the sensory feedback now available. For whatever reason a voluntary contraction is no longer possible or as easy as previously. Another situation when a therapist may need to choose between using EMG and electrical stimulation is when they wish to retrain a muscle that the person is not usually able to contract voluntarily, perhaps because the muscle and attached tendon have been transplanted and its new actions have to be learned.

One guideline is that if there is no voluntary action, use electrical stimulation and encourage the patient to work with it. As they can produce more MUAPs voluntarily, gradually decrease the intensity of stimulation used and then consider using EMG biofeedback to further encourage voluntary activation. Using EMG biofeedback too early can lead to excessive frustration if the patient is unable to achieve even minimal goals. Once they can reliably contract the affected muscles or produce the required activity, consider introducing EMG biofeedback. An example of this sequencing is evident in a case study of a patient who had not recovered in the expected manner after a lateral release of her patella. Electrical stimulation of her vastus medialis was used initially and biofeedback later, only once she had an increased level of activation of that muscle and mobility of her patella (Robertson and Ward, 2002).

The nexus between EMG and electrical stimulation is also evident in EMG triggered stimulators. This equipment is designed to encourage voluntary contraction prior to stimulation being applied. The therapist sets the threshold EMG level required for the stimulation to commence. Assuming improvement in the strength of the EMG signal as the patient improves, the threshold is gradually increased by the therapist so that more voluntary activity is required before stimulation starts. One study compared the outcomes of using EMG-triggered stimulation in stroke patients to those following a standard therapy approach. Both were used for 30-minute individual sessions daily and the EMG-triggered electrical stimulation resulted in greater functional gains (Fransisco, 1998).

A further commonality is that both EMG apparatus and electrical stimulators have a direct electrical connection to the patient through the electrodes. There is thus a heightened risk of electric shock, particularly if the equipment is mains powered. The issue of electrical safety with electromedical equipment is discussed in chapter 7.

CONCLUSION

With all biofeedback, perhaps the critical element is the use of reliable feedback. If reliable, sensitive and contiguous with an action, feedback is clearly an essential contributor to learning. Biofeedback equipment can more reliably provide feedback than can most clinicians who, unlike the equipment, cannot respond instantly, tire and have other commitments and obligations in the course of a day. Biofeedback is also user dependent: the user must want to use it, must understand what is required of them and must be able to work to goals they can set using the feedback equipment. Aspects of the potential of biofeedback have yet to be fully explored. As computer interfacing of equipment becomes easier and more transducers of different types are developed, the role of biofeedback is likely to increase. This is the future of biofeedback, one needing more technological development and considerably more research to identify which users are likely to be successful and under which conditions.

References

Araujo, R., Duarte, M., Amadio, A. (2000). On the inter- and intra-subject variability of the electromyographic signal in isometric contractions. Electromyog Clin Neurophysiol, **40**, 225–229.

Armagan, O., Tascioglu, F., Oner, C. (2003). Electromyographic biofeedback in the treatment of the hemiplegic hand: a placebo-controlled study. Am J Phys Med Rehabil, **82**, 856–861.

Biedermann, H., Hemingway, M. (1996). Electromyography and chronic pain: do current electromyographic diagnostic techniques discriminate against injured female workers? Perceptual Motor Skills, **83**, 28–30.

Brucker, B. (1996). Biofeedback effect on electromyography responses in patients with spinal cord injury. Arch Phys Med Rehabil, **77**, 133–137.

Cairns, M., Harrison, K., Wright, C. (2000). Pressure biofeedback: a useful tool in the quantification of abdominal muscular dysfunction? Physiotherapy, **86**, 127–138.

Coleman, K., Harry, J. (2002). Development and testing of a novel EMG feedback technology to induce movement. Neurol Report, **26**, 94–100.

Cowan, S., Bennell, K., Hodges, P. (2000). The test-retest reliability of the onset of concentric and eccentric vastus medialis obliquus and vastus lateralis electromyographic activity in a stair stepping task. Phys Ther Sport, **1**, 129–136.

Dursun, M., Dursun, E., Kilic, Z. (2001). Electromyographic biofeedback – controlled exercise versus conservative care for patellofemoral pain syndrome. Arch Phys Med Rehabil, **82**, 1692–1695.

Fransisco, G. (1998). Electromyogram-triggered neuromuscular stimulation for improving the arm function of stroke survivors: a randomized pilot study. Arch Phys Med Rehabil, **79**, 570–575.

Frost, N., Clarke, J. (2004). Ultrasound for biofeedback in physiotherapy. Soundeffects, 10–13.

Geiger, R., Allen, J., O'Keefe, J., Hicks, R. (2001). Balance and mobility following stroke: effects of physical therapy interventions with and without biofeedback/forceplate training. Phys Ther, **81**, 995–1005.

Gilliland, R., Heymen, J., Altomare, D. et al. (1997). Biofeedback for intractable rectal pain: outcome and predictors of success. Dis Colon Rectum, **40**, 190–196.

Glavind, K. (1996). Biofeedback and physiotherapy versus physiotherapy alone in the treatment of genuine stress urinary incontinence. Int Urogynecol J Pelvic Floor Dysfunction, **7**, 339–343.

Glavind, K. (1998). Efficacy of biofeedback in the treatment of urinary stress incontinence. Int Urogynecol J Pelvic Floor Dysfunction, **9**, 151–153.

Hanke, T. (1999). Therapeutic uses of biofeedback. In R. Nelson, K. Hayes, D. P. Currier (eds.), Clinical Electrotherapy, 3rd edn, pp. 489–522. Stamford: Appleton & Lange.

Hartveld, A., Hegarty, J., Blurton, A. (1996). Tools to give computer feedback to movement. Physiotherapy, **82**, 509–513.

Henderson, R., Hart, M., Lal, S, Hunyor, S. (1998). The effect of home training with direct blood pressure biofeedback of hypertensives: a placebo-controlled study. J Hypertension, **16**, 771–778.

Heymen, S. (1999). A prospectve, randomized trial comparing four biofeedback techniques for patients with constipation. Dis Colon Rectum, **42**, 1388–1393.

Heymen, S., Jones, K., Ringel, Y. et al. (2001). Biofeedback treatment of fecal incontinence: a critical review. Dis Colon Rectum, **44**, 728–736.

Heymen, S., Jones, K., Scarlett, Y., Whitehead, W. (2003). Biofeedback treatment of constipation: a critical review. Dis Colon Rectum, **46**, 1208–1217.

Hides, J., Richardson, C., Gull, G. (1995). Use of real-time ultrasound for feedback in rehabilitation. Aust J Physiother, **41**, 187–193.

Hiraoka, K. (2001). Rehabilitation effort to improve upper extremity function in post-stroke patients: a meta-analysis. J Phys Ther Sci, **13**, 5–9.

Hodges, P., Richardson, C., Jull, G. (1996). Evaluation of the relationship between laboratory and clinical tests of TA function. Physiother Res Internatl, **1**, 30–40.

Holliday, J., Veremakis, C. (1999). Reduction in ventilator response to CO_2 with relaxation feedback during CO_2 rebreathing in normal adults. Chest, **115**, 1285–1292.

Jundt, K., Peschers, U., Dimpfl, T. (2002). Long-term efficacy of pelvic floor re-education with EMG-controlled biofeedback. Eur J Obstet Gynecol Reprod Biol, **105**, 181–185.

Klose, K., Needham, B., Schmidt, D. et al. (1993). An assessment of the contribution of electromyographic feedback as an adjunct therapy in the physical training of spinal cord injured persons. Arch Phys Med Rehabil, **74**, 453–456.

Laycock, J., Brown, J., Cusack, C. et al. (2001). Pelvic floor reeducation for stress incontinence: comparing three methods. Br J Commun Nurs, **6**, 230–237.

Leahy, A., Clayman, C., Mason, I. et al. (1998). Computerised biofeedback games: a new method for teaching stress management and its use in irritable bowel syndrome. J R Coll Phys Lond, **32**, 552–556.

Marcer, D. (1986). Biofeedback and Related Therapies in Clinical Practice. London: Croom Helm.

Middaugh, S., Haythornthwaite, J., Thompson, B. et al. (2001). The Raynaud's Treatment Study: biofeedback protocols and acquisition of temperature biofeedback skills. Appl Psychophysiol Biofeedback, **26**, 251–278.

Moreland, J., Thomson, M. (1994). Efficacy of electromyographic biofeedback compared with conventional physical therapy for upper extremity function in patients following a stroke: a research overview and meta-analysis. Phys Ther, **74**, 534–543.

Moreland, J., Thomson, M., Fuoco, A. (1998). Electromyographic biofeedback to improve lower extremity function after stroke: a meta-analysis. Arch Phys Med Rehabil, **79**, 134–140.

Morris, M., Matyas, T., Bach, T. et al. (1991). The effect of electromyographic feedback on knee hyperextension following stroke. Paper presented at the WCPT 11th International Congress Proceedings, London.

Morrish, M. (1999). Surface electromyography: methods of analysis, reliability, and main applications. Crit Rev Phys Rehab Med, **11**, 171–205.

Neblett, R., Gatchel, R., Mayer, T. (2003). A clinical guide to surface-EMG-assisted stretching as an adjunct to chronic musculoskeletal pain rehabilitation. Appl Psychophysiol Biofeedback, **28**, 147–160.

Norton, C. (2001). Anal sphincter biofeedback and pelvic floor exercises for faecal incontinence in adults – a systematic review. Aliment Pharmacol Ther, **15**, 1147–1154.

Norton, C., Chelvanayagam, S., Wilson-Barnett, J. et al. (2003). Randomized controlled trial of biofeedback for fecal incontinence. Gastroenterology, **125**, 1320–1329.

Palmerud, G., Kadefors, R., Sporrong, H. et al. (1995). Voluntary redistribution of muscle activity in human shoulder muscles. Ergonomics, **38**, 806–815.

Patankar, S. (1997). Electromyographic assessment of biofeedback training for fecal incontinence and chronic constipation. Dis Colon Rectum, **40**, 907–911.

Richardson, C., Jull, G. (1995). Muscle control – pain control. What exercises would you prescribe? Manual Ther, **1**, 2–10.

Robertson, V., Ward, A. (2002). Vastus medialis electrical stimulation to improve lower extremity function following a lateral patellar retinacular release. J Orthop Sports Phys Ther, **32**, 437–445.

Ross, B., Nedzelski, J., McLean, J. (1991). Efficacy of feedback training in long-standing facial nerve paresis. Paper presented at the WCPT 11th International Congress Proceedings, London.

Sedlacek, K., Taub, E. (1996). Biofeedback treatment of Raynaud's disease. Prof Psychol: Res Practice, **27**, 548–553.

Soderberg, G., Knutson, L. (2000). A guide for use and interpretation of kinesiologic electromyographic data. Phys Ther, **80**, 485–498.

Spence, S., Sharpe, L., Newton-John, T., Champion, D. (1995). Effect of EMG biofeedback compared to applied relaxation training with chronic, upper extremity cumulative trauma disorders. Pain, **63**, 199–206.

Storheim, K., Bo, K., Pederstad, O., Jahnsen, R. (2002). Intra-tester reproducibility of pressure biofeedback in measurement of transversus abdominis function. Physiother Res Int, **7**, 239–249.

Teasell, R., Bhogal, S., Foley, N., Speechley, M. (2003). Gait retraining post stroke. Topics Stroke Rehabil, **10**, 34–65.

Toner, L., Cook, K., Elder, G. (1998). Improved ankle function in children with cerebral palsy after computer-assisted motor learning. Dev Med Child Neurol, **40**, 829–835.

Truijen, G., Wyndaele, J., Weyler, J. (2001). Conservative treatment of stress urinary incontinence in women: who will benefit? Int Urogynecol J, **12**, 386–390.

Wiener, N. (1948). Cybernetics or Control and Communication in the Animal and the Machine. New York: Wiley.

Ultrasound

Ultrasound is not strictly electrotherapy because it is mechanical vibration, albeit produced electrically. In the context of patient treatment it has sometimes been described as micro-massage because it is the mechanical vibration of tissue.

This chapter deals first with the nature and, briefly, the production of ultrasound. Attention is given to the important matter of the way in which a beam of sonic energy behaves in the tissues. The physiological and therapeutic effects of this therapy are considered and some uses, including phonophoresis are discussed. The principles of application are described and this is followed by a description of the dosage parameters and some discussion of the possible dangers and contraindications. The chapter concludes with a brief overview of diagnostic ultrasound and its use for evaluating the musculoskeletal system.

Ultrasound refers to mechanical vibrations which are essentially the same as sound waves but of a higher frequency. Such waves are beyond the range of human hearing and can therefore be called ultrasonic.

Vibration merges with sound at frequencies around 20 Hz; vibration below this frequency is often called infrasound or infrasonic radiation and is felt, rather than heard. Frequencies in the range 20 Hz to about 20 kHz are described as sound waves, because the human ear detects them. The upper limit of frequency for human hearing, and hence the range of frequencies defined as sound, varies considerably. It is higher in children (about 20 kHz) and lower in old age (typically 14 kHz). Most of the frequencies involved in speech and music lie in the range of 30 to 4000 Hz. Ultrasonic energy or ultrasound describes any vibration at a frequency above the sound range, but it is frequencies of a few megahertz that are typically used therapeutically: several different frequencies are employed in the range from 0.5 to 5 MHz (Table 9.1). The terms 'sonic' and 'sound' are often used interchangeably, a practice followed here, but strictly sound refers to audible frequencies.

While ultrasound may be described as 'micro-massage', the 'massage' is a mechanical push and pull at much higher frequencies than normal, human-delivered massage so there is a limited analogy.

Infants can typically hear sounds with frequencies approaching 20 kHz. The upper limit drops so that at about age 35, the average upper limit has dropped to less than 15 kHz.

Figure 9.1 A sonic wave travelling through matter. The diagram shows the position of the wave at three successive time instants.

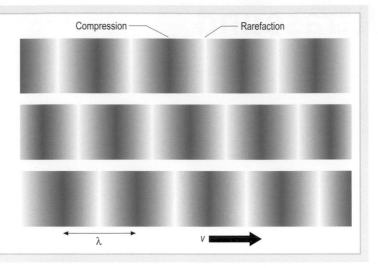

Compression —   Rarefaction

λ v

Table 9.1 Frequency and wavelength of ultrasound at $1500\,\mathrm{m.s^{-1}}$

Frequency (MHz)	Wavelength (mm)	Period (μs)
0.5	3.0	2
0.75	2.0	1.33
0.87	1.72	1.15
1.5	1.0	0.66
2.0	0.75	0.5
3.0	0.5	0.35
5.0	0.3	0.2

THE NATURE OF SONIC WAVES

Sonic waves are a series of mechanical compressions and rarefactions in the direction of travel of the wave, hence they are called longitudinal waves. They can occur in solids, liquids and gases and are due to regular compression and separation of molecules. This is illustrated in Figure 9.1 where deep blue indicates regions of compression and white, regions of rarefaction. Oscillatory compressions are applied at regular intervals and the resulting disturbance is propagated (travels) at a fixed speed, which depends on the nature of the medium.

Wavelength and wave velocity

Regions of compression are separated by a fixed distance, the wavelength (symbol λ). The compressive disturbance travels through the medium at a constant velocity, v, measured in metres per second ($\mathrm{m\,s^{-1}}$). Figure 9.1 shows the position of the wave at three successive time instants.

The passage of these waves of compression through matter is normally invisible because the amount of compression is small. When they can be seen, the impression is often a blur because the vibrations are often faster than the eye can register. When a stringed instrument is plucked, the movement of the object producing the sound (the string) is seen as a blur. The sound waves produced, travelling through air, are not seen in this case as the air is transparent.

An important thing to note is that sound is matter vibrating and molecules vibrate about their average position as a result of a sonic wave but do not, on average, go anywhere (just as a string vibrates about its mean position when plucked). Energy is transmitted by molecules pushing on their neighbours in an oscillatory manner and it is the disturbance which is propagated and which transmits the energy.

If a flag could be attached to a molecule in the medium, the flag would be seen to oscillate back and forth as a result of the sonic wave, but the oscillations would centre on a fixed point.

The wave equation

For any wave, there is a fixed relationship between the wave velocity, its frequency and its wavelength. The wave equation:

$$v = f.\lambda$$

relates frequency, f, wavelength, λ and wave velocity, v.

In water and soft tissues such as muscle and fatty tissue, sonic waves travel at a velocity close to 1500 metres per second ($m\,s^{-1}$), regardless of their frequency. This means that the wave frequency and wavelength are inversely related as the product, $f.\lambda$ is the velocity, which is constant.

Table 9.1 lists some examples of frequencies and wavelengths of ultrasound travelling at $1500\,m\,s^{-1}$. The inverse relationship is readily apparent.

Sound waves pass more rapidly through material in which the molecules are close together, so their velocity is higher in solids and liquids than in gases. Sound waves in air, for example, have a velocity of $340\,m\,s^{-1}$. In bone the velocity is approximately $2800\,m\,s^{-1}$ and in steel, $5850\,m\,s^{-1}$.

Wave absorption

As a sound wave passes through any material the energy is dissipated or attenuated. Sometimes the energy is absorbed rapidly; sometimes the sound wave passes with almost no loss.

The molecules of all matter are in constant random motion; the amount of molecular agitation is what is measured as heat – the greater the molecular movement, the greater the heat or thermal motion (see chapter 10).

As the molecules jostle and collide with one another energy will be transferred from one to another, so that some will oscillate at higher frequencies and with greater amplitude because they have gained

Thermal motion is partly oscillatory, for instance the whole molecule may move or rotate to and fro, or it may change shape in an oscillatory way and this may occur at many different frequencies. The motion also includes linear movement with the paths of the molecules following a zig-zag as a result of sudden collisions which result in a change of direction.

energy, while others will be at lower frequencies and amplitudes because their energy has been transferred by collision. Linear movement is affected in the same way. A molecule may collide, losing or gaining energy, which is transferred to or gained from another molecule which then moves faster or slower. This continual interchange of molecular energy is a fundamental feature of the heat energy of an object.

When sonic vibration is applied to a material it is superimposed on the existing motions and will add to them. A consequence is that the regular sonic wave energy tends to become randomized as the energy it gives to particular molecular motions becomes spread out in collisions with other molecules. In this way the sonic energy is steadily converted to heat energy.

The rate at which this exchange occurs will depend on both the nature of the material, i.e. the way the molecules oscillate and move about, and the frequency of the sonic wave. Thus the ratio of transmission to absorption of sonic waves differs in different materials and varies with the frequency of the sonic energy.

PRODUCTION OF THERAPEUTIC ULTRASOUND

Sound and ultrasound waves are produced by mechanically vibrating a material medium, either solid, liquid or gas. To produce the high-frequency ultrasound waves used therapeutically (and diagnostically), mechanical oscillation frequencies in the range from about 1 to 3 MHz are needed.

Piezoelectrical crystals are crystalline solids which have as a special property that they change in thickness in response to an applied voltage. If an alternating voltage is applied to a piezoelectric crystal, its thickness will change in an oscillatory manner. In other words, the crystal will vibrate at the frequency of the alternating voltage. The natural or best oscillating frequency is determined by the exact thickness of the crystal. Crystals are therefore cut in thickness so as to naturally vibrate at a particular desired frequency.

Many types of crystal can be used to produce therapeutic ultrasound but the most favoured are quartz, which occurs naturally, and some synthetic ceramic materials such as barium titanate and lead zirconate titanate (PZT).

All therapeutic ultrasound generators have a hand-held probe with a treatment head, within which a piezoelectric crystal is mounted (Figure 9.2). Vibrations of the piezoelectric crystal are transmitted from the crystal to the metal housing and thence to any solid or liquid to which it is applied. If the treatment head is not in contact with a solid or liquid, but simply in air, little energy is transmitted to the air and the confinement and concentration of ultrasound energy in the treatment head can destroy the crystal. For this reason, most modern ultrasound machines have a contact sensor which cuts-off power to the treatment head if it is not in contact with a dense medium.

When objects in the everyday world vibrate, the vibration frequency is normally sonic or subsonic so sound or infrasound is produced, but rarely ultrasound.

For more information on piezoelectric crystals and the piezoelectric effect see chapter 10 of the book 'Biophysical Bases of Electrotherapy' on the CD which comes with this book.

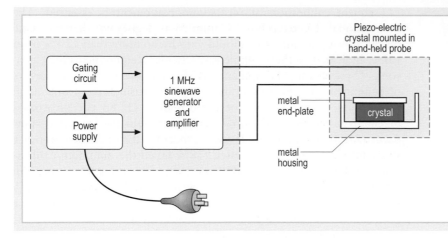

Figure 9.2 The components of a therapeutic ultrasound generator.

The other essential parts of a therapeutic ultrasound generator are a power supply circuit to provide electrical energy for the apparatus, an oscillator (sine wave generator) circuit to produce oscillating voltages to drive the transducer and a controlling (gating) circuit, which can turn the oscillator on and off to give a pulsed output.

Suitable circuitry can maintain a constant alternating voltage to cause the piezoelectric crystal to change shape at the same frequency and so drive the metal plate backwards and forwards also at the same high frequency, producing a train of sonic compression waves in any medium with which it is in contact.

An intensity control in the oscillator circuit controls the amplitude of the alternating voltage applied to the crystal which in turn controls the magnitude of the mechanical vibration of the crystal and hence the amplitude and energy of the sonic wave. Therapeutic ultrasound machines have a display which shows the ultrasound output intensity. The intensity is the energy crossing unit area in unit time perpendicular to the sonic beam. It is measured in watts per square centimetre ($W\,cm^{-2}$). Some machines also display the power output in watts.

Current supplied to the oscillator circuit can be automatically switched on and off to produce a pulsed output, typically giving ratios in the range 1:1 to 1:10. With 1:1 pulsing the average power is one half of the peak power. With 1:10 pulsing it is one eleventh.

The displayed output intensity is often an unreliable indicator of the true output intensity. This is because the number displayed is determined by the voltage applied to the crystal, not the actual output intensity. Machines are normally calibrated by the manufacturer so that when the display reads, say, 2.5 the output intensity is $2.5\,W\,cm^{-2}$, but the calibration can change with time. If the crystal is cracked or otherwise damaged, the calibration can change markedly. The crystal is glued to the metal housing of the treatment head and it is not unusual for the joint to be damaged so the crystal is only firmly adhered over part of its surface.

The power is the rate of production of energy, measured in watts (W). Energy is measured in joules and 1 watt is 1 joule per second ($J\,s^{-1}$).

It is very easy to measure and display the voltage applied to a piezoelectric crystal. To measure the actual output intensity requires external apparatus which can directly measure the intensity of the ultrasound beam.

Frequent calibration of ultrasound equipment is essential. The International Electrotechnic Commission legislated that acoustic output power and intensity should vary by no more than ±20% from values indicated on the equipment (Particular Requirements for Ultrasonic Physiotherapy Equipment, 2000). Despite this, most surveys of equipment in use by therapists indicate considerable problems in maintaining even this level of performance. Of 83 currently used machines tested in 2000, 39% were not within the legislated standards (Artho et al., 2002). Of more concern is the findings of another study in which of 45 units tested, 38% failed the minimum calibration standards but 16% failed to meet the electrical safety inspection (Daniel and Rupert, 2003). Although not new (Rivest et al., 1987; Pye, 1996) these ongoing defects highlight the need for standards for both calibration and electrical safety testing on at least an annual basis or as legislated. These findings also help explain some of the difficulties in establishing effective treatment dosages as the actual dosage may differ considerably from the indicated one on uncalibrated equipment (Robertson, 2003).

The ultrasound beam

The metal plate of the treatment head moves backwards and forwards to generate a stream of compression waves that forms the sonic beam. Because the wavelength of these waves is much smaller than the face of transducer (the treatment head), the sonic beam is roughly cylindrical and of the same diameter as the transducer (Williams, 1987). Even the smallest therapeutic transducers are 2 or 3 cm across and, as can be seen from Table 9.1, wavelengths are only a few millimetres.

This beam of ultrasound emitted from the transducer is by no means uniform even in a homogeneous medium. Waves emitted from the different places on the face of the transducer will travel to the same point in space in front of the transducer face by different paths and hence arrive out of phase. Some waves cancel out, others reinforce so that the net result is a very irregular pattern of sonic waves in the region close to the transducer face, called the near field or Fresnel zone (Figure 9.3). On average, there is more energy in the central part of the cross-section of the beam.

In the region beyond this, the far field or Fraunhofer zone, the sonic field spreads out somewhat and becomes much more regular because the differing path lengths from points on the transducer become insignificant at greater distances.

The length of the near field depends on:

- the size of the transducer face. Specifically it varies directly with the square of the transducer radius
- the wavelength. The length of the near field depends inversely on the wavelength.

For audible sound with wavelengths much larger than the source producing them – about 1.34 m for middle C – the sound waves spread out in all directions so that sound can be heard equally well at all places equidistant from the source.

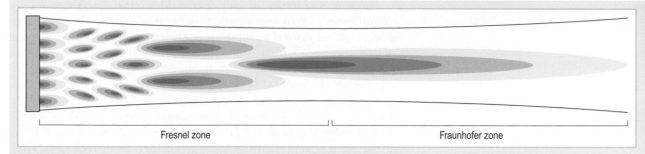

Figure 9.3 The variation in ultrasound intensity with distance from a therapeutic ultrasound transducer. Deeper shading indicates higher intensity.

Table 9.2 Length of near (Fresnel) zone in cm for different sized transducers at various frequencies

Transducer diameter (cm)	Frequency (MHz)			
	0.75	1	1.5	3
2	5 cm	6.7 cm	10 cm	20 cm
3	11 cm	15 cm	23 cm	45 cm
5	31 cm	41 cm	63 cm	125 cm

Thus: length of Fresnel zone $= \dfrac{r^2}{\lambda}$

For example, a 3 cm diameter transducer working at 1 MHz in water, or soft tissues, would have a near field stretching 15 cm from the treatment head. This is because for 1 MHz ultrasound in water, $\lambda = 1.5$ mm (Table 9.1). If the transducer radius, r, is 15 mm then $r^2 = 225$ mm^2 and

$$\frac{r^2}{\lambda} = \frac{225}{1.5} = 150\,\text{mm} = 15\,\text{cm}$$

Table 9.2 shows other examples.

The *beam non-uniformity ratio (BNR)* is the ratio between peak intensity and average intensity in the beam. The lower the BNR the more uniform the beam. This is an important measure because of the irregularity of the areas of intensity in the ultrasound beam as, for all practical purposes, therapeutic ultrasound utilizes the near field. The near-field irregularity is 'ironed out' to some extent by continuous movement of the treatment head during therapy.

The actual BNR of therapeutic equipment ranges up to 14, although the limit is now 8 (Pye, 1996). Ideally machines should have a BNR of 5 to 6 or lower. Even at those levels the peak spatial intensity will be between 15 and 18 W cm^{-2} when the nominal (average) intensity is set to 3 W cm^{-2} (peak intensity = BNR × average intensity).

The non-uniformity of the near field means that the intensity cannot be expressed in a simple way because it varies from place to place in the ultrasonic beam. Instead the *spatial peak intensity* or the *spatial average intensity* is specified. Further, if the output is pulsed the intensity over time varies so it can either be expressed as temporal average or temporal peak. Thus the intensity can be described in four ways: spatial average temporal average (SATA), spatial peak temporal average (SPTA), spatial peak temporal peak (SPTP) or spatial average temporal peak (SATP). It is usual for spatial average to be given, but it is important to ascertain whether the meter is displaying temporal average or temporal peak intensity.

Summary

A beam of therapeutic ultrasonic waves emitted from a transducer has these characteristics:

- roughly cylindrical
- very irregular in the near zone, more uniform in the far field
- near zone is defined by r^2/λ and is the region of therapy
- BNR expresses the spatial peak intensity in a field and should be 5 to 6 or less
- overall spatial intensity is described as spatial average intensity
- pulsing intensities can be described by the temporal peak and temporal average intensities.

TRANSMISSION OF SONIC WAVES

Boundaries between media

As has already been explained, a wave is a transfer of energy. Sonic waves involve vibratory motion of molecules and there is a characteristic velocity of wave progression for each particular medium. The velocity depends on the density and elasticity of the medium and together these specify what is known as the acoustic impedance of the medium.

The energy carried by a wave also depends on its frequency (the higher the frequency, the greater the energy) and its amplitude (the larger the amplitude, the greater the energy). Most of us have experienced this when standing in the sea; the higher and more frequent the waves, the harder it is to keep on our feet!

When sonic waves come to a boundary, various changes occur:

- They must travel in the new medium at a velocity characteristic of that medium and related to its acoustic impedance.
- The frequency remains the same so the wavelength must change. The new wavelength can be calculated using the wave equation, $v = f.\lambda$ which relates frequency, f, wavelength, λ and wave velocity, v.

The acoustic impedance describes the nature of the material, i.e. how easily the molecules move in relation to one another, so it is not surprising that the velocity of sonic waves in that medium is related to it.

- Some of the energy is reflected back. The amount of energy reflected is proportional to the difference in acoustic impedance between the two media. This applies to waves that strike boundaries at or near right angles.

- If the wave front strikes the boundary at some other angle the reflected wave will travel away from the boundary at the same angle; i.e. the angle of incidence of a beam equals the angle of reflection and is in the same plane (see Figure 14.4).

- *Refraction* also occurs with sonic waves due to the difference in acoustic impedance. The beam of sonic energy that passes into the second medium does not continue in the same straight line as the incident wave but changes direction at the boundary because of the different velocities in the two media. If the boundary between air and water is considered, a sonic wave travelling in air at $340\,\mathrm{m\,s^{-1}}$ striking the water surface at an angle of incidence of about $10°$ would be refracted in water through an angle of about $50°$ (see Figure 14.4). If the acoustic impedances are closely matched little refraction will occur.

- The turning back of a wave in the same medium has a further consequence. Two waves, the original and the reflected, are travelling in opposite directions so they will interfere. At some points they will reinforce, producing a greater amplitude and hence wave energy, and at other points they will cancel one another out. This produces a stationary wave pattern of maximum and minimum wave intensity, called a *standing wave*. Such waves are certainly generated in the tissues by therapeutic ultrasound but are unlikely to have significant consequences as reflection is only partial so the energy maxima and minima do not differ a lot.

In summary, the transmission of ultrasound through differing media, like the tissues, with many boundaries, or interfaces as they are often called, can alter both the direction and intensity of the beam by reflection and refraction.

Absorption of sonic waves in a parallel beam

As described already, ultrasound will increase the motion of molecules causing more molecular vibration and molecular collisions, resulting in heat. Thus kinetic energy is converted to heat energy as the wave passes through the material. The energy will decrease exponentially with distance from the source in a homogeneous material (Figure 9.4). In an exponential decrease, a fixed proportion of the energy is absorbed at each unit distance so that the remaining amount will become a smaller and smaller percentage of the initial energy (see Figures 9.4 and 14.7). This means that if half the energy is absorbed in a distance x, one half of one half (one quarter) will remain at a distance $2x$, one eighth at distance $3x$ and so on. Thus if a beam of ultrasound is passed through the tissues it will be steadily reduced in intensity in the manner shown in Figure 9.4.

Water and glass have rather different acoustic impedances and over 63% of the incident sonic energy is reflected at the interface. Water and soft tissue, on the other hand, have very similar impedance so that only 0.2% is reflected (Williams, 1987).

For more information on the topics refraction and standing waves see chapter 9 of the book 'Biophysical Bases of Electrotherapy' on the CD which comes with this book.

More information on penetration and exponential absorption is also to be found in chapter 9 of the book 'Biophysical Bases of Electrotherapy' on the CD which comes with this book.

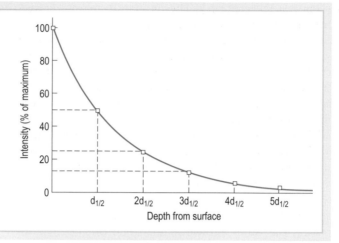

Figure 9.4 An exponential decrease in ultrasound energy with depth.

Table 9.3 Half-value depth in mm of 1 MHz and 3 MHz ultrasound in different tissues

Frequency (MHz)	Tissue		
	Fat	Muscle	Bone
1	50	12	1.5
3	17	4	0.5

Half-value depth

There is no depth at which all the energy has been absorbed. The energy just reduces by some fraction with equal distances in the medium. It gets smaller and smaller but never reaches zero. A 'depth for complete absorption' does not exist. For this reason a half-value depth is specified. The half-value depth is the distance at which half the initial energy has been absorbed. It can be used to describe the exponential curve of energy transmitted against distance penetrated (see also the description of penetration depth in chapter 14).

Since the conversion of sonic energy to heat is due to increased molecular motion, it follows that the amount converted will depend on the nature of those molecules and on the frequency/wavelength of the ultrasound. Thus the half-value depth is different in different tissues for any given ultrasound frequency (Table 9.3).

Note that the values shown are approximate only. Authors differ in their stated 'best estimate' values of half-value depth (Ward, 1986; ter Haar, 1996; Dowsett et al., 1998). Values measured for muscle, in particular, also depend on the origin of the test specimen and the alignment of muscle fibres in the ultrasound beam. Hoogland (1989) states that in the line of the muscle fibres (not the usual direction of clinical application), measured half-value depths are almost three times higher than when the beam is at right-angles to the fibre direction. The values shown in Table 9.3 are those quoted by Dowsett et al. (1998) which are similar to values given by ter Haar (1996).

The absorption of sonic energy is greatest in tissues with the largest amounts of structural protein and lowest water content (Frizzel and Dunn, 1982). This should not be interpreted as meaning that protein molecules, as such, are good absorbers. It is more likely that the structures which they form, which are comparable in size to the ultrasound wavelength, are responsible for ultrasound energy absorption. Thus ultrasound with a shorter wavelength is absorbed more easily and this is obvious when considering the different rates of absorption of 1 MHz and 3 MHz frequency ultrasound; 3 MHz ultrasound with the smaller wavelength is absorbed in a considerably shorter distance than 1 MHz frequency ultrasound with the larger wavelength.

For example, collagen molecules are poor absorbers of ultrasound but collagen fibres in connective tissue are good absorbers.

Absorption of energy in different tissues

For tissues in combination, e.g. the fat/muscle/bone combination in the limbs, the rate of absorption of ultrasound energy in a particular tissue depends on two factors: the half-value depth and the amount of reflection at the tissue boundaries.

- The half-value depth indicates the decrease in energy with depth in a tissue as the wave travels through it. It depends both on the rate of absorption of energy with distance and the amount of scattering as the wave travels through the tissue. Scattered waves will be absorbed at the same rate as those transmitted unhindered but because they are absorbed more superficially, the measured half-value depth is less.
- When wave energy is reflected at tissue boundaries, the reflected waves travel back through the tissue and are progressively absorbed. This adds to the rate of heating in the more superficially located tissues.

Figure 9.5a shows the relative rate of heating predicted for a fat/muscle/bone combination when 1 MHz ultrasound is applied. The tissue combination assumed has a 1 cm thick layer of fatty tissue, 6 cm of muscle and then bone. The variation shown takes into account reflection and absorption. The half-value depths listed in Table 9.3 are used for the calculations and it is assumed that 25% of the incident energy is reflected at the muscle/bone boundary (Ward, 2004).

The value of 1 MHz ultrasound for selective heating of muscle underlying fatty tissue is quite apparent and is relevant when there is a thick layer of soft tissue overlying the bone, such as when treating the quadriceps.

Figure 9.5b shows the corresponding rate of heating when the tissue thicknesses are different. A lower thickness of muscle (1 cm) is assumed. In this case, the risk of periosteal burning is highlighted. A maximal rate of heating is produced at the bone surface. This introduces the risk that periosteal burns could be produced at intensities which produce moderate heating of the overlying musculature.

Figure 9.5 Proportional heating produced by 1 and 3 MHz ultrasound travelling through a fat-muscle-bone tissue combination. Values are scaled to a maximum of 1.0 at any point in the tissue volume.

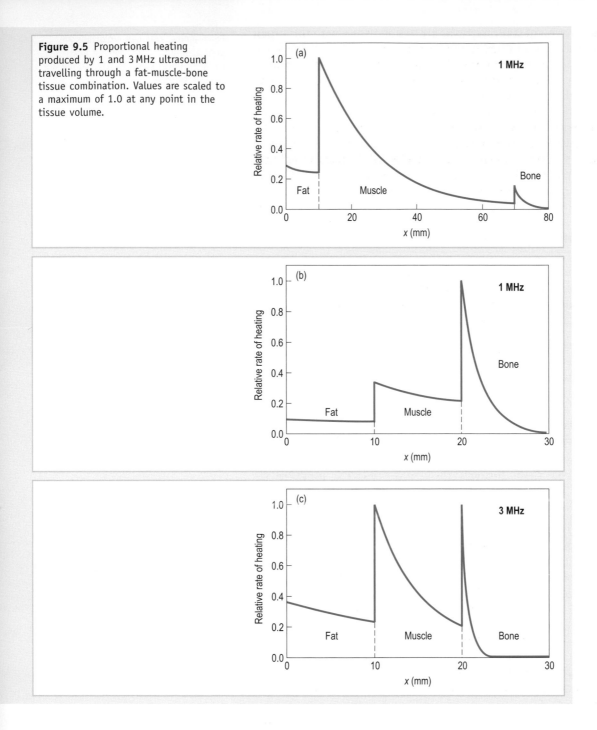

Alternatively, if the intensity is below that which produces periosteal burns, the heating of muscle would likely be inadequate.

The problem is the very rapid absorption of ultrasound energy in bone. In Figure 9.5a, where the bone has an overlying soft tissue thickness of 70 mm, rapid absorption of energy in the bone is of little consequence as hardly any energy (about 3%) reaches the bone so even though rapid absorption occurs, the relative rate of heating is small. In Figure 9.5b, about half of the incident energy reaches the bone and the high rate of absorption results in excessive heating of the bone surface.

Figure 9.5c shows the corresponding rate of heating at an ultrasound frequency of 3 MHz when the tissue dimensions are the same as in Figure 9.5b. At the higher frequency, the half-value depths in each tissue are smaller so less energy (about 10%) reaches the bone. In this example there is no excess periosteal heating.

The analysis above suggests that an ultrasound frequency of 1 MHz is preferable when treating large soft-tissue volumes where the bone is deeply located. If the overlying tissue thickness is small, i.e. the bone is more superficially located, one option is to use a frequency of 3 MHz and the other is a lower intensity of 1 MHz than if the bone had more overlying muscle.

While 1 MHz ultrasound is preferable for heating deeper tissues, the depth efficiency of heating is not as great as implied in Figure 9.5. The reason is that the graphs are simplified. They show the relative rate of absorption of ultrasound energy in homogeneous, flat layers of tissue exposed to a uniform ultrasound beam. This is far from the clinical reality. Curvature of the underlying tissues will increase the amount of reflection at each boundary and tissue inhomogeneity will result in scattering of the ultrasound beam. This leads to less energy being transmitted to deeper tissues, reducing the amount of wave energy available for conversion into heat energy at depth. The net result is less deep heating than implied by Figure 9.5.

Summary

At MHz frequencies:

- the ultrasound beam is pencil-shaped (has little divergence)
- the beam has a 'near field' where the energy distribution is very non-uniform and a 'far field' where the distribution is uniform. Clinical treatment uses the near field
- the rate of absorption depends on the tissue type and the ultrasound frequency
- the half-value depth of fatty tissue is high, muscle is lower and bone is lowest
- half-value depths are lower at 3 MHz than 1 MHz.
- the rate of heating at depth also depends on tissue curvature and homogeneity.

Temperature elevation in tissues due to ultrasound

Figure 9.5 shows the relative rate of wave energy absorption predicted for different thickness fat-muscle-bone combinations exposed to

1 MHz and 3 MHz ultrasound. The rate of temperature increase and the amount of temperature elevation produced in each tissue depends not just on the rate of energy absorption but also on the properties of the tissue. Three properties are most important:

Heat capacity is the amount of heat energy required to raise the temperature of 1 kg of the substance by 1 degree.

- the *heat capacity* of the tissue. Muscle has a higher heat capacity than fatty tissue and bone so its temperature increase, for the same amount of heat energy, is less. In general, the higher the water content, the higher the heat capacity.
- *heat transfer* within and from the tissue. Blood flow provides an efficient means of dissipating heat and so reducing the temperature increase. Highly vascularized tissue, such as muscle will be cooled more rapidly than more poorly vascularized tissue and will thus have less of a temperature increase than might otherwise have been expected. Less vascular tissue, such as dense connective tissue in the form of tendon or ligament, may thus experience a relatively greater temperature rise. Conduction of heat from 'hot spots' to adjacent, cooler regions will reduce the peaks and troughs of the heating rate patterns (see Figure 9.5) and result in less extreme temperature increases than the graphs might suggest.
- *tissue distribution and shape*. The actual depth of fat, skin thickness, muscle depth, fascial planes and the shape of each of these and the presence of bone (or air or fluid) will all affect the actual temperature increase in a specific area (Demmink et al., 2003).

Yet another factor determining tissue temperature increase is the tissue temperature before the ultrasound application. Applying a hot pack prior to 1 MHz ultrasound results in a greater tissue temperature increase at depth in a shorter time than if no pre-heating is done (Draper et al., 1998a). Similarly, moderate heating of the gel can improve tissue heating (Oshikoya et al., 2003). Conversely, applying a bag of crushed ice for 5 minutes prior to applying ultrasound limits the extent of heating at depth (Draper et al., 1995).

The variation shown in Figure 9.5 is thus only indicative as there are other factors that influence the heating rate of tissue. One other important complicating factor is that *shear waves* can be formed at tissue interfaces (Williams, 1987). This occurs when waves are refracted to an angle near 90°, i.e. so that the refracted wave travels very close to the boundary. At the boundary, tissue stresses are large as one side is being oscillated at high frequency while the other is stationary. The refracted wave produces a shear wave at the boundary. The shear wave is absorbed very rapidly, resulting in greater heating at the tissue interface.

As noted earlier, moving the transducer head during treatment is important to smooth out the irregularities in intensity of the near field. Another effect is that this reduces some of the irregularities in absorption that might occur due to reflection at interfaces, refraction and

Table 9.4 Mark:space ratios and duty cycles for 50 Hz bursts of ultrasound with different pulse durations

Pulse	Interval	Mark:space ratio	Ratio of pulse to total period	Duty cycle
10 ms	10 ms	1:1	1 in 2	50%
4 ms	16 ms	1:4	1 in 5	20%
2 ms	8 ms	1:4	1 in 5	20%
2 ms	18 ms	1:9	1 in 10	10%

shear wave production. Thus the resulting heating pattern is likely to be more even than implied by Figure 9.5.

PULSED ULTRASOUND

To pulse the ultrasound beam, a circuit in the ultrasonic generator (see Figure 9.2) is arranged to turn the ultrasound on in short bursts or pulses. This reduces the time averaged intensity and hence the amount of energy available to heat the tissues while ensuring that the energy available in each pulse (pulse averaged intensity) is high. This means that any mechanical effects due to tissue stress are still produced but direct thermal effects are reduced (see also discussion, chapter 10).

Many therapeutic ultrasound generators produce 2 ms pulses and vary the intervals between pulses. This can be expressed either as:

- the mark:space ratio, which is the ratio of the pulse length to the interval
- the duty cycle, which is the ratio of the pulse duration to the total time of the pulse plus interval, expressed as a percentage.

Table 9.4 illustrates the relationship between these different ways of expressing the pulse characteristics using, as an example, 50 Hz bursts of ultrasound. At 50 Hz the period (pulse + interval duration) is 1/50th of a second or 20 ms.

Some ultrasound machines produce a 12.5 ms pulse at a frequency of 16 Hz, hence a duty cycle of 20%. Sixteen Hz is argued to be a fundamental frequency of the intracellular calcium system and is therefore claimed to be more effective. The argument for this claim is, to say the least, questionable.

Effects of pulsing

If pulsed ultrasound is applied at a mark:space ratio of 1:9, the amount of introduced energy is one-tenth of that which would be introduced by continuous ultrasound applied for the same length of time and at the same intensity. To introduce the same amount of energy, the pulsed ultrasound could be applied for ten times the length of time or at ten times the peak intensity of the continuous treatment. But the effects of each will differ.

If the ultrasound is pulsed with a 10% duty cycle and the treatment time is ten times longer than with continuous treatment, the same amount of energy will be delivered but the physiological effects will be much less as the temperature elevation throughout treatment will be much lower. This is because heat is continually dissipated by conduction between and within the tissues and to the circulating blood.

If the peak intensity for pulsed treatment were increased by ten times, the average heating would be the same as with continuous treatment. However, there would be the risk of mechanical damage to tissue as the applied high-intensity bursts would produce a 'shock wave' effect in the tissue.

Pulsed ultrasound treatment is usually applied at the same peak intensity as used with continuous ultrasound. This effectively reduces heating while applying peak mechanical stresses which are the same as with continuous application but not high enough to cause appreciable mechanical damage. This may be therapeutically beneficial. While the argument is plausible, there is little actual evidence, as yet, in support.

Research using in vitro models shows that applications of ultrasound can increase rates of ion diffusion across cell membranes (Dyson, 1985); this could be due to increased particle movement on either side of the membrane and increased motion of the phospholipids and proteins that form the membrane. There has also been some conjecture that short bursts of more vigorous agitation, as produced by pulsing ultrasound, have different, more significant and potentially beneficial effects (Dyson and Suckling, 1978). Dyson and Pond (1970) found that short pulses at high peak intensity can result in tissue damage even when the average power is not excessive. This stresses the importance of peak, not just average, intensity. Whether beneficial effects are produced by pulsing remains a question.

PHYSICAL AND PHYSIOLOGICAL EFFECTS OF ULTRASOUND

The result of absorption of ultrasound in the tissues, as has already been discussed, is the oscillation of particles about their mean position. This oscillation, or sonic energy, is converted into heat energy which is proportional to the intensity of the ultrasound. If all this heat is not rapidly and efficiently dissipated by normal physiological means a local rise in temperature will occur and thermal effects will result. There may also be other effects, non-thermal (mechanical), on structures comparable in size to the ultrasound wavelength due to the back-and-forth oscillations of the particles and the consequent stresses

---

The assumtion here is that mechanical effects have some threshold which, if exceeded, produces physical damage.

If pulsed ultrasound is of value it must be capable of producing better therapeutic outcomes than continuous ultrasound. Although this is plausible, it has yet to be demonstrated clinically.

The study by Dyson and Pond (1970) clearly demonstrates that short duration, high intensity pulses can be damaging. The study did not find evidence of potentially beneficial effects.

produced in the tissue. By pulsing the ultrasound output but keeping the peak intensity constant, thermal effects will be reduced but mechanical effects will still be achieved.

Thermal effects

If the local temperature is raised to between 40 and 45°C hyperaemia will result (Lehmann and Guy, 1972). Temperatures above 45°C are destructive. To achieve a useful therapeutic effect the tissue temperature has to be maintained between these values for at least 5 minutes (Lehmann and deLateur, 1982).

Mild heating (in the chronic phase of injury) is known to reduce pain and muscle spasm and to promote healing processes. The pain and muscle spasm is a direct neurophysiological effect. A promotion of healing processes would be expected if the temperature elevation was not excessive, due to increased cellular metabolism and, consequently, cellular activity.

It has been shown that temporary increases in range of movement are produced by ultrasound treatment (Draper et al., 1998b; Knight et al., 2001). Collagenous tissue such as tendon, ligament and joint capsule does not change appreciably in stiffness or extensibility if heated in the therapeutic range. This suggests that the benefits observed are more to do with modulation of pain fibre activity than changes in tissue mechanical properties.

Non-thermal effects

Cavitation

Many of the non-thermal effects attributed to ultrasound in early studies were subsequently identified as due to cavitation (Nyborg, 2001). Cavitation only occurs at high ultrasound intensities and is the formation of tiny gas bubbles in the tissues as a result of ultrasound vibration. These bubbles are generally a micron (10^{-6} m) or so in diameter (ter Haar, 1987), although they can grow much larger under some circumstances.

Cavitation is thought to be unlikely in intact living mammalian tissue at therapeutic levels of intensity, particularly $1\,\mathrm{W\,cm}^{-2}$ or less (Frenkel et al., 2000; Nyborg, 2001). The clinical relevance of cavitation appears minimal except during subaqueous applications of ultrasound, when bubbles forming on and between the treatment head and skin can block transmission (Monk, 1996; Ward and Robertson, 1996).

At higher intensities cavitation has been reported in cat brains ($100\,\mathrm{W\,cm}^{-2}$) and in the lungs of mice ($180\,\mathrm{W\,cm}^{-2}$) (Frenkel et al.,2000). Its clinical relevance appears minimal.

Standing waves

Standing waves have already been described as being due to reflected waves being superimposed on the incident waves. The result is a set

The effect of standing wave production in the clinical application of ultrasound is probably negligible.

of standing or stationary waves with peaks of high pressure (anti-nodes), half a wavelength apart, between which are zones of low pressure (nodes). In in vitro studies, this pressure pattern has been shown to cause stasis of cells in blood vessels at the pressure nodes (Dyson and Pond, 1973). The endothelium of the blood vessels exposed to standing waves can also be damaged leading to thrombus formation (Dyson et al., 1974). The clinical relevance of this is limited for two reasons: a standing wave formation is unlikely in living tissue given the shapes of the underlying structures, which are more likely to reflect and absorb most of the incident energy and, more importantly, moving the treatment head means that standing waves would not 'stand' for any appreciable length of time but would be moved around in the tissues. This would prevent hot spots from forming.

Acoustic streaming

When a beam of sound waves travel through an absorbing medium, radiation pressure, acting along the beam axis, is produced. There is also pressure generated on any structures which reflect the sound energy. This results in a flow or streaming, and there are two types: bulk and microstreaming (Baker et al., 2001). Bulk streaming is the movement of fluid that is visible when testing the output of ultrasound equipment and that can occur in any fluid being insonated.

Microstreaming is streaming at the microscopic (cellular) level. It can exert stress on the cell membrane but more importantly it washes away ions and molecules that have accumulated outside the cell due to cellular activity and membrane transport (secretion). Evidence from in vitro studies has identified: increased secretion from mast cells (Fyfe and Chahl, 1982), increased calcium uptake (Mortimer and Dyson, 1988) and greater growth factor production by macrophages (Young and Dyson, 1990).

> Microstreaming has the potential to be clinically beneficial but there is no hard scientific or clinical evidence to indicate that it occurs.

Whether these findings are clinically significant is yet to be established. Cavitation will not occur in biological tissues at therapeutic intensities and its absence implies that microstreaming will not occur (Baker et al., 2001). What is probably more relevant though is the pressure changes that are exerted on the cell, the microscopic vibration, when ultrasound is applied.

Micromassage

The rapidly changing pressures on the cells and tissue structures being insonated probably have some important effects. This has been called micromassage. The differentials in pressure between cell layers and at tissue boundaries would certainly produce mechanical effects. The implications of these effects in mammalian tissue are unknown.

Summary

Absorption of ultrasound energy in tissue results in tissue heating and the rate and extent of the associated temperature increase depends on:

- the rate of energy absorption in the particular tissue
- the heat capacity of the particular tissue
- the rate of heat transfer to adjacent tissues and to the bloodstream.

In addition to thermal effects, ultrasound absorption also produces non-thermal (mechanical) effects. These are:

- cavitation, which is damaging but unlikely to be produced using therapeutic ultrasound equipment
- standing wave effects which are potentially damaging but also unlikely to be produced in normal clinical applications of ultrasound
- acoustic streaming and micromassage, the clinical benefits of which need further investigation.

Pulsing the ultrasound beam reduces the rate of heating while allowing the same peak intensity to be used. This favours mechanical effects over thermal effects.

Therapeutic mechanisms

Two schools of thought have developed concerning the therapeutic mechanisms of ultrasound (Fyfe and Bullock, 1985). One considers heating to be the only effect. This view is found in much of the American writing on the subject. High doses are recommended and little value is seen in low-intensity and pulsed treatments. This might be described as the 'factual' or 'evidence-based' school of thought. The term 'ultrasonic diathermy' is often used, which emphasizes the heating effect. The other school of thought, largely European, is more concerned with the possibility of low average intensities causing important mechanical or biological effects with pulsed treatments.

Many uncertainties remain concerning ultrasound. The part played by heat versus mechanical effects is an area which is yet to be fully explored. One way of examining the effectiveness of ultrasound is via clinical studies and ascertaining which types of dosages consistently produce better outcomes. Another is to look for evidence of a clear dose–response relationship (especially in non-clinical but more tightly controlled in vitro studies) which can provide evidence of what dosages effect which types of changes and when.

The roles of acoustic streaming and cavitation are also uncertain. They appear to increase calcium ion diffusion across the cell membrane (Mortimer and Dyson, 1988). While demonstrated in

As indicated earlier, cavitation and microstreaming are unlikely to occur in tissues at therapeutic intensities and frequencies, though they have been demonstrated by in vitro studies.

vitro, there is little evidence that this occurs *in vivo* and a therapeutic link has not been properly established.

A problem with in vitro studies is producing doses which are comparable to those produced in vivo. When ultrasound is applied in vitro, i.e. to a thin layer of cells coating the bottom of a small dish with a few millilitres of liquid above, the changes which occur are not necessarily the same as might occur when ultrasound is applied to the body, where a much larger volume of tissue is treated. In vitro exposure typically involves most of the energy being confined to, and absorbed in, a very small volume so the power density is much higher than produced in vivo. For this reason the effects demonstrated in vitro might not occur at power levels used therapeutically.

Changes identified in vitro are included here as they may be relevant to clinical effectiveness but, as noted above, the links are tenuous.

Effects of ultrasound on inflammation and repair processes

The inflammation and repair processes that occur after tissue injury were described in chapter 2. Most of the following research concerns laboratory or animal studies. This enables the necessary precise control over ultrasound and investigating its effects on different tissues. Care must be taken, however, in assuming that human responses are necessarily the same. Species differ in their responses, some have a different innate susceptibility and in others it relates to the tissue distribution in treated areas (AIUM Bioeffects Report, 2000). Also, as noted above, it is difficult to compare the power levels used therapeutically with the power levels of in vitro studies or animal experimentation as the volume treated is so different as are the consequent power densities.

Acute stage

One claimed effect of therapeutic ultrasound is an increased local blood flow. However, one acute effect of ultrasound can be vasoconstriction of the small arterioles, resulting in a local decrease in blood flow (Rubin et al., 1990).

In vitro, ultrasound has effects on the production and release of wound-healing factors. These include the release of histamine from mast cells and factors from macrophages (Young and Dyson, 1990). If this also occurs in vivo, ultrasound could increase the normal rate of healing. While demonstrated in vitro, there is little evidence that the same effects occur in vivo.

Proliferative (granulation) stage

This begins approximately 3 days after injury and is the stage at which the connective tissue framework is laid down by fibroblasts prior to invasion by new blood vessels. When exposed to ultrasound during repair, fibroblasts produce more collagen. Not only is more collagen formed but it also has a greater tensile strength after ultrasound treatment, as shown in studies where damaged Achilles tendons in rats (Enwemeka, 1989; Jackson et al., 1991) and extensor tendons in chickens (Gan et al., 1995) were insonated during healing.

Higher dosages, such as the $2.5\,W\,cm^{-2}$ applied to rats' Achilles tendons, using the direct contact method, retarded healing (da Cunha et al., 2001). This is not surprising, given the very small volume of tissue treated. At a lower dose, $0.5\,W\,cm^{-2}$ (SATA), ultrasound produced better organized and aggregated collagen bundles. Similar effects are seen in studies of the use of ultrasound to treat damage to medial collateral ligaments in rats (Leung et al., 2004).

One study (Karnes and Burton, 2002) found that ultrasound accelerates the rate of repair of contraction induced skeletal muscle damage in rats. Another (Rantanen et al., 1999) found that, although ultrasound stimulates the proliferation of both satellite cells and fibroblasts, it does not appear to affect the rate of muscle fibre regeneration following contusion injury. The different findings might reflect the different nature of the injuries or the different way of assessing the effectiveness of ultrasound exposure.

One unanswered concern is whether ultrasound, by stimulating fibroblasts so effectively, can increase the amount of scar production (Rantanen et al., 1999).

Remodelling stage

This stage can last months or years until the new tissue is as near in structure as possible to the original tissue. It has not been established whether ultrasound treatment during the remodelling stage is beneficial but the biophysical evidence suggests that it could be, particularly if combined with stretch.

Repair of articular cartilage

A possible area of future development is the use of ultrasound for repair of long-standing or acute articular cartilage damage (Cook et al., 2001). A study of the effects of 40 minutes daily for 4 to 52 weeks on cartilage in rabbits' patellae showed considerable improvements in the first 4 to 8 weeks. The equipment and dosage used were the same as that described later in the section on fracture healing with a very low output and BNR. Similar results have been obtained in rats, where ultrasound appears to promote healing of damaged articular cartilage in rats with induced osteoarthritis. Specifically, it decreases signs that indicate the severity of damage such as the extent of fibrillation of the cartilage (Huang et al., 1997).

Wound healing

There are several studies on animals that show that ultrasound at therapeutic intensities facilitates wound healing. One well-executed study on pigs (Byl et al., 1992) reported that ultrasound significantly increased the strength and rate of closure of wounds. Although all wounds appeared similar, the treated ones had a higher tensile strength (24% more than controls), a higher level of collagen deposition (29% more), and more degranulation of mast cells. Similar effects were demonstrated in another study (Byl et al., 1993), which compared $1.5\,W\,cm^{-2}$ and $0.1\,W\,cm^{-2}$ (SATA) dosages with controls. After the first 10 days, the wounds treated with the lower dosage had a higher breaking strength and greater collagen depostion than the high dose or controls.

A study of laser-caused burn injuries in rats (Cambier and Vanderstraeten, 1997), found that there was no evidence that using ultrasound, SATA $0.25\,W\,cm^{-2}$ (pulsed), or $0.3\,W\,cm^{-2}$ (continuous) enhanced the rate of repair. The study, however, did not include sham or control rats.

For an authoritative account of the influence of ultrasound on tissue healing, particularly the in vitro effects, see Young (1996).

DISCUSSION OF THERAPEUTIC USES

Therapeutic ultrasound has been applied to a wide range of conditions with claims of successful outcomes. These include acute and subacute traumatic and inflammatory conditions, chronic rheumatoid and arthritic conditions, scar and excessive fibrous tissue and for pain relief. This section starts by considering some of the major reviews of clinical ultrasound.

Reviews

After over 60 years of clinical use of ultrasound and many different studies there are still difficulties in establishing with any certainty when ultrasound is effective and if there is dose-response relationship. Some recent studies, reporting the treatment of fractures and other collagenous tissues with ultrasound, are methodologically sound and have positive findings which are discussed later. Evidence for other clinical uses has received considerable attention in reviews and is summarized below.

Most reviews of therapeutic ultrasound in the past decade or so have reported that there is little evidence of clinical effectiveness (Holmes and Rudland, 1991; Gam and Johannsen, 1995; van der Heijden et al., 1997; van der Windt et al., 1999, 2002; Robertson and Baker, 2001; Robertson, 2003). Some of these reviews have focused on the use of ultrasound to treat a particular region such as the shoulder (van der Heijden et al., 1997) or a condition, e.g. ankle sprains (van der Windt et al., 2002). Others have used a range of inclusion criteria to examine a body of literature on clinical uses of ultrasound. A common finding of the reviews was the lack of methodologically acceptable trials on the use of ultrasound. A problem with such

An important point to note is that the reviews do not conclude that ultrasound is ineffective, but rather that the studies reviewed could not be regarded as conclusive. The question of clinical effectiveness is thus unanswered rather than answered in the negative.

reviews is that the reader could well conclude that ultrasound is ineffective, when in fact there is no sound evidence base for any such conclusion. The problem is compounded if 'non-clinical', i.e. laboratory-based scientific evidence is ignored or discounted.

One recent review identified two studies which both were methodologically convincing and identified clear changes following treatment by ultrasound (Robertson and Baker, 2001). The first of these used ultrasound to treat carpal tunnel syndrome (Ebenbichler et al., 1998) and the other, shoulders with a diagnosed calcific tendinitis (Ebenbichler et al., 1999). Both studies had the same leading researcher who subsequently agreed that ultrasound may not have been the optimal treatment for carpal tunnel syndrome because of the risk of a relapse (Ebenbichler, 1998). Nevertheless, the results showed a clear benefit of ultrasound for quite different conditions.

Another problem concerns dosage (Robertson, 2003). Not all studies provide evidence that equipment has been calibrated and if it has, after how many uses. A considerable level of drift may occur with some machines so that a purported output of $1\,W\,cm^{-2}$ may well not be that.

Yet another problem is that even if the power applied is known, the dosage actually delivered to the target tissues is not, so it is not possible to report with any certainty that a positive outcome can be obtained with a set dosage. This is part of the reason there is still no known dose-response relation.

> This means that it is not possible to predict with any certainty the response of any tissue to a dosage of, for example, $1\,W\,cm^{-2}$ for a subacute lesion at a depth of 2 cm.

Cochrane reviews have been published on the use of ultrasound for a range of conditions. For example, the effect of using ultrasound to treat rheumatoid arthritis is not clear but it may assist with some joints (Casimiro et al., 2004). For treating osteoarthritis of the knee it appears to have no benefits over shortwave (Welch et al., 2004). Similarly, it has little effect on patellofemoral joint pain (Brosseau et al., 2004).

Besides a considerable overlap in authors the Cochrane reviews described here have another major commonality: all indicate the low methodological quality of existing trials of ultrasound on the topic they reviewed. This suggests that the findings, as with those of the reviews noted above, have to be considered with caution. As higher quality research studies are published it will become possible to say with more certainty when ultrasound is effective and when not. The questions remain open.

The remainder of this section considers specific studies and the evidence they provide. This needs to be read with caution as a rigorous methodological review of each study has not necessarily been conducted. The section starts with studies with a clearly beneficial outcome.

Fracture healing

The benefit of applying ultrasound to both delayed union and non-union fractures are clear (Mayr et al., 2000; Nolte et al, 2001; Takikawa

The important point is that ultrasound used for fracture healing is effective but the equipment used is purpose designed and different from the usual therapeutic ultrasound equipment.

et al., 2001; Busse et al., 2002). The rate of union is higher than otherwise expected. In one study the healing rate was 89% (of 1317 chronic, non-uniting fractures) in 131 days of treatment with ultrasound (Mayr et al., 2000), a success rate well above that of controls. The ultrasound which has been shown to be effective for fracture healing in humans to date is, however, different to that used by therapists. The equipment used for fracture healing has a BNR of 2.16, a frequency of 1.5 MHz, an ERA of typically $4\,cm^2$ and a SATA output of $0.03\,W\,cm^{-2}$. It is normally pulsed at a frequency of 1 kHz (Hadjiargyrou, 1998; Warden et al., 2000). Another difference concerns the method of use: a stationary applicator for 20 minutes per day. The combination of both very low SATA intensity and BNR (usually 5 to 6 in therapeutic equipment) permits this different method of application.

Articular cartilage repair

The extent of the effects of ultrasound on chronic arthritis or its precursors is unknown. Studies with animals, discussed earlier, suggest it might be effective. One case study also attributed the healing of a grade II tear of the posterior horn of a medial meniscus to the use of ultrasound (Muche, 2003). However, as no repeat visualization of the meniscus was conducted after treatment this claim is not adequately justified.

Wound healing

Identifying the type of wound is important, if acute, surgically caused or not, if chronic and if any other comorbidities that might affect the outcome are also present. One study of the effects of ultrasound on pressure ulcers in humans showed little difference between those insonated and non-insonated (ter Riet et al., 1996). In this study the sham group had larger ulcers that, on medical grounds, were probably less likely to recover. That no significant difference was found despite the bias against the sham group, suggests that ultrasound is ineffective for treating pressure ulcers.

The conclusions of ter Riet et al. (1996), however, contrast with those of Callam et al. (1987) who found that insonated ulcers healed 20% more in 12 weeks than controls.

A single case study in which pulsed low intensity ultrasound and sham were applied on alternate weeks to a stage III pressure ulcer over a sacrum (Selkowitz et al., 2002) found that the rate of healing was faster in the baseline period than in the low ultrasound and slowest in the sham ultrasound period. The negative effect of sham ultrasound could possibly be due to microtrauma with the movement of the applicator over the wound even using a gel pad.

Whether ultrasound improves the rate of healing of wounds remains an open question. Often important details are omitted, such as the methods of assessing wound change and other concurrent care, as well as of the dosage and calibration. The results to date with wounds do not provide a sound and convincing evidence base for future treatments using ultrasound.

This summary is consistent with that of a Cochrane review of the effects of therapeutic ultrasound for venous leg ulcers (Flemming and Cullum, 2004).

Soft tissue injuries

Recent research indicates that ultrasound applied after acute ankle sprains (van der Windt et al., 2002) or chronic shoulder disorders (Gursel et al., 2004) does not improve the outcomes. A possible reason for this is that small increases in the rate of otherwise normal healing might not be identifiable given the usual outcome measures which focus on gross function such as range of movement, pain or strength. That is, if it takes 7 days for healing normally, an improvement of 0.5 of a day is unlikely to be easily identified, except with very sensitive measures.

An issue with soft tissue lesions is obtaining sufficient subjects with similar problems, often leading to the use of a heterogeneous group of subjects and a negative outcome, not because the effects were not different nor of clinical importance, but rather that the standard deviation of the outcome measures was large. This highlights the need for tightly controlled research, perhaps laboratory rather than clinically based, to establish which types of tissue injuries are likely to benefit from ultrasound. The choice of subsequent clinical tests could then be restricted to those likely to be successful on the basis of hard scientific evidence and plausibility.

Another use of ultrasound is to treat muscle soreness. There is little evidence that it is effective as currently used (Craig et al., 1999; Plaskett et al., 1999). Similarly, used for patellar tendinopathy, there is no evidence that ultrasound or transverse frictions are as effective as an exercise programme (Stasinopoulos and Stasinopoulos, 2004).

Whether ultrasound might improve the rate of healing of soft tissue injuries remains an open question. The limited clinical evidence available does not provide a sufficient evidence base. While clinical evidence is the ultimate 'proof of the pudding', there is anecdotal evidence that heating during the acute phase may be detrimental and that heating during the chronic phase can be beneficial. Such anecdotal evidence has a sound physiological basis and should therefore be accorded some weight.

Pain relief

Few studies report using ultrasound to treat pain per se. Most aim to treat soft tissue damage and consequently to reduce pain by promoting healing and resolving inflammation.

Scar tissue

Evidence of the effects of ultrasound on changing the extensibility of scar tissue is predominantly anecdotal, although it is sometimes used by physiotherapists in the UK for this purpose (Kitchen and Partridge, 1996). No comparative studies of the effects of hot packs or other types of superficial heat and ultrasound on scar tissue were identified.

Blood flow

Considerable differences have been reported. Using 1 MHz ultrasound at 1 to 1.5 $W cm^{-2}$ for 5 to 15 minutes over the calf muscles produced a change in one study (Fabrizio et al., 1996). A similar dosage increased hand circulation in people both with or without rheumatoid arthritis (Berliner and Piegsa, 1997). By contrast, an investigation of the effect of continuous ultrasound on blood flow (Robinson and Buono, 1995) using a dose of 1.5 $W cm^{-2}$ for 5 minutes applied to the forearm found no change in skeletal muscle blood flow.

A complication is that the rate of movement of the sound head has a major effect on local tissue heating. Slow movement evokes a greater response as the heat is more localized and prolonged. This would have a big effect on reflex vasodilation and consequent blood flow.

Diagnosis of stress fractures

Ultrasound has long been used clinically to identify stress fractures (Lowden, 1986). If one is present, anecdotally, ultrasound over the surface causes considerable pain and discomfort. The one study identified which evaluated this use of 1 MHz ultrasound showed that it was not a reliable method of identifying stress fractures of the tibia (Romani et al., 2000). Ultrasound with increasing intensities, ranging up to 2.9 $W cm^{-2}$ was applied with direct contact over the possible tibial stress fracture site (26 subjects, 16 MRI grade 2 or 3 stress fractures on affected legs). Only 40% of subjects (legs) were correctly classified as having a stress fracture or not. This suggests that the method used, or 1 MHz ultrasound, has a very low rate of predictive success with recent stress fractures (symptoms having started within 2 weeks of being tested).

Future clinical trials

This paucity of controlled trials of ultrasound is a little surprising in view of the fact that it is relatively easy to arrange a double-blind trial, as the patient is usually unaware of any sensation at most therapeutic intensities. The functioning of the machine is not always easily concealed from the therapist but it can be managed, especially with direct contact ultrasound (McLachlan, 1991). Ideally, studies of ultrasound should have sham and active treatment groups as well as a control group. This removes doubts regarding any effect of the massage over the skin from the applicator as well as any placebo effect.

Summary

The principal therapeutic uses of ultrasound include promoting the:

- healing of chronic ulcers
- healing of acute soft tissue injuries
- improvement of scar tissue.

Judged by 'Evidenced Based Practice' standards, there is little evidence of any therapeutic benefit of ultrasound. Both hard scientific and anecdotal evidence, however, indicate that ultrasound treatment may be beneficial. The therapeutic benefits are thus plausible but unproven.

PRINCIPLES OF APPLICATION

Couplant

Adequate transmission of ultrasonic energy to the tissues depends on having a couplant that provides a good match of acoustic impedance between the metal of the transducer head and the skin. There is virtually no transmission of ultrasound from the transducer to air; the energy is reflected back and causes heating of, and possibly damage to, the transducer itself. Water is a good couplant (see below) but has to be held in place between the treatment head and the tissues in some way. It is therefore made into a gel or a gel pad, held in a plastic or rubber bag or the body part is immersed in water with the treatment head (Figure 9.6). All three methods are in use but the direct contact method, in which water-based gel is interposed between the sound head and the tissue, is the most common.

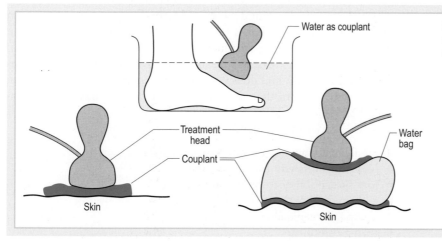

Figure 9.6 Immersion, direct contact and water bag applications of ultrasound.

Continuous movement of the treatment head

With all methods and for both continuous and pulsed outputs, the treatment head must be moved continuously relative to the tissues for the following reasons:

- the ultrasound beam is very irregular in the near zone (see Figure 9.3) so a stationary applicator could produce hot spots in the patient's tissue
- at high intensities excess local heating can occur and cause tissue damage. Figure 9.5b indicates the risk of damage to the bone and periosteum when the soft tissue layers overlying bone are thin.

Steady movement of the treatment head means that the ultrasound energy reaching the bone is not localized but distributed over a larger bone surface area. At the same time, the dose delivered to the overlying soft tissue is more evenly spread as the local high-intensity regions (see Figure 9.3) are moved around during treatment and so do not produce 'hot spots' in the treated tissue.

Despite the precaution of movement of the treatment head, there is still the risk of exacerbating discomfort if any regions are heated excessively. If the patient complains of any increased pain or discomfort during treatment, the ultrasound application should be terminated.

Method of application

With all methods of application, a coupling medium must be used between the sound head and the treated tissue. Water is an adequate coupling medium but thixotropic gels, in practical terms, are superior.

Direct contact application

With 'direct contact' application, the ultrasound energy is transferred to tissue by a coupling medium which is usually a thixotropic gel. Thixotropic gels make ideal couplants for ultrasound. They are thick gels when sitting on the skin but become thin and liquid-like when vibrated by the ultrasound beam. The thixotropic properties mean that in the ultrasound beam the gel will flow and easily fill the gap between the skin and the treatment head. Flow is necessary as the gap will vary while the treatment head is moving. Gel outside the ultrasound beam is thick and does not run. This minimizes mess and, more importantly, ensures that the moving head always has a thick surrounding region of gel.

The essential requirements of a couplant are that it has:

- an acoustic impedance similar to the tissues
- high transmissivity for ultrasound
- low susceptibility to bubble formation
- a chemically inactive nature
- a hypoallergenic character
- relative sterility.

Water immersion application

A water immersion application uses water as the only couplant. Water and ultrasound gel are similar in all of the above listed 'essential requirements' except susceptibility to bubble formation. Water is less desirable in this regard. Unless the water is degassed (and this is unlikely to be practicable), the air in solution will tend to form bubbles on the treatment head and the skin. These bubbles block and reflect ultrasound unless manually removed as soon as they are visible to the operator.

Water bag application

As noted above, water is a good couplant provided that air bubbles do not form, so a water bag application has merit. If a soft plastic bag is used, the bag will deform and mould to the skin and treatment head contours, ensuring efficient transmission of ultrasound energy. A thin layer of couplant should be used, between the skin and the bag and also between the treatment head and the bag, to eliminate any air gaps.

Coupling agents

Besides water, gel and gel pads, the most common coupling agents are oils, either mineral or vegetable. While degassed water, gel and gel pads have similar transmission coefficients, oils have lower ones (Griffin, 1980; Casarotto et al., 2004) and so will heat more and feel warmer to the patient. Not too much importance should be attached to the transmittivity of different couplants with direct contact application as a thin layer is used so the amount of energy absorbed is small, even for poor couplants. Providing that no bubbles form (which would completely reflect the ultrasound beam), the proportion of the energy transmitted is high.

Method of application

The following stages relate specifically to direct contact application, however, the principles and precautions also apply to water immersion and water bag applications.

Stages

Patient

Explanation: the nature and duration of the treatment and the need for a couplant are explained to the patient. What the patient should expect to feel and what they should not feel must also be described along with an explanation of how ultrasound is expected to promote their recovery.

Examination and testing: the skin surface to be treated should be inspected; treatment over inflammatory skin conditions should be avoided.

Apparatus

Prior to any treatment, check that there is an output from the machine. Position the treatment head just below the water surface, so the head is angled but fully covered, in a suitable container such as a small metal basin. Observe the disturbance which appears in the water as the intensity is rapidly increased to near maximal output using a continuous wave (CW) and immediately decreased. This method minimizes any risks to the crystal while indicating the presence of an output. To quantify the output reliably a radiation balance is required. Periodical testing for electrical safety and proper functioning of the apparatus should include a radiation balance check of the output. As discussed earlier, many machines are not calibrated sufficiently frequently and may not be producing the stated output.

Preparation of part

Clean the area and apply couplant to the skin surface.

A practical point: position the patient so that they and the therapist are both comfortable and the therapist has clear access throughout to the area being treated with ultrasound and to the machine.

Setting up

The therapist's position should enable clear access so the treatment head can be kept in full contact with the skin for the entire treatment time. After applying the couplant, rest the weight of the treatment head on the part with sufficient pressure only to ensure close contact throughout the treatment, to maximize transmission of the ultrasound energy. Then turn on the output while the treatment head is in contact with the skin and being moved. This is an important part of avoiding damage to the transducer and even burning of the patient's skin, which can occur if sufficient energy is reflected back into the treatment head. Some machines have a monitoring system to indicate if the quality of the contact between the skin and treatment head is not optimal. If it is not, typically, the output reduces and some sort of warning light or sound is provided. Users should not rely on the equipment for this type of feedback but endeavour to develop a technique which always optimizes the treatment head to skin contact for direct applications. On completion of a treatment, turn the output down and off, while still moving the treatment head and before lifting it off. Again, this reduces risks to the patient and the equipment.

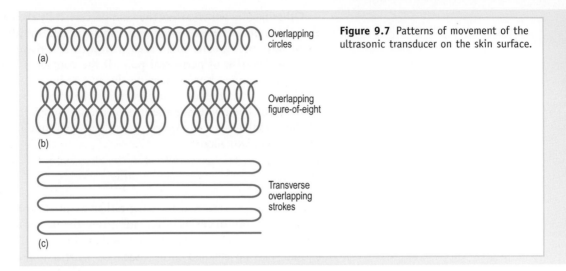

Figure 9.7 Patterns of movement of the ultrasonic transducer on the skin surface.

(a) Overlapping circles

(b) Overlapping figure-of-eight

(c) Transverse overlapping strokes

Instructions and warnings

The patient is asked to keep the part being treated still and relaxed and to report any increase in pain or other changed sensations immediately.

Application

Most ultrasound machines have a switch associated with the timer. The output commences only after the time has been set and output ceases once the set time has expired.

The treatment head is moved continuously over the surface with an even pressure for both continuous and pulsed outputs. The emitting surface must always be kept parallel to the skin surface to reduce reflection and pressed sufficiently firmly to exclude any air. The rate of movement must be slow enough to allow the tissues to deform and thus remain in complete contact with the rigid treatment head but fast enough to prevent 'hot spots' developing when using a higher-intensity treatment. A standard speed is $4\,cm\,s^{-1}$ but this is not practical in some areas and not easy to measure clinically. The pattern of movement can be a series of overlapping parallel strokes, circles or figures-of-eight (Figure 9.7).

Patient reports of the level of heating during an application are not a reliable indicator of the intensity used as it is dependent upon a number of factors. If the aim is to increase the level of patient perceived heat, the following steps are recommended:

- decrease the size of area insonated – smaller is better
- use an oil as the couplant – rather than gel, gel pad or water
- warm the couplant before insonation
- use a higher SATA output intensity
- decrease the speed of movement of the applicator – a slower speed increases the local temperature

Other factors which affect the heat perceived by the patient include the depth of soft tissue over bone and the quality of contact. Soft tissue heating is greater in an area with little soft tissue cover but this increases the risk of periosteal pain. If the contact is poor, the treatment head can get hot, increasing the risk of burns.

Conversely, to reduce heat perception the above factors need to be considered. The point is, patient perception is not a reliable indicator of the actual output of equipment as these factors all contribute to what they might report.

Termination

The intensity is returned to zero, either manually or automatically, before the transducer is removed from the water bath or tissue contact. The skin is cleaned of couplant or dried. The transducer should also be cleaned after each use with a non-corrosive, non-abrasive antiseptic solution containing alcohol, chlorine or glutaraldehyde as recommended by the manufacturer or relevant legislation or guidelines.

Recording

The following should be recorded: date, machine used, SATA or SATP intensity, frequency, pulse mode, insonation time, couplant, region and size of area of insonation and response to treatment.

Water bath application

When direct contact is not possible because of the irregular shape of the part (e.g. malleoli), or because of local tenderness, a water bath may be used. This is really only useful for treating the hand, forearm, foot or ankle.

Procedure

Test the output of the machine and inspect the part to be treated, as above.

Seat the patient comfortably and immerse the part in water at a comfortable temperature.

Put the treatment head in the water, which should be degassed, and move it parallel to the surface of the part being treated at a distance of 1 to 2 cm.

When non-degassed water (such as tap water) is used, bubbles normally form on the treatment head and skin. These must be removed immediately by wiping, otherwise the bubbles will reflect much of the ultrasound.

When ultrasound is applied by water immersion and a plastic water bath is used, the tissue dosage is markedly reduced by comparison with direct contact application. With a 1 to 2 cm distance between the treatment head and skin it is necessary to increase the output intensity by 30 to 50% to achieve the same dosage as direct contact application (Ward and Robertson, 1996).

The type of water basin used is important (Robertson and Ward, 1995). The implications of metal and plastic basins were compared while using a 2 cm distance between the treatment head and skin. The rate and amount of heating was more than 50% greater if a metal basin was used. This finding suggests that a great deal of energy is reflected at the water/skin interface. A plastic basin absorbs this reflected energy but a metal basin does not: rather the energy is reflected by the metal, back to the part. This means that the dosage only needs correcting if a plastic bath is used. A metal basin confines, but does not absorb the energy to any significant extent.

Yet another aspect of using a water bath is that the therapist should not leave their hand in the water while the equipment is operating, unless essential, and then only for the shortest time possible (e.g. to dislodge air bubbles on the treatment head or part). An option is to use a knitted or mesh glove inside a rubber glove to ensure little or no ultrasound energy is absorbed by the operator's hand.

Water bag application

A way of applying ultrasound to irregular surfaces which cannot conveniently be placed in a water bath is to use a plastic or rubber bag filled with water. This forms a water cushion between the treatment head and the skin (see Figure 9.6). The water bag is preferably a self-sealing plastic bag or a condom (as the rubber is thin and of good quality). The bag should be filled with warm water, preferably degassed, and all air should be squeezed out before sealing the bag. Cover the bag surface and the skin with a couplant, preferably gel. The bag is then held in place over the irregular surface to be treated and the treatment head is then pressed firmly against the gel covered bag with a layer of water about 1 cm thick to separate it from the skin. The treatment head is then moved mainly by deforming the bag, although it can also be moved over the surface of the bag.

A study comparing plastic bags, condoms and balloons found that plastic bags and condoms transmit ultrasound energy efficiently but that balloons impede energy transmission (Monk, 1996). For plastic bags and condoms, the energy transmitted through the enclosed water was found to depend on the distance through water in the same way observed with immersion application in a plastic bath (Ward and Robertson, 1996). With balloons, however, the transmitted energy was about 25% of that transmitted by the condoms and plastic bags. This is probably due to the greater thickness of the balloon rubber (0.23 mm) than condom rubber (0.065 mm) or plastic (0.083 mm).

If the reason for water bath application is the presence of bony prominences which produce surface irregularity, a high intensity should be avoided in order to minimize the risk of periosteal burns.

The condom and plastic layer are apparently transparent as far as the ultrasound beam is concerned, because they are so thin.

Gel pads and plastic films as couplants

Ultrasound treatment should not be directly applied over open wounds or injured skin because of the risk of transmitting infection and causing further damage with a moving treatment applicator. One solution is to use a polyacrylamide or agar gel pad as a couplant. These materials are transparent, normally about 3 mm thick and are designed to be used for areas where direct contact ultrasound is not desirable. Although designed to be used directly over the wound or skin, it helps to add a little sterile saline or ultrasound gel to exclude any air bubbles that might prevent transmission. Applied to the outside of the pad too, the water or gel excludes air and allows smoother movement of the treatment head over the surface of the pad.

Polyurethane film dressings are used in the same way. These and similar wound dressings have high ultrasound transmissivity (Pringle, 1995) and allow more efficient energy transfer than water immersion application. Interposing a layer of plastic or condom rubber between the sound head and tissue does not make any appreciable change to the energy delivered (Monk, 1996).

Summary

Therapeutic ultrasound may be applied to the tissues:

- by direct contact using coupling gel
- in a water bath
- through a water bag (either a condom or plastic bag)
- via a gel pad, plastic film or thin layer of rubber.

DOSAGE

Three factors must be considered when deciding what ultrasound dosage to use (Figure 9.8):

- the *size* of the area to be treated
- the *depth* of the lesion from the surface
- the *nature* and staging of the lesion

The parameters which influence dosage include:

- the *mode*, whether continuous or pulsed
- the *frequency*, usually 1 or 3 MHz
- the *intensity*
- *other factors* such as the specific equipment used, the effective radiating area (ERA) of the treatment head and the duration, frequency and total number of treatments.

There is no certain way of knowing how much energy is absorbed in any particular tissue. Graphs such as those shown in Figure 9.5 give an indication but factors such as the location, orientation and

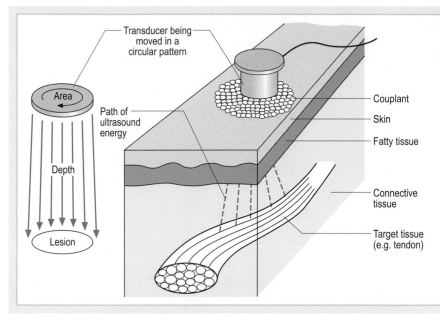

Figure 9.8 Some determinants of ultrasound dosage: the size of area to be treated, the depth of the lesion from the surface, the nature and staging of the lesion and the particular location being treated.

shape of different tissues will influence the amount of reflection so dosage becomes, to some extent, a matter of judgement. This judgement must be based on the known factors governing absorption and reflection of ultrasound. The dosage applied at the surface is only a rough indication of the dose at the target tissue.

The dosage is more reliably known when ultrasound is applied directly over a wound but even then is uncertain as it depends on reflection from underlying tissues (particularly bone).

Mode – continuous or pulsed output

Continuous mode will produce heat in the tissues if the intensity is high enough, whereas pulsed ultrasound at the same instantaneous intensity has a much lower time-averaged intensity, and hence lower or even negligible heating (e.g. $0.5\,W\,cm^{-2}$ pulsed at 1:4 will deliver the same energy as $0.1\,W\,cm^{-2}$ on continuous mode).

The usual basis for deciding between continuous and pulsed is how acute is the problem being treated. More acute soft tissue injuries, for example, are usually treated with pulsed ultrasound to reduce the risk of local heating. Conversely, more chronic lesions are treated with continuous or higher intensities of pulsed ultrasound.

Frequency

Ultrasound attenuation increases with rising frequency so lower frequencies penetrate further (see Table 9.3) and have greater effect at depth. Thus a higher percentage of the energy carried in 3 MHz

Whether there are grounds for believing that pulsed ultrasound is of value for acute-phase injuries is questionable. What is unquestionable is that heating is undesirable, but it is not obvious whether brief 'hammer-blows' or even 'gentle taps' of acoustic energy might assist the acute phase response to injury.

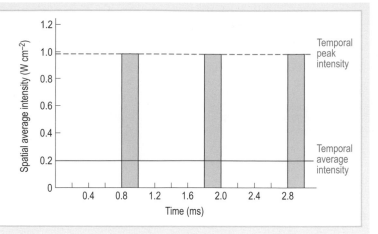

Figure 9.9 The relationship between temporal peak and temporal averaged intensity for ultrasound SATP output of $1\,W\,cm^{-2}$, pulsed 2 ms on and 8 ms off.

ultrasound is absorbed in the superficial tissues, whereas 1 MHz ultrasound penetrates more deeply through the tissue. As a general principle, for superficial tissue heating use 3 MHz ultrasound and for greater depth efficiency use 1 MHz ultrasound.

One implication of the high rate of absorption of 3 MHz ultrasound in the superficial tissues is that care must be taken in selecting the intensity to be applied. A rule of thumb is to divide the intensity by the frequency so, if a 1 MHz frequency ultrasound was to be applied at $1\,W\,cm^{-2}$ (SATA), using the 3 MHz frequency means reducing the intensity to $0.3\,W\,cm^{-2}$.

Intensity

Power, the total energy per second supplied by the machine, is measured in watts. Since this is spread over the whole face of the transducer, and transducers are of different sizes, it is more useful to give the intensity in $W\,cm^{-2}$. Most therapeutic sources emit a maximum spatial average of $2–3\,W\,cm^{-2}$.

Time-averaged intensity is an important value in pulsed treatments. The intensity shown on the meter is usually the peak intensity, more correctly described as the space averaged temporal peak (SATP) intensity. During pulsed treatments the average (SATA) intensity is obviously much lower (Figure 9.9 and Table 9.5). It is worth noting that a SATP intensity of $2\,W\,cm^{-2}$ at a 1:4 pulse ratio is equivalent to a SATA intensity (continuous mode) of $0.4\,W\,cm^{-2}$. Conversely, a SATA intensity of $0.1\,W\,cm^{-2}$ is equivalent to a SATP intensity at 1:4 pulse ratio of $0.5\,W\,cm^{-2}$.

To compare the dosages used in treating different sized lesions, a measure called energy density can be used. Energy density is the total energy (SATA intensity $[W\,cm^{-2}] \times$ ERA $[cm^2] \times$ time [s]) applied per unit area of skin surface treated. It is measured in $J\,cm^{-2}$ (Robertson and Baker, 2001).

Table 9.5 Examples of SATA outputs from an ultrasound source with a temporal peak display meter and maximum output of $3\,W\,cm^{-2}$

SATA intensity ($W\,cm^{-2}$) at transducer face	Intensity shown on meter ($W\,cm^{-2}$)		
	Continuous	Pulsed 1:1	Pulsed 1:4
0.1	0.1	0.2	0.5
0.2	0.2	0.4	1.0
0.5	0.5	1.0	2.5
1.0	1.0	2.0	–
1.5	1.5	3.0	–
2.0	2.0	–	–
3.0	3.0	–	–

The beam non-uniformity ratio (BNR) is another factor affecting intensity. Given the irregularity of the ultrasound beam, BNR is used to indicate peak intensity in the beam. The average intensity of the peaks and troughs of the sonic field over a specific area, usually the transducer face, is the space-averaged intensity (SA). A pressure balance measures total power output from the transducer and hydrophone scanning measures the beam profiles. From the total power output and the beam profile, the effective radiating area and the beam non-uniformity ratio (BNR) can be calculated. The lower the BNR, the lower the high intensity peaks in the Fresnel zone.

Irrespective of the uncertainties in dosages, it is clearly necessary to increase the intensity to compensate for absorption and scattering in the overlying tissue when treating more deeply placed targets. By estimating the depth of the target tissue from the surface and knowing the half-value depth, a reasonable intensity can be selected. For example, the intensity required to treat a lesion situated at the half-value depth of the ultrasound would be twice that needed for a similar surface lesion. The intensity required to treat a lesion situated at double the half-value depth would be four times that needed for a similar surface lesion.

How ultrasound is applied affects the dose rate of the underlying tissue. When tested, the extent of heating was found to be higher and last longer if the size of the area is twice, rather than four times, the effective radiating area of the applicator (Chan et al., 1998). Not all therapists keep the applicator in the recommended area, twice the treatment head area. A study of how physiotherapists applied ultrasound to a model showed considerable inter-therapist variation and much lower actual dose per unit area than predicted (Grey, 2003). The median dosages were 0.3 to 0.9 times the planned average local dosages. This was because most therapists exceeded a designated treatment area of $10\,cm^2$ (with a beam $5\,cm^2$) so that the average energy per unit area was lower. This study demonstrates that a critical component of selecting the dosage is user technique: their ability to apply ultrasound to a predetermined area or to compensate by increasing the intensity in a commensurate manner.

A practical limitation of these simple calculations is that the intensity required may well produce excessive heating of the overlying tissues. It may also exceed the maximum power output of the ultrasound machine.

Dosage records should provide details of the applied intensity, specifying whether it is SATA or SATP intensity, and the duty cycle if pulsed. The tissue volume treated should also be described in terms of, for example, the particular area treated, depth of underlying bone and thicknesses of overlying tissues.

Factors affecting the intensity applied to a tissue

- A factor determining the intensity which should be applied to a lesion is whether it is acute or chronic, i.e. the staging of the lesion. A high intensity is inappropriate for an acute lesion. In practical terms, this means a SATA of $0.1\,W\,cm^{-2}$ to 0.5 or $0.8\,W\,cm^{-2}$ if acute to subacute and 0.8 to $3\,W\,cm^{-2}$ if chronic.
- Frequency. If using a higher frequency, also use a lower intensity to compensate for the higher rate of absorption in a tissue volume.
- Depth of lesion being treated. If deeper, increase the intensity to compensate for more absorption of ultrasound energy in the overlying tissues.
- If using pulsed, increase the pulsing ratio to decrease the average intensity (SATA). Increasing the pulse ratio from 1 : 1 to 1 : 2 then 1 : 4 decreases the dosage to 50% then 20%.
- Size of treatment area actually insonated. If large, the energy per unit area is reduced. This depends on the size of area treated and the therapist's technique.
- Tissues underneath. If there is little depth to bone, always use a low intensity (less than $0.5\,W\,cm^{-2}$). If there is considerable depth, select the intensity according to the depth of lesion and type of overlying tissue.

As for any form of treatment, the lowest intensity required to produce the desired therapeutic effect should be used.

When increasing the intensity to heat a deeply located structure, be careful to avoid excessive heating of the overlying tissues.

If there is a thick muscle layer, even with 1 MHz frequency ultrasound little energy will be left at 4 cm depth through the muscle, overlying fat and skin.

Specific equipment used

Machines that are apparently identical are not necessarily so. This means that records of dosage should indicate which machine was used and if it was the same or a series of them, during a course of treatment. Unless the machine has been tested and calibrated there is no guarantee that the intensity displayed on the output meter is an accurate or even approximate indication of the actual dose rate.

Effective radiating area (ERA) and actual area of treatment head

The ERA is usually smaller than the actual face of the treatment head. This is the area moved by the crystal, the effective radiating surface. In clinical practice it is often assumed to be the same as the actual area of the face of the treatment head, but the ERA is normally 85–95% of the actual area. Manufacturers provide this information for each ultrasound unit.

The size of the area to which ultrasound is applied also affects the extent of heating at a location. As noted previously, some therapists have difficulty in limiting applications to the size of area treated. This can mean a considerable reduction in energy delivered per unit volume of treated tissue.

A 5 cm^2 treatment head offers more congruence with the skin than a 10 cm^2 one, especially on limbs. Using a 1 or 2 cm^2 one is preferable in small areas such as over a temporomandibular joint. If a smaller head is used at the same intensity (W cm^{-2}), the total energy delivered will be less but the energy per unit volume will not be: it is just that the volume treated will be less. If the structure treated is small, this factor is relatively unimportant.

The area of the treatment head affects the beam: there is less divergence with a 5 cm^2 than a 1 or 2 cm^2 applicator, but in practice, beam divergence would be relatively inconsequential at MHz frequencies and would make little difference clinically.

Duration, frequency and total number of treatments

The amount of energy applied to the tissues depends not only on the intensity but also on the length of time for which it is applied (the treatment duration). The usual treatment time is 5 to 10 minutes per treatment area (twice the area of the treatment head face) but this figure seems to be based on the economic concept of 20 minutes of treatment being an upper limit, rather than it being an established optimum treatment time. While it has been established that temperature increases generally plateau at about 20 minutes, this is hardly an argument for ceasing the treatment, since the temperature will then decrease back to normal.

The effects of ultrasound on bone and collagenous materials suggest that longer times daily may be more effective than the traditional times (Mayr et al., 2000; Cook et al., 2001) or the times used in many studies (Draper, 2002).

The ideal treatment frequency for any particular condition at a certain stage is unknown. More acute lesions are often treated at least once daily, and chronic on alternate days until sufficient improvement is obtained. Whether this is ideal is unknown and again it seems that current practice is probably often dictated by economic considerations.

Progression and timing

Progression is based on the outcome of previous treatment. If there is subjective and objective improvement the treatment should be continued at the same dose. If the symptoms are unpredictably worse the treatment should be reduced or discontinued. If there is no change when one would be expected, the dosage should be reconsidered and changed or ultrasound should be discontinued.

Summary

Dosage parameters:

- mode – pulsing gives less power than continuous output
- frequency – lower frequency gives greater depth of penetration
- intensity – measured in $W\,cm^{-2}$ and usually as the SATA intensity
- time – duration of each treatment, in minutes, related to the size of area being treated
- size of area treated
- treatment repetition – once or twice per day for acute lesions, less frequently for chronic.

Possible dangers

Apart from an instance of extreme abuse with self-administered treatment (Levenson and Weissberg, 1983) there is little reported evidence of damage due directly to therapeutic ultrasound. This possibly represents an underreporting for medico-legal reasons as, anecdotally, injuries, especially burns, occur under some conditions.

- Burns can occur if the heat applied exceeds the physiological ability of the tissue to dissipate it. Typically this is due to poor technique such as occurs with insufficient movement, only partial contact or an inadequate couplant to treatment head contact or to a reduced dissipation capacity of the tissue.
- Tissue destruction from transient cavitation has been demonstrated in laboratory experiments using small animals or tissue samples. Damage can occur in capillaries near large air masses at sufficiently high intensities. There is no evidence related to humans to date but it is likely to be a clinical non-issue as the intensities produced by existing commercial therapeutic equipment are too low.
- Blood cell stasis and endothelial damage have also been demonstrated in in vitro studies. Again, in a living human this is unlikely as a shallowly located reflecting surface is needed (metal or glass) and the treatment head must be stationary.

If the patient feels any changes in pain or the development of some aching or prickling during the application, this signals actual or potential tissue damage and the intensity should be reduced immediately or the treatment terminated.

Extraneous radiation from the transducer into the therapist's hand is minimized by good equipment design and by users always holding the non-metal sections of the treatment head. There is, however, evidence from a small sample of frequent users of 1 MHz ultrasound that a reduced vibration sensitivity in the fingers may be a consequence (Lundstrom, 1985).

Research with small animals shows that cavitation damage can occur when air is within or near the tissues, such as with the lungs (Barnett et al., 2000) or gut (Rapid Response Group, 1999) or immediately following surgery. This is presumably due to almost complete reflection of wave energy at the tissue–air boundary.

CONTRAINDICATIONS AND RISKS

The distinctions between contraindications and risks are not always obvious. They require agreement on precisely when a risk is worth taking (risk) and when it is never worth taking (contraindication). Some of the resultant inconsistencies were described in a study of the contraindications usually described for heating and ultrasound (Batavia, 2004). Evidence to substantiate the claims made in the following section is provided when possible. Otherwise an attempt is made to indicate the likely level of risk. However, changing the dosage can alter the risks considerably, making a previously acceptable situation now contraindicated as the risks are more likely to be realized.

Rapidly dividing tissue

Tumours

Applications of therapeutic levels of ultrasound have been shown to increase the rate of tumour growth in mice (Maxwell, 1995; Sicard-Rosenbaum et al., 1995, 1998). With gel as a couplant, 3 minute pulsed or continuous applications daily for 6 days also produced a slightly higher incidence of metastases than in those treated with sham ultrasound or no ultrasound (Maxwell, 1995). With a matched SATA intensity, the results seemed similar whether the ultrasound was pulsed or continuous (Sicard-Rosenbaum et al., 1998). This suggests that ultrasound, even at very low doses, should never be applied over a tumour or a possible tumour site.

> The exception is the use of focused ultrasound for tumour ablation. This requires a much higher focused, albeit brief, intensity designed to ensure tissue destruction and is not directly comparable to therapeutic ultrasound.

Pregnant uterus

Avoid applying ultrasound over a pregnant uterus. There is a possible risk to the rapidly dividing and differentiating cells of the embryo and fetus. A study of the effect on mouse fetal limb development after treatment by ultrasound found a dose-related response to ultrasound: as the intensity increased the percentage of non-viable limbs also increased (Houghton and Radman, 2000). The caveats in assuming that the same effects necessarily hold for humans concern the method used: a volume of approximately 20 ml of fluid was treated with ultrasound. This bears little relationship to the possible fetal dose in utero, a much bigger tissue volume and depth that might safely absorb sufficient ultrasound energy and reduce the risk to near zero. Consistent with this, diagnostic ultrasound is believed to be safe for mammalian tissues at levels, in vivo, below $0.1 \, W \, cm^{-2}$ (Barnett et al., 2000): an intensity which at times approximates low doses of therapeutic ultrasound.

> In the absence of incontrovertible evidence of safety, therapists are well advised not to use therapeutic level doses of ultrasound over the uterus when pregnancy is a possibility.

small increase in the concentration in fat tissue, approximately $2\,\text{ng}\,\text{mg}^{-1}$, irrespective of the method used. The other interesting outcome was that the increase in plasma levels was only slight and occurred with pulsed ultrasound only. An important implication of this study is that methods used to assay a drug in a living human may not be optimal and may explain some of the apparent relative lack of effectiveness compared to phonophoresis in animals. Another implication is that using pulsed ultrasound may have a considerable advantage as the lower level of heating increases tolerance of this method over continuous ultrasound.

A range of drugs has been delivered using phonophoresis. They include steroids, anti-inflammatories and local anaesthetics.

Summary

In phonophoresis:

- ultrasound facilitates the passage of some drugs into and through the skin
- the effects are due both to absorption of the drug and to the ultrasound
- lower ultrasound frequencies appear to lead to a more effective drug penetration
- pulsing the ultrasound improves the drug penetration and reduces skin heating
- the quantity of drug entering the skin is proportional, in general, to the time and intensity of ultrasound application.

Application

The drug to be driven into the tissues is combined with a suitable gel or cream which forms the couplant. It is smeared onto the part, using a spatula so that it is not applied to the therapist's fingers. The treatment head is moved over the skin in the usual manner. Relatively high intensities of 1 and $1.5\,\text{W}\,\text{cm}^{-2}$ have been used with either a continuous or pulsed output. The depth of the target tissue determines the frequency used. The time of treatment depends on the area over which phonophoresis is to be applied; 1 minute treatment for every $10\,\text{cm}^2$ area is reasonable, although Griffin et al. (1967) suggest 5 minutes for each $25\,\text{in}^2$, i.e. about 1 minute for $30\,\text{cm}^2$. The pulsed mode appears to be more effective, as noted above.

When treatment is completed the remaining couplant, containing the drug, should be removed from both the patient's skin and the ultrasound transducer. Otherwise any remaining drug may be inadvertently and inappropriately applied to the next person treated.

As the cream or gel containing the drug is also the couplant, it is important that it transmits ultrasound adequately. This was investigated for a number of different products and identified wide variations and several with poor transmissivity (Benson and McElnay, 1988, 1994). Measured transmissivities, compared to water as the couplant, ranged from zero to 120%. Transmissivity depends on three factors: the half-value depth in the couplant, the amount of reflection at the sound-head/couplant interface and the couplant/skin interface and the thickness of the couplant layer. Of these three, the thickness of the couplant layer is most important. Unfortunately, the thickness was not measured or controlled in these studies. In clinical practice too, the thickness would not be known and would be difficult to control.

Two valid conclusions can be drawn from the cited studies. Gels are generally more efficient coupling agents than creams, particularly for higher (1.5 and 3 MHz) frequency ultrasound. This is probably because gels are able to form thin layers compared to thicker, more viscous creams. The problem with creams is compounded by the fact that they are emulsions, consisting of tiny oil bubbles suspended in water. Energy is reflected and scattered at each bubble surface, resulting in greater absorption of ultrasound energy in the couplant.

> If the thickness of the couplant layer is much smaller than the ultrasound wavelength, the layer is transparent to the ultrasound. In practice this means a layer less than a few tenths of a millimetre in thickness – easily achieved with most gels.

Contraindications

The same considerations apply when using phonophoresis as ultrasound. The effect of the drug must also be considered, e.g. anti-inflammatory drugs may suppress necessary inflammatory reactions, and responses to local skin infections, allowing them to become more serious. If local skin anaesthetizing drugs are being used, the person's capacity to detect heat from the ultrasound under the treatment head will gradually be lost: pulsing is preferable in this instance. As noted earlier, pulsing may be a more effective mechanism as mechanical vibration may facilitate transmission more effectively than temperature elevation as such.

LONGWAVE ULTRASOUND

This chapter has considered therapeutic ultrasound at megahertz frequencies, but there are machines with lower frequency outputs of 45 kHz. The wavelength of 3.3 cm is, therefore, some twenty times that of 1 MHz ultrasound, hence it is called 'longwave' ultrasound. At this frequency the ultrasonic beam diverges considerably in the tissues and is much less rapidly attenuated than MHz frequency ultrasound. A consequence of this marked divergence and a greater reflection from the irradiated surface is that strong, superficial energy absorption occurs and, in spite of the greater penetration depth, considerable heating occurs in a few millimetres of surface tissue, as with infrared radiation or a hot pack (Robertson and Ward, 1997).

The particle displacement at 45 kHz is far greater than at 1 MHz at the same acoustic pressure and this is said to be one of the key issues in the effectiveness of longwave ultrasound (Dyson et al., 1999).

Therapeutic benefit beyond that due to MHz ultrasound has been claimed for treatment with longwave ultrasound (Bradnock et al., 1996), but the major supporting study has been heavily criticized (Robertson and Ward, 1997).

COMBINATION THERAPY

The application of two therapeutic modalities at the same time, and to the same site, is described as combination therapy. The most widely used combinations are those of ultrasound with some form of nerve and muscle stimulating current (e.g. ultrasound and interferential). This is possible because the ultrasonic transducer can provide low-resistance electrical contact with the skin.

An important factor with combination therapy is that the couplant used should transmit both forms of energy. Thus an ultrasound gel used also for electrical stimulation should be a good electrical conductor.

Ward (1984) compared the electrical conductivities of a number of gels and found that some ultrasound gels had very poor electrical conductivity.

The production, application and therapeutic effects are those of the individual therapies as described in this text. The justification for using combination therapy is principally that the benefits of both modalities may be achieved at the same time, making the therapy time efficient for the therapist and patient. A second justification is a possible enhancing effect of one therapy upon the other, making the combination more effective than each therapy alone. At present there is no evidence to support the second claim.

There are, however, some risks with applying two modalities either concurrently or sequentially. Using any modality that alters cutaneous sensation by heating or cooling the skin or changing pressure/light touch perception can increase the risks when using another modality. There is currently neither supporting evidence for any clinical benefit nor evidence of any enhancing effects of combination therapies in their present form.

DIAGNOSTIC ULTRASOUND

The previous section has discussed what ultrasound is, its effects on tissues and clinical uses of therapeutic ultrasound. The focus of this section is ultrasound for imaging, where ultrasound is used to visualize the arrangement and composition of tissue at depth.

Biophysical principles

The major differences between therapeutic and diagnostic ultrasound lie in the equipment used and the aims of applying it. Diagnostic equipment differs from therapeutic in one major respect: the transducer is more complex and is designed to detect ultrasound energy reflected from the tissues as well as supplying it. The transducer emits bursts of MHz frequency ultrasound. This is similar to pulsed ultrasound but the bursts are of very short duration and the interval between bursts is long. When the ultrasound wave strikes a boundary, some of the energy is reflected back to the transducer. The amount of energy reflected depends on the difference in impedance. Thus reflection at the fat/muscle boundary is small (about 1%) while at a soft tissue/bone boundary it is larger (about 25%). Since only a small amount of energy is reflected at soft tissue interfaces, the detectors in the transducer must be very sensitive and they can only be used in the interval between bursts, otherwise the ultrasound energy produced by the transducer would swamp the tiny reflected signals which are typically 1/1000 times smaller.

Ultrasound imaging apparatus is able to construct an image of deep tissue by measuring the time delay between the emitted and reflected bursts. When a reflected signal is detected, the time delay is used to calculate the distance of the reflecting interface from the transducer. If only a single detector is used, the time delay indicates how deep the reflecting boundary is, but gives no information about the shape of the tissue surface. If a number of detectors are used, each in a different location, the time delay between the detected reflected pulses can be used to generate a three-dimensional map of the tissue volume. Signals reflected from the different tissue interfaces are thus sufficient to indicate the shape, nature and location of the underlying tissues in a graphic image when multiple detectors are used.

The reflected signals are amplified and modified so they can form screen images and be stored electronically. At this stage, some of the very weak reflected signals and electronic 'noise' are deleted to optimize the images. The final image produced is not as clear and as detailed as an MRI (magnetic resonance image) or CAT (computerized axial tomography) scan. Despite this, diagnostic ultrasound apparatus has some advantages over the equipment used for MRI or CAT scans: it is comparatively cheap and can be portable. It also avoids the X-ray exposure of a CAT scan.

Changes at the cellular level are not visible with ultrasound. This is because cells (and anything smaller) are not visible as they are much smaller than one wavelength. For example, 4 MHz ultrasound with a wave velocity in soft tissue of $1500 \, \text{m s}^{-1}$ has a wavelength given by the wave equation, $v = f\lambda$ so:

$$\lambda = \frac{v}{f} = \frac{1500}{4 \times 10^6} \approx 4 \times 10^{-4} \text{m or } 0.4 \, \text{mm}$$

so anything which is a lot smaller than 0.4 mm is 'transparent' in the sense that it is too small to reflect 4 MHz ultrasound appreciably. The ultrasound wavelength thus dictates the size of the structures which can be detected and visualized.

Air cavities and bone block the ultrasound beam: ultrasound is not transmitted. Consequently, diagnostic ultrasound is not useful where

Penetration depth and absorption of energy in tissues are also an issue. A low penetration depth will mean appreciable absorption of ultrasound energy and this will further reduce the amount of reflected energy reaching the detectors.

CAT is an acronym for computerized axial tomography, which uses bursts of X-rays sequentially beamed from several directions to generate a 3-D image of tissue structures.

Gas in the bowel and lungs can limit the value of doing some ultrasound scans. Inside joints, ultrasound is of no use for visualization.

bone or gas is lying between the probe and the area of interest. The reason that air-filled cavities are a problem is that when ultrasound travelling through soft tissue strikes an air boundary, the difference in impedance is so great that almost all of the ultrasound energy is reflected. The result of the strong reflection is a sharp and clear image of the top surface of the air-filled cavity but no view of the opposite surface or underlying tissues. The reason that bone is a problem is that the penetration depth of ultrasound in bone is so small (see Table 9.3) that the amount of ultrasound energy penetrating bone and reaching the underlying tissue is negligible.

This brief outline describes the major categories of equipment that are currently used and issues in interpreting ultrasound images. To become a proficient user requires both an understanding of the physics of ultrasound and a knowledge of the equipment and anatomy which is beyond the scope of this text. Books such as Dowsett et al. (1998) provide a good introduction.

The focus of this section is relatively narrow and is on some aspects of the use of ultrasound for imaging the musculoskeletal system rather than the more widely known use, imaging of the fetus in utero.

Types of diagnostic ultrasound

A familiar example of the Doppler effect is the sound heard by someone standing near a railway line as a train passes with its horn sounding. As the train approaches, the sound heard is high-pitched (a higher frequency than actually produced by the horn). When the train passes the sound changes from high to low pitch (a lower frequency).

The two main types of diagnostic ultrasound now used are real-time and Doppler ultrasound. Real time ultrasound gives rapidly changing scans of tissue in which new images are presented so quickly that there is the illusion of continuous or 'real time' movement. Real-time imaging thus generates a seemingly continuous display of moving tissue such as a contracting muscle or a fetus. Doppler ultrasound exploits the Doppler effect, whereby if a reflecting surface is moving towards or away from the detector, the frequency is changed. The changed frequency is used to produce ultrasound images which emphasize movement such as occurs with blood flow.

An important change over time is the increase in the output of diagnostic ultrasound machines. In the past their output was orders of magnitude smaller than therapeutic ultrasound machines. This is now not so as a comparison of the heating produced by the following three types of ultrasound units shows (Atkins and Duck, 2003): Scanner A, a 4.8 MHz curved array with both pulsed Doppler and colour Doppler modes; Scanner B, a more recent 3 MHz pulsed Doppler scanner with an output among the highest of commercially available diagnostic scanners, and a 3 MHz frequency therapeutic ultrasound machine used at a spatial average output of $1 \, W \, cm^{-2}$ with a 1:4 pulsing regimen and an effective radiating area (ERA) of the transducer of $5 \, cm^2$. A 10 minute period of insonation by the therapeutic equipment produced a 1°C temperature rise at the transducer and for Scanner B, 3.2°C. At depth in the tissue model used, Scanner B again produced a higher temperature rise, 2.8°C at 10 cm compared to 0.4°C for Scanner A at 4 cm and 0.8°C at 1 cm for the therapeutic equipment.

At the depth of the bone the rise was even higher for Scanner B, 6.4°C versus 2.5°C for the therapy equipment and 1.4°C for Scanner A. This study highlights the issue of temperature rise at the transducer (transducer self-heating) and the extent of heating that is possible in tissue when using pulsed Doppler ultrasound.

A risk of the higher output intensities used for diagnostic ultrasound is that they might cause excessive heating and adverse biological effects. Three major potential sites of heating are of interest: at the transducer face, at depth within tissue, and at the bone interface.

Some aspects of real-time ultrasound and Doppler ultrasound (including their risks) are briefly described, along with factors that affect the images they produce.

Real-time ultrasound

Real-time ultrasound provides visualization of moving structures (such as contracting muscle, heart or a fetus). As the scanner is moved over soft tissues the images are provided on a continuing basis. The rate of image production is sufficiently fast that they appear instantaneous as well as flicker free. Contractions of individual muscles or the movement of fetal limbs can then be seen by a viewer either as a moving image or a series of fixed images.

Different types of transducers are used to produce real-time images. The main ones are the phased, linear and curved arrays. The importance of the array is that its shape and size affect the image obtained, the quality of resolution and the size and depth of the view.

Factors affecting the image

The quality of the image will be affected by a range of factors including the properties of the ultrasound applied and of the arrangement and types of underlying structures. Both types of factors are described below.

The *frequency* affects the penetration of ultrasound in the tissues and consequently the image obtainable. To visualize more superficial tissues a frequency of between 7 to 15 MHz is usually used (Dowsett et al., 1998). This includes many superficial musculoskeletal structures as well as the scrotum and thyroid. For deeper structures the frequency has to be lower and is usually between 2 and 5 MHz for abdominal, pelvic and obstetric scans.

The level of *power*, and therefore intensity, applied also affects the possible viewing depth. Applying a higher level of power means that more energy is available at a greater depth. It can also increase the number of artefacts and the brightness of the image as more energy is available for reflection.

Properties of underlying tissues are important as the extent of the reflection (echo) from a structure will depend on its composition and shape. Acoustic shadowing, for example, occurs when ultrasound

A viewer must be aware not only of the properties of ultrasound but also of the cross-sectional anatomy to interpret accurately some of the images.

The 'secondary' reflections produced by air occur because the tissue–air boundary is almost completely reflective, unlike bone and gallstones, which are partly reflective but block transmission by rapidly absorbing the ultrasound.

does not penetrate through a structure. Instead, the beam is largely absorbed or reflected (Dogra and Rubens, 2004). For example, stones in a gall bladder are effectively ultrasound opaque, causing a shadowing effect on the distal side. Similarly bone and air in the gut or lungs will form a shadow and limit the viewing of structures on their other side. Air will also produce secondary reflections and a 'dirty' shadowing (Middleton et al., 2004). The following list gives examples of some of the major types of artefacts due to the different properties of the tissues and their relationships to others:

● *echogenecity* – a hyperechoic structure, such as gas or metal, will reflect all or most of the signal back. Conversely, a structure can be hypoechoic (or echopenic) and produce very few reflections relative to others in the area. The extreme of this is an anechoic structure which fully absorbs and attenuates ultrasound energy.

● *enhancement* – the image of a structure underlying a weakly attenuating layer will be relatively enhanced. Fluid, for example, does not attenuate ultrasound as much as adjacent structures might. Structures on the other side of a collection of fluid, such as a cyst, might appear brighter than if it was a solid tissue because there is less absorption in the fluid (Middleton et al., 2004).

● *mirror imaging* – flat surfaces and gas can act as a mirror and reflect an image. The base of the right lung can be used to reflect the image of the liver and diaphragm, as can the trachea during neck scans (Middleton et al., 2004).

Refraction only occurs if a beam strikes a boundary at an angle other than 90°. This is inevitable in ultrasonography as the tissue structures are invariably curved.

● *refraction* – ultrasound reflections are redirected (refracted) by an interface between acoustically different structures. This occurs, for example, at the junction of the muscle, rectus abdominus, and the fat of the abdominal wall (Middleton et al., 2004). As a result the image from a midline scan can show a duplication of the deeper abdominal and pelvic structures.

● *ring down* – gas and metal in the area are hyperechoic and can produce bright echoes deep to them because of the reflection back to the transducer of the signal.

● *side-lobe* – rarely, the weaker side lobes (the off-axis peaks in the Fresnel zone, see Figure 9.3) can be reflected by a strong reflector and be detected (Middleton et al., 2004).

● *beam width effect* – given a beam width will often be smaller than the structure being examined, only parts will be seen in any one image.

For a clear picture of the tendon structure, the applicator should be at 90°. At other angles the fibrillar structure may be less evident and any pathology may be masked.

● *angle at which energy is applied* – if a tissue is anisotropic, its echogenicity may vary with the orientation of the structure to the beam (Middleton et al., 2004). Thus the nature and quality of the image may depend on the angle at which energy is applied. For example, a tendon comprises a number of fibres that, when imaged at 90°, produces a clear fibrillar pattern: a set of closely spaced and parallel lines which represent the fibres of the tendon.

Musculoskeletal imaging

The main musculoskeletal structures visualized using ultrasound have high levels of attenuation. Consequently they appear as follows (Middleton et al., 2004):

- tendons and ligaments, hypoechoic unless visualized at 90° when they produce fibrillar images
- muscles, hypoechoic
- articular cartilage, either anechoic or hypoechoic
- fibrocartilage, anechoic to hypoechoic
- peripheral nerves, hypoechoic.

Musculoskeletal ultrasound imaging has a range of uses, diagnostic, research and during treatment (Stokes et al 1997). These uses include the following:

- To investigate:
  - the integrity of ligaments, muscles and tendons and to grade the extent of any damage
  - if an avulsion of a ligament or tendon has occurred
  - the extent and location of bleeding within tissues
  - any changes in a bursa
  - changes in the structure or location of fat pads
  - changes in muscle bulk, hypertrophy or atrophy and measuring them (Perkin et al., 2003; Chi-Fishman et al., 2004)
  - the location and identification of foreign bodies (Middleton et al., 2004)
  - masses to ascertain if cystic, solid or complex, its source and vascularity (Middleton et al., 2004).
- To diagnose differentially the following:
  - changes in tendons, such as an Achilles tendinopathy
  - complex lesions such as involve the rotator cuff muscles and subacromial area
  - what an intramuscular mass is.
- For accurately locating an injection site
  - for aspirating a joint or bursa
  - for injecting a steroid or local anaesthetic.
- For feedback
  - identifying if and when a muscle is contracting, such as particular spinal muscles that are too deep to be palpated or pelvic muscle activity (Whittaker, 2004)
  - on changes in muscle bulk following exercise or electrical stimulation.

Doppler ultrasound

Dopper ultrasound is often used to visualize blood flow. The Doppler effect means that as an erythrocyte moves it reflects successive ultrasound signals at a changing frequency. By including information on this change in frequency, the Doppler frequency shift, another dimension of information, is added to that used in real-time ultrasonography.

The three common types of Doppler ultrasound units are briefly described below. As noted above, one problem with this type of equipment is that it often produces a reasonable level of tissue heating owing to the high energy. Given that the extent of sensitivity of fetal tissue to ultrasound is unknown, Doppler is not recommended for use in early pregnancy (Barnett et al., 1997).

Duplex (pulsed) Doppler

Equipment which has a pulsed Doppler output and produces grey-scale images, enhanced to indicate areas where movement is occurring, is called duplex Doppler (Middleton et al., 2004). Duplex Doppler is particularly useful for identifying flow in even quite small vessels and for detecting arterial stenosis.

Colour Doppler

Colour Doppler provides a real-time image but with the blood flow in colour and the other tissues in grey (Middleton et al., 2004). This type of ultrasound is the one most commonly used to assess blood flow to an area and its direction of flow. Vessel contents moving towards the scanner are assigned blue, and those moving away, red. This type of ultrasound is used primarily to identify vessels, especially small ones, and any areas where flow is obstructed or changed.

Power Doppler

Power Doppler is used to indicate the level of flow in blood vessels. However, it does not show the direction of flow or indicate the velocity as does colour Doppler. This type is generally used less frequently than the other two types.

For information on problems with imaging when using Doppler ultrasound and for details of examinations of particular areas in the body, readers are referred to appropriate texts on the subject (e.g. Dowsett et al., 1998; Middleton et al., 2004) as both are beyond the scope of the present book.

Dangers and contraindications

The issues of the dangers of diagnostic ultrasound have been thoroughly investigated owing to its frequent use for in utero examination of a fetus. Consequently, there are many papers discussing the issues including the sensitivity of biological tissue to ultrasound and making appropriate recommendations for its use (Barnett et al., 1997,

2000). At present, there is no convincing epidemiological evidence (Duck and Shaw, 2003) that diagnostic ultrasound used for fetal development is a hazard for the following:

- causing low birth weight
- an increase in childhood malignancies
- altering speech or neurological development.

The level of risk is controlled largely by the following:

- keeping the ultrasound intensity to a safe value
- the quality of manufacture of equipment and appropriate ongoing maintenance and testing (quality assurance)
- selection and use of appropriate equipment and parameters
- suitably trained users and operators.

References

AIUM Bioeffects Report. (2000). Selected biological properties of tissues: potential determinants of susceptibility to ultrasound-induced bioeffects. J Ultrasound Med, **19**, 85–96.

Anderson, T., Wakim, K., Herrick, J. et al. (1951). An experimental study of the effects of ultrasonic energy on the lower part of the spinal cord and peripheral nerves. Arch Phys Med, **32**, 71–83.

Artho, P., Thyne, J., Warring, B. et al. (2002). A calibration study of therapeutic ultrasound units. Phys Ther, **82**, 257–263.

Atkins, T., Duck, F. (2003). Heating caused by selected Doppler and physiotherapy ultrasound beams measured using thermal test objects. Eur J Ultrasound, **16**, 243–252.

Baker, K., Robertson, V., Duck, F. (2001). A review of therapeutic ultrasound: Biophysical effects. Phys Ther, **81**, 1351–1358.

Bare, A., McAnaw, M., Pritchard, A. et al. (1996). Phonophoretic delivery of 10% hydrocortisone through the epidermis of humans as determined by serum cortisol concentrations. Phys Ther, **76**, 738–749.

Barnett, S., Rott, H., ter Haar, G. (1997). The sensitivity of biological tissue to ultrasound. Ultrasound Med Biol, **23**, 805–812.

Barnett, S., ter Haar, G., Ziskin, M. et al. (2000). International recommendations and guidelines for the safe use of diagnostic ultrasound in medicine. Ultrasound Med Biol, **26**, 355–366.

Batavia, M. (2004). Contraindications for superficial heat and therapeutic ultrasound: Do sources agree. Arch Phys Med Rehabil, **85**, 1006–1012.

Benson, H., McElnay, J. (1988). Transmission of ultrasound energy through pharmaceutical products. Physiotherapy, **74**, 587–589.

Benson, H., McElnay, J. (1994). Topical non-steroidal anti-inflammatory products as ultrasound couplants: their potential in phonophoresis. Physiotherapy, **80**, 74–76.

Berliner, M., Piegsa, M. (1997). Effects of therapeutic ultrasound in a water bath on skin microcirculation and skin temperature in rheumatoid arthritis. Eur J Med Rehabil, **7**, 46–49.

Bishop, S., Draper, D., Knight, K. et al. (2004). Human tissue-temperature rise during ultrasound treatments with the Aquaflex gel pad. J Athletic Training, **39**, 126–131.

Bradnock, B., Law, H., Roscoe, K. (1996). A quantitative comparative assessment of the immediate response to high frequency ultrasound and low frequency ultrasound ('longwave therapy') in the treatment of acute ankle sprains. Physiotherapy, **82**, 78–84.

Brosseau, L., Casimiro, L., Robinson, V. et al. (2004). Therapeutic ultrasound for treating patellofemoral pain syndrome (Cochrane Review). In The Cochrane Library, Issue 3. Chichester, UK: John Wiley & Sons, Ltd.

Busse, J., Bhandari, M., Kulkarni, A., Tunks, E. (2002). The effect of low-intensity pulsed ultrasound therapy on time to fracture healing: a meta-analysis. Can Med Assoc J, **166**, 437–441.

Byl, N., McKenzie, A., Wong, T. et al. (1993). Incisional wound healing: A controlled study of low and high dose ultrasound. J Orthop Sports Phys Ther, **18**, 619–628.

Byl, N., McKenzie, A., West, J. et al. (1992). Low dose ultrasound effects on wound healing: a controlled study with Yucatan pigs. Arch Phys Med Rehabil, **73**, 656–664.

Cagnie, B., Vinck, E., Rimbaut, S., Vanderstraeten, G. (2003). Phonophoresis versus topical application of ketoprofen: comparison between tissue and plasma levels. Phys Ther, **83**, 701–712.

Callam, M., Harper, D., Dale, J. et al. (1987). A controlled trial of weekly ultrasound therapy in chronic leg ulceration. Lancet, July 25, 204–206.

Cambier, D., Vanderstraeten, G. (1997). Failure of therapeutic ultrasound in healing burn injuries. Burns, **23**, 248–249.

Casarotto, R., Adamowski, J., Fallopa, F. (2004). Coupling agents in therapeutic ultrasound: acoustic and thermal behavior. Arch Phys Med Rehabil, **85**, 162–165.

Casimiro, L., Brosseau, L., Robinson, V. et al. (2004). Therapeutic ultrasound for the treatment of rheumatoid arthritis (Cochrane Review). In The Cochrane Library, Issue 3. Chichester, UK: John Wiley & Sons, Ltd.

Chan, A., Myrer, J., Measom, G., Draper, D. (1998). Temperature changes in human patellar tendon in response to therapeutic ultrasound. J Athletic Training, **33**, 130–135.

Chi-Fishman, G., Hicks, J., Cintas, H. et al. (2004). Ultrasound imaging distinguishes between normal and weak muscle. Arch Phys Med Rehabil, **85**, 980–986.

Cook, S., Salkeld, S., Popich-Patron, L. et al. (2001). Improved cartilage repair after treatment with low-intensity pulsed ultrasound. Clin Orthop Rel Res, **391** Suppl, S231–243.

Craig, J., Bradley, J., Walsh, D. et al. (1999). Delayed onset muscle soreness: lack of effect of therapeutic ultrasound in humans. Arch Phys Med Rehabil, **80**, 318–323.

da Cunha, A., Parizotto, N., Vida, B. (2001). The effect of therapeutic ultrasound on repair of the achilles tendon (tendo calcaneus) of the rat. Ultrasound Med Biol, **27**, 1691–1696.

Daniel, D., Rupert, R. (2003). Calibration and electrical safety status of therapeutic ultrasound used by chiropractic physicians. J Manip Physiol Ther, **26**, 171–175.

De Forest, R., Herrick, J., Janes, J., Krusen, F. (1953). Effects of ultrasound on growing bone. Arch Phys Med Rehabil, **34**, 21–31.

Demmink, J., Helders, P., Hobaek, H., Enwemeka, C. (2003). The variation of heating depth with therapeutic ultrasound frequency in physiotherapy. Ultrasound Med Biol, **29**, 113–118.

Dogra, V., Rubens, D. (2004). Ultrasound secrets. Philadelphia: Hanley & Belfus.

Dowsett, D., Kenny, P., Johnston, R. (1998). The Physics of Diagnostic Imaging. New York: Chapman & Hall Medical.

Draper, D. (2002). Don't disregard ultrasound yet – the jury is still out. Phys Ther, **82**, 190.

Draper, D., Anderson, C., Schulthies, S., Ricard, M. (1998b). Immediate and residual changes in dorsiflexion range of motion using an ultrasound heat and stretch routine. J Athletic Training, **33**, 141–144.

Draper, D., Harris, S., Schulthies, S. et al. (1998a). Hot-pack and 1-MHz ultrasound treatments have an additive effect on muscle temperature increase. J Athletic Training, **33**, 21–24.

Draper, D., Schulthies, S., Sorvisto, P., Hautala, A. (1995). Temperature changes in deep muscles of humans during ice and ultrasound therapies: An in vivo study. J Orthop Sports Phys Ther, **21**, 153–157.

Duck, F., Shaw, A. (2003). Safety of diagnostic ultrasound. In P. Hoskins, A. Thrush, K. Martin, T. Whittingham (eds), Diagnostic ultrasound, pp. 179–203. London: Greenwich Medical Media Ltd.

Dyson, M. (1985). Therapeutic applications of ultrasound. In W. Nyborg, M. Ziskin (eds), Biological Effects of Ultrasound. London: Churchill Livingstone.

Dyson, M., Pond, J., Woodward, B. et al. (1974). The production of blood cell stasis and endothelial cell damage in the blood vessels of chick embryos treated with ultrasound in a stationary wavefield. Ultrasound Med Biol, **1**, 133–148.

Dyson, M., Pond J. (1970). The effect of pulsed ultrasound on tissue regeneration. Physiotherapy, **56**, 136–142.

Dyson, M., Pond, J. (1973). The effects of ultrasound on circulation. Physiotherapy, **59**, 284–287.

Dyson, M., Preston, R., Woledge, R., Kitchen, S. (1999). Longwave ultrasound. Physiotherapy, **85**, 40–49.

Dyson, M., Suckling, J. (1978). Stimulation of tissue repair by ultrasound: a survey of the mechanisms involved. Physiotherapy, **64**, 105–108.

Ebenbichler, G. (1998). Author's reply. Br Med J, **317**, 601.

Ebenbichler, G., Erdogmus, C., Resch, K. et al. (1999). Ultrasound therapy for calcific tendinitis of the shoulder. New Engl J Med, **340**, 1533–1538.

Ebenbichler, G., Resch, K., Nicolakis, P. et al. (1998). Ultrasound treatment for treating the carpal tunnel syndrome: randomised 'sham' controlled trial. Br Med J, **316**, 731–735.

Enwemeka, C. (1989). The effects of therapeutic ultrasound on tendon healing. Am J Phys Med Rehabil, **68**, 283–287.

Fabrizio, P., Schmidt, J., Clemente, F. et al. (1996). Acute effects of therapeutic ultrasound delivered at varying parameters on the blood flow velocity in a muscular distribution artery. J Orthop Sports Phys Ther, **24**, 294–302.

Flemming, K., Cullum, N. (2004). Therapeutic ultrasound for pressure sores (Cochrane Review). In The Cochrane Library, Issue 3. Chichester, UK: John Wiley & Sons, Ltd.

Frenkel, V., Kimmel, E., Iger, Y. (2000). Ultrasound induced intercellular space widening in fish epidermis. Ultrasound Med Biol, **26**, 473–480.

Frizzel L., Dunn F. (1982). Biophysics of ultrasound. In J. F. Lehmann, (ed.), Therapeutic Heat and Cold. Baltimore: Williams & Wilkins.

Fyfe, M., Bullock, M. (1985). Therapeutic ultrasound: Some historical background and development in knowledge of its effect on healing. Aust J Physiother, **31**, 220–224.

Fyfe, M., Chahl, I. (1982). Mast cell degradation: A possible mechanism of action of therapeutic ultrasound. Ultrasound Med Biol, 1 Suppl, 62.

Gam, A., Johannsen, F. (1995). Ultrasound therapy in musculoskeletal disorders: a meta-analysis. Pain, **63**, 85–91.

Gan, B., Huys, S., Sherebrin, M., Scilley, C. (1995). The effects of ultrasound treatment on flexor tendon healing in the chicken limb. J Hand Surgery, **20B**, 809–814.

Grey, K. (2003). Distribution of treatment time in physiotherapeutic application of ultrasound. Physiotherapy, **89**(12), 696–707.

Griffin, J. (1980). Transmissiveness of ultrasound through tap water, glycerin and mineral oil. Phys Ther, **60**, 1010–1016.

Griffin, J., Echternach, J., Price, R., et al. (1967). Patients treated with ultrasonic driven hydrocortisone and with ultrasound alone. Phys Ther, **74**, 594–601.

Gursel, Y., Ulus, Y., Bilgic, G., van der Heijden, G. (2004). Adding ultrasound in the management of soft tissue disorders of the shoulder: a randomized placebo-controlled trial. Phys Ther, **84**, 336–343.

Hadjiargyrou, M., McLeod, K., Ryaby, J., Rubin, C. (1998). Enhancement of fracture healing by low-intensity ultrasound. Clin Orthop, **355** (Suppl 2), 216–229.

Holmes, M., Rudland, J. (1991). Clinical trials of ultrasound treatment in soft tissue injury: A review and critique. Physiother Theory Pract, **7**, 163–175.

Hoogland, R. (1989). Ultrasound Therapy. Delft, Holland: Enraf-Nonius.

Houghton, P., Radman, A. (2000). Effects of therapeutic ultrasound on fetal limb development in an organ culture system. Physiother Theory Pract, **16**, 119–134.

Huang, M., Ding, H., Chai, C. et al. (1997). Effects of sonication on articular cartilage in experimental osteoarthritis. J Rheumatol, **24**, 1978–1984.

Jackson, B., Schwane, J., Starcher, B. (1991). Effect of ultrasound therapy on the repair of Achilles tendon injuries in rats. Med Sci Sports Exerc, **23**, 171–176.

Karnes, J., Burton, H. (2002). Continuous therapeutic ultrasound accelerates repair of contraction-induced skeletal muscle damage in rats. Arch Phys Med Rehabil, **83**, 1–4.

Kitchen, S., Partridge, C. (1996). A survey to examine the clinical use of ultrasound, shortwave diathermy and laser in England. Br J Ther Rehabil, **3**, 644–650.

Knight, C., Rutledge, C., Cox, M. et al. (2001). Effect of superficial heat, deep heat, and active exercise warm-up on the extensibility of the plantar flexors. Phys Ther, **81**, 1206–1214.

Kuehn, K., Ege, W., Gopp, U. (2005). Acrylic bone cements: mechanical and physical properties. Orthop Clin N Am, **36**, 29–39.

Kumar, D., Papini, R., Tillman, R. (2001). Partial growth plate fusion caused by burn. Burns, **27**, 664–667.

Lehmann, J., de Lateur, B. (1982). Therapeutic heat. In J. F. Lehmann (ed.), Therapeutic Heat and Cold, 3rd edn. Baltimore: Williams & Wilkins.

Lehmann J., Guy, A. (1972). Ultrasonic therapy in interaction of ultrasound and biological tissues. In J. M. Reid, M. R. Sikov (eds). Workshop Proceedings, pp. 141–152. US Dept of Health Education and Welfare publication (FDA) 73-8008,

Leung, M., Ng, G., Yip, K. (2004). Effect of ultrasound on acute inflammation of transected medial collateral ligaments. Arch Phys Med Rehabil, **85**, 963–966.

Levenson, J., Weissberg, M. (1983). Ultrasound abuse: a case report. Arch Phys Med Rehabil, **64**, 90–91.

Lowden, A. (1986). Application of ultrasound to assess stress fractures. Physiotherapy, **72**, 160–161.

Lowe, A., Walker, M., Cowan, R., Baxter, G. (2001). Therapeutic ultrasound and wound closure: lack of healing effect on x-ray irradiated wounds in murine skin. Arch Phys Med Rehabil, **82**, 1507–1511.

Lundstrom, R. (1985). Effects of local vibration transmitted from ultrasonic devices on vibrotactile perception in the hands of therapists. Ultrasonics, **28**, 793–803.

Lyon, R., Liu, X., Meier, J. (2003). The effects of therapeutic vs high-intensity ultrasound on the rabbit growth plate. J Orthop Res, **21**, 865–871.

Machet, L., Boucaud, A. (2002). Phonophoresis: efficiency, mechanisms and skin tolerance. Int J Pharma, **243**, 1–15.

Maxwell, L. (1995). Therapeutic ultrasound and the metastasis of a solid tumor. J Sport Rehabil, **4**, 273–281.

Mayr, E., Frankel, V., Ruter, A. (2000). Ultrasound – an alternative healing method for nonunions? Arch Orthop Trauma Surg, **120**, 1–8.

McLachlan, Z. (1991). Ultrasound treatment for breast engorgement: a randomised double blind trial. Aust J Physiother, **37**, 23–28.

Merrick, M., Bernard, K., Devor, S., Williams, J. (2003). Identical 3-MHz ultrasound treatments with different devices produce different intramuscular temperatures. J Orthop Sports Phys Ther, **33**, 379–385.

Merrick, M., Mihalyov, M., Roethemeier, J. et al. (2002). A comparison of intramuscular temperatures during ultrasound treatments with coupling gel or gel pads. J Orthop Sports Phys Ther, **32**, 216–220.

Middleton, W., Kurtz, A., Hertzberg, B. (2004). Ultrasound, 2nd edn. Missouri: Elsevier.

Monk, M. (1996). The application of 1 MHz ultrasound through applicator bags. Honours thesis, School of Physiotherapy, LaTrobe University, Australia.

Mortimer, A., Dyson, M. (1988). The effect of therapeutic ultrasound on calcium uptake in fibrinoblasts. Ultrasound Med Biol, **14**, 499–506.

Muche, J. A. (2003). Efficacy of therapeutic ultrasound treatment of a meniscus tear in a severely disabled patient: a case report. Arch Phys Med Rehabil, **84**, 1558–1559.

Nolte, P., van der Krans, A., Patka, P. et al. (2001). Low-intensity pulsed ultrasound in the treatment of nonunions. J Trauma Injury Infect Crit Care, **51**, 693–702; discussion 702–693.

Nyborg, W. (2001). Biological effects of ultrasound: development of safety guidelines. Part II: general review. Ultrasound Med Biol, **27**, 301–333.

Oshikoya, C., Shultz, S., Mistry, D. et al. (2003). Effect of coupling medium temperature on rate of intramuscular temperature rise using continuous ultrasound. J Athletic Training, **35**, 417–421.

Particular Requirements for Ultrasonic Physiotherapy Equipment. (2000). International Electrotechnical Commission, Geneva, Switzerland: IEC publication 60601-2-5 (2000-07).

Perkin, H., Bond, E., Thompson, J. et al. (2003). Real time ultrasound: an objective measure of skeletal muscle. Phys Ther Reviews, **8**, 99–108.

Plaskett, C., Tiidus, P., Livingston, L. (1999). Ultrasound treatment does not affect postexercise muscle strength recovery or soreness. J Sport Rehabil, **8**, 1–9.

Pringle, D. (1995). Therapeutic ultrasound: acoustic transmissiveness of wound dressings. Abstract from Physiotherapy Research Workshop at Manchester Royal Infirmary, Nov. 94. Physiotherapy, 81, 240.

Pye, S. (1996). Ultrasound therapy equipment – does it perform? Physiotherapy, **82**, 39–44.

Rantanen, J., Thorssen, O., Wollmer, P. et al. (1999). Effects of therapeutic ultrasound on the regeneration of skeletal myofibers after experimental muscle injury. Am J Sports Med, **27**, 54–62.

Rapid Response Group (1999). Ultrasound-induced morphological changes in the murine small intestine. Ultrasound Obstet Gynecol, **14**, 78.

Rivest, M., Girardi, C., Seaborne, D., Lambert, J. (1987). Evaluation of therapeutic ultrasound devices: performance stability over 44 weeks of clinical use. Physiother Can, **39**, 77–86.

Robertson, V. (2003). Therapeutic ultrasound: re-evaluating the evidence. Physiother Singapore, **6**, 114–121.

Robertson, V., Baker, K. (2001). A review of therapeutic ultrasound: effectiveness studies. Phys Ther, **81**, 1339–1350.

Robertson, V., Ward, A. (1997). Longwave (45 kHz) ultrasound reviewed and reconsidered. Physiotherapy, **83**, 123–130.

Robertson, V., Ward, A. (1995). Subaqueous ultrasound: 45 kHz and 1 MHz machines compared. Arch Phys Med Rehabil, **76**, 569–575.

Robinson, S., Buono, M. (1995). Effect of continuous-wave ultrasound on blood flow in skeletal muscle. Phys Ther, **75**, 145–150.

Romani, W., Perrin, D., Dussault, R. et al. (2000). Identification of tibial stress fractures using therapeutic continuous ultrasound. J Orthop Sports Phys Ther, **30**, 444–452.

Rubin, M., Etchison, M., Condra, K. et al. (1990). Acute effects of ultrasound on skeletal muscle oxygen tension, blood flow and capillary density. Ultrasound Med Biol, **16**, 271–277.

Selkowitz, D., Cameron, M., Mainzer, A., Wolfe, R. (2002). Efficacy of pulsed low-intensity ultrasound in wound healing: a single-case design. Ostomy Wound Management, **48**, 40–50.

Sicard-Rosenbaum, L., Danoff, J., Guthrie, J., Eckhaus, M. (1998). Effects of energy-matched pulsed and continuous ultrasound on tumor growth in mice. Phys Ther, **78**, 271–277.

Sicard-Rosenbaum, L., Lord, D., Danoff, J. et al. (1995). Effects of continuous therapeutic ultrasound on growth and metastasis of subcutaneous murine tumors. Phys Ther, **75**, 3–13.

Stasinopoulos, D., Stasinopoulos, I. (2004). Comparison of effects of exercise programme, pulsed ultrasound and transverse friction in the treatment of chronic patellar tendinopathy. Clin Rehabil, **18**, 347–352.

Stokes, M., Hides, J., Nassiri, D. (1997). Musculoskeletal ultrasound imaging: diagnostic and treatment aid in rehabilitation. Phys Ther Rev, **2**, 73–92.

Takikawa, S., Matsui, N., Kokubu, T. et al. (2001). Low-intensity pulsed ultrasound initiates bone healing in rat nonunion fracture model. J Ultrasound Med, **20**, 197–205.

ter Haar, G. (1987). Basic physics of therapeutic ultrasound. Physiotherapy, **73**, 110–113.

ter Haar G. (1996). Electrophysical principles. In S. Kitchen, S. Bazin, (eds), Clayton's Electrotherapy, 10th edn. Philadelphia: W. B. Saunders.

ter Riet, G., Kessels, A., Knipschild, P. (1996). A randomised clinical trial of ultraound in the treatment of pressure ulcers. Phys Ther, **76**, 1301–1311.

van der Heijden, G, van der Windt, D., de Winter, A. (1997). Physiotherapy for patients with soft tissue shoulder disorders: a systematic review of randomised clinical trials. Br Med J, **315**, 25–29.

van der Windt, D., van der Heijden, G., Van Den Berg, S. et al. (1999). Ultrasound therapy for musculoskeletal disorders: a systematic review. Pain, **81**, 257–271.

van der Windt, D., van der Heijden, G., Van Den Berg, S. et al. (2002). Ultrasound therapy for acute ankle sprains. Cochrane Database Syst Rev, (1), CD001250.

Ward, A. (1984). Electrode coupling media for transcutaneous electrical nerve stimulation. Aust J Physiother, **30**, 82–85.

Ward, A. (1986). Electricity fields and waves in therapy. Marrickville: Science Press.

Ward, A. (2004) Biophysical bases of electrotherapy. Mount Waverley: Excell Biomedical Publications. (On the CD accompanying this text.)

Ward, A., Robertson, V. (1996). Dosage factors for the subaqueous application of 1 MHz ultrasound. Arch Phys Med Rehabil, **77**, 1167–1172.

Warden, S., Bennell, K., McMeeken, J., Wark, J. (2000). Accelerations of fresh fracture repair using the sonic accelerated fracture healing system (SAFHS): a review. Calcif Tissue Int, **66**, 157–163.

Welch, V., Brosseau, L., Peterson, J. et al. (2004). Therapeutic ultrasound for osteoarthritis of the knee (Cochrane Review). In The Cochrane Library, Issue 3. Chichester, UK: John Wiley & Sons, Ltd.

Whittaker, J. (2004). Abdominal ultrasound imaging of pelvic floor muscle function in individuals with low back pain. J Manual Manipulative Ther, **12**, 44–49.

Williams, R. (1987). Production and transmission of ultrasound. Physiotherapy, **73**, 113–116.

Young, S. (1996). Ultrasound therapy. In S. Kitchen & S. Bazin (eds), Clayton's Electrotherapy (10th edn, pp. 243–267). Philadelphia: WB Saunders.

Young, S., Dyson, M. (1990). Macrophage responsiveness to therapeutic ultrasound. Ultrasound Med Biol, **16**, 261–269.

Heat and cold

Heat and cold are probably the oldest of all physical therapies; in one form or another, both have been applied to the body for healing throughout recorded history.

This chapter deals with the underlying basic concepts associated with heat and cold. Therapeutic applications of heat and cold to the body surface are considered in chapters 11 and 12 and deep heating in chapters 9, 13 and 15.

To this end the general principles, including the meaning of temperature, quantity of heat, heat transfer and energy conversions, are all considered at the beginning of the chapter. The thermal regulatory mechanisms of the body are described and explained, with the physiological consequences of temperature changes at the body surface. This forms the bulk of the chapter. Finally, the therapeutic effects of local tissue heating, but not cooling, are addressed.

It should be noted that therapeutic modalities that produce tissue heating differ in their effects more because of the tissue volume, site and magnitude of tissue heating rather than any difference in its nature. This chapter therefore focuses on the general effects of local tissue heating. The particular features of different heating modalities are described in later chapters, as is cooling.

Despite the fact that heat and cold are very familiar ideas, the fundamental nature of heat is often not well understood. A study of the basic science of heat is central to recognizing the way in which therapy works.

GENERAL PRINCIPLES

To understand what happens when matter becomes hot it is necessary to consider the microstructure of matter.

Solids are formed of collections of atoms or molecules bonded together in a regular pattern and packed very closely, so that each can only move a short distance. The atoms or molecules vibrate about their equilibrium positions and it is the movement energy – kinetic energy – which is recognized as heat. If more heat energy is added the amount of motion increases and usually (but not in all circumstances) the matter becomes hotter, i.e. the temperature increases.

In *liquids* the atoms or molecules have a rather greater amplitude of vibration and can briefly overcome the interatomic forces of their immediate neighbours which keep them in position. The atoms are

Adding heat energy does not always increase the temperature. At the melting point, heat is absorbed and the energy is used to convert the solid to a liquid. In this special circumstance the temperature does not increase.

thus able to move and change position randomly, even though still being tightly packed, as in a solid. It is this ability to jump positions which allows flow in liquids. The molecules have greater average speed and this is measured as an increased temperature.

In *gases* the atoms are widely spaced and move randomly over much larger distances. Adding heat causes more rapid motion so the movement (kinetic) energy of the molecules is increased and a temperature increase is registered. The average separation of the atoms increases as the matter expands. Expansion with increasing temperature is very evident in gases but less obvious in liquids and solids where bonding between molecules holds them together and limits expansion.

Temperature and thermometers

Temperature is a measure of the level of heat. Humans assess this level through special temperature receptors in the skin. The judgement made by the central nervous system is not absolute; rather it is a comparison of skin temperatures. If the right hand is immersed in hot and the left in cold water and both hands are then placed in tepid water it feels cold to the right hand and hot to the left. This illustrates a general feature of perception in the nervous system which tends to recognize contrasts.

To measure temperature two fixed points, the melting point of ice and the boiling point of water, are found and the region between them divided into 100 parts, called degrees. Such a scale, in which 0°C is the freezing point of water and 100°C is its boiling point, is known as the Celsius scale, abbreviated to °C.

As temperature is due to the kinetic energy of atoms and molecules there is no upper limit, but there is a definite lower limit where no motion occurs at all. This point is called absolute zero, and is −273.2°C. For much scientific work the more logical Kelvin scale is used; this is the SI (international system) unit of temperature. This treats absolute zero as 0 K and uses the same degrees as the Celsius scale so that the freezing point of water becomes 273 K and its boiling point 373 K.

A thermometer is an instrument that measures temperature. It may utilize any physical change that correlates with heating and cooling. By far the most familiar is the mercury-in-glass thermometer. This device depends on the expansion of mercury, which is much greater than that of glass when both are heated. The mercury-filled bulb is heated and the expansion is made visible because a thin line of mercury is forced along a narrow glass capillary tube. A typical clinical thermometer with a range of 30–45°C has a constriction in the capillary tube which breaks the mercury thread, preventing its return to the bulb as cooling occurs. This allows an accurate reading of the maximum temperature reached. The glass cylinder acts as a lens to enlarge the view of the mercury thread. These thermometers can

Contrast recognition results from the adaptation of sensory receptors. If the skin is suddenly heated or cooled, the relevant sensory fibres fire at high frequency, signalling the change in temperature, but quickly adapt and fire at lower frequencies at the new temperature.

The Fahrenheit scale was formerly used. Its use was discontinued in most parts of the world in the mid-twentieth century.

Alcohol-in-glass thermometers work in the same way as their mercury counterparts. They are usually larger and can be made easier to read by colouring the alcohol. They are often used for checking room or waterbath temperatures.

be extremely accurate: when new the vast majority are accurate to within 0.1°C (Cetas, 1982).

Another widely used thermometer (the bimetal strip thermometer) depends on the difference in expansion of two metals when they are heated. Such devices are sturdy but often inaccurate and are normally used as a thermostat to open or close a switch at a pre-set temperature. This kind of system is found controlling the temperature of domestic water heaters, room temperature, electric blankets, electric heater pads and the paraffin wax baths used in clinics, as well as many other situations.

Other thermometers use different effects. In the thermistor, which is a semiconductor, the electrical resistance decreases with rise in temperature. They can be manufactured to be very small – a tiny bead on the end of two fine wires – and are relatively accurate. For these reasons they are used as thermal probes (inserted using hypodermic needles) for testing temperature deep in the tissues. Infrared photodiodes are diodes whose conduction properties change when exposed to infrared radiation. They are used in modern digital thermometers and their speed, ease of use, non-invasiveness and safety has made them more popular for clinical use than mercury or alcohol thermometers.

Note: digital thermometers are no more accurate, and sometimes less reliable, than the mercury-in-glass type originally developed over 300 years ago (Cetas, 1982).

Quantity of heat

If a kettleful of boiling water is poured into a bath of tepid water the bath water may become perceptibly warmer but not nearly as hot as the water in the kettle. Clearly when a small quantity of water is added it carries a small quantity of heat which when spread throughout the larger volumes leads to little rise in temperature. To describe the quantity of heat a unit called the calorie was formerly used. This is the amount of heat needed to raise the temperature of 1 g of water by 1°C; but since it is an energy measurement the appropriate SI unit (the joule, abbreviated J) is now used.

In dietetics the kilocalorie is still widely used and is confusingly called the Calorie (with a capital C); this is equal to 4.18 kJ.

Heat capacity

The same amount of heat energy, applied to different materials, will produce different temperature increases. For example, 10 kJ of heat energy applied to 1 kg of iron will increase its temperature by 22°C. The same amount of energy applied to 1 kg of water will cause a temperature increase of only 2.4°. Water has a much higher heat capacity than iron. Heat capacity is defined as the amount of heat required to raise the temperature of 1 kg of a material by 1° (Celsius or Kelvin). This used to be called the 'specific heat' of a substance.

Water has a much greater heat capacity than other common materials (Table 10.1) so that it takes a great deal of heat energy to raise

Table 10.1 Heat capacity of different materials

	Heat capacity ($kJ\,K^{-1}\,kg^{-1}$)
Water	4.18
Air	1.01
Aluminium	0.90
Copper	0.40
Mercury	0.14
Glass	0.77
Paraffin wax	about 2.7
Rubber	2.0
Whole human body	3.6
Skin	3.8
Fat	2.3
Muscle	3.8
Bone	1.6
Whole blood	3.6

Data from Sekins and Emery (1982).

the temperature of water and conversely hot water stores much heat per unit mass.

The heat capacity of the human body is close to $3.6\,kJ\,K^{-1}\,kg^{-1}$ (Sekins and Emery, 1982) which is not surprising since it is 70% water. To raise the temperature of a 50 kg woman by 2°C it takes 360 kJ of energy ($50 \times 3.6 \times 2$). Notice that this would be additional to the energy continuously being generated in the body. In fact, even at rest the basal metabolic rate leads to the emission of heat.

The addition of heat

When heat is added to matter it can cause expansion (an increase in volume or, if the volume is restricted, an increase in pressure), it may change the physical state of the material, by melting or vaporizing it, it may cause a temperature rise in the material, or any combination of these. When water boils a change of state occurs in which the liquid is changed into gas. The heat energy is used in separating molecules, disrupting the bonding forces and changing the state from liquid to gas, rather than increasing the kinetic energy; therefore there is no rise of temperature during the process. Exactly the same thing happens when the solid form, i.e. ice, is melted to water and when any other substance is vaporized or melted.

In solids atoms are more strictly confined by neighbouring atoms so that the addition of heat leads to each atom oscillating more vigorously, increasing the average separation from other atoms, and hence expanding the whole material. When heat energy is added it not only goes to increasing the kinetic motion of the molecules, thus raising the temperature, but also to increasing the intramolecular and intra-atomic energies.

Liquids have rather more space between molecules than solids but much less than in gases. Almost all liquid states are therefore less dense than the solid states. Water is exceptional in that the molecules are more closely packed together at around 4°C than when the crystalline solid, ice, is formed; thus ice will float on water. Increasing the energy of the microstructure of matter will lead to many other effects, notably the acceleration of chemical reactions (Van't Hoff's law) and the production of electromagnetic radiation, described in chapter 14. The viscosity of fluids is reduced, since the increased molecular motion diminishes the cohesive attraction.

Summary

Heating of matter may lead to:

- expansion
- a change of state: solids melting, liquids vaporizing
- an increased rate of chemical reaction
- production of electromagnetic radiation
- reduced viscosity in fluids.

Energy conversions

Heat, the energy of the microstructure of matter, can be converted to other forms of energy, but not with 100% efficiency. Similarly, if one form of energy is converted to another, say chemical to mechanical, there is always some part converted to heat in the material so that such conversions can never be 100% efficient. Of course, the general law of conservation of energy – energy can neither be created nor destroyed – holds true for the total energy exchange. Since all energy ultimately ends as heat in the structure of matter it is sometimes described as the basic form of energy, but it is simply the tendency to randomization.

Heat transfer

Conduction – One method of transferring heat from place to place is by the kinetic motion of atoms and molecules being passed from one to the next, well described as 'atoms jostling one another'. This is called conduction and is easily demonstrated, especially in metals; if one end of a metal bar is heated the other end becomes hotter in time. (This concept is familiar to most of us as a consequence of leaving metal spoons and forks in the cooking pot!)

Metals make good heat conductors while liquids and gases are much less effective. Notice that if two different materials are in contact heat can be transferred from one to the other in the same way,

Conduction is an inevitable consequence of molecular and atomic motion in the microstructure of any material and it would be expected that 'jostling' would be more effective in transmitting energy if the molecules are closer together, as happens in solids, and this is generally the case.

Table 10.2 Causes of heat gain and loss	
Causes of heat gain	**Causes of heat loss**
Basal metabolism	Radiation to the environment
Metabolism of muscle contraction	Conduction to cooler objects
Metabolism of other tissues beyond basal, e.g. digestion	Conduction to air, continually removed by convection
Absorption of radiation from the environment	Evaporation of water from skin – 'insensible perspiration' – vapour carried away by convection
Conduction from hotter objects	Evaporation of sweat – water vapour carried away by convection
	Exhaled warm air – forced convection
	Excretion of urine, faeces and other fluids

very efficient method of heat loss as the evaporation of each gram of sweat at body temperature takes some 2.5 kJ of heat energy. Under suitable conditions an adult human can lose 1 kg of sweat per hour, thus achieving a cooling rate of nearly 700 W (2300 J × 1000 g/3600 s = 694.4 W; Holwill and Silvester, 1973).

The difference between the core temperature and the normally lower body surface temperature is critical in controlling heat loss from the body. The reason is that the rate at which heat can be lost from the body surface depends on the temperature difference between the surface and the environment. A large temperature difference can be maintained between the core and the outer shell of the body because of the low thermal conductivity of tissue, especially fat tissue. The flow of heat from the deep tissue to the skin is largely due to the blood flow – forced convection. Heat is thus transmitted through the thermal barrier provided by the subcutaneous fat. This concept of a temperature gradient between the core and surface can be expressed schematically by the isothermal lines shown in Figure 10.1 and the tissue temperature gradients shown in Figure 12.1. There are variations of skin temperature on different areas of the body. The forehead skin is often at a higher temperature and there tends to be a progressive fall in temperature towards the periphery so that at toe-level skin temperature can be the same as room temperature.

When the body is exposed to cold the loss of heat can be limited and controlled by vasoconstriction which greatly reduces the blood flow to the extremities and skin of the trunk, allowing skin and subcutaneous tissue temperatures to fall. Conversely, if the body retains too much heat vasodilation of skin vessels vastly increases the blood flow and hence the skin temperature. The isothermic lines are close to the surface, showing that there is now less difference between the surface and the core temperature (Figure 10.1).

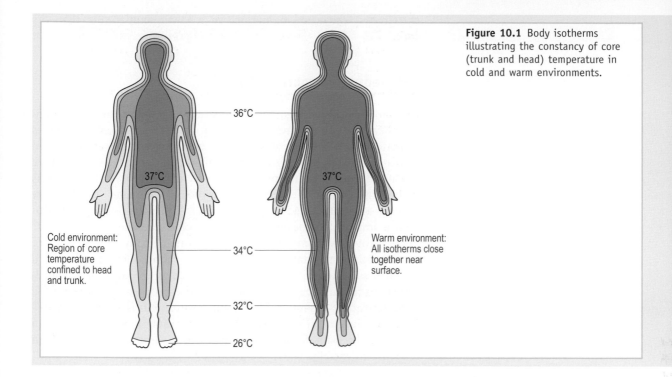

Figure 10.1 Body isotherms illustrating the constancy of core (trunk and head) temperature in cold and warm environments.

36°C

37°C   37°C

Cold environment: Region of core temperature confined to head and trunk.

Warm environment: All isotherms close together near surface.

34°C

32°C

26°C

The thicker layer of subcutaneous fat in women gives them better thermal control than men. At low environmental temperatures their skin is colder but becomes warmer in hotter environments (Hardy, 1982). Thus the internal body temperature is less affected by changes in the environmental temperature while the skin temperature is more markedly affected. It also appears that sweating starts earlier and tends to be more extensive in men. This is consistent with lesser shielding by fatty tissue and a greater reliance on neural control mechanisms.

Counter-current heat exchange

Counter-current heat exchange is another aspect of thermal regulation in the body. Heat can be exchanged between the warm arterial blood moving from the body core to the periphery and the cooler venous blood returning from the extremities. If arteries and veins lie close together, as in the limbs, where the venae comitantes are situated on each side of a medium artery, heat can pass from the warmer artery to the cooler vein. Since arterial blood loses heat as it passes to the periphery and venous blood gains heat as it moves centrally, the heat gradient between them is reduced; heat exchange continues throughout the length of the vessels. The value of this arrangement is that body core heat in the arterial blood is conserved in the central parts by being used to heat the incoming venous blood instead of the

While this counter-current mechanism is of great importance in some animals its effectiveness in humans has been questioned. Estimates of the heat savings vary from a negligible 5% to a significant 50% (Hardy, 1982).

extremities which are maintained at a lower temperature than the core.

Cutaneous thermoreceptors

Receptors in the skin signal temperature changes; some are heat receptors but many more are cold receptors. Heat and cold receptors respond to a change in temperature by firing rapidly at first, then slowing if the temperature change is maintained. In other words there is a rapid sensory adjustment to the new temperature. This happens within the 'tolerable', i.e. 'no physiological damage' temperature range – about 15 to 45°C (Figure 10.2). Outside this range physiological impairment occurs and non-specific pain nerve endings (C fibres; group IV unmyelinated) are activated, mainly as a result of accumulation of metabolites or molecules released as a result of cell breakdown. Thus below 15°C, a deep, aching sensation is invoked, similar to that associated with a bad bruise because the pattern of C fibre activation is similar. High-temperature pain is subjectively different because a different pattern of activation is involved, though many of the pain fibres activated are the same ones activated in response to extreme cold.

Thermal perception thus involves interpretation of the impulses from cold, warm and pain receptors by the central nervous system.

Cutaneous thermoreceptors have two roles:

- to signal temperature sensation, which is the conscious perception of whether the skin is being warmed or cooled – this requires measurement of the temperature change
- to contribute to the control of body temperature, which is unconscious – this requires measurement of absolute skin temperature.

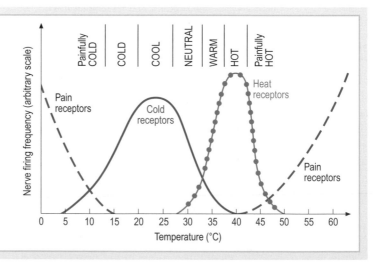

Figure 10.2 Response of thermal receptors in the skin at different temperatures.

The perception of thermal sensation is also influenced by the size of the area stimulated and, importantly, by the rate of change of the stimulation.

The continuous discharge of receptors shown in Figure 10.2 depends on the absolute skin temperature as shown but, if the skin is suddenly heated, there is an abrupt decrease in cold receptor activity and a corresponding increased frequency of warm receptor discharge. Both frequencies slowly return to the frequency appropriate for the new absolute skin temperature. Thus information from these receptors is used to perceive skin temperature and temperature changes as well as to contribute to subconscious temperature regulation (Fischer and Solomon, 1965). The perception of temperature change on the skin is extraordinarily sensitive. At skin temperatures around 30°C changes of as little as 1°C can be recognized under some conditions. At colder or hotter skin temperatures, and if the change is slow, larger changes of 5 or 10°C are needed before temperature change is recognized.

The usual method of testing thermal sensitivity by applying warm and cold water-filled test tubes to the skin, being about 10°C above and below skin temperature respectively, should thus allow easy recognition of the temperatures unless there is a significant sensory deficit (see details later).

The sensations associated with different surface temperatures are shown in Table 10.3 but it must be realized that this is a very subjective matter.

Table 10.3 Temperature ranges

Environmental temperature	Temperature (°C)	Skin surface temperatures	
		Subjective feeling	Effect
	60		
Behavioural regulation	55		Tissue damage
	50		
	45	Pain	
	40	Very hot	
	35	Hot	
Region of physiological temperature regulation	30	Warm neutral	
	Region of 25	Cool	
	thermal 20	Cold	
	comfort 15		
	10	Very cold	
	5	Pain	
Behavioural regulation	0		
	−5		Tissue damage
	−10		

THERMAL REGULATION

There are two facets of human heat regulation:

- *physiological*, controlled by the hypothalamus, which is itself sensitive to blood temperature – this involves metabolic, vasomotor and sweating responses
- *behavioural*, controlled in the higher centres and concerned with aversion responses.

Metabolic control

When much heat is being lost from the body some restoration can be made by increasing the metabolic activity. The most evident form this takes is shivering, in which irregular muscle contractions are provoked by stimulation of the sympathetic nervous system. Over short periods shivering can produce quite good heating but for several hours of cold exposure it can only double the resting metabolism on average (Hardy, 1982).

Brown adipose tissue is fatty tissue with more than the usual vascularity, hence making it look brown. It is found in a number of sites in the trunk close to the heart and kidney and between the scapulae. Fat metabolism can occur locally in this tissue in a way that releases energy entirely as heat.

At rest most body heat (about 70%) is produced in the viscera within the trunk and in the brain. On activity most of the heat (about 90%) is produced by the muscles. This heat is mostly transferred to the skin via the bloodstream, which moves the sites of major heat production nearer to the surface and to the extremities (Hardy, 1982). The increased blood flow needed to maintain oxygenation and nutrition to sustain continuous muscle contraction serves to dissipate heat from the working muscles to the rest of the body.

> While important in newborn infants the value of brown adipose tissue metabolism in adults is uncertain. It is stimulated by adrenalin release.

Vasomotor control

The blood flow in the skin has a nutritional role and acts as a heat transfer system. Arterioles feed capillary loops in the dermis forming papillae which drain via venules to a network of small veins. Rather larger venous plexuses are slightly more deeply placed: blood moving through these transfers heat to the overlying skin (Figure 10.3). Over most of the skin surface the blood flow is regulated by the lumen of the arteriole which is under the control of the sympathetic nervous system. In the skin of the hands, feet, ears, lips and some mucous membrane surfaces arteriovenous anastomoses are present between the arteriole and the large venous plexuses. These are regulated by vasoconstrictor impulses from the sympathetic nervous system so that when closed, in cold conditions, the flow of blood in the veins is

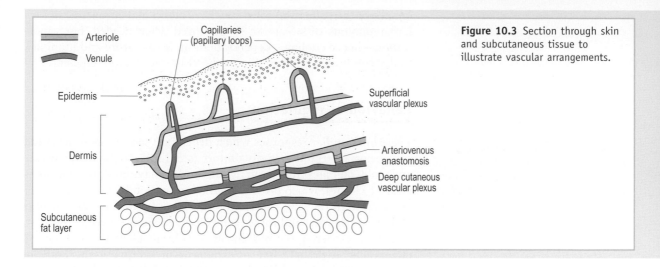

Figure 10.3 Section through skin and subcutaneous tissue to illustrate vascular arrangements.

reduced to almost nothing, but the nutritive blood flow through the papillae is maintained. On dilation they allow a large flow of venous blood through plexuses causing a marked rise in skin temperature and thus loss of heat from the surface.

At rest the skin contains some 20 times more blood than is needed for nutrition alone. Under cold conditions the blood flow to each 100 g of skin can be reduced to as little as 1 ml min^{-1}, whereas in hot conditions this can rise to 150 ml min^{-1} (Hubbard and Mechan, 1987).

Sweating

As noted earlier, water evaporation from the skin surface is a very efficient way of losing heat; in fact it is the only way when the environmental temperature is the same as, or even greater than, the skin temperature. It is not difficult to see why so much energy (2.5 kJ g^{-1}) is used since the energy leads to increased movement of the water molecules, giving them a range of kinetic energies. The ones with the highest kinetic energy will be 'thrown off' the water surface to form vapour which moves away from the skin surface by convection. At all times, under all circumstances, the body is losing heat by evaporation (about 500 g per day for a 1.5 m^2 surface area, e.g. the 50 kg woman considered previously). About half of this is the water vapour of expired air while the remainder is due to the steady transpiration of water through the skin, the so-called insensible perspiration. This is more or less constant at environmental temperatures below about 30°C but at higher temperatures, or when metabolic heat is produced by vigorous exercise, active sweating occurs and the amount of sweat vaporized increases with temperature.

There is an enormous number of eccrine sweat glands in the skin under sympathetic nervous system control via cholinergic nerves (glands of the palms and soles may have additional adrenergic fibres). Large amounts of sweat can be produced when needed, but vaporization – hence cooling – depends both on temperature and humidity. In dry conditions body cooling is therefore much more efficient.

Behavioural regulation

The effectiveness of trapped air as an insulator is noticed when clothes become wet and immediately feel much colder. This occurs because the thermal conductivity of water is nearly 25 times that of air.

These are familiar responses which depend on sensations of heat and cold being interpreted as discomfort (see Table 10.3). In temperate and cold climates the main method of behavioural regulation is wearing clothes, which provide thermal insulation by trapping a layer of air close to the skin surface. In other words, clothes prevent heat loss due to thermal and forced convection of air warmed by the skin. Similarly, restricting the movement of cold air close to the body by maintaining a draught-free environment or wrapping the body in blankets acts in the same way. Using a material that reflects infrared radiation (survival sleeping bags) reduces the heat loss further by blocking radiation emission from the body. Vigorous voluntary muscular activity is also used to increase metabolic heat.

Opposite behaviours encourage heat loss in a hot environment. Remaining in the shade and limiting activity in hot environments helps to control body temperature. Air trapping is reduced by wearing light loose-fitting clothing which reduces the absorption of radiation while allowing air convection currents close to the skin. Applying a steady draught of air by a fan or other means further assists cooling.

Temperature regulation

Small temporary changes of core temperature, such as occur with exercise, are physiologically normal.

Temperature regulation is largely controlled by the hypothalamus which is effectively a thermostat. It responds to lowered blood temperatures by initiating heat-generating and conserving mechanisms and acts in the opposite way to raised blood temperatures. Signals from heat-sensitive neurons in the anterior hypothalamus, affected by blood temperature, are integrated in the posterior hypothalamus with signals from peripheral receptors, to provide overall control (Guyton and Hall, 1997). Adrenalin release is an important endocrine response to cooling. As indicated above, higher centres in the brain also become involved.

Bacterial or viral infections of sufficient virulence lead to the release of substances which, in some ill-understood way, reset the thermostat of the temperature-regulating centre. Thus the patient shivers and feels cold and the heat-conserving mechanisms come into play despite the elevated temperature. Consequently the core temperature rises to a new, higher level for a time. When the infection has been overcome, possibly aided by the higher metabolic rate and consequent increased activity of the immune system, the central nervous system thermostat is reset to normal and the patient feels hot. Cutaneous vasodilation occurs with sweating to bring the body temperature down.

Body temperature regulation is helped by the high heat capacity of the human body ($3.6\,kJ\,K^{-1}\,kg^{-1}$; see Table 10.1) which means that it takes a large quantity of heat to raise, or heat loss to lower, the body temperature.

Since the principal source of heat is metabolism, which depends on tissue mass, and the principal source of heat loss is from the whole of the skin, which depends on the surface area, it is evident that body size will have an important effect. Babies have a larger surface area in proportion to their mass than adults, so they are at more risk from excessive heat loss. They appear to compensate by maintaining a higher metabolic rate and also by brown adipose tissue metabolism (when necessary).

Summary

Thermal regulation is brought about by:

- Inputs from
  - temperature of blood perfusing hypothalamus
  - peripheral cutaneous receptors
- Control via
  - hypothalamus
  - higher centres, i.e. behavioural
  - hormonal (adrenaline) response
- Output, regulation
  Involuntary (physiological)
  - metabolic control: shivering; metabolism of brown adipose tissue in babies
  - vasomotor control: blood flow in skin is varied
  - sweating: evaporation from skin is varied
  Voluntary
  - insulation of body surface varied: clothes; shelter
  - voluntary increase/avoidance of metabolic activity: muscle contraction or inactivity
  - seeking or avoiding environmental heat.

Hyperthermia and hypothermia

Even in healthy subjects the heat-regulating mechanisms can become overwhelmed by extremes of heat (hyperthermia) or cold (hypothermia). Both extremes have effects ranging from mild to severe (fatal).

Deaths from hypothermia often occur in the cold weather and should generally be preventable (Anonymous, 2003). The causes include a loss of heat, a reduced heat production or an impaired

During hard work at high outside temperatures, body temperature is controlled by sweating and if water and salt are not replaced, muscle cramps and fatigue result.

thermoregulatory system. Death occurs most often in those aged under 3 or over 65 years or is associated with alcohol abuse (Anonymous, 2003). The elderly population is particularly vulnerable to hypothermia due both to a reduced capacity to thermoregulate and often to social factors associated with poverty. A Scottish study found peaks in hypothermic presentations to an accident and emergency department were associated with periods of particularly cold weather (Pedley et al., 2002).

The effects of hypothermia, a reduced oxygen demand and lower metabolic rate are routinely used in controlled circumstances as part of medical treatment. For example, during some major surgery cooling is used. Similarly following severe neurological trauma, such as an acute stroke or traumatic brain injury, induced hypothermia may be used.

Hyperthermia is the outcome of an excessive level of core heating. It may occur following prolonged and intensive physical activity such as running a marathon, result from a metabolic disorder or be a response to various toxins or the ingestion of certain chemicals. When during heat stroke heat regulation fails, the person stops sweating and body temperature starts to rise. Urgent treatment to cool the patient and maintain body fluids is required.

Mortality rates rise during heatwaves and very cold spells, particularly among the elderly and those with chronic cardiovascular disease. Hypothermia is generally more prevalent, particularly among elderly people living alone. In addition, in some medical conditions, exposure to extremes of heat or cold may lead to particular difficulties. For example, cystic fibrosis is associated with inefficient production of sweat and hence inadequate control in extreme heat.

> The use of cocaine, for example, can cause hyperthermia. Cocaine causes an elevated body temperature while reducing the taker's awareness of heat stress (Crandall et al., 2002).

PHYSIOLOGICAL EFFECTS OF TEMPERATURE CHANGE ON BODY TISSUES

Any form of local body tissue heating causes a complex set of physiological changes which then interact and produce more complex responses. These merge with the systemic changes needed to maintain thermal homeostasis that have just been considered.

It has already been noted that the terms 'heating' and 'cooling' are based on human perceptions, so that a skin temperature raised to 35°C would be considered warming, whereas lowering the deep tissue temperature to the same level is cooling. Cooling the tissues has effects which are not the simple reverse of those due to heating. The effects of tissue cooling are considered separately in chapter 12.

> These ideas are developed further in chapters discussing: ultrasound (chapter 9); conduction heating (chapter 11); cooling (chapter 12); shortwave diathermy (chapter 13); microwave diathermy (chapter 15); infrared therapy (chapter 16).

Living tissue is affected by temperature changes in three interdependent ways:

- temperature dependent biological and biochemical changes, due to changes in metabolic rate and consequently, metabolite concentrations

- changes in the pattern of neural activity which affect perceptions of discomfort or pain
- physiological changes needed for regulation to protect the body from damage, such as in the vascular and nervous systems.

All three invoke changes in neural activity. There is a direct effect of temperature on nerve fibre activity, an effect due to changes in metabolite concentrations which may hypersensitize or desensitize receptors and regulatory changes which may involve suppression or sensitization. The neural response to temperature changes and the rate of temperature change are important factors determining the therapeutic effects of heating and cooling.

Metabolic activity

The rate of any simple chemical reaction is increased by a temperature rise (Van't Hoff's law). Metabolism, being a series of chemical reactions, will increase with a rise and decrease with a fall of temperature. The actual change is about one-eighth for each 1°C, so increasing the tissue temperature by, say, 4°C would increase the metabolic rate by some four eighths or 50%. In the living organism increasing temperature can denature proteins and thus interfere with the enzyme (protein) controlled metabolic processes. Thus after some increased activity an optimum temperature is reached at which metabolic activity is maximally stimulated by the heat and yet not sufficiently hot to destroy the necessary enzymes. This temperature will differ for different enzymes. At temperatures above 45°C so much protein damage occurs that there is destruction of cells and tissues. At low temperatures metabolism is progressively reduced and tissue destruction occurs if the intra- or extracellular fluid becomes frozen.

From a therapeutic point of view the local temperature changes that can, or should, be achieved are limited in the deeper tissues to about 5 or 6°C above or below core temperature. For skin and subcutaneous tissue much lower temperatures can safely and usefully be achieved by cooling.

With an appropriate rise in temperature, all cell activity increases, including cell motility and the synthesis and release of chemical mediators. Furthermore, the rate of cellular interactions, such as phagocytosis or growth, is accelerated.

Viscosity

The resistance to flow in a blood vessel depends directly on the viscosity of the fluid and inversely on the fourth power of the radius of the vessel. This striking dependence of blood flow on the diameter of the blood vessel is the reason why autonomic control of the arteriole diameter regulates the tissue blood flow so effectively. Less dramatic is the effect of viscosity. This property of moving fluids is sometimes described as friction between the moving particles. It is temperature dependent, so raising the temperature in liquids, but not gases, lowers

Joint stiffness has been found to be reduced by heating (Wright and Johns, 1961); on cooling, joint stiffness is increased. The effects are more likely to be of neurophysiological origin than due to changes in tissue extensibility or fluid viscosity.

the viscosity. Viscosity changes affect not only the fluids in narrow vessels (blood and lymph), but also fluid movement within and throughout the tissue spaces. Thus, although the effect is quite small, it is widespread. Whether changes in viscosity are clinically significant has not been established.

Collagenous tissue changes

Changes occur in collagen due to heating. At the extreme, cooking meat renders the collagenous parts jelly-like, making it more tender. Collagen suddenly melts at a temperature close to 60°C (Mason and Ward, 1972). At temperatures within a therapeutically applicable range (40 to 45°C), the extensibility of collagen tissue has been shown to increase slightly (Lehmann et al., 1970). This only occurs if the tissue is simultaneously stretched and requires temperatures near the therapeutic limit, but it is possibly an important therapeutic effect. The clinical relevance is unknown largely because it is not clear how much heating of collagen tissue occurs within a living person nor whether increased range of movement ('extensibility') is a mechanical or a neurophysiological effect.

Nerve stimulation

Neural activity is markedly affected by changes in temperature. There is a direct effect on thermoreceptors and a secondary effect due to changes in metabolic activity and consequently changes in metabolite concentrations.

As far as the primary effect is concerned, heat and cold stimulate the sensory receptors of the skin as both sensations can be recognized and distinguished (see earlier). These receptors also pass information to the heat-regulating centres, contributing to the control of body temperature.

Stimulating afferent nerves by heating may act on the gate control mechanism in the same way as the mechanoreceptors do (see chapter 6). This mechanism would account for the analgesic effects of local heating. Similarly, heating the secondary afferent muscle spindle nerve endings and Golgi tendon endings may be the mechanism by which muscle spasm is reduced by heating (Lehmann and de Lateur, 1982).

Cooling has marked effects on peripheral nerves. Initially cold receptors are stimulated, adding to the overall sensory input, but at lower temperatures firing rates are depressed. This occurs at first in the small myelinated fibres and later in large myelinated fibres. With sufficient cooling some nerve conduction is abolished so that numbness occurs. The therapeutic implications are considered in chapter 12.

Secondary effects occur because changes in metabolite concentration can change the local pH, which affects neural excitability. There are also changes in neural activity which are metabolite-specific.

Blood vessel changes

Heat and cold applied to the skin have obvious effects. With heating the skin surface reddens, i.e. an erythema is produced, and with cooling it initially becomes pale due to vasoconstriction, although subsequent reddening, due to vasodilation, may occur (see chapter 12).

Vasodilation distributes the additional heat around the body, allowing compensatory heat loss from other regions, and it also protects the heated skin. This is important because when the skin surface is heated externally, heat conduction is not effective through the subcutaneous fat.

Vasodilation due to heat is thought to be caused by several mechanisms:

- a direct effect on capillaries, arterioles and venules, causing them to dilate (Lehmann and de Lateur, 1982); the nature of this mechanism is not understood
- an axon reflex triggered by stimulation of polymodal receptors is an important cause of the vasodilation; in this mechanism only the peripheral branches of the afferent nerve fibres are involved
- increased metabolism which will lead to further release of carbon dioxide and lactic acid, leading to greater acidity of the heated tissues, which tends to provoke dilation
- an inflammatory reaction. If excessive heating occurs it can damage proteins and this may initiate the release of histamine-like substances and bradykinins which evoke vasodilation (Lehmann and de Lateur, 1982).

The foregoing accounts for the area being heated; other skin areas may well show cutaneous vasodilation to lose heat in response to signals from the heat-regulating centre. Note also that the above refers to heat-induced vasodilation. Cold-induced vasodilation is somewhat different and the mechanisms are discussed in chapter 12.

The striking cutaneous hyperaemia due to heat leads to the idea that similar effects occur in other tissues but this is not the case. As noted already, the skin is specially adapted for heat regulation and what is being seen is a heat-blocking response.

Blood and tissue fluid

As a consequence of the increased metabolic activity, decreased fluid viscosity and arteriole and capillary dilation (leading to a rise in capillary blood pressure and flow), there is an inevitable increase in fluid exchange across capillary walls and cell membranes. The acidity of the blood rises (pH falls) and both carbon dioxide and oxygen tensions increase. There is an increase in lymph formation and a higher blood leucocyte count.

> **Summary of the physiological effects of temperature change**
>
> **Physical changes**
>
> - Metabolic rate raised by heating (about 13% per 1°C) and lowered by cooling (Van't Hoff's law).
> - Proteins denatured by sufficient heat, generally irreversible damage if maintained over 45°C.
> - Freezing of fluids leads to tissue destruction.
> - Blood and tissue fluid viscosity lowered by heating and raised by cooling.
> - Softening of collagen due to heating.
>
> **Physiological changes**
>
> - Stimulation of sensory nerves by both heat and cold.
> - Lowered nerve conduction due to sufficient cooling.
> - Immediate skin arteriole vasodilation due to heating and vasoconstriction due to cooling.
> - Subsequent skin vasodilation in some areas due to cooling (see chapter 12).
> - Increased blood flow and tissue fluid exchange due to heating.

THERAPEUTIC EFFECTS OF LOCAL TISSUE HEATING

Tissue healing

Although the comments above suggest that any condition in which increased metabolic rate, cell activity and local blood flow might be beneficial could be appropriately treated by mild heating, there is little hard evidence of this. There is general agreement though that the application of heat to inflammatory injuries in the early stages is unlikely to be beneficial. Very mild or subperceptual levels of heating, such as that produced using pulsed shortwave diathermy, are used to promote healing after the immediate risk of further bleeding has abated. Most research on this topic is older but it is consistent with low levels of heating providing some stimulus to earlier repair. The amount and duration of heating is likely to be quite important. Chronic inflammatory states and the stages of repair and regeneration are all appropriately treated with mild to moderate levels of heating. In these instances heating is usually used in association with exercises and stretches to facilitate regaining of movement. All forms of therapeutic heating are applied to a wide range of chronic and post-traumatic conditions including the arthritides, soft tissue lesions and post-surgical healing.

Relief of pain

Therapeutic heat is widely used for the relief of pain. Anecdotally heat ranks highly among patients, after analgesics, as a way of controlling or managing pain. Consistent with this the non-analgesic method used by 68% of cancer patients to control pain was heat (Barbour et al., 1986). Also, heat, and not cold, reduced the spontaneous pain behaviours in rats with induced acute arthritis of a knee (Sluka et al., 1999).

Changes in a physiological indicator of pain, the sympathetic skin response, indicated that using superficial heat, hot packs, significantly reduced the sympathetic palmar sweating response to painful electrical stimulation of a distant region (On et al., 1997). Other methods of applying heat have also been reported as having similar effects and are discussed in the following chapters on superficial and deep methods of clinical heating.

Most therapeutic heating is of the skin. This suggests that the major pain relieving effects are mainly reflex, possibly an activation of the pain gate mechanism. Pain is also possibly relieved by heat reducing the level of muscle spasm usually associated with it. The pathways by which local tissue heating may alleviate pain are illustrated in simplified form in Figure 10.4.

Vascular changes could also reduce local pain. The increased blood flow that has been observed (Lehmann and de Lateur, 1982) would help remove some of the pain provoking metabolites resulting from tissue injury. These include prostaglandins and bradykinin.

Reduction of muscle spasm

Part of the relief of pain provided by heat may be because of its effect on muscle spasm. Heat may reduce muscle spasm by reducing the

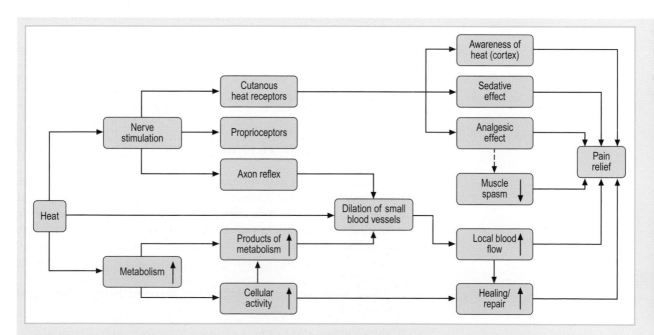

Figure 10.4 A simplified diagrammatic illustration of the pathways by which local tissue heating may alleviate pain.

levels of ischaemia associated with prolonged contraction in affected muscles (Wright and Sluka, 2001). Another possibility is that increasing the muscle temperature to about 42°C changes the output of both the muscle spindle and the type 1b Golgi tendon organ afferent fibres. The net result is an inhibition of the motor neuron pool and a reduced level of muscle excitation (Lehmann and de Lateur, 1982). While this effect has been demonstrated by applying heat directly to nerves in the cat, it does not necessarily follow that this is a mechanism that operates in humans. Since pain and muscle spasm are interdependent, a reduction in one will cause a reduction in the other.

Sedative effect

A rather unspecific sedative effect has been observed. During and after heat treatments patients have been found to sleep more readily. While this might be simply a consequence of pain relief it has been noted that skin temperatures rise just before the onset of sleep so that this sedative effect of superficial heat could be a reflex phenomenon (Lehmann and de Lateur, 1982).

Despite the widespread use of therapeutic heat for pain relief across many cultures and throughout recorded history, there is not yet a satisfactory explanation of why, anecdotally, it appears so effective. However, despite the dearth of supportive clinical studies, there is still considerable acceptance of the use of heat for pain relief. The possible decline in the clinical use of heat over the last few decades is consistent with a greater focus on medications, and on evidence based practice and possibly even on changes in the time allowed for most treatments.

It is well to remember the association of warmth with comfort and relaxation. This may lead to feelings of well-being when the body surface is warmed, which is a psychosomatic effect. Compare this with comments on cold in chapter 12.

Increase of range of joint motion

Used in conjunction with different types of stretching, an increase in joint range is obtained (Peres et al., 2002; Draper et al., 2004). Heat is also often used in conjunction with exercises to treat chronic musculoskeletal problems such as knee osteoarthritis. A problem with establishing the extent of its contribution to a generally successful outcome is the lack of methodological quality of many studies (Marks et al., 1999).

There seem to be two mechanisms involved here – neural and mechanical:

- the analgesic effect of heat allows greater tolerance of stretching; a comparison of the effects of heat, stretch or heating and stretching on increasing hip flexion, abduction and external rotation shows that heating and stretching produced more improvements that were sustained longer (Henricson et al., 1984)

- the deformability of the tissues increases with heating. Viscous (time dependent) effects occur more rapidly (Wright and Johns, 1961) and collagen tissue extensibility increases slightly at higher temperatures (Lehmann et al., 1970).

Only small changes in the mechanical properties of tissue have been found at increased temperatures within the physiologically tolerable range.

Despite this, heat is used prior to passive stretching and exercise to increase joint movement or lengthen scars or contractures, and in conditions in which fibrosis is a marked feature. Similarly, heat is often applied prior to stretching superficial scarring in the skin or subcutaneous tissues. The discussion above also suggests that applying heat concurrent with stretching might offer greater benefits.

A point to consider is that the studies of the effects of heat and stretching typically investigate intact, undamaged tissue in subjects with normal or near normal range of movement. Repairing tissue might respond differently to modest temperature increases. There is indirect evidence of a greater effect. Collagen molecules in solution denature at only 1 or 2 degrees above body (core) temperature. By contrast, collagen fibres do not denature unless the temperature is more than 20 degrees above core temperature. An implication is that free, loosely bound or badly incorporated collagen molecules in repairing connective tissue are more susceptible to heat denaturation. When denatured the collagen would be mopped-up as protein debris. A similar argument might apply to poorly incorporated collagen fibrils associated with early stages of repair. Heat with stretching may thus not only result in tissue elongation but also a better overall alignment of the fibres. Although this effect is plausible, it does not yet seem to have been demonstrated experimentally. The other issue, the use of subjects with normal or near normal range, means that many evaluations of the contribution made by heating to increasing tissue extensibility may underestimate its effects considerably (Robertson et al., 2005).

> Of the two, the analgesic mechanism is probably the major factor. Increased deformability and time dependent effects have been demonstrated in vitro but the effects are small and their clinical importance is questionable.

Infection

The role of heat in the therapeutic control of infection by microorganisms is not clear cut. In so far as the defence mechanisms are enhanced by heat there is obvious benefit but, at the same time, heating may promote bacterial or viral growth and replication (Van't Hoff's law) thus negating any advantage. Historically, home heat treatments such as poultices have been widely used. Applications of heat to the surrounding healthy tissues of infected wounds were also used in the past. However, the availability of effective antibiotics has

> All methods of enhancing the natural defence mechanisms, including heat, may be needed in the future.

made this largely irrelevant over the past 50 to 60 years. Superficial heating can, however, be used in some instances to dry skin to limit bacterial and fungal colonizations as these occur more readily on moist skin.

As a precursor of other treatment

Heat treatment is often used prior to other forms of treatment, e.g. muscle stretching, joint mobilization, massage or traction, to assist muscle relaxation and to reduce pain. It is also used prior to exercise therapy for the pain-relieving effect and because it may contribute to muscle 'warm-up' or preparedness for activity.

Summary

The therapeutic effects of local tissue heating include:

- acceleration of healing
- pain relief and sedation
- reduction of muscle spasm
- facilitation of joint motion.

SITES OF TISSUE HEATING

Clearly the effects of local therapeutic heating will depend on the extent of heating – the volume of tissue heated and temperature reached – and on the particular tissues heated. The former is largely a matter of application and is determined by the extent and nature of the lesion to be treated. The latter is dependent on the modality used for heating. Thus modalities in which the energy is absorbed almost entirely at the surface, such as infrared radiation or conduction heating, will affect the skin and immediately underlying tissues, whereas diathermies (shortwave, microwave and ultrasound) spread energy more deeply in the tissues. The details of energy distribution in the tissue are discussed with each modality in the appropriate chapter. Another consideration is the spread of heat in the tissues. This occurs in two ways:

- conduction through the surrounding tissues (similar in most soft tissues to the conduction rate in water but notably less in fat and epidermis). This is modest with the small temperature differences applied in therapy. The temperature of the epidermis has been shown to rise in an area only a few millimetres beyond the heated region (e.g. see Cervero et al., 1993)
- dispersion of the heated blood accounts for most of the spread of energy in the tissues (i.e. thermal convection due to the blood flow).

The increased blood flow in the dermis, a consequence of heating the skin surface, is apparent as an erythema. It has a protective function, dissipating heat from the skin to prevent a damaging skin temperature rise.

Ultimately, the raised systemic blood temperature and signals from skin thermoreceptors will trigger reflex activity in the hypothalamus to stimulate the heat loss mechanisms of the body. This will cause vasodilation of other parts. Theoretically this effect might be usable clinically. However, the volume change with most forms of external heating, certainly the superficial ones, is probably less than that achieved by voluntary exercise. Local pathophysiology can also reduce the extent of changes in local perfusion if, for example, the proximal part of a limb was heated with the intent of a reflex increase in flow distally.

Table 10.4 Methods of heating and modes of heat transfer to the tissues

Method	Mode of transfer
Superficial heating	
Heat from outside transferred to skin by conduction, convection or radiation – does not pass the thermal barrier	Hot water bottle
	Hot pack
	Hydrocollator
	Hot water bath
	Hot muds
	Wax bath
	Electric heat pad
	Fluidotherapy
	Hot air/hairdrier
	Hydrotherapy
	Infrared radiation
Deep heating	
One form of energy converted to heat in the tissues – avoids the thermal barrier	Ultrasound
	Shortwave diathermy
	Microwave

TISSUE DAMAGE DUE TO EXCESS LOCAL HEAT – BURNS

Burns are of considerable importance in medicine. Permanent skin damage or loss is a serious disability if anything more than a tiny area is involved.

Skin temperatures over 45°C can cause tissue damage, depending on the duration of exposure as well as the temperature. The sensation of heat becomes one of pain at this same temperature; the pain increases in intensity with rising temperature. Both injury and the resulting pain are a result of permanent damage of basal skin cells.

The relationship between time, temperature and skin damage is important. Thus a skin temperature around 45°C can be tolerated for, perhaps, an hour or so before damage occurs but with higher temperatures the period shortens so that 50°C can be tolerated for about 1 minute or so and 65°C about 1 s or so (Hardy, 1982). Many much hotter objects can be touched for short periods without causing a burn as they do not necessarily lead to sufficient heat transfer to raise the skin to the same temperature. Most people have experience of touching a very hot object, say a saucepan of boiling water with a temperature about 100°C, yet because the hand is removed very quickly no damage occurs, except a transient erythema. This has important implications in the immediate treatment of burns. The damaged area should be cooled as quickly as possible. Cold water should be applied at once; a scalded hand should be plunged immediately into cold water.

Testing thermal sensation

This is important for the safe application of most heat treatments and essential where it is the only way of ascertaining heat distribution (e.g. shortwave and microwave). The customary method is to apply two dry test-tubes of water at 40 to 45°C and 15 to 20°C randomly to the area, asking the patient to identify which is which while their eyes remain shut. The temperature difference between the tubes falls during the test so that patients are actually discriminating between only a few degrees Celsius. Temperatures over 45°C or much below 15°C should not be used because these may test pain rather than thermal sensations. Also, the tester should be aware of different levels of thermal sensitivity on different parts of the body when conducting a test.

Summary

Therapeutic heating can thus be divided into:

- superficial heating due to heat conduction or infrared radiation being produced by hot packs and similar means, as described in chapter 11, and infrared lamps, as described in chapter 16.
- deep heating, also referred to as conversion or conversive heating, due to the conversion of energy passing through the tissues to heat, as with ultrasound (chapter 9), shortwave (chapter 13) and microwave diathermy (chapter 15). (Strictly speaking, infrared radiation is also conversion heating.)

The distinction between these two groups is important; the skin and subcutaneous fat act as a thermal barrier to conduction and much radiation heating, thus limiting the heating of deeper tissues. There are, of course, indirect effects on deeper tissues mediated through the nervous system or due to the heated blood being carried to other parts. In contrast, the conversive methods, or diathermies, are able to generate heat in both superficial and deep tissues, as explained in chapters 9, 13 and 15, much like metabolic heating (Table 10.4).

References

Anonymous. (2003). Hypothermia-related deaths – Philadelphia, 2001, and United States, 1999. MMWR – Morbid Mortal Wkly Rep, **52**, 86–87.

Barbour, L., McGuire, D., Kirchott, K. (1986). Non-analgesic methods of pain control used by cancer outpatients. Oncol Nursing Forum, **13**, 56–60.

Cervero, F., Gilbert, R., Hammond, R. et al. (1993). Development of secondary hyperalgesia following non-painful thermal stimulation of the skin: a psychophysical study in man. Pain, **54**, 181–189.

Cetas, T. (1982). Thermometry. In J. F. Lehmann (ed.), Therapeutic Heat and Cold, pp. 35–69. Baltimore: Williams & Wilkins.

Crandall, C., Vongpatanasin, W., Victor, R. (2002). Mechanism of cocaine-induced hyperthermia in humans. Ann Int Med, **136**, 785–791.

Draper, D., Castro, J., Feland, B. et al. (2004). Shortwave diathermy and prolonged stretching increase hamstring flexibility more than prolonged stretching alone. J Orthop Sports Phys Ther, **34**, 413–420.

Fischer, E., Solomon, S. (1965). Physiological responses to heat and cold. In S. Licht (ed.), Therapeutic Heat and Cold, pp. 126–169. Baltimore: Waverley Press.

Guyton, A., Hall, J. (1997). Human Physiology and Mechanisms of Disease. Philadelphia: W. B. Saunders.

Hardy, J. (1982). Temperature regulation, exposure to heat and cold and effects of hypothermia. In J. F. Lehmann (ed.), Therapeutic Heat and Cold, pp. 172–198. Baltimore: Williams & Wilkins.

Henricson, A., Fredriksson, K., Persson, I. et al. (1984). The effect of heat and stretching on the range of hip motion. J Orthop Sports Phys Ther, **6**, 110–115.

Holwill, M., Silvester, N. (1973). Introduction to Biological Physics. London: John Wiley.

Hubbard, J., Mechan, D. (1987). Physiology for Health Care Students. Edinburgh: Churchill Livingstone.

Lehmann, J., de Lateur, B. (1982). Therapeutic heat. In J. F. Lehmann (ed.), Therapeutic Heat and Cold, pp. 404–562. Baltimore: Williams & Wilkins.

Lehmann, J., Masock, A., Warren, C. et al. (1970). Effect of therapeutic temperatures on tendon extensibility. Arch Phys Med Rehabil, **51**, 481–487.

Marks, R., Ghassemi, M., Duarte, M., Van Nguyen, J. (1999). A review of the literature on shortwave diathermy as applied to osteoarthritis of the knee. Physiotherapy, **85**, 304–316.

Mason, P., Ward, A. (1972). Viscoelastic studies of the structure of collagen: dependence on temperature and pH. J Conn Tiss Res, **1**, 195–203.

On, A., Colakoglu, M., Hepguler, M., Aksit, R. (1997). Local heat effect on sympathetic skin responses after pain of electrical stimulus. Arch Phys Med Rehabil, **78**, 1196–1199.

Pedley, D., Paterson, B., Morrison, W. (2002). Hypothermia in elderly patients presenting to accident & emergency during the onset of winter. Scottish Med J, **47**, 10–11.

Peres, E., Draper, D., Knight, K., Ricard, M. (2002). Pulsed shortwave diathermy and prolonged long-duration stretching increase dorsiflexion range of motion more than identical stretching with diathermy. J Athletic Training, **37**, 43–50.

Robertson, V., Ward, A., Jung, P. (2005). The contribution of heating to tissue extensibility: a comparison of deep and superficial heating. Arch Phys Med Rehabil, **86**, 819–825.

Sekins, K., Emery, A. (1982). Thermal science for physical medicine. In J. F. Lehmann (ed.), Therapeutic Heat and Cold J. F., pp. 70–132. Baltimore: Williams & Wilkins.

Sluka, K., Christy, M., Peterson, W. et al. (1999). Reduction of pain-related behaviours with either cold or heat treatment in an animal model of acute arthritis. Arch Phys Med Rehabil, **80**, 313–317.

Wright, A., Sluka, K. (2001). Nonpharmacological treatments for musculoskeletal pain. Clin J Pain, **17**, 33–46.

Wright, W., Johns, R. (1961). Quantitative and qualitative analysis of joint stiffness in normal subjects and in patients with connective tissue diseases. Ann Rheum Dis, **20**, 36–46.

Therapeutic conduction heating

Body surface warming – a comforting warmth – is perhaps the most primitive panacea for pain. The therapeutic application of heated substances directly to the skin is the subject of this chapter.

The transfer of heat to the body surface is largely by conduction, hence the title, but there is also some transfer by radiation since all heated bodies emit some infrared radiation. Although the effects are very similar, it seems sensible to describe pure infrared heating separately in chapter 16.

First, some general points concerning tissue temperature changes as a consequence of local surface heating are discussed. A list of superficial heating methods was given in Table 10.4 previously. Some of those that involve conduction heating are then considered, together with their method of application.

The chapter concludes with some further consideration of the effects and therapeutic uses of conduction heating.

Conduction heating using paraffin wax, hot packs including hydrocollator packs, contrast and whirlpool baths, hot air treatment and electric heater pads are considered in this chapter.

THE EFFECTS OF CONDUCTION HEATING

When local heating is applied to the body it does not normally cause a rise in core temperature. As explained in the previous chapter, the heat added in one place is dispersed throughout the body – by conduction and convection – to be lost at other surfaces. Thus local temperature rises will be a balance between heat input and dispersion. As noted previously, if the temperature is high enough to cause tissue damage, i.e. above 45°C, the time in which this damage occurs becomes shorter at higher temperatures. In the therapeutic situation such high skin temperatures are not applied so that after a local rise in temperature the dispersion mechanism can keep pace with the heat input. This allows local heat to be applied indefinitely without producing tissue damage.

The rate of temperature rise at any given point in the tissues due to local heating depends on a combination of the following factors:

- the initial temperature of both the heat source and the part being heated

- whether the heat source is constant temperature (e.g. heat pad) or cooling during treatment (e.g. hot pack)
- any barriers to heating (e.g. layers of towelling, thickness of subcutaneous fat)
- the size of the area heated (which affects the extent of heating of the body)
- the thermal conductivity of the substance used and the tissues being heated (see discussion of wax immersion which is very different from methods using water, a better thermal conductor)
- the method used for a particular type of superficial heating (e.g. for wax if 'dip and leave' or 'dip and wrap')
- the duration of the exposure.

Epithelium and fat have lower thermal conductivities than the higher water content tissues, such as muscle or blood. Consequently heat will flow more readily through tissues deeper than the skin and the superficial fat layer (Sekins and Emery, 1982). However, heat transfer by conduction within the tissues will be obstructed by the subcutaneous fat layer and the temperature increase will tend to be confined to the area of skin heated. With a thicker subcutaneous fat layer the effect is more pronounced, which accounts for the slightly higher skin temperature found in women at environmental temperatures above 30°C.

Figure 11.1 illustrates the temperature increase likely to be expected with conductive heating. It is clear that greatest effect will be produced at depths less than about 1 to 2 mm.

An important feature of the dermis and epidermis is the abundance of sensory nerve fibres and receptors. An immediate effect of conductive heating is stimulation of sensory receptors, in particular heat receptors.

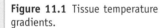

With conduction heating the skin (epidermis and dermis) gets hot while the deeper tissues are less affected.

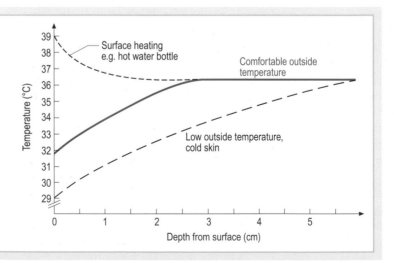

Figure 11.1 Tissue temperature gradients.

Most, if not all, of the effects of conductive heating are directly due to superficial heat production and the consequent stimulation of sensory nerve fibres. As noted previously, in the context of electrical stimulation, activation of sensory (A-β) fibres has a gating or partial blocking effect on transmission of C (pain) fibre signals. Warmth is thus associated with a sedatory, i.e. pain-relieving, effect.

Superficial heating will also trigger reflex vasodilation and so produce a greater blood flow through the dermis.

The main way in which heat is moved through tissues underneath the epidermis is by convection, due to blood flow. Reflex vasodilation helps to prevent excessive heating of the dermis and epidermis. Blood flowing through the dermis is warmed and carries heat into the deeper tissues on its return from capillaries to venules and veins. Consequently, cutaneous dilation will markedly increase heat transfer to the deeper tissues (see Figure 10.3 previously). Although heat transfer to the deeper tissues produces some heating, most of the heat is widely dispersed by the bloodstream. Tissue beneath the dermis thus does not suffer a large temperature rise with superficial heating but does experience an increased blood flow. The increased blood flow may have an effect on the resolution of some chronic conditions as it will increase the flow of metabolites to and from cells and so could accelerate the rate of healing. There is little evidence to support this belief but, used in conjunction with activity, heating may promote recovery from some chronic conditions.

Local tissue heating is, of course, superimposed on the existing tissue temperature gradient, described in chapter 10 in terms of temperature 'shells' (see Figure 10.1). Application of heat to the surface of the body or part being treated will reverse this gradient locally (Figure 11.1, first 1 to 2 cm).

The rise in subcutaneous tissue temperature does not occur instantly. As would be expected the skin temperature rises first, the subcutaneous tissue temperature rises more slowly, and even a very small change in superficial muscle temperature (of 1°C or so) takes as long as 20 or 25 minutes to occur. This is illustrated in Figure 11.2, which shows the temperature of various tissues against time: these data are based on studies by Lehmann et al. (1966) using hydrocollator hot packs. The pattern would be similar whatever form of superficial heat was applied for as long as the heat source remained warmer than the skin and body tissues. To overcome the cooling of the hot packs over the 30-minute test period, Lehmann et al. (1966) used new ones every 10 minutes. In clinical practice most forms of superficial heating are not constant heat sources, instead, they are cooling from the moment of placement. This reduces the extent of heating obtained.

The marked rise in skin temperature of some 10°C (Figure 11.2) contrasts with the trivial rise in deep-tissue (e.g. muscle) temperature of 1°C or so.

Convection is when heat is transferred from one region to another by movement of a hot fluid. The important idea is that heat is transferred by physical movement of the fluid.

One experimental study (on dogs) has demonstrated rather higher muscle temperature increases of 4.7°C, when using hot packs on the skin (McMeeken and Bell, 1990), but whether the results are generalizable to humans is arguable because of the very different limb volumes and tissue layer thicknesses. The dogs were also anaesthetized so there was no overt indication of excessive skin heating or pain.

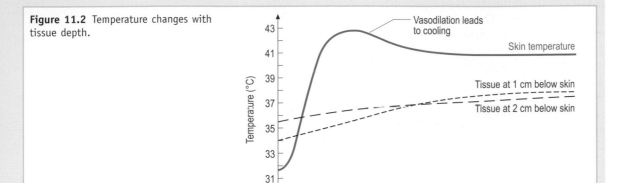

Figure 11.2 Temperature changes with tissue depth.

The skin temperature may actually decrease after some minutes, as shown, because the increased blood flow due to cutaneous vasodilation cools the skin. More importantly, unless a constant source of heating is used, the source will also be cooler. After 15 to 20 minutes the temperatures of the source and part have stabilized and continuing heating leads to no further change. This is why heat treatments are usually for a maximum of 20–30 minutes. After removal of the heat source the tissue temperatures slowly return to normal, skin more rapidly than deeper tissues.

Summary

Local conduction heating of the skin surface leads to:

- a marked and rapid rise in skin temperature (sometimes followed by a slight fall) over some minutes – then a steady skin temperature is maintained if a constant source of heating is used, if not, the skin temperature will slowly start to fall along with the temperature of the heat source
- marked cutaneous vasodilation evidenced by an erythema
- a slight rise in deep tissue temperature reaching a steady state in some 15 to 20 minutes or so
- dissipation to, and heat loss from, other parts to maintain heat balance.

PARAFFIN WAX BATHS

Paraffin wax melts at around 54°C, but this point can be lowered by the addition of mineral oil (liquid paraffin). Most wax baths are kept at temperatures between 42 and 52°C, often at the higher range for hand treatments and lower for the feet. The wax is maintained molten in stainless steel or enamelled baths which are electrically heated; the temperature is kept constant by a thermostat. Some baths are contained within a heated outer water bath. There may be a fixed thermometer to check the temperature and a means of adjusting the thermostat setting to alter the temperature. Even if a thermometer is not an integral part of the bath the temperature of the wax must still be checked.

The more modern designs of wax bath can be adjusted for height. They are light, with a stainless steel bowl and outer fibreglass shell. Initial heating is quicker with this type because there is no water-jacket to be heated.

Method of application

The most widely used method of application is 'dip and wrap'. This can only be used for the extremities – hands, wrists, feet and ankles. Repeated dipping is used so that the wax solidifies between dips and a thick layer of warm, solid wax builds-up.

Stages

Patient

The nature of wax treatment is explained and the area to be treated is inspected for contraindications.

Apparatus

The temperature of the wax is checked with a thermometer in the deeper central part of the bath or manually with the clinician's index finger.

Preparation of the part

The part is washed and thoroughly dried to keep water and skin flakes out of the wax bath. The patient is positioned to dip the part in the wax in a convenient and comfortable way.

Application

The part is immersed for a second or so in the wax, withdrawn and allowed to cool for 2 or 3s and then re-immersed. Re-immersions must be brief otherwise the outermost coating melts off and the thickness of wax does not build. The procedure is repeated six to eight times to produce a coating of wax 2 or 3mm thick over the body part. The part is then put into a plastic bag or paper cover and wrapped in a blanket or towel to limit the rate of heat loss to the air. If oedema formation is likely, the part should be elevated and kept above the level of the heart. Otherwise, heating will tend to exacerbate any swelling of the extremities.

Termination

The wax 'glove' is normally left in place for 15 minutes by which time the wax is completely solid, although still malleable, and removed in one piece.

To achieve a higher skin temperature for longer periods the 'dip and leave in' method can be used. After a suitably thick layer of wax has been built up by a succession of dips the part is left in the wax bath for 15 or 20 minutes; this method can produce a much greater increase in tissue temperature (Abramson et al., 1964), but it necessitates the hand or foot remaining dependent throughout the treatment, which can lead to an increase in oedema.

If the part cannot be immersed in wax, it is possible to coat the surface by either painting the wax on using a large brush, or ladling it over the part with a suitably large bowl placed beneath. Alternatively, bandages of a suitable size and mesh can be soaked in the hot wax and then wrapped around the limb; additional wax can be brushed over the bandage. These latter methods are rarely used because they are time-consuming and messy. After use the wax is cleaned in a purifier and reused.

Mode of action of paraffin wax heating

Despite the fact that skin temperatures above 45°C can lead to damage it is possible to put the hand comfortably in a bath of wax at some 50°C. Water at the same temperature would be uncomfortably hot and ultimately cause damage. This is because wax in contact with the skin cools and solidifies. Thus a thin layer of solid wax is formed on the skin surface. The thermal conductivity of solid wax is low so the solid wax acts to insulate the skin from the hotter surrounding liquid: some air may be trapped between this solidified layer and the skin, adding to the insulating effect (Griffin and Karselis, 1988).

The wax transmits heat energy to the tissues by giving up energy as it solidifies – the latent heat of fusion. This amount of energy is quite small: about $35\,kJ\,kg^{-1}$ (Sekins and Emery, 1982). Although the temperature of the thin layer of wax on the tissues falls quite quickly if its outside surface is exposed to air at room temperature, the low thermal conductivity prevents much heat loss from the skin surface. It also prevents any evaporation of water from the skin, further improving the insulating qualities.

Thus the wax provides a modest amount of direct heating as it solidifies but it also dramatically reduces normal heat loss. The net effect is to provide remarkably effective low-temperature heating of the part.

A consequence of preventing water loss from the surface of the skin is that a wax treatment tends to leave the skin with more moisture and feeling soft and pliable. This may be therapeutically valuable if the skin is dry.

Practical point

A way of achieving the benefits of prolonged higher temperatures coupled with elevation is to place the wax-covered part in a loose-fitting plastic bag. This is then wrapped with towelling and elevated for 15 minutes. Alternatively, the part is left elevated in a warm-air cabinet (simple heat cradle or infrared lamp will work); air temperature of about 70°C. This latter method can be combined with active exercise while the limb is elevated. The wax may fall away as it cools but a thin layer usually remains even as the fingers are moved.

Effective low-temperature heating with paraffin wax is enhanced in the hand or foot by the large surface area to volume ratio and the small amount of subcutaneous tissue separating the joints from the skin.

There is widespread support among patients with painful and stiff joints for this form of heat. There is, however, little hard evidence supporting this clinical practice (Ayling and Marks, 2000). Combined with exercise, for patients with rheumatoid arthritis there is at least a short-term benefit of using wax (Robinson et al., 2004). This is consistent with most clinical usage of wax, as an adjunctive treatment, not a sole treatment.

Contraindications and dangers

- Wax is sterile as no organisms can live in pure oil. Wax should not, however, be allowed to enter an open wound since it will set in the tissues acting as an inert foreign body and may delay healing.
- Large pieces of dirt in the wax bath may harbour organisms but it is extremely unlikely that these would lead to infection.
- Patients with skin infections or acute inflammation of underlying joints should not usually be treated with wax as heat may increase the inflammatory activity and could cause tissue damage.
- Some individuals may become allergic to the wax with extended and prolonged treatments but this is rare.
- Acute dermatitis may be made worse by wax, or indeed any form of heat on the skin.
- Circumstances in which there is defective thermal sensation coupled with deficient cutaneous circulation, as occurs with recently healed skin grafts, should not be treated.

Wax is highly inflammable if it becomes overheated so should only be used when a fire blanket and suitable carbon dioxide or foam extinguisher are available.

Wax spilt on the floor makes it very slippery and must be dealt with promptly.

Pouring water on blazing wax is ineffective and dangerous because the wax floats on the water surface.

HOT PACKS

There are two categories of hot packs: reusable and disposable. The reusable category includes hydrocollator packs and microwavable packs. The two types of hydrocollator packs are dry and moist (described below). The dry packs typically have a plastic covering with a paraffin wax mixture inside and provide an almost dry form of heating. The moist hydrocollator packs contain a silicate gel and, as the name suggests, provide moist heating. The rate of tissue heating and heat transfer for both types is the same but some patients prefer moist (Poindexter et al., 2002). The other type of reusable pack is microwavable and includes gel packs and wheat packs. These are easily obtained but care must be taken to limit their level of heating, especially the wheat packs.

Single-use hot packs appear to be wasteful and more environmentally unfriendly than their reusable counterparts. There also appears to be no evidence of any greater clinical benefit.

The second category of hot packs contains a range of disposable packs. These are single-use items as heat is produced by chemicals reacting inside the pack. The chemical reactions are exothermic (release heat) so they are sometimes called exothermic hot packs, indicating the heating is the result of an irreversible chemical reaction usually triggered by pulling a tab. They come in a variety of shapes and sizes from 'wraps' to hand warmers initially designed for skiers.

HYDROCOLLATOR PACKS

These consist of a silicate gel, such as bentonite, enclosed in a canvas cover. This gel can absorb large quantities of water which, if it is hot, provides a considerable store of heat energy. The gel is contained in a set of separated fabric pockets, like a duvet, so that the whole pack is flexible and the gel confined. The packs are made in various sizes to fit different body areas. They are heated by being placed in a special tank of water warmed to 75–80°C by an electric heater controlled by a thermostat. The packs, usually supported on racks in the tank, take from 30 minutes to 2 hours to become fully heated from cold, depending on the power rating of the hydrocollator.

The method of application follows the usual format, as described above, of explanation, preparation of patient and apparatus and the necessary checking for contraindications. This latter should include thermal sensitivity because, unlike wax treatment, the application is often at a temperature that could cause tissue damage if the insulation is not adequate.

The hot packs are wrapped so 1–2 cm of towelling is between the pack and the skin. This provides thermal insulation, largely because of the air in the towelling, so that although the pack is at about 75°C the skin temperature does not rise above 42°C or so. It takes some time (about 8 minutes) for the skin temperature to reach its maximum (Lehmann et al., 1966). During this time the pack temperature is falling but the towelling and pack prevent the skin surface from losing heat so that the skin and superficial tissue temperature rises, as indicated in Figures 11.1 and 11.2. For this reason, the therapist should check the patient's response and skin colour under the pack at approximately 10 minutes after placing it. Skin colour alone is not a reliable indicator of temperature change (Fyfe, 1982); verbal feedback is essential. The packs are normally left in place for 15 to 20 minutes.

Practical point
Using a fresh hot pack every 10 minutes may prolong the heating, but it makes no difference to the temperature reached in the subcutaneous tissues in a 20 minute treatment (Lehmann et al., 1966). This lends justification to the common practice of not changing packs during a treatment.

CONTRAST BATHS

Contrast baths involve alternate immersion in hot and cold water producing marked hyperaemia of the skin. The temperatures in the subcutaneous tissue just below the skin can fluctuate from 8°C to 14°C when using contrast bathing, but little change, 0.5°C, occurs at a 1 cm depth intramuscularly (Myrer et al., 1997). By contrast, ice packs produced intramuscular temperature drops of approximately 7°C and subcutaneous tissue drops of 17°C.

Contrast baths are used because of the considerable sensory stimulation they produce as the cutaneous hot and cold receptors are alternately activated. This stimulation is relatively vigorous because each time neural accommodation starts to occur the temperature stimulation is reversed. This strong sensory stimulation may act to suppress pain by means of a gating mechanism (see chapter 6) and account for the subjective relief of pain that occurs in patients receiving this treatment. There is no evidence, however, that contrast baths help to reduce local oedema by promoting alternate vasodilation and vasoconstriction. Instead, contrast baths may actually increase oedema, perhaps because this treatment usually requires the treated limb to be dependent.

Method of application

An explanation and examination are given in the usual way and thermal sensitivity of skin tested.

Two suitably sized baths are filled, the hot at 40–45°C and the cold at 15–20°C (water from the cold tap is usually in this range). Treatment usually starts and finishes with immersion in the hot water. Immersion in the hot water is longer – 3 or 4 minutes – while immersion in the cold water is kept to 1 minute. This cycle is repeated three or four times so that the whole treatment lasts from 15 to 25 minutes. An initial hot immersion of 10 minutes has been recommended to achieve hyperaemia (Lehmann and de Lateur, 1982).

During the treatment the hot water will cool and the cold will be warmed, partly due to the transfer of the warm/cold wet limb from one bath to the other. It might be necessary to top up both baths during treatment with hot or cold water to maintain the required temperatures. A thermometer should be available to monitor the water temperature.

HYDROTHERAPY

Warm water has been used for therapeutic purposes since ancient times, particularly where the presence of natural warm water has provided an opportunity for the development of spas. In thermal areas in some parts of the world such as Iceland or New Zealand, the water appears as geysers or bubbles up in hot mud. Such sources often contain sulphur and other minerals. Ground water can be forced to the surface after permeating deeply placed, and hence hotter, rock formations. In some limestone areas, e.g. the Mendips, water is carried deeply in porous rock to become heated; it emerges at Bath (in the UK) at about 46°C.

Swimming and exercising in warm water have beneficial effects which were often ascribed to the minerals dissolved in the water. These effects could well be due to the warmth itself.

As the whole body is immersed and the major therapeutic effect is considered to be due to the exercise rather than the water temperature or chemicals present, hydrotherapy is outside the scope of this book and current texts on hydrotherapy should be consulted.

WHIRLPOOL BATHS

Whirlpool baths are stainless-steel tanks or baths of various sizes. The smaller ones are made to accommodate one limb, while larger ones allow the patient to sit. The 'whirlpool' refers to turbulence produced by a jet of air produced by an electric pump which mixes air and water into a jetstream. This water agitation can be varied in force by controls on the pump (or turbine) and air pressure. The direction of the stream can be altered by changing the position of the output nozzle. A mixing tap allows any desired water temperature; temperatures between 36 and 41°C are usually employed.

The agitation of the water, the whirlpool effect, serves to stimulate the skin surface mechanically. This stimulation of large-diameter mechanoreceptors together with thermoreceptors may account for analgesic effects (Walsh, 1996) due to the gating mechanism discussed in chapter 6. The mechanical effect can also be used in the cleaning of open wounds – gentle debridement of dirt and necrotic tissue. Vigorous action can destroy the delicate granulation. In circumstances where healing is slow, such as varicose ulcers, the mechanical effect is considered to provoke granulation tissue formation by increasing the local blood flow.

There is evidence that the temperature of the subcutaneous tissues rises with whirlpool bath treatment, as with any other form of conduction heating (Borrel et al., 1980), and thus there is some increase in blood flow. There is also evidence that treatment in the bath increases oedema; an increased tissue volume was found both in patients and in healthy subjects (Magness et al., 1970). If oedema is a likely problem it would be reasonable to modify the treatment so that it is followed by a period of warmth and/or exercise with the limb in elevation.

Treatment is usually for 20 minutes. Longer treatments confer no greater benefit, at least in so far as tissue heating is concerned. Prolonged immersion in hot water leads to temporary wrinkling of the skin which, in healthy skin, recovers rapidly on drying. However, repeated soaking tends to increase the risk of skin infection and exacerbate any infection already present; atrophic skin is particularly at risk.

CONSIDERATIONS AND CONTRAINDICATIONS TO TREATMENTS WITH HOT WATER

There is very little chance of damage with these treatments since mild heat and simple, familiar materials are used:

Although the water in whirlpool baths is changed for each patient, it is often advisable to add an antibacterial agent to the water. Sodium hypochlorite (bleach) in a 1 to 20 to 1 to 100 dilution is recommended (Walsh, 1996).

An increase in oedema is unsurprising since, again, the extremities will be dependent during immersion in the warm water.

- *Poor treatment technique or accidents*: local burns can occur if very hot water contacts the skin; this would require a careless application of a hydrocollator pack or malfunction of the apparatus used for most other forms of superficial heating. With most types of superficial heat treatments it is advisable to check the patient's level of cutaneous thermal sensitivity in the treated area. This means a suitable technique can be selected or modified as necessary.

- *Any ischaemic disease that reduces the local circulation*. Local thermal regulation depends on an increased cutaneous blood flow in response to heating. If this cannot occur the tissue may be at risk of local burns and subsequent necrosis.

- *Altered heat loss mechanisms*: in this case, immersion of the whole body, or large segments in water above the core temperature means there is no way of losing heat from the areas under the water. Those with any deficiency of the cardiovascular system or heat-regulating mechanisms may be at risk in these circumstances.

- *Infections, especially fungal*, often thrive in moisture. Examples include tinea pedis (athlete's foot) and paronychia. Use a form or dry heating or a plastic barrier when thermal effects that do not wet the skin are required.

- *Exacerbations of acute dermatitis or eczema*: heat, especially immersion in hot or warm water, can exacerbate these conditions. Similarly, superficial heat should not be used following applications of cutaneous chemical irritants, and for at least 6 months following radiotherapy.

- *Dependent limb following trauma*: this should be avoided, an important consideration with some forms of superficial heating in which it is not avoidable.

HEATED AIR TREATMENT

Both simple hot, dry air and a mixture of air and water vapour are described as hot air baths. Small hot air cabinets – a metal box fitted with an electric fan or element heater, both thermostatically controlled – are useful for hand injuries with oedema and open wounds as the hand can be exercised in elevation and nothing but warm air comes in contact with the tissues. Temperature in the metal cabinet should be about 70°C, but because of the low thermal conductivity of air, the skin temperature is kept much lower.

Small fan heaters, such as hairdriers, are occasionally used to give mild heating to open wounds such as bedsores. Although there is no hard evidence as yet, the accompanying drying effect could be detrimental to the healing process.

Hot or hot moist air can also be applied by enclosing the whole body in special cabinets. This can produce a small rise in body core temperature and needs strict control and adequate body fluid replacement.

ELECTRIC HEATING PADS

These vary from small pads about 30 by 30 cm to electric blankets. Electric resistance wire is contained in a suitable fabric and the current flow is controlled and selectable so that the pad produces various levels of heating when placed against the skin. These pads are particularly useful for treatment at home and for producing muscle relaxation prior to other treatments such as exercise or mobilization.

HEATING AND COOLING APPARATUS

A heating and cooling flow unit is another option for superficial heating. These units circulate thermostatically controlled warm or cool water through a sealed bag held in contact with the skin. The units are described in more detail in the chapter on cold, in the section on 'Cryotherapy flow units'.

Summary

Therapeutic thermal conduction methods:

- wax baths – heating and moistening skin
- hot packs –moist or dry heating
- contrast baths – heating and cooling
- whirlpool baths – heating and mechanical stimulation
- hot air – heating
- electrical heating pads – heating
- cryotherapy flow units – heating and cooling.

THE EFFECTS OF SUPERFICIAL HEAT ON TISSUES

Superficial heating is usually used in conjunction with other types of treatment such as exercise, mobilization or massage and rarely as a sole treatment. As explained above, tissues above the fatty tissue layer, which contain an abundance of sensory receptors, are heated appreciably so sensory fibre activity increases markedly. Temperature elevation in the fatty tissue and underlying tissue is less for two reasons: first that fat is a good insulator and second, that heat is rapidly conducted away by the circulating blood.

Applying heat to the skin leads to reflex vasodilation which helps to dissipate the local heat. The local vasodilation in the heated skin subsequently extends to nearby areas of the skin, and increases the heat loss from the body. As noted above, little direct heating of the deeper tissues occurs as they are shielded by the thermal insulation provided by the subcutaneous fat. Vasodilation results in increased blood flow which conducts heat away from both superficial and more deeply located tissue. These effects are consistent with studies of the effectiveness of clinical uses of superficial heating.

Most studies examining the effectiveness of superficial heating investigate either the changes in the blood flow (a quantitative measure) or pain (a qualitative and so more subjective and less reliable but essential outcome measure). Also, the effects of treatment packages that contain superficial heating as one component have been examined.

Changes to blood flow with superficial heating can range from a baseline flow of $50\,ml\,min^{-1}$ to an extreme of 2 to $3\,l\,min^{-1}$: an increase of about fifty-fold. Homeostatic mechanisms in the body limit the local effects as the heat is transferred by convection, i.e. transfer of heat via the bloodstream, to deeper and adjacent tissues. If local perfusion is limited, for example, by compression or pathological obstruction of the vascular system there is a risk of skin damage if the local tissue temperature becomes too high. For this reason patients should never lie on sources of heat that are either hot (e.g. hydrocollator packs, at least initially) or where the temperature is not thermostatically limited to a safe level.

The main clinical indicators for using superficial heating are for pain reduction and increasing range of movement. A number of studies show that superficial heating is an effective way of relieving some forms of pain. Superficial heating with hydrocollator packs can reduce a physiological response to pain, the sympathetic skin response. The reduced pain response continues for at least 15 minutes after removing the hot pack (On et al., 1997). Similarly, heat wrap, a longer lasting method of superficial heating has been shown to produce extended periods of pain relief and a faster resolution of muscle stiffness (spasm) for patients with non-specific low back pain (Nadler et al., 2003). Superficial heating using a heated gel pack can also reduce pain following exercise-induced soreness. When compared to the pain relief offered by a cold gel pack, a room temperature gel pack or no treatment, Sumida et al. (2003) found that a heated gel pack was considerably more effective.

What is described as 'increased tissue extensibility' prior to stretching is the other main clinical indication for using superficial heating. The term 'increased tissue extensibility' should not be interpreted as meaning that the mechanical properties of deep tissue are changed by superficial heating but rather that the CNS activity produced by stretch is reduced. Heating has a palliative effect which allows greater stretch without discomfort, not greater stretch because the tissue is softer.

Research findings suggest some clinical benefit of superficial heating but the effects are not always sufficient to be statistically significant (Lentell et al., 1992; Taylor et al, 1995; Robertson et al, 2004). Possible explanations for the 'insignificant' findings are either that the heating was not deep enough (Sawyer et al., 2003) or that the resulting temperature increase was insufficient.

A more common way of using heat for pain relief is as part of a treatment package. For example, it may be used with stretching and cold spray or electrical stimulation to treat myofascial and trigger point pain (Hou et al., 2002). Similarly it may be used with exercise to treat various forms of arthritis.

Cochrane reviews of the effectiveness of thermotherapy for treating rheumatoid arthritis (Robinson et al., 2004) and osteoarthritis (Brosseau et al., 2004) highlight the lack of well designed studies on the topic and so cannot provide conclusive recommendations.

Studies of changes in intra-articular temperatures have shown that some changes occur with superficial heating but the greater the depth the less the change.

The extent of heat transfer is evident in a study which measured changes in the intra-articular and skin temperatures following an application of hot packs at 42°C for 30 minutes. The five patients tested each had bilateral effusions and the intra-articular temperature in only the treated knees increased by a statistically significant amount, albeit after the skin temperature (Weinberger et al., 1989). This indicates that some conduction to the local deep tissues does occur and it is for this reason that superficial heat is used to treat such structures; for example, applying hot packs to a knee as part of treatment of chronic arthritis. There is, however, little evidence of how clinically effective this is.

Some other interesting uses of superficial heating include it as a way of increasing exercise tolerance for patients with advanced cardiac disease. For those with a limited exercise tolerance due to chronic heart failure, superficial heating of exercising leg muscles by hot packs can increase exercise tolerance (Yamanouchi et al., 1996). Hot packs also seem to slow the extent of signs of fatigue associated with repetitive exercise (Nadler et al., 2001). The clinical significance of this is unknown.

Hot packs have also been used prior to ultrasound to increase the depth and extent of intramuscular heating. A 15 minute application effectively reduces the time needed to apply ultrasound to reach a particular level of heating (Draper et al., 1998; Holcomb, 2003). The main advantage is the longer time available for active treatment as, while the rate of temperature increase and decrease will be similar, the higher initial temperature extends the effective treatment time.

In another interesting study, applications of hot packs to the forearm and hand produced a small increase in finger tapping speed which persisted for at least 30 minutes (Kauranen and Vanharanta, 1997). Hot packs also, rather curiously, were found to delay reaction time; an effect ascribed by the authors to diminished mental alertness as a consequence of greater relaxation induced by the warmth.

THE THERAPEUTIC USES OF SUPERFICIAL HEATING

Various forms of superficial heating are widely used for pain relief; the mechanisms have been discussed in chapter 10. Since the effects are largely confined to the skin it is reasonable to propose that the major pain-relieving effects are due to a form of pain-gating. The other therapeutic effects, discussed in chapter 10 and illustrated in Figure 10.4, are attributable to conduction heating which is limited by the insulation properties of fatty tissue.

The lack of convincing evidence supporting the clinical effectiveness of superficial heating is consistent with its rarely being used as a sole treatment. Instead, superficial heating is usually used as part of a treatment package for the long accepted and major benefits it can offer patients, pain reduction and increased range of movement.

Summary

Therapeutic uses of superficial heat:

- the relief of pain
- the relief of muscle spasm
- increase tissue extensibility (i.e. the range of joint movement)
- acceleration of healing/resolution of chronic inflammatory states
- increase exercise tolerance in some patients
- facilitation of fine movements.

References

Abramson, D., Tuck, S., Chu, L. et al. (1964). Effect of paraffin bath and hot fomentations on local tissue temperature. Arch Phys Med Rehabil **45**, 87–94.

Ayling, J., Marks, R. (2000). Efficacy of paraffin wax baths for rheumatoid arthritic hands. Physiotherapy, **86**, 190–201.

Borrell, P., Parker, R., Henley, E. et al. (1980). Comparison of 'in vivo' temperatures produced by hydrotherapy, paraffin wax treatment and fluidotherapy. Phys Ther, **60**, 1273–1276.

Brosseau, L., Yonge, K., Robinson, V. et al. (2004). Thermotherapy for treatment of osteoarthritis (Cochrane Review). In The Cochrane Library, Issue 1. Chichester, UK: John Wiley & Sons, Ltd.

Draper, D. O., Harris, S. T., Schulthies, S. et al. (1998). Hot-pack and 1-MHz ultrasound treatments have an additive effect on muscle temperature increase. J Athletic Training, **33**, 21–24.

Fyfe, M. (1982). Skin temperature, colour, and warmth felt, in hydrocollator pack applications to the lumbar region. Aust J Physiother, **28**, 12–15.

Griffin, J., Karselis, T. (1988). Physical Agents for Physical Therapists, 3rd edn. Springfield, USA: Charles C. Thomas.

Holcomb, W. (2003). The effects of superficial heating before 1-MHz ultrasound on tissue temperature. J Sport Rehabil, **12**, 95–103.

Hou, C., Tsai, L., Cheng, K. et al. (2002). Immediate effects of various physical therapeutic modalities on cervical myofascial pain and trigger-point sensitivity. Arch Phys Med Rehabil, **83**, 1406–1414.

Kauranen, K., Vanharanta, H. (1997). Effects of hot and cold packs on motor performance of normal hands. Physiotherapy, **83**, 340–344.

Lehmann, J., de Lateur, B. (1982). Therapeutic heat. In J. Lehmann (ed.), Therapeutic Heat and Cold, pp. 404–562. Baltimore: Williams & Wilkins.

Lehmann, J., Silvermann, D., Baum, B. et al. (1966). Temperature distribution in the human thigh produced by infra-red, hot pack and microwave applications. Arch Phys Med Rehabil, **47**, 291–299.

Lentell, G., Hetherington, T., Eagan, J., Morgan, M. (1992). The use of thermal agents to influence the effectiveness of a low-load prolonged stretch. J Orthop Sports Phys Ther, **16**, 200–207.

Magness, J., Garret, T., Erickson, D. (1970). Swelling of the upper extremity during whirlpool baths. Arch Phys Med Rehabil, **51**, 297.

McMeeken, J., Bell, C. (1990). Effects of selective blood and tissue heating on blood flow in the dog hind limb. Exp Physiol, **75**, 355–366.

Myrer, J. W., Measom, G., Durrant, E., Fellingham, G. W. (1997). Cold- and hot-pack contrast therapy: subcutaneous and intramuscular temperature change. J Athletic Training, **32**, 238–241.

Nadler, S., Steiner, D., Erasala, G. et al. (2003). Continuous low-level heatwrap therapy for treating acute nonspecific low back pain. Arch Phys Med Rehabil, **84**, 329–334.

Nadler, S. F., Feinberg, J. H., Reisman, S. et al. (2001). Effect of topical heat on electromyographic power density spectrum in subjects with myofascial pain and normal controls: a pilot study. Am J Phys Med Rehabil, **80**, 809–815.

On, A. Y., Colakoglu, Z., Hepguler, S., Aksit, R. (1997). Local heat effect on sympathetic skin responses after pain of electrical stimulus. Arch Phys Med Rehabil, **78**, 1196–1199.

Poindexter, R., Wright, E., Murchison, D. (2002). Comparison of moist and dry heat penetration through orofacial tissues. J Craniomandibular Pract, **20**, 28–33.

Robertson, V., Ward, A., Jung, P. (2005). The contribution of heating to tissue extensibility: a comparison of deep and superficial heating. Arch Phys Med Rehabil, **86**, 819–825.

Robinson, V., Brosseau, L., Casimiro, L. et al. (2004). Thermotherapy for treating rheumatoid arthritis (Cochrane Review). In The Cochrane Library (Vol. Issue 1). Chichester, UK: John Wiley & Sons, Ltd.

Sawyer, P. C., Uhl, T. L., Mattacola, C. G. et al. (2003). Effects of moist heat on hamstring flexibility and muscle temperature. J Strength Conditioning Res, **17**, 285–290.

Sekins, K., Emery, A. (1982). Thermal science for physical medicine. In J. Lehmann (ed.), Therapeutic Heat and Cold, pp. 70–132. Baltimore: Williams & Wilkins.

Sumida, K., Greenberg, M., Hill, J. (2003). Hot gel packs and reduction of delayed-onset muscle soreness 30 minutes after treatment. J Sport Rehabil, **12**, 221–228.

Taylor, B. F., Waring, C. A., Brashear, T. A. (1995). The effects of therapeutic application of heat or cold followed by static stretch on hamstring muscle length. J Orthop Sports Phys Ther, **21**, 283–286.

Walsh, M. (1996). Hydrotherapy: The use of water as a therapeutic agent. In S. Michlovitz (ed.), Thermal Agents in Rehabilitation, 3rd edn, pp. 139–167. Philadelphia: F.A.Davis Company.

Weinberger, A., Fadilah, R., Lev, A. et al. (1989). Intra-articular temperature measurements after superficial heating. Scand J Rehabil Med, **21**, 55–57.

Yamanouchi, T., Ajisaka, R., Sakamoto, K. et al. (1996). Effect of warming of exercising legs on exercise capacity in patients with impaired exercise tolerance. Jpnese Heart J, **37**, 855–863.

Cold therapy

Cold therapy or cryotherapy refers to the use of local or general body cooling for therapeutic purposes. The latter is of importance for major cardiothoracic surgery or neurosurgery but it is the former – local cooling or cryotherapy – that is the subject of this chapter. The effects of cooling the surface of the skin are dealt with first, followed by discussion of the therapeutic uses of cold therapy. Major methods of applying cold are then described, including immersion, cold packs, ice towels, ice massage and evaporating sprays. Finally, dangers and contraindications are discussed.

EFFECTS OF COOLING THE SKIN

Cooling the body surface is simply the transfer of energy away from that region. This lowers the local tissue temperature and provokes a range of thermoregulatory responses described in chapter 10. Although cooling can be achieved in different ways, including evaporating liquids off the skin or blowing cold air over it, the majority of cold treatments use crushed ice. Heat is thus transferred by conduction from the skin and the energy is used in changing solid ice to water. It takes a great deal of energy to melt ice ($333\,kJ\,kg^{-1}$).

The extent of temperature changes in the tissues will depend on both the rate and amount of heat energy removed. In practice, this means the changes in temperature in tissue due to local cooling will depend on the following factors:

- the difference in temperature between the cooling source and the part being cooled
- whether the cooling source has a constant temperature (e.g. ice bath with cooling system) or is gradually warming (e.g. uncovered cooled gel pack)
- whether there are barriers to cooling (e.g. layers of towelling or the presence of oil, dry towelling or paper covering and protecting bony areas such as malleoli)

More than twice as much energy is needed to melt 1 g of ice than is needed to raise the temperature of 1 g of water from 0°C to 37°C.

The normal layer of subcutaneous fat serves as thermal insulation so that heat loss from the underlying tissue depends on the fatty tissue thickness and blood flow through this fatty layer.

- the size of area cooled (which affects the extent of cooling of the body so that the larger the area being cooled, the more heat energy is lost from the body)
- the thermal conductivity of the substance used and the tissues being cooled (e.g. the properties of gel and ice packs are very different and affect the extent of cooling). Similarly, the thermal conductivity varies between different body areas – it is higher in water-rich tissues such as muscle, and less in fat and skin
- the volume rate of flow of blood through the tissue as it transfers heat from the rest of the body and so reduces the rate and extent of temperature drop
- the method used for a particular type of cooling (e.g. for ice packs if covered with a dry or a damp towel and, placement of compression bandages directly on the skin or over the ice pack)
- the duration of the exposure. The temperature falls until the energy lost at the surface is balanced by heat energy supplied from the rest of the body, at which point the temperature becomes constant.

While the skin temperature can be changed abruptly and markedly with the application of cold the deeper tissues are cooled much less and much more slowly. This has been demonstrated by several investigators. Figure 12.1 illustrates this point. In this example it takes some 30 minutes to lower the muscle temperature at a depth of 4 cm by 3.5°C or so. Muscle tissue at 2.5 cm can take up to 20 minutes or longer to drop 5°C (Palastanga, 1988).

Similarly the application of a 3 kg bag of ice chips for 30 minutes to the front of the knee caused the intra-articular temperature of the knee joint to fall by an average of 9.4°C (Oosterveld et al., 1992). This remarkably low intra-articular temperature was associated with a fall of 16.4°C in the knee skin temperature of these normal subjects.

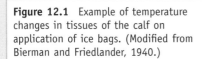

Figure 12.1 Example of temperature changes in tissues of the calf on application of ice bags. (Modified from Bierman and Friedlander, 1940.)

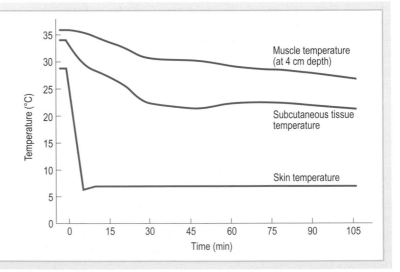

The paucity of subcutaneous fat over the knee joint may account for the lower than expected intra-articular temperatures.

PHYSIOLOGICAL CHANGES

Cooling the skin surface leads to rapid local changes at the cooled site. A range of other changes happens, more gradually, as the temperature of the deeper tissue decreases and the heat regulating mechanisms of the body are activated (see Figure 12.1).

The local effects

On cutaneous blood vessels

There is immediate vasoconstriction of cutaneous blood vessels, shown by the blanching that occurs. This restricts the blood flow in the skin so that heat loss is minimized. The speed with which this vasoconstriction occurs indicates that it is an autonomic nervous system reflex triggered by the stimulation of thermal receptors in the skin. This vasoconstriction leads to a dramatic decrease in blood flow through the skin, and hence limits the conduction of heat to the body surface. Blood viscosity increases due to cooling and this also contributes to the reduced local blood perfusion.

After some minutes the vasoconstriction may give way to a marked vasodilation which itself may last some 15 minutes before being replaced by another episode of vasoconstriction. This alternation of constriction and dilation is called the Lewis 'hunting reaction' (Lewis, 1930), in the sense that the vessel 'hunts' or oscillates about its mean degree of constriction. This cold-induced vasodilation occurs most easily when the rest of the body is relatively warm and is largely confined to certain body areas. It occurs most readily and most rapidly in the face, especially the nose and ears, but also in the hands, feet, patella region, olecranon, buttocks and some parts of the chest wall (Fox and Wyatt, 1962). The response varies from person to person and does not always show the clear-cut cycling effect.

This curious hunting response to cold protects tissues, especially those in exposed and activity-compressed areas, from damage due to prolonged cooling and relative ischaemia.

On deeper tissue blood flow

What is known about the effects on deeper tissue blood flow comes from both animal and human studies. At the microvascular level in the striated muscles of hamsters the arteriolar diameters decrease by up to 43% over 30 minutes of local hypothermia at 8°C (Thorlacius et al., 1998). As expected, this causes a marked reduction in blood flow rate, of up to 80%. The marked reduction in local blood flow might be expected to cause local tissue damage because of ischaemia. This does not occur and the lack of tissue damage produced by cooling is attributed to a decreased rate of cellular metabolism and possibly

This indicates that due consideration must be given to the anatomical properties of each area when local cooling is applied. For example, a reduction in blood flow sufficient to cause skin damage is possible over areas with limited soft tissue coverage.

This again emphasizes the need for users to consider the area being cooled and what factors might increase or decrease effectiveness and any risks of damage through applying local cooling.

to changes in prostaglandin synthesis (Thorlacius et al., 1998). The same effects in humans suggest the same, or very similar, microvascular responses occur to cold.

Cooling applied to the skin also affects blood flow at deeper levels, including in the bone (Ho et al., 1995). A drop of as much as 5% in skeletal blood flow can occur after 5 minutes of continuous surface cooling. This increases to 20% after 25 minutes. The extent of change is affected by the depth of soft tissue. In this example, relatively superficial bony areas (knees) were cooled. For areas covered with a greater depth of soft tissue the extent of the changes in bone would be less.

The temperatures in the subacromial space and glenohumeral joint have been shown barely to change in response to skin cooling using a continuous flow system (Levy et al., 1997). Large muscles envelope this area versus the relatively small cover over the knee region. Also, the relative size of the area cooled is less over the shoulder as a circumferential method is not possible, unlike with the knee or ankle region. Again this highlights the importance of considering the anatomy of the region being treated and the possible effects of different methods of cooling.

The thickness of the overlying adipose tissue also, of course, affects the extent of temperature change in deeper soft tissues. Myrer et al. (2001) report that the difference in temperature change is approximately three times less at depths of both 1 and 3 cm if the skinfold thickness is 20 mm or more compared to 8 mm or less. This difference at both 1 and 3 cm depths illustrates the extent of the contribution of the adipose layer to insulating deeper structures against temperature changes.

Deeper tissues tend to cool and re-warm more slowly than the skin and superficial 1 cm or so of tissues. At 2 and 3 cm depth, the temperature usually drops minimally during a 20 minute application of a cold pack (Enwemeka et al., 2002). However, it continues to fall, even after the cold pack is removed and the skin and superficial tissues have re-warmed. Presumably the heat from deeper tissues is transferred more superficially to re-warm the overlying (but still relatively deeply located) tissues which have not rapidly re-warmed.

The lower rate of temperature change in deeper tissues has implications for users of local cooling. A longer time to cool at depth suggests that 20 minutes is a more appropriate time for deeper cooling than 5 minutes. To ensure and maintain deep cooling the application should be repeated within another 40 to 60 minutes. This was demonstrated in studies involving sheep both with and without local trauma (Walton et al., 1986). Twenty minute applications of cold packs repeated after 20 minutes without continued to reduce the deeper tissue temperatures while the skin and superficial tissue substantially reverted to near-initial temperatures during the 20 minute 'pack off' periods.

Cooling also decreases the microvascular permeability and motility and adherence of leucocytes in rats (Deal et al., 2002) and hamsters (Thorlacius et al., 1998). Presumably the same effects occur in humans as local cooling is known to decrease or at least reduce the extent of oedema formation following acute trauma.

On tissue metabolism

A major reason for cooling living tissue is to reduce the local metabolic rate. With an acute injury there are two sources of damage: from the primary injury and from secondary hypoxia and post-trauma enzyme activity (Merrick et al., 1999). Superficial cooling of affected tissues should therefore increase their chances of survival if applied soon enough after trauma.

The primary injury produces cell death and disruption of the micro-architecture including the blood supply. Cells which survived the immediate injury may be deprived of their usual rate of oxygen supply and suffer hypoxic death. The reduced metabolic demand and rate of necrotic enzyme release and activity at lower temperatures enhances the chances of survival of these vulnerable cells.

A reduction in oedema, due partly to less tissue damage and also to decreased diffusion rates at lower temperatures, also reduces secondary damage. Swelling would increase the distance of cells from their usual supply vessels and possibly occlude some smaller ones. This would further reduce the rate of oxygen transport through affected areas and cause greater local cell necrosis. By using cooling to limit swelling, secondary damage and thus total damage is reduced.

On the peripheral nervous system

The direct effects of cooling on peripheral nerve fibres are reasonably well understood but their relationship to the observed physiological effects of cooling is less well established. If the hand is immersed in ice-cold water, there is an immediate perception of coldness. The sensation gradually fades and numbness sets in. This is accompanied or followed by a deep, aching pain sensation.

The primary sensation of cold is produced by the activation of cold receptors (see Figure 10.2), which generate activity (action potentials) in small-diameter, myelinated A-δ fibres. The perception of cold, particularly the initial perception, is also due to a change (often a decrease) in activity of other, larger-diameter, myelinated sensory fibres (A-β fibres). The delayed-onset, deep aching is produced by the activation of nociceptors; the fine nerve-endings of C fibres. C fibre nocioceptor activity is generated by the chemical debris, the toxins released by dead and damaged cells.

If nerve fibres are cooled sufficiently, conduction block occurs. Nerve fibres are not all equally affected in this way. C fibres, because they are unmyelinated are relatively unaffected. Comparing the myelinated fibres, the smaller the diameter, the greater the effect. A-δ fibres

C fibre activity is not in response to the actual temperature decrease, as such, but rather in response to the resulting damage to cells.

Table 12.1 Peripheral nerve fibres affected by cooling		
Most affected by cold	**Moderately affected by cold**	**Least affected by cold**
A-β Intrafusal muscle fibres Low-threshold mechanoreceptors	A-α Extrafusal muscle fibres Cutaneous, joint and muscle receptors	B Preganglionic efferent autonomic C Postganglionic efferent autonomic
A-γ Intrafusal muscle fibres		Slow pain, polymodal nociceptors
A-δ Fast pain High-threshold mechanoreceptors Cold receptors		Warm receptors

are the most susceptible to cold. A-γ and A-β fibres are less, but still markedly, affected. A-α fibres are affected to a lesser extent. This explains why the initial sensation of coldness disappears (A-δ blocking) and numbness sets in (blocking of larger, sensory neurons). It also explains why the deep aching persists, despite the numbness.

Table 12.1, derived from Douglas and Malcolm (1955) summarizes the susceptibility of the different nerve fibre types to conduction block by hypothermia.

With the temperature drops to be expected in clinical applications of cooling, the decrease in B and C fibre function would be negligible. The major effect would be on A-δ fibre activity and, to a lesser extent, that of A-β and A-γ fibres.

This helps to explain why icing is of value with an acute injury. Sharp pain (A-δ activity) is reduced. Low threshold mechanoreceptor activity (activated by pressure increases in damaged tissue due to swelling) is also reduced as is intrafusal muscle fibre activity. This is partly due to blocking of the fibres and also due to reduced pressure and swelling as a consequence of the decreased metabolic activity of the tissues at lower temperatures and thus less initiation of nerve fibre activity. The amount of C fibre activity would also be less, not directly because of the cooling, but because the lower temperatures result in a reduced rate of secondary cell damage and consequently a reduced rate of production of chemical irritants.

This also helps to explain why icing is of little value for the treatment of most chronic pain syndromes, where C fibre activity is predominant and a lower temperature would not necessarily reduce the levels of irritants causing fibre activity.

A conclusion from Douglas and Malcolm's pioneering work is that pain reduction due to cooling is not a consequence of reduced C-fibre transmission (though it could result from decreased C-fibre activation). Nor is pain reduction likely to be due to gating of the pain signals, as this would need increased A-fibre activity. Cooling

This helps explain the relief of chronic pain by heating. Heat will stimulate sensory fibre activity and produce gating of C fibre pain signals.

affects the sharp/acute pain associated with A-δ activity and indirectly affect the deep, aching pain sensation conveyed by C fibre activity by lowering the levels of chemical irritants.

On the motor system

Locally applied cold (ice towels, for example) has been shown to increase the isometric strength and endurance of the quadriceps (Sanya and Bello, 1999). The effect is limited to low amounts of cooling and has a short duration as muscle activity markedly increases the rate of re-warming of deeper tissues after cooling (Myrer et al., 2000). If cooling is either greater or prolonged, the outcome is a reduction in muscle strength. Thermoregulatory effects on blood flow may, in part, explain these effects. Modest cooling would result in reflex vasodilation and increased blood flow. Greater cooling would induce protective vasoconstriction and a consequent reduction in the supply of nutrients and removal of waste products.

Tremor is an inseparable part of muscle contraction. In youth, the fluctuations in muscle force which produce tremor are usually small so the tremor is unnoticeable. With normal ageing, tremor increases. In conditions such as Parkinson's and Alzheimer's disease, tremor is markedly increased. Cooling reduces tremor. The cooling effect has been used to improve hand function in patients with clinically significant tremor (Cooper et al., 2000) and to reduce spasticity (Allison and Abraham, 2001). It may be that slower nerve conduction as a result of cooling has a dampening effect on the neural feedback loops which produce tremor.

> Tremor is accentuated markedly by stimulants such as caffeine and is reduced by depressants such as barbiturates and alcohol.

Motor skills are diminished by local cooling. Voluntary movement is slowed and there is a loss in dexterity. An ice pack applied for 15 minues to the forearm causes a significant decrease in the velocity of movement and finger tapping speed (Kauranen and Vanharanta, 1997). These effects could be due to slowed nerve conduction (which would increase the cycling time of neural feedback loops and reflex arcs), a direct slowing of muscle contraction or a combination of such factors.

Cooling has also been shown to reverse the conduction block associated with demyelination of peripheral nerve fibres. Local damage to the myelin sheath of peripheral nerves can result from compression or inflammation, preventing transmission of action potentials. Heating the region of injury will usually exacerbate the block. Cooling has the opposite effect (Rutkove, 2001).

> Cooling can produce conduction block in undamaged nerve but can facilitate transmission in demyelinated nerve fibres.

It is evident that the effects of cooling on the motor system depend on the amount and duration of cooling and may differ if there is pathology. The duration and method used will affect the depth and extent of cooling. If greater cooling for longer, the effect is more likely to be a decreased activation. If less cooling then the effect might be an increased activation. This difference should suggest to users how they might vary treatment to meet different patient requirements.

Summary

The local effects of cooling include:

- Immediate perception of cold and pain:
  - cold receptors are stimulated
  - pain receptors responding to cold may be stimulated
- Immediate vasoconstriction of cutaneous vessels followed by cold-induced vasodilation in some areas, which may continue in a cyclical manner
- Reduced local deep blood volume and flow rate:
  - depends on area cooled, local depth of soft tissue
  - deeper effects are less if thickness of overlying adipose tissue is greater
  - deeper tissues cool and re-warm more slowly than superficial ones
- Reduced local metabolic rate:
  - reduced oxygen requirement
  - reduced cellular activity
- Effects on peripheral nervous system:
  - initial strong sensory stimulus
  - eventual suppression or reduction of pain
- Variable effect on motor system:
  - can increase muscle strength and endurance
  - can reduce motor activity and fine skill performance.

General effects of cooling

Cooling applied to the skin immediately stimulates cold receptors which are more numerous than heat receptors in any given area. Although some of these cold receptors are firing at normal skin temperatures their activity increases greatly as cooling occurs, diminishing somewhat when cooling becomes steady, i.e. they show adaptation. Extreme cold is experienced as pain, involving pain receptors (see chapter 10). Both pain and temperature neurons synapse in the posterior horn of the spinal cord; the subsequent neuron ascends in the spinothalamic tract of the opposite side. Apart from a synapse in the thalamus with a neuron to the sensory cortex, giving awareness of cold, there are many collateral paths, particularly to the hypothalamus.

As explained in chapter 10, the hypothalamus acts as a thermostat to maintain core temperature. The posterior hypothalamus is concerned with the response to body cooling, being affected by nervous input from the skin and probably other receptors as well as the blood temperature. To conserve heat the response, via the vasomotor centre, is cutaneous vasoconstriction. The degree of general vasoconstriction that occurs is dependent on the extent of the cooling. Further, if the temperature drop is great enough shivering will occur. This increases

The skin blood flow can be increased (see Figure 10.3) by vasodilation much more readily than it can be diminished (Hubbard and Mechan, 1987), indicating that humans are better adapted to a hot environment; this is also evidenced by the efficiency of the sweating response.

the rate of metabolism, and hence heat production, by irregular muscle contractions. The resting metabolic rate can be doubled by shivering over periods of several hours and rather more over shorter periods (Hardy, 1982). However, it is expensive in physiological terms in that energy is being expended. As noted in chapter 10, brown adipose tissue in neonates is able to produce heat by directly metabolizing but this does not seem to occur significantly in adults. Shivering in the muscles of mastication gives rise to the familiar teeth chattering with cold. Awareness of cold leads to behavioural responses to maintain body temperature, such as increased activity or putting on more clothes.

THERAPEUTIC USES OF COOLING

Recent injuries

In response to injury, vascular tissues undergo three distinct but overlapping processes: necrosis, inflammation and repair. Consider, for example, a slip with a kitchen knife resulting in a flesh wound. The initial laceration produces little tissue damage or cell death. Far greater damage occurs secondarily. Blood clotting is essential to prevent blood loss, but an unfortunate consequence is that many more cells die due to lack of oxygen (hypoxia). This is the necrotic phase which results from the injured area being sealed-off. Necrosis is compounded by the effects of proteolytic enzymes released from ruptured cells.

Necrosis is followed by an inflammatory phase where blood flow in the surrounding region is increased, there is dilation of the vascular walls and increased permeability of the vessel walls as part of the process of cleaning up the damage. As described in chapter 2, oedema production is an integral part of the inflammatory process. The third phase, repair, involves the laying down of fibrous tissue which is then invaded by new blood vessels. Fibrous repair tissue, scar tissue which is predominantly collagen, is laid down and then undergoes a prolonged period of remodelling.

Cold is widely used in the treatment of recent injuries. Applied to the skin, cold causes immediate vasoconstriction and makes the blood more viscid; both diminish the flow. Combined with pressure over the wound such treatment leads to haemostasis. However, the cooling must not be so intense or so prolonged as to delay blood coagulation – clotting time is lengthened by cooling. When bleeding occurs deep in the tissues, forming an intramuscular haematoma, for example, the same principle would apply but much longer periods of cold application would be needed to achieve cooling at this depth, as illustrated in Figure 12.1 and noted earlier.

The immediate treatment of cutaneous heat burns requires rapid cooling of the area, as described in chapter 10. Prompt cooling lowers the tissue temperature and thus limits tissue damage. There is

Many of the chemicals released from ruptured cells are irritants, provoking the nocioceptor activity invariably associated with injury.

The study by Farry et al. (1980) also showed that some swelling occurred in the subcutaneous tissues after removal of the ice in both injured and uninjured joints. The significance of this finding and whether it occurs in humans is not known.

histological evidence that cooling can lessen the inflammatory reaction: experiments on pigs investigating the effects of ice on injured ligaments showed less inflammation and secondary damage when the ligaments were cooled compared to controls (Farry et al., 1980).

Soft tissue injuries of all kinds are almost universally treated by cold in the early stages. The amount of pain relates to the rate and extent of the inflammatory response. Cooling will diminish oedema formation and the production of irritants and alleviate the pain. Compression and elevation of the part will also limit oedema formation. The initial treatment of traumatic injuries is summarized in the acronym RICE, standing for Rest, Ice, Compression and Elevation (see below).

Pain

Pain can be alleviated in several ways by the application of cold. The reduction of oedema and the decreased release of pain-inducing irritants are two important aspects. The efficacy of cooling is apparent in a comparison of the effects of the application of different methods of cold and an anti-inflammatory steroid-based foam to the perineum following postnatal trauma. Treatment with cold produced less bruising and pain (Steen et al., 2000). The mechanism was presumably a reduction in the extent of local inflammation by the cold, and possibly also by the blocking effect of cold on transmission of 'fast' pain signals, carried by A-δ fibres.

Palastanga (1988) suggests that because cold induces deep aching pain signals conveyed by C fibre activity it could contribute to pain reduction by stimulating the release of endorphins and encephalins.

Another way that cold can reduce pain is via a direct effect on nocioceptors. Although cold has little effect on the conduction of action potentials in C fibres (see Table 12.1), it can reduce the rate of firing of nocioceptors, i.e. the rate at which pain signalling action potentials are produced by reducing the rate of production of pain-inducing irritants.

Postoperative uses

Different methods of cooling are used, particularly post-orthopaedic surgery involving the limbs. The results of using cooling to the knee region following a total knee arthroplasty suggest it may reduce the pain and level of analgesics required, reduce the extent of wound drainage (Webb et al., 1998), produce a faster rate of regaining movement (Morsi, 2002) and increase the rate of mobilization and discharge (Scarcella and Cohn, 1995). Similar results have been obtained with hip arthroplasties: those treated with cooling being discharged earlier, suggesting they regained their mobility earlier (Scarcella and Cohn, 1995). Measuring recovery by discharge timing assumes a consistent policy, thus introducing a potentially confounding variable. This means the evidence offered by the results is not as strong as it might be. Similarly, there is no standardization in how cooling is applied nor of the duration of use (Barry et al., 2003).

Cryotherapy is often used post-arthroscopic reconstructions of the anterior cruciate ligament (ACL). A comparison of the outcomes of two different methods, continuous flow cooling and ice packs, suggests the former is considerably better (Barber, 2000). Further, a comparison of continuous flow cooling with a no-cooling group showed that the cooling produced significantly less pain following an ACL repair (Barber et al., 1998). This was improved if an intra-articular injection of bupivacaine and morphine was given on completion of surgery (Brandson et al., 1996). The use of a continuous flow cooling system with or without the postoperative analgesia produced a greater level of pain control than a placebo condition of a saline injection and no cooling. Without a sham treatment group, however, it is not possible to be sure of the extent to which other factors, such as the compression in the no-cooling group in the Barber et al. study, might also have helped or whether the changes were due to the cold alone.

Patients with carpal tunnel release were treated with cooling using one of two methods: controlled cold method or ice packs. Those who had the controlled cold system reported less postoperative pain, swelling and analgesic use on day 3 than those who used the ice packs (Hochberg, 2001).

> The consistency of clinical findings with predictions from physiological studies lends confidence to the conclusion that cooling is beneficial for the treatment of postoperative and other forms of acute pain.

Muscle spasm

Muscle spasm is linked to pain in that the pain of an injury appears to provoke muscle spasm as a protective measure. One possible consequence is that the ischaemia from a prolonged muscle contraction itself causes more pain and muscle spasm, a self-perpetuating cycle. The application of cold is used to break the vicious cycle, so reducing muscle spasm and discomfort and producing two benefits: an increase in the range of movement and possibly a higher rate of tissue healing.

Spasticity

Cooling has been used clinically for many years to reduce muscle spasticity. An early study showed cold produced a marked decrease in ankle clonus (Peterjan and Watts, 1962). Such effects have been studied extensively but the mechanism remains unknown. A complete explanation is likely to be complex, as the effects are, no doubt, due to both neurological changes and changes happening at the local level of the muscle fibres.

There is inconsistency in clinical reports of the effectiveness of cooling in treating spasticity. This is possibly a consequence of the

Normal tremor and spasticity may be closely linked as they are both pertubations in neural activity though they differ in degree and timing. Since normal tremor is reduced by cooling it might be expected that spasticity would also be reduced.

extent and amount of cooling. The effects of local cooling applied briefly may be quite different from more prolonged cooling that affects deeper muscles (see Figure 12.1). The extent of cooling is also important: a partial immersion in a cold water bath at 24°C for 20 minutes would produce less deep cooling than an ice pack at 10°C for the same time. It has been reported that spasticity in multiple sclerosis patients was increased by cold-water immersion in one study (Chiara et al., 1998). This contrasts with the decreased clonus found in another (Peterjan and Watts, 1962). More systematic and controlled studies of the effects on spasticity are clearly needed to assist clinicians in deciding how and when to use cooling.

Muscle strengthening

There is evidence that cooling the skin surface can lead to greater strength of the underlying muscles, although there are also conflicting reports of a strength decrease following cryotherapy. The different findings may be due to differences in the amount and depth of cooling involved.

Sanya and Bello (1999) found an increase of around 16% in the strength of the quadriceps immediately after 5 minutes of ice-towel cooling of the anterior aspect of the thigh; 10 minutes post cooling the difference (10%) was still significant.

The muscle strength increase has been ascribed to a facilitatory effect on the α-motoneuron pool, at least in the short term. Sympathetic system stimulation has also been suggested as the mechanism for greater immediate muscle strength; cold stress has a potent effect on the sympathetic system and catecholamine release. On the other hand, if the muscle tissue itself, which is more deeply located, is cooled there will be a reduction in metabolic activity of the muscle fibres and thus a potential decrease in strength. The contradictory findings may thus be reflecting a difference in the degree of cooling in different investigations; the shorter applications stimulating the nervous system, while prolonged intensive cooling affects muscle metabolism leading to weakness.

These differences suggest that clinical users of cooling need to consider carefully the method and the duration for which it is used. Otherwise, the risk is that movement is inhibited or less force is produced, an opposite outcome to that planned.

Chronic inflammatory conditions

Pain reduction by cooling in acute inflammatory conditions would be expected due to reduced metabolic activity and hence reduced stimulation of pain receptors.

The use of cold therapy for acute inflammatory conditions is both rational and supported by clinical experience and research evidence. For example, after an application of cold, rats with an acute arthritis respond less to additional pain (Sluka et al., 1999). This suggests not that it affected their arthritis per se but that it reduced pain fibre activity. Positive effects of cold on acute inflammation, however, do not necessarily imply similar effects on chronic inflammation, which has different microscopic dynamics.

Two Cochrane reports investigated the effects of thermotherapy on osteoarthritis (Brosseau et al., 2004) and on rheumatoid arthritis (Robinson et al., 2004). Neither reported the actual effect on arthritis per se. They reported on the effects of heat and cold on the symptoms. With osteoarthritis, the evidence suggests that cold can improve knee range, function and strength. Cold can also reduce swelling but does not appear to significantly affect pain. With rheumatoid arthritis the researchers had problems in drawing conclusions beyond saying that cold can be used palliatively.

Chronic oedema and joint effusions

Cold reduces the extent of oedema produced and also appears to assist in the reduction of some existing oedema. The mechanisms are not fully understood but cold does reduce the permeability of the very small blood vessels (Deal et al., 2002). In addition, it reduces the changes in leucocyte motility and adhesion that are precursors to their migration into the interstitial spaces.

As well as interstitial oedema, inflammatory joint effusions benefit from cooling. This must be contrasted with the application of cold for obstructive oedema, such as that due to deep vein thrombosis. Such treatment for the latter condition is questionable and not recommended.

Cold is also used to treat chronic oedema. This effect was quantified in nine hemiplegic patients whose swollen hands were intermittently immersed in water at around 10°C for 30 minutes (Moon and Grangnani, 1989). Although hand volumes are variable, both between subjects and at different times in the same subject, the hand volume reduced in all patients. The change was statistically significant in eight of them. During both treatment and measurement the hands were dependent. Given that gravitational pressures might increase oedema in a dependent limb, this suggests a different method, one that permitted treatment with the hand elevated, might have produced even better results.

> The application of ice and a compression bandage for an acute joint effusion are almost universally recognized and accepted treatments.

Summary of the therapeutic uses of cold

- Applied to recent injuries and post surgery:
  - limits bleeding by vasoconstriction and increased blood viscosity
  - limits pain by reducing the rate and extent of oedema formation and production of pain nerve irritants
  - reduces the local metabolic rate and hence secondary cell ischaemia and possible cell necrosis
  - reduces oedema and joint effusions.

- Reduction of pain:
  - as a consequence of above processes
  - reduces the conduction of some pain nerves in skin
  - provides sensory stimulation, a pain gate mechanism
  - possibly also facilitates release of endorphins and encephalins.
- Reduction of muscle spasm:
  - by reducing pain component of the pain-spasm cycle.
- Changes muscle spasticity:
  - can increase spasticity
  - with more prolonged cooling can decrease spasticity.
- Changes muscle responses:
  - can facilitate muscle activity
  - with more prolonged cooling can inhibit and limit muscle activity.

METHODS OF APPLYING COLD THERAPY

Cooling of the body surface may be achieved by:

- the application of a substance at a lower temperature, thus conducting heat energy away from the surface
- evaporating a chemical of low boiling point from the tissue surface.

The former is by far the most widely used and the majority of cold treatments use melting ice. Using flaked (or crushed) ice in particular is convenient and efficient for cooling any but the smallest body region since it provides a large surface area of ice from which melting can occur. By contrast, ice blocks exert pressure locally and so can impede circulation. Flaked ice machines can produce a continuous supply of consistently sized flakes which can then be stored in a large container. These machines work on the same principle as an ordinary domestic electric refrigerator and are usually plumbed into the water supply.

Technique of application of cold therapy

For all the different methods considered below the general features of the technique of application follows the format set out in chapter 1.

Stages

Patient

Explanation: Explain the reasons for, and nature of, the cold treatment to the patient.

Examination: Examine the area to be treated carefully to exclude all specific contraindications and, if necessary, test the patient's local cutaneous response to ice (ice reaction test, see chapter 7).

Apparatus

Prepare the means of applying cold and thoroughly dampen the towelling to be used between the pack and skin.

Preparation of part

Position the patient so they are comfortable. Select the position according to whether the part is to be immersed or have a pack applied, and if elevation is required. Apply oil or dry towelling to the skin if bony areas need protection from possible excessive local cooling.

Instructions for the patient

Advise the patient what they should expect to feel and warn them of any relevant risks and to indicate immediately if they experience any increased pain or discomfort.

Application

Check the skin under the cold pack immediately after applying it (or any other method) and again after 5 minutes. Look for adverse or allergic reactions or unusual changes in skin colour.

Termination

Remove the cold source and dry and inspect the skin carefully.

Cold packs

Treatment using cold packs normally follows one of two protocols which have the acronyms RICE and CRIE. Both protocols represent basic first aid for an acute injury involving soft tissue damage that is causing pain and swelling. The difference is the timing and emphasis placed on compression.

- *R* is for rest. This means stopping activity to limit the extent of trauma and of any bleeding into the tissues.
- *I* is for ice, which can actually be any appropriate method of local cooling. Most commonly it will be one of the types of ice packs described below but it can also be the immersion method or a continuous cooling system, for example.

The order is determined by the nature of the injury. In general, immediate injury should be treated with the CRIE protocol. Treatment applied longer after the injury but still in the acute phase might more appropriately follow the RICE sequence.

- *C* is for compression. This is arguably the most important element if bleeding is continuing or likely, or a considerable degree of protein leakage from vessels into the interstitial spaces is occurring. Applying external pressure reduces the extent of extravasation from vessels into tissue.
- *E* represents elevation. This assists the compression to reduce the extent of loss from blood vessels into the adjacent tissues following trauma.

Ice packs

Flaked ice is folded into damp terry-towelling or put into bags made of the same material (previously dampened) and applied directly to the skin. These packs may be held in place by dry towelling, bandages or a plastic sheet wrapped around the part and the pack. Placing the pack beneath the part is not advisable unless the limb is supported in elevation because the weight of the limb on the pack can limit the circulation enough to cause excessive local cooling and even an ice burn. Rolls of towelling can be positioned either side of the treatment area to support the weight of the limb to minimize any risk of tissue compression by the ice pack.

Skin cooling is quite rapid at first as the ice-cold water seeps through the damp towelling but after a minute or so the layer of water in contact with the skin warms up a little so that these packs are quite tolerable for some 20 minutes or so. While an ice pack remains stationary, a thin layer of water on the skin surface tends to be held at a higher temperature than that of the ice pack. This means that the skin temperature is usually above the 0°C of melting ice, often around 5–10°C. If the pack is removed after a few minutes and immediately reapplied, a fresh cold surface is produced by stirring the warm water layer with the cooler ice beneath. When applied to the skin, greater and more rapid cooling is achieved. However, this strategy has more risks as very rapid cooling can sometimes lead to skin damage (see below) and so should not be routinely used.

Flaked ice may also be tied in a suitably sized polythene bag to reduce the mess as the ice melts. A damp towel is again used to separate the bag from the skin. The extent of cooling after 15 minutes if the ice is contained in a plastic bag is a little less (a drop of 9.9°C versus 12°C if no bag) (Belitsky et al., 1987). Even so, the extent of cooling is greater than when a cooled gel pack is used (which produced only a 7.3°C drop).

Areas that need protection, such as bony prominences, are separated from the packs either by dry towelling or, less usually, oil and paper towelling on the skin. The difference is marked. In one study the skin under an ice bag reached 12.5°C (Tsang et al., 1997). With a dry towel in between, the skin temperature reached 23.5°C. Similarly, compression applied with the ice bag affects the extent of temperature drop. After approximately 10 minutes of cooling the skin under a compressed region was, on average, about 5°C cooler than under a region compressed by the weight of the pack alone (Barlas et al., 1996). This has important implications for deciding which method of cooling is appropriate in a situation and how an ice pack is to be applied.

With all treatments using ice packs the bag should be removed after a minute to inspect the underlying skin to determine the response, and if it is considered abnormal the pack is not replaced. This should be repeated after 5 minutes if no abnormal reactions, requiring termination of treatment, were obvious in the initial inspection.

Commercial cold packs

Commercial cold packs come in two forms: reusable, store in fridge, gel-packs and single-use packs which do not need prior refrigeration and rely on an endothermic chemical reaction for cooling. The advantage of both types of pack is their convenience. The disadvantage of gel-packs is that their rate of re-warming is usually greater than flaked ice packs. The disadvantage of endothermic packs is their cost and non-reusability. For these reasons, gel packs are more commonly used.

Gel-packs are plastic (often vinyl) bags filled with a gel that does not freeze when cooled; so the pack remains flexible and can be moulded to the body part. Commercial cold packs come in various sizes, usually small enough to store in the freezer compartment of a domestic refrigerator. The pack will therefore be stored at a temperature below 0°C, typically between −10°C and −20°C. Consequently, these packs are initially at a lower temperature than flaked ice packs and can therefore cool the skin very rapidly. These packs should always be applied over a damp towel to prevent ice burns. As long as the towel remains damp and not frozen, the surface in contact with the skin will not be below 0°C. The temperature of a gel pack rises more rapidly on application than an ice pack. Consequently, gel-packs usually provide adequate cooling for less than 20 minutes.

Gel compression packs are a commercial variation on the gel-pack theme. A gel-pack is contained within a compression pack that can be inflated as required to set the amount of compression of the pack on a limb. Ideally, the inner surface should be covered by towelling or cotton that is damped first. These packs are usually designed to fit either areas such as ankles or knees or circumferentially for small, medium or large sized body parts. Their limitation is that their shape and size can mean a 'fit' is not always easy. The extent of compression is usually limited by a pressure sensitive valve to reduce any risks to the patient.

Interestingly, it has been shown that bags of frozen peas provide a useful and cheap home alternative to gel-packs (Chesterton et al., 2002). Bags of frozen peas cooled the skin considerably more than a gel-pack during a 20 minute application over a layer of damp cotton (towelling). As with all other types of cold pack, the frozen pea pack was wrapped in a damp towel to prevent any excessive cooling of the skin.

Practical point

Skin temperature can be varied according to how a pack is applied. A firm application, especially with overlying compression, will lead to very low temperatures, especially if the pack is disturbed during the treatment (this will move the otherwise static layer of water). Very low skin temperatures of 0°C for example, must be avoided as they can cause skin damage. By contrast, a loosely applied pack or one with compression under it or where the towelling against the skin is dry, will not produce particularly low skin temperatures. Air pockets will remain, providing greater insulation and hence less skin cooling.

Traditional gel packs are filled with wet silica-gel. Modern cold packs use a more efficient, high thermal capacity, cellulose-based material combined with propylene glycol.

Chesterton et al. (2002) found that with 20 minutes of cooling a skin temperature of 10.8°C was obtained using frozen peas versus 14.4°C with a gel pack and 26.1°C for the control group.

Endothermic or chemical packs are single use cold packs. A tab is pulled or container broken to mix the chemicals within the pack. If one of these packs is accidentally ruptured the contents should be washed off the skin immediately as some are strongly corrosive and can cause effects ranging from irritation (with short exposure) to major tissue damage (with longer exposure).

Cryotherapy flow units

Users often label different forms of cryotherapy with their manufacturer's name, but the types are described here and, so as to avoid potential confusion due to national differences, trade names are not used.

These comprise a water reservoir to which water is added and that is then connected, via an insulated tube, to a sleeve or sealed bag-like unit. The water circulates through the bag which covers the area being treated. Depending on the unit, the water is kept at a thermostatically preset temperature (controlled temperature flow) or flaked ice is added to the water in the reservoir so water at or close to 0°C is circulated. The water is either pumped through continuously by an electric pump (continuous flow) or is circulated by flushing it back through the reservoir every 15 minutes or so (intermittent flow).

Most research indicates that the effectiveness of cryotherapy flow units is greater than other methods. This is true following a carpal tunnel release in which they were found to be preferable to ice packs (Hochberg, 2001), and after knee (Scarcella and Cohn, 1995; Webb et al., 1998; Morsi, 2002) and hip arthroplasties (Scarcella and Cohn, 1995). Similarly they appear to be more effective than no cold (Brandson et al., 1996; Barber et al., 1998) or an ice pack (Barber, 2000) after an arthroscopic patellar tendon autograft reconstruction of the anterior cruciate ligament (ACL). The cooling post-ACL repair, as shown using intra-articular thermocouple probes, was marked (Glenn et al., 2004).

The incidence of frostbite injuries post-pedal surgery is extremely low at 0.00224 over a 5-year period (Wilke and Weiner, 2003), i.e. two per thousand treatments. However, there is some evidence that the additional compression of a brace or strap over a flow bag can increase the risk of skin damage (Konrath et al., 1996). Users should be aware of this issue and ensure that whenever there is an increased risk of compression of blood vessels, be it by equipment or body weight, additional care is taken to prevent skin damage.

Local immersion

This is the simplest method of all. The part to be cooled is placed in a container of iced water or in a whirlpool bath. Flaked ice is mixed with water from the cold tap. The temperature is controlled by varying the amount of ice used. At temperatures around 16–18°C continuous immersion can usually be tolerated for 15 to 20 minutes (Lee et al., 1978). At lower temperatures, such as around 10°C, continuous immersion is uncomfortable, so an intermittent application is usually given: the part is left in the water for only 1 minute or so at a time.

Clearly, such treatment can only be conveniently applied to the extremities – hand, forearm, foot and leg – which can be placed in a water bath if the part can be left dependent for the required time. It is also necessary to agitate the water occasionally because the layer of water in contact with the skin tends to warm up and the water temperature should be checked as it will also gradually become warm and adding more ice may be necessary.

The extent of intramuscular cooling in a cold whirlpool is slightly less at 20 minutes (a decrease of 5.1°C) than if an ice pack is used (a 7.1°C decrease) (Myrer et al., 1998). A more important difference is that the temperature at depth continues to decrease for up to 30 minutes post-whirlpool treatment (a further drop of 1.8°C) while the intramuscular temperature after the ice pack was removed increased by 2°C in the same time. The effect, presumably, is due partly to the difference in surface area cooled and partly due to the extent of cooling. Users of local cooling need to remember this practical difference.

Surface area is important because if a bigger surface area is cooled, the central region will only be able to rewarm by absorbing heat from deeper tissues. A small area will rewarm by absorbing heat from both the deeper tissues and the surrounding warm tissue.

Ice towels

A towel is placed in a mixture of flaked ice and water and then wrung out. Much of the chipped ice adheres to the cloth which is used to cover a large area, such as a leg or arm, to provide immediate surface cooling. The first towel is replaced by another after 2 or 3 minutes to continue the cooling, for, say, 20 minutes in total. An advantage of this technique is that it allows movement and/or exercise to be performed while cold therapy is being applied. For example, as discussed above, using this method produced a significant increase in isometric force of the quadriceps (Sanya and Bello, 1999). A disadvantage is that it is a messy method of cooling.

Ice massage

A solid piece of ice, either as an ice cube wrapped in paper or cloth or an ice 'lollipop' on a wooden stick is used to massage a small area.

Ice massage is used for the following:

- the relief of pain: the ice block is moved over a small area using a slow circular motion for 5 to 10 minutes. During this time the patient will feel local cold, burning and then aching sensations before the area finally becomes numb
- neurological facilitation: the ice should be applied briefly, either dabbing for about 4 s at a time or using short strokes. The application should be over the dermatome supplied by the same nerve roots as those of the muscle that is to be stimulated.

An 'ice lollipop' is made by putting a wooden tongue depressor (spatula) upright in a small plastic cup of water in the freezer. Being larger, the lollipop lasts longer and is easier to handle than the usual size of ice cube.

The rate of local intramuscular cooling produced using ice massage is greater than if an ice pack is used. One study found that the lowest temperature took approximately 18 minutes to reach with ice massage but 28 minutes with an ice bag (Zemke, 1998). This suggests an advantage of this method for treating acute onset local pain. This disadvantage of this method is that it is labour intensive and messy.

Evaporating sprays

Spraying a rapidly evaporating liquid on the skin causes local cooling as the heat energy is removed. Modern sprays, e.g. fluorimethane, are non-flammable. The liquid is sprayed on the area to be cooled in a series of short strokes of about 5 s each with a few seconds' interval between each. The nozzle of the spray is held about 45 cm from the skin surface and close to perpendicular. Cooling from such sprays is very rapid but does not last long. If used near the face care should be taken to avoid the eyes and prevent the vapour from being inhaled.

Evaporating spray is very easy to use but not without risk. Skin burns can be produced if an excessive amount of spray is applied to a small area from close-up. Frost formation on the skin is a clear sign that excessive cooling has been produced and tissue damage (frostbite) is likely.

Ice wrap

A more recent method of applying cooling to the skin is another evaporative system. A crepe bandage is soaked in a solution and then wrapped over the skin. The liquid evaporates more slowly than the spray and the level of cooling is less but can be effective for a longer duration.

Unfortunately, the term 'ice wrap' is used for two different techniques. One uses a wrap-on bandage, wetted with a rapidly evaporating coolant, as described here. The other uses a bandage which holds a gel-pack (or packs) in place.

Fluorimethane is the trade name for a mixture of chlorofluorocarbons (CFCs) with low boiling points. These are powerful ozone-depleting substances so there are concerns about their continued use.

Summary of methods of application of cold therapy

Conduction cooling:

- cold packs
  - flaked ice packs
  - commercial cold packs, reusable and single use
- cryotherapy flow units
  - continuous flow
  - intermittent flow
- local immersion
- ice towels
- ice massage

Evaporative cooling:

- evaporating spray
- ice wrap.

CHOOSING BETWEEN HEAT AND COLD

As heating the tissues adds energy and cooling extracts energy these are obviously opposite treatments. However, many chronic conditions appear to benefit equally well from either thermotherapy or cryotherapy. This is not a contradiction as some of the effects are indirect and the total effect on the tissues is complex. The apparent paradox has spawned several studies of superficial heat and cold applied to the same condition for comparison.

Acute conditions respond better to cold. Adding heat to an area in which bleeding is still occurring and oedema is still forming means both will continue to increase. In addition, the local metabolic rate is increased, risking a more extensive secondary cell anoxia and eventual necrosis. Heat should consequently not be added in the initial period, the precise time depending on the extent of the injury.

For chronic conditions the choice is not always so obvious. Some conditions in some patients respond well to cold. Cold can facilitate increasing the range of movement in a joint. In one study a greater range was obtained using cold packs than hot packs (Lin, 2003).

This suggests that users need to consider the requirements and preferences of individual patients. If their condition has responded more favourably in the past to cold, then perhaps it should be used again. This also highlights the need for more research to detail the factors a user needs to consider to optimize their selection of heat or cold in a given instance.

Another practical factor is the time and cost of buying and setting up equipment. A comparison of the effects on oedema reduction post-calcaneal fracture of using pulsed shortwave diathermy (SWD) and an intermittent flow cryotherapy unit did not identify a significant difference (Buzzard et al., 2003). While there was no sham group and the subject numbers were relatively small, so was the size of the effect and its clinical relevance probably also insignificant. These findings suggest that using cooling can be a better option than pulsed SWD because of the costs and time involved. These factors must also be considered by therapists choosing between two modalities of equal effectiveness.

The Cochrane studies of the effects of thermotherapy on osteoarthritis and rheumatoid arthritis were discussed earlier (Brosseau et al., 2004; Robinson et al., 2004). In both instances cold was effective, but so was heat for treating other aspects of the patients' problems.

Summary

- Both heat and cold can relieve pain and muscle spasm.
- Cooling can increase and decrease spasticity.
- Recent trauma benefits from immediate cooling to reduce bleeding and the rate and extent of oedema formation, and pain.
- Later, the same injury will benefit from mild heating to increase metabolism and gently increase the healing processes; continued use of cold can slow healing.
- Skilled movements are impaired by cooling.
- Muscle activity can be facilitated by brief local cooling.
- Joint stiffness is decreased by heating and increased by cooling.

DANGERS AND CONTRAINDICATIONS

There are two ways in which tissue injury might occur:

- excessive local cold causing damage to normal tissues
- normal local cooling causing damage due to some predisposing pathological condition.

Damage in either circumstance in the clinical context is rare.

Excessive local cold on normal tissue

Ice burns with fatty necrosis are rare and are said to occur in areas which are underlain by thick subcutaneous fat and which have been cooled rapidly.

The mildest form causes the appearance of erythema and tenderness of the skin a few hours after the application of ice, subsiding in a day or two; this is called an ice burn. A more severe form, an ice burn with fatty necrosis, shows bruising as well as more tenderness and can last up to 3 weeks (Lee et al., 1978). Inadequately crushed ice can lead to a large piece being held against the skin for a long time, which increases the possibility of an ice burn. There have also been some reports of peripheral nerve damage due to locally applied cold (Covington and Basselt, 1993). These have occurred in situations where the affected nerve is superficial, such as the common peroneal at the neck of the fibula.

With extreme cold, freezing of the tissues can occur but this is extremely unlikely with the treatment methods described above. What happens depends on the rate of cooling; if it is rapid ice crystals can form in the cells which may lead to cell death, whereas slower cooling tends to cause freezing of the extracellular fluid and withdrawal of water from the cells. This is referred to as 'frostbite' and only occurs if the body suffers extreme exposure; similar prolonged exposure to low temperatures without freezing the tissues, 'immersion foot' for example, can also produce severe tissue damage.

Certain pathological conditions

Reduced peripheral vascular supply, cold sensitivity and hypertension present risks which must be assessed in deciding whether to use local cooling.

Reduced peripheral vascular supply

Any condition which restricts the blood supply to an area being treated with cryotherapy increases the risk of local tissue damage. This includes pathological changes in blood vessels ranging from vasospasm to blockages to peripheral vascular disease to the pressure caused by resting a limb on an ice pack. In each instance the rate of perfusion of an area can be reduced sufficiently that oxygenation of the cells can be adversely affected, even with the reduced oxygen requirements associated with cooling.

Cold sensitivity

Vasospasm – Raynaud's phenomenon is a condition often associated with connective tissue disorders in which excessive vasoconstriction, triggered by cold, occurs in the digital arteries. Obviously cold treatment should not be used if it might provoke vascular spasm. Some other vascular conditions may have an element of vasospasm as well as obstruction, such as thromboangiitis obliterans (Buerger's disease), and should therefore also not be treated with cold.

Cryoglobinaemia – An abnormal protein is present in the blood; it can form a precipitate at low temperatures blocking blood vessels and thus causing local ischaemia. Although not common, this condition can also be found in association with some of the connective tissue disorders such as systemic lupus erythematosus and rheumatoid arthritis.

Cold urticaria – Cold causes the release of histamine from mast cells leading to a local weal and erythema and sometimes general (systemic) symptoms such as lowered blood pressure and raised pulse rate. The skin under all types of cryotherapy should be checked immediately after application and again 5 minutes later for this type of response as, although rare, it can be serious.

With vascular disorders which are primarily obstructive, such as arteriosclerosis, cold treatments are considered unsuitable by some, but the reasons are unclear. Since cold reduces the metabolic rate it is difficult to see what harm can occur as the tissues are already partly ischaemic; in fact cooling can temporarily relieve the pain.

Cardiac disease

Coronary thrombosis and anginal pain have sometimes been provoked by cold, leading to injunctions to avoid ice treatment, especially of the left shoulder. There is little supporting evidence to justify this advice.

Arterial blood pressure

Cooling larger areas, such as a limb segment, can lead to a transient rise in arterial blood pressure. This could be dangerous for some hypertensive patients or those with especially labile blood pressure. Monitoring the blood pressure during and for a short time after treatment would be advisable if large areas are to be cooled and there is uncertainty regarding the patient's likely response.

Summary

Contraindications to cold therapy:

- vasospasm
- cryoglobinaemia
- cold urticaria

Special care with:

- applications under splints or a limb or any other form of external compression
- areas with deeper layers of subcutaneous fat
- areas overlying superficial nerves.

Sensory deficiency

Cooling can lead to partial sensory loss and it can be safely applied to an anaesthetic area (Lee and Warren, 1974) so this might suggest there is little need for sensory testing prior to cryotherapy. However, if there is a sensory impairment, there are greater risks of tissue damage occurring: there is even less possibility of any awareness of it happening and a more protracted healing process if it does as the normal circulatory response is altered if the autonomic nerves are affected. Accordingly, some users recommend thermal sensation testing prior to cryotherapy. Observing that normal vasoconstriction has taken place early in treatment – the autonomic response – is a sensible precaution as is testing of the rate of capillary return if there is any suggestion of a restricted local blood supply.

It should also be noted that the neurological effects of cooling, such as pain control and the facilitation of muscle contraction, require intact sensory (afferent) nerves so that if there is a sensory impairment, there may be no point in treatment.

Emotional and psychological features

Some patients may have a strong aversion to cold in any form or to local cold applications in particular. This may be partly due to cultural factors since our language abounds with metaphors in which 'cold' has some unpleasant connotations, e.g. in cold blood, cold-hearted. There is an obviously physiological association with fear – cold feet and cold sweat. Both cold and fear stimulate the sympathetic system. There is also an emotional link and the connection of cold with death is also well recognized.

Pale grew thy cheek and cold,
Colder thy kiss
Truly that hour foretold
Sorrow to this!

Byron: 'When we two parted'

References

Allison, S., Abraham, L. (2001). Sensitivity of qualitative and quantitative spasticity measures to clinical treatment with cryotherapy. Int J Rehabil Res, **24**, 15–24.

Barber, F. (2000). A comparison of crushed ice and continuous flow cold therapy. Am J Knee Surg, **13**, 97–101.

Barber, F., McGuire, D., Click, S. (1998). Continuous-flow cold therapy for outpatient anterior cruciate ligament reconstruction. Arthroscopy, **14**, 130–135.

Barlas, D., Homan, C., Thode, H. (1996). In vivo tissue temperature comparison of cryotherapy with and without external compression. Ann Emerg Med, **28**, 436–439.

Barry, S., Wallace, L., Lamb, S. (2003). Cryotherapy after total knee replacement: a survey of current practice. Physiother Res Int, **8**, 111–120.

Belitsky, R., Odam, S., Hubley-Kozey, C. (1987). Evaluation of the effectiveness of wet ice, dry ice, and cryogen packs in reducing skin temperature. Phys Ther, **67**, 1080–1084.

Bierman, W., Friedlander, M. (1940). The penetrative effects of cold. Arch Phys Ther, **21**, 585–591.

Brandson, S., Rydgren, B., Hedner, N. et al. (1996). Postoperative analgesic effects of an external cooling system and intra-articular bupivicaine/morphine after arthroscopic cruciate ligament surgery. Knee Surg Sports Traumatol Arthrosc, **4**, 200–225.

Brosseau, L., Yonge, K., Robinson, V. et al. (2004). Thermotherapy for treatment of osteoarthritis (Cochrane Review). In The Cochrane Library, Issue 1. Chichester, UK: John Wiley & Sons, Ltd.

Buzzard, B., Pratt, R., Briggs, P. et al. (2003). Is pulsed shortwave diathermy better than ice therapy for the reduction of oedema following calcaneal fractures? Physiotherapy, **89**, 734–742.

Chesterton, L., Foster, N., Ross, L. (2002). Skin temperature response to cryotherapy. Arch Phys Med Rehabil, **83**, 543–549.

Chiara, T., Carlos, J., Martin, D. et al. (1998). Cold effect of oxygen uptake, perceived exertion and spasticity in patients with MS. Arch Phys Med Rehabil, **79**, 523–528.

Cooper, C., Evidente, V., Hentz, J. et al. (2000). The effect of temperature on hand function in patients with tremor. J Hand Therapy, **13**, 276–288.

Covington, D., Basselt, F. (1993). When cryotherapy injures. Physician Sports Med, **21**, 78–93.

Deal, D., Tipton, J., Rosencrance, E. et al. (2002). Ice decreases edema: a study or microvascular permeability in rats. J Bone Jt Surg (Am), **84**, 1573–1578.

Douglas, W., Malcolm, J. (1955). The effect of localised cooling on cat nerves. J Physiol, **130**, 53.

Enwemeka, C., Allen, C., Avila, P. et al. (2002). Soft tissue thermodynamics before, during, and after cold pack therapy. Med Sci Sports Exerc, **34**, 45–50.

Farry, P., Prentice, N., Hunter, A., Wakelin, C. (1980). Ice treatment of injured ligaments: an experimental model. N Z Med J, **91**, 14–16.

Fox, R., Wyatt, H. (1962). Cold induced vasodilation in various areas of the body surface in man. J Physiol, **162**, 289–297.

Glenn, R., Spindler, K., Warren, T. et al. (2004). Cryotherapy decreases intraarticular temperature after ACL reconstruction. Clin Orthop Related Res, **421**, 268–272.

Hardy, J. (1982). Temperature regulation, exposure to heat and cold and effects of hypothermia. In J. Lehmann (ed.), Therapeutic Heat and Cold, pp. 172–196. Baltimore: Williams & Wilkins.

Ho, S., Illegen, R., Meyer, R. et al. (1995). Comparison of various icing times in decreasing bone metabolism and blood flow in the knee. Am J Sports Med, **23**, 74–76.

Hochberg, J. (2001). A randomized prospective study to assess the efficacy of two cold-therapy treatments following carpal tunnel release. J Hand Ther, **14**, 208–215.

Hubbard, J., Mechan, D. (1987). Physiology for Health Care Students. Edinburgh: Churchill Livingstone.

Kauranen, K., Vanharanta, H. (1997). Effects of hot and cold packs on motor performance of normal hands. Physiotherapy, **83**, 340–344.

Konrath, G., Lock, T., Goitz, H., Scheidler, J. (1996). The use of cold therapy after anterior cruciate ligament reconstruction. A prospective, randomized study and literature review. Am J Sports Med, **24**, 629–633.

Lee, J., Warren, M. (1974). Cold Therapy in Rehabilitation. London: Bell and Hyman.

Lee, J., Warren, M., Mason, S. (1978). Effects of ice on nerve conduction velocity. Physiotherapy, **64**, 2–6.

Levy, A., Kelly, B., Lintner, S., Speer, K. (1997). Penetration of cryotherapy in treatment after shoulder arthroscopy. Arthroscopy, **13**, 461–464.

Lewis, T. (1930). Observation upon the reactions of the vessels of the human skin to cold. Heart, **15**, 177–208.

Lin, Y. (2003). Effects of thermal therapy in improving the passive range of knee motion: comparison of cold and superficial heat applications. Clin Rehabil, **17**, 618–623.

Merrick, M., Rankin, J., Andres, F., Hinman, C. (1999). A preliminary examination of cryotherapy and secondary injury in skeletal muscle. Med Sci Sports Exerc, **31**, 1516–1521.

Moon, A., Grangnani, J. (1989). Cold water immersion for the oedematous hand in stroke patients. Clin Rehabil, 97–101.

Morsi, E. (2002). Continuous-flow cold therapy after total knee arthroplasty. J Arthroplasty, **17**, 718–722.

Myrer, J., Measom, G., Fellingham, G. (1998). Temperature changes in the human leg during and after two methods of cryotherapy. J Athletic Training, **33**, 25–29.

Myrer, J., Myrer, K., Measom, G. et al. (2001). Muscle temperature is affected by overlying adipose when cryotherapy is administered. J Athletic Training, **36**, 32–36.

Myrer, J., Measom, G., Fellingham, G. (2000). Exercise after cryotherapy greatly enhances intramuscular rewarming. J Athletic Training, **35**, 412–416.

Oosterveld, F., Rasker, J., Jacobs, J., Overmars, H. (1992). The effect of local heat and cold therapy on the intraarticular and skin surface temperature of the knee. Arth Rheum, **35**, 146–151.

Palastanga, N. P. (1988). Heat and cold. In P. Wells, V. Frampton, D. Bowsher (eds), Pain: Management and Control in Physiotherapy, pp. 169–180. London: Heinemann Medical Books.

Peterjan, R., Watts, N. (1962). Effects of cooling on the triceps surae reflex. Am J Phys Med, **41**, 240–251.

Robinson, V., Brosseau, L., Casimiro, L. et al. (2004). Thermotherapy for treating rheumatoid arthritis (Cochrane Review). In The Cochrane Library (Vol. Issue 1). Chichester, UK: John Wiley & Sons, Ltd.

Rutkove, S. (2001). Focal cooling improves neuronal conduction in peroneal neuropathy at the fibular neck. Musc Nerve, **24**, 1622–1626.

Sanya, A., Bello, A. (1999). Effects of cold application on isometric strength and endurance of quadriceps femoris muscle. Afr J Med Med Sci, **28**, 195–198.

Scarcella, J., Cohn, B. (1995). The effect of cold therapy on the postoperative course of total hip and knee arthroplasty patients. Am J Orthop **24**, 847–852.

Sluka, K., Christy, M., Peterson, W. et al. (1999). Reduction of pain-related behaviours with either cold or heat treatment in an animal model of acute arthritis. Arch Phys Med Rehabil, **80**, 313–317.

Steen, M., Cooper, K., Marchant, P. et al. (2000). A randomised controlled trial to compare the effectiveness of ice-packs and Epifoam with cooling maternity gel pads at alleviating postnatal perineal trauma. Midwifery, **16**, 48–55.

Thorlacius, H., Vollmar, B., Westermann, S. et al. (1998). Effects of local cooling on microvascular hemodynamics and leukocyte adhesion in the striated muscle of hamsters. J Trauma Injury Infect Crit Care, **45**, 715–719.

Tsang, K., Buxton, B., Guion, W. et al. (1997). The effect of cryotherapy applied through various barriers. J Sports Rehabil, **6**, 343–354.

Walton, M., Roestenburg, M., Hallwright, S., Sutherland, J. (1986). Effects of ice packs on tissue temperatures at various depths before and after quadriceps hematoma: studies using sheep. J Orthop Sports Phys Ther, **15**, 294–300.

Webb, J., Williams, D., Ivory, J. et al. (1998). The use of cold compression dressings after total knee replacements: a randomised controlled trial. Orthopedics, **21**, 59–61.

Wilke, B., Weiner, R. (2003). Postoperative cryotherapy: risks versus benefits of continuous-flow cryotherapy units. Clin Pod Med Surg, **20**, 307–322.

Zemke, J. (1998). Intramuscular temperature responses in the human leg to two forms of cryotherapy: ice massage and ice bag. J Orthop Sports Phys Ther, **27**, 301–307.

Electromagnetic fields: shortwave

A more informative title for this chapter would be 'electromagnetic fields: shortwave diathermy, pulsed electromagnetic energy and magnetic therapies'. Although explanatory, it is too long for a title and detracts from the main emphasis, which is shortwave therapy.

As often occurs in electrotherapy, the topic is plagued by a profusion and confusion of names. The term 'shortwave therapy' has little to do with short waves, which are a form of electromagnetic radiation (considered in later chapters) normally used for radio transmissions. Rather it has to do with the effects of alternating electric or magnetic fields on the body. The electric and magnetic fields used clinically alternate at shortwave radio frequencies (normally 27.12 MHz), hence the confusing terms 'shortwave diathermy' and 'pulsed shortwave'.

The basic therapeutic mechanism being considered here is the induction of relatively high-frequency currents in the body by alternating electric or magnetic fields. This produces heating in both deep and superficial tissues. When the average intensity is low, due to pulsing of the field intensity, no overall heating may be evident. The consequences of such low average energy treatments are considered by some to be due to effects other than heating and explicable in terms of high intensity 'shock' effects of the transient bursts of energy delivered by the pulses.

When appreciable heating of deeply located tissue occurs it is called 'diathermy' (a word, coined from the Greek, meaning 'through heating'), hence shortwave diathermy refers to deep heating produced by electric or magnetic fields which alternate at high (shortwave radio) frequencies. Otherwise names such as pulsed electromagnetic energy (PEME) or pulsed shortwave are used. A description of these two entities forms the bulk of this chapter. First, the nature and production of electric and magnetic fields are briefly considered, followed by the way in which these fields induce a flow of current in tissue. Next is a description of how induced high-frequency currents affect the tissues. The principles of application are explored, including the important effects of varying the size, position and relationship of electrodes to the tissues on the heating pattern. The technique of application of

In shortwave therapy, electromagnetic radiation is produced as a byproduct of the alternating electric or magnetic fields which are used, but the radiation is not an important part of the treatment.

Ultrasound and microwaves can also produce deep heating, so they are classed, along with shortwave, as 'diathermic modalities'.

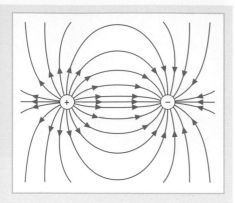

Figure 13.1 The electric field between two small, charged objects.

For more information on electric and magnetic fields and forces see chapter 6 of the book 'Biophysical Bases of Electrotherapy' on the CD which comes with this book.

continuous shortwave diathermy is then described together with dosage and potential dangers.

Pulsed shortwave is then considered, with comment on its application, dosage and contraindications. The chapter concludes with some reference to low-power high frequency energy, Indiba therapy and the use of magnetism in therapy. Finally, there is some comment on the current concern with the safety of all kinds of electromagnetic fields.

NATURE

Electromagnetic energy can be considered from three aspects:

- *Electrostatic forces* between stationary electric charges. There is an attraction between opposite charges and a repulsion of like charges. These forces act between any charges and their strength and direction can be described by drawing lines called lines of electric force. The area in which this force acts is called an *electric field* and the lines are often simply referred to as electric field lines. The electric field between two small, spherical charged objects is shown in Figure 13.1.
- When charges move, the movement constitutes an *electric current*. An inevitable consequence of constantly moving charges is the formation of a *magnetic field*. Figure 13.2 shows the pattern of magnetic field lines produced when a current (I) flows through a cylindrical coil of wire (an inductor). The field can be mapped with iron filings or a compass.
- If an electric charge is accelerated it causes the production of *electromagnetic radiation*. This radiates away from the moving charge and once generated is independent of the charge. If electric currents are made to oscillate, the rapid acceleration of charges causes the production of electromagnetic radiation whose wavelength and frequency are determined by the frequency of oscillation. Radio waves are just one example of electromagnetic radiation produced by high-frequency oscillating currents. The nature and production of electromagnetic radiation is further described in chapter 14.

If a material is placed in an electric field, charges within the material will experience an electric force. The direction of the force is along the electric field lines. The amount of force depends on the electric field intensity, which is indicated by the density of electric field lines. Thus in Figure 13.1, areas where the field lines are close together are regions of high field intensity and high force production.

Magnetic fields are rather different to electric fields in that the direction of the associated force is not along magnetic field lines but at right-angles. As with electric fields, however, the force is proportional to the magnetic field intensity, again indicated by the density of field lines. Thus in Figure 13.2, the magnetic field intensity is greater inside than outside the coil.

Forces acting on charges, whether electric or magnetic forces, will result in charges moving: in other words, a flow of current. Thus when a body part is placed in an alternating electric or magnetic field, as in shortwave treatment, an alternating current flow is induced in the tissues.

The question is, why should appreciable heating occur when high frequency currents are induced in tissues, since it was pointed out in chapter 4 that therapeutic low-frequency currents produce negligible heating. The answer lies in the fact that much higher currents flow in the tissues with diathermy. Since the heating rate depends on the square of the current, a higher current will lead to a disproportionate, very much higher, level of tissue heating. The low-frequency currents of chapter 4 were generally at milliampere level, whereas diathermy heating can involve total currents of 0.5–1 A, although it is the current density (current per unit area) that matters.

The importance of current density is evident in surgical diathermy. Here heating is produced by high frequency alternating current which flows between two quite differently sized electrodes which, unlike shortwave diathermy, are in direct contact with tissue. The electrosurgical knife (an electrode) is much smaller than the other electrode, so the current density around the knife blade is very high. The associated heating is great enough to cauterize and seal blood vessels.

The reason why large currents can flow in tissues without directly stimulating nerve or muscle is that if they are oscillating rapidly enough, i.e. have a high enough frequency, there is not enough time at each oscillation for nerve or muscle tissue to be affected. Excitable tissue is affected by altering the ionic balance across the membrane, as explained in chapter 2. Single pulses (phases) of voltage need to pass for about 0.1 ms to stimulate a nerve with minimal voltage. Shorter pulses would need higher voltages. At the usual shortwave diathermy frequency of 27.12 MHz the voltage phases are less than 1/50th of a microsecond so no excitatory effect on muscle or nerve can occur.

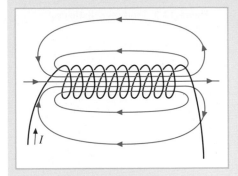

Figure 13.2 The magnetic field around a current-carrying coil of wire.

> When current flows through a resistor, the rate at which electrical energy is converted to heat energy is given by Joule's law, $P = I^2R$ where P is the power or rate of energy conversion, I is the current and R is the resistance.

SHORTWAVE DIATHERMY APPARATUS

Shortwave diathermy apparatus produces electric or magnetic fields which alternate at high frequency and it is the rapidly alternating fields which produce the physiological effects and therapeutic benefits. A side-effect of electric or magnetic field production is that stray electromagnetic radiation is produced. The amount of electromagnetic radiation is small and the physiological effects are negligible but such radiation can interfere with radio, television and other forms of data transmission. For this reason, specific frequency bands have been allocated by international agreement for industrial, scientific and medical purposes to prevent interference with communications. These frequencies and their wavelengths are shown in Table 13.1. Of these the 27.12 MHz frequency is by far the most widely used because it has

Figure 13.3 Shortwave diathermy apparatus.

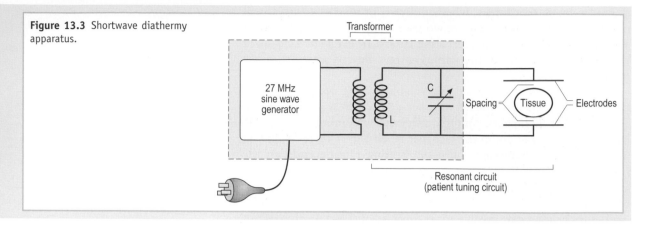

Table 13.1 Assigned frequencies and wavelengths	
Frequency (MHz)	Wavelength (m)
13.56 (±6.25 kHz)	22.12
27.12 (±160 kHz)	11.06
40.68 (±20 kHz)	7.38

the widest frequency band; that is to say, the extent to which it is allowed to drift off the assigned frequency is much greater than the others.

Shortwave diathermy apparatus consists of a sine wave generator circuit which produces alternating current with a frequency of 27.12 MHz and a resonator: a resonant circuit which can be tuned to exactly the same frequency. The sine wave generator supplies energy to the resonant circuit (the patient circuit) by transformer action. Figure 13.3 illustrates the arrangement.

A resonant circuit is made by combining an inductor and a capacitor. The frequency (f) at which such a circuit will naturally oscillate or resonate depends only on its electrical properties, i.e. the capacitance (C) and inductance (L). The resonant frequency can be calculated using the formula:

$$f = \frac{1}{2\pi\sqrt{LC}}$$

The capacitance of the patient tuning circuit will vary because the pair of electrodes with tissue in between acts as a capacitor and so contributes to the total capacitance. The variable capacitor (C in Figure 13.3) must be adjusted to make the resonant frequency equal to that of the sine wave generator. This tuning can either be done manually, using the excursion of a meter or brightness of a light to indicate resonance, or automatically. In this latter case a motor drives the tuning capacitor and is itself regulated by the output from the resonator circuit. This automatic mechanism, an example of negative feedback, keeps the machine tuned even if the patient moves a little.

Once tuned, the heating of the tissues is controlled by regulating the power output of the sine wave generator. This is done by operator adjustment of the output control of the machine.

The output of the shortwave apparatus may be coupled to the patient in two ways:

- using a capacitive method as in Figure 13.3. A pair of electrodes is connected to the output of the machine and the part of the patient to be treated is positioned between the electrodes. The tissues are affected principally by the oscillating electric field produced between the electrodes.
- using an inductive coil method. One way to do this is to wind a coil of wire (see Figure 13.2), actually an insulated cable, around the part of the patient to be treated. More commonly a monode is used: a drum-shaped applicator which contains a flat helical metal coil (see Figure 13.18). The tissues are affected mainly by the oscillating magnetic field which induces oscillating currents in the tissues; see later discussion.

INDUCTION OF HIGH-FREQUENCY CURRENTS IN TISSUES

When the kind of low- and medium-frequency currents discussed in chapters 3 and 4 are used for stimulation of nerve and muscle, it is necessary to apply conducting electrodes to the skin surface. Even with oscillations approaching 1 MHz this method is still needed if appreciable current is to flow in tissue (surgical diathermy is an example). For higher frequencies, i.e. shortwave, electric or magnetic field effects are dominant. It no longer matters that there is an insulator separating the electrodes and the tissue. The air, being an insulator, blocks the flow of current but the field induces a flow of current in tissue.

Currents around and just below 1 MHz heat the tissues they pass through quite efficiently and were used extensively by physiotherapists some 50 years ago and known as longwave diathermy.

Effects of high-frequency currents on the tissues

The major effect of induced currents of sufficient intensity at frequencies above 1 MHz is to cause heating. The nature of heat was considered in chapter 10 and it will be recalled that heat is energy, basically the amount of random molecular and atomic motion in a material. Anything that increases the internal kinetic energy of matter causes heating, accompanied by a temperature rise in the material.

Vibration of ions

Tissues contain large numbers of ions, which are charge carriers which move, producing a flow of current. If an electric field is applied first in one direction and then in the other the ions will be accelerated first

The dielectric constant of familiar insulators is much lower than that of water. Polythene (2.2) and glass (about 9) are examples: they are much less polarizable than water.

For a fuller description of the pattern of electric and magnetic fields in tissues see chapter 6 of the book 'Biophysical Bases of Electrotherapy' on the CD which comes with this book.

to one, but substances that polarize strongly have high dielectric constants, e.g. pure water at 81.

If an electric field is applied across a homogeneous material it will be relatively uniform, but if there is a boundary between materials with different dielectric constants and/or different conductivities the electric field lines are refracted at the boundary. This is much the same as the refraction that occurs when visible radiation (or any wave motion) passes from one medium to another. In general, those tissues that have a high dielectric constant are good conductors, e.g. water and tissues with a high water content. The reverse is also evident; fatty tissues have a low dielectric constant and low conductivity. Thus the electric field lines in the tissues tend to be refracted at various interfaces both at the surface and between various tissue layers. The overall effect is to spread the field within the tissues.

Some simplified illustrations of the effects of different sizes and orientations of electrodes are shown in Figure 13.5. The shape of the part being heated will also have an effect.

To provide sufficient energy for heating in the tissues it is necessary to concentrate the field in the particular area to be treated. Equally it is important not to allow the field to be so concentrated as to produce excessive heating and hence damage. The following points

Figure 13.5 The effect of positioning electrodes on the electric field through tissues using a contraplanar technique.

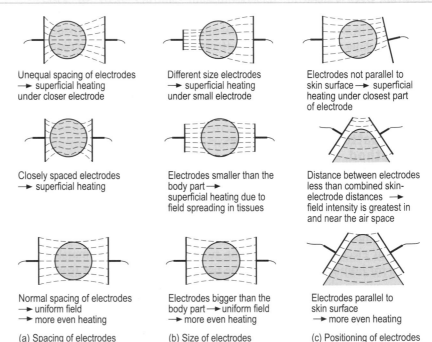

Unequal spacing of electrodes → superficial heating under closer electrode

Different size electrodes → superficial heating under small electrode

Electrodes not parallel to skin surface → superficial heating under closest part of electrode

Closely spaced electrodes → superficial heating

Electrodes smaller than the body part → superficial heating due to field spreading in tissues

Distance between electrodes less than combined skin-electrode distances → field intensity is greatest in and near the air space

Normal spacing of electrodes → uniform field → more even heating

Electrodes bigger than the body part → uniform field → more even heating

Electrodes parallel to skin surface → more even heating

(a) Spacing of electrodes

(b) Size of electrodes

(c) Positioning of electrodes relative to tissues

should be considered in conjunction with Figure 13.5. The aim is to achieve a uniform field in the tissues.

Spacing of electrodes

- 2–4 cm skin–electrode distance is advisable.
- Wide spacing gives the most uniform field in the tissues (Figure 13.6).
- More temperature increase is generated in and near the skin than in the deeper tissues. This ensures the safety of shortwave diathermy since the skin is highly sensitive to temperature changes.

Size of electrodes

- Electrodes should be a little larger than the part to achieve a uniform electric field through the tissues.
- Different sized electrodes can be used to localize treatment. The field will be concentrated under the smaller electrode.

Positioning of electrodes relative to the tissues

- Electrodes should be parallel to the skin surface so that skin–electrode distance is as constant as possible.
- The field takes the shortest pathway and will preferentially pass through the material of least impedance, i.e. tissue rather than air.
- The distance between the electrodes must be greater than the combined skin–electrode distance of the two electrodes or the field will

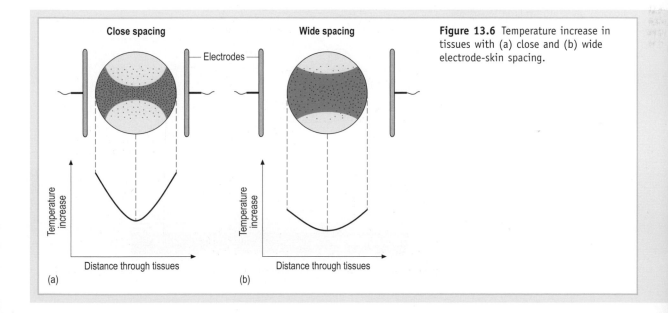

Figure 13.6 Temperature increase in tissues with (a) close and (b) wide electrode-skin spacing.

pass through the air between the electrodes rather than through the tissues.

- Uneven spacing leads to concentration of field at the closest point.
- Closer spacing of one electrode leads to concentration of the field on that side.

Nature of the tissues and electrode positioning

The two factors that are most important in determining the rate of temperature increase in a particular tissue are the electrical properties of, and the electric field intensity in, the tissue. The field intensity is influenced by both the electrode positioning and the electrical properties of the particular tissue. Electrode positioning was covered above. What of the electrical properties of the tissue?

- Tissues of high water content are heated more rapidly than others. Figure 13.7 shows a coplanar electrode positioning, such as might be used for treating spinal musculature. In the region between (but not directly under) the electrodes, fatty tissue, muscle and bone are in parallel and some current is induced in each. The highest current is induced in the water-filled tissues, such as muscle and blood vessels, because these have the lowest impedances (highest ion contents). The current induced in fatty tissue and bone is less. On this

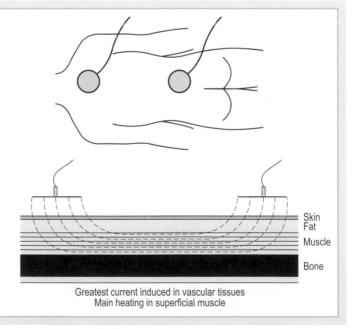

Figure 13.7 The coplanar technique produces greater heating in superficial muscle and tissue close to the electrodes.

Skin
Fat
Muscle
Bone

Greatest current induced in vascular tissues
Main heating in superficial muscle

basis it would be predicted that greater heating of muscle would occur than fat or bone, i.e. a selective deep heating of muscle.

- Nonetheless, the rate of temperature increase in fatty tissue is usually greater than in muscle in the shortwave field (Schwan, 1965). There are three reasons for this. First, because with most electrode configurations, the field intensity is highest close to the electrodes and drops quite markedly with distance (see Figure 13.6). Second, muscle is cooled more efficiently than fatty tissue by heat transfer to the vascular system. Third, because the heat capacity of muscle is much higher than fatty tissue. A higher heat capacity means that for the same amount of heat energy delivered, the temperature increase is less.

Within fatty tissue, induced currents are highest in the narrow vascular channels because they are low-impedance compared with the fat. This means that even if the overall heating of the fatty tissue is not excessive, it is still possible that selective heating of blood vessels could result in tissue damage. The lack of reports of tissue damage could be due to the sensory apparatus of the human body responding efficiently to the temperature increase, thus alerting the patient and clinician to the impending harm and allowing adverse consequences to be avoided.

If the shortwave field is passed through the long axis of a limb (Figure 13.8, longitudinal setup), there is marked heating in the vascular channels and muscle and negligible heating in the bone and fat lying in parallel. In other words, along the long axis of the limb, muscle would be heated preferentially to fatty tissue or bone. This is similar to the coplanar electrode arrangement shown in Figure 13.7. As with the coplanar arrangement, there is significant heating of the skin and fatty tissue immediately beneath the electrodes which would place limits on the total amount of heating. Although this could be therapeutically disadvantageous, it would also ensure protection against deep tissue burns.

A way to reduce excessive heating of superficial tissues while still heating deeper tissues is to use the 'crossfire' technique, depicted in Figure 13.9. The transverse method (also called contraplanar) is shown. Half of the treatment is given with electrodes in one position (Figure 13.9a). The electrodes are then moved so that the new elec-

For a fuller description of the pattern of electric and magnetic fields in tissues see chapter 6 of the book 'Biophysical Bases of Electrotherapy' on the CD which comes with this book.

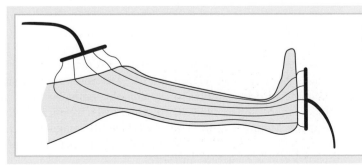

Figure 13.8 The shortwave electric field applied along the long axis of a limb.

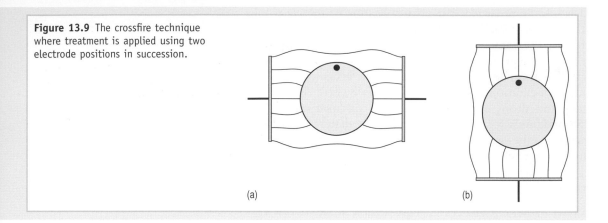

Figure 13.9 The crossfire technique where treatment is applied using two electrode positions in succession.

(a)   (b)

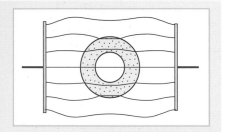

Figure 13.10 The field pattern for a dielectric which has an air-filled hollow.

tric field is at right angles to the old one (Figure 13.9b) and the treatment is continued. In this way deeply located tissue receives treatment for twice as long as the skin. The cross-fire treatment may be used, for example, on the knee joint or pelvic organs. It is also particularly useful for treating the walls of cavities within a structure, for example the sinuses.

Figure 13.10 shows the field pattern obtained with an object of high dielectric constant which has an air-filled hollow at its centre. The field lines are concentrated in the dielectric resulting in uneven heating of the walls of the cavity. Crossfire treatment ensures that all of the cavity wall area is treated.

Heating pattern in the tissues – inductothermy

Heating by inductothermy is due to currents flowing in circular paths and the currents are sometimes referred to as 'eddy currents'. The difference between inductothermy and the capacitor field method lies in the way energy is introduced into the tissues leading to a different pattern of heating. The magnetic field is a result of electron movement (i.e. current) in a cable or metal coil and the current flow induced in tissue is parallel to the current flowing in the coil. Thus, when a coil is wrapped around a limb as shown in Figure 13.11a, the induced current flows in circular pathways (Figure 13.11b).

An alternative method of applying inductothermy is by using a flat 'pancake' spiral called a helix. The spiral is placed parallel to the skin surface as shown in Figure 13.12. The induced current flows in circular pathways parallel to the coils of the helix. Heat production occurs more superficially with a pancake applicator than a coil wrapped around a limb. This is because the magnetic field intensity decreases quite rapidly with distance from the helix, whereas the field inside a coil is relatively uniform.

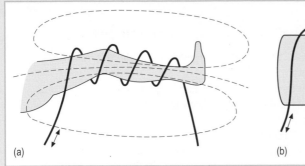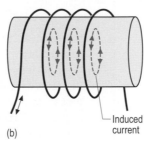

Figure 13.11 (a) A coil wrapped around a limb and the resulting magnetic field pattern. (b) Current flow induced in tissue as a result of the high frequency alternating magnetic field.

If this were the whole story, inductothermy, particularly using a coil wrapped around a limb, would be a very efficient way selectively to heat muscle with negligible heating in the bone and fatty tissue. In practice there is greater superficial heating than would be expected from the alternating magnetic field alone. The explanation is that, in addition to the magnetic field, there is also an electric field effect between adjacent turns of the coil. This is illustrated in Figure 13.13.

A consequence is that additional heating occurs, due to an electric field which is most intense close to the wire of the coil. This limits the amount of deep heating with inductothermy. Superficial heating due to electric field effects provides a sensory indication of the total amount of heating which acts as a protective mechanism against excessive heating of deep tissue.

The capacitative heating effect can be eliminated if an electrostatic screen (a wire mesh often called a faradic screen) is placed between the coil and the tissues; it will eliminate the electric field and leave only the magnetic field. When this is done experimentally, heating diminishes dramatically, showing that capacitive heating accounts for much of the heating due to the coil. Some drum-type electrodes have such a screen built in, so that only the magnetic field is applied.

If a cable is used it must be kept at a distance of 2–3 cm from the skin surface, otherwise electric field effects will dominate and deep, inductive heating would be compromised. This is achieved partly by the rubber insulation of the cable and partly by applying the cable over a minimum of 1 cm thickness of towelling or other suitable material. It is also important that adjacent turns of the coil are evenly separated from each other by insulating material to avoid concentration of the field and overheating of the cable. Wooden or perspex spacers are provided for this purpose.

The plastic casing of a drum electrode ensures suitable spacing but an additional air gap is also needed to achieve adequate depth heating (Lehmann and de Lateur, 1982); 1–2 cm is an appropriate minimum distance from the electrode to the skin; 4 cm is probably ideal and 6 cm the maximum to ensure an even heating.

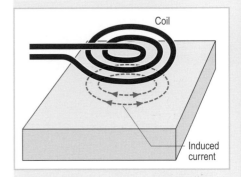

Figure 13.12 A spiral coil or helix, used for more localized treatment.

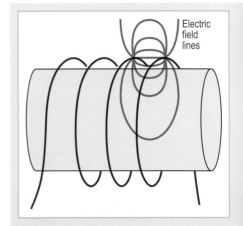

Figure 13.13 The electric field produced between adjacent turns of an inductive coil.

Summary

Several factors affect the heating pattern in the tissues:

- The nature of tissues involved – dielectric constant and conductivity.
- The field intensity within the particular tissue.
- The capacitive field is influenced by:
  - spacing of electrodes
  - size of electrodes
  - relationship of electrodes to skin surface.
- The inductive field is influenced by:
  - relationship of the coil to the tissues
  - proximity of the coil to the skin surface.
- In both cases the greatest rate of temperature increase is normally produced in fatty tissue, with the effect normally being greatest in capacitive applications.

Technique of application

Stages

Patient

Explanation: describe the nature of the treatment, identify possible contraindications and advise the patient of the following: the risks, the expected levels of heating of the part that should be experienced and what is not to occur (touching or moving operating equipment or allowing the level of heating to become more than comfortably warm).

Examination: expose the area to be treated adequately and do not pass the field through clothing. The clothing may:

- be made of unsuitable synthetic material
- contain metal fastenings
- be damp or conceal dampness on the skin
- constrict circulation to the part.

In addition, exposure of the area enables identification of possible risks including those associated with any local pathologies or previous surgery, local blood return rate, and metal in the vicinity.

Test and record thermal sensation at least prior to the first treatment.

Apparatus

Assemble the machine and apparatus. Therapist testing of the apparatus is not advised. Having the therapist place their hand in the field to assess the level of heating is inappropriate as it is unreliable and potentially hazardous to the therapist. The output indicator of the machine provides a guide to the power output of the machine but the most reliable indicator of the dose received by tissues is via patient report and knowledge of the properties of SWD.

Preparation of the part

Position: the area to be treated (and the patient as a whole) must be safely and comfortably positioned for the treatment. Movement should be minimized to optimize tuning. Remove all metal objects and synthetic materials within a minimum of 30 cm. Dry the skin if it is moist. Any skin surfaces in contact with each other must be separated by some absorbent material such as towelling.

Setting up

Select the method: capacitor field or inductothermy.

The capacitor field method may be applied in different ways:

- Transverse (contraplanar) (see Figure 13.6): place electrodes on opposite sides of the part, parallel to the part and not each other, to treat deeply placed structures, e.g. joints.
- Coplanar (see Figure 13.7): place electrodes on the same side of the part to treat more superficial structures, e.g. the spinal musculature. They must be separated by a gap at least twice their distance from the skin.
- Crossfire (see Figure 13.9): give half the treatment with the electrodes in one contraplanar position and for the second half reposition the electrodes at right angles. This technique may be used to achieve more uniform heating of the tissues and particularly the walls of air-filled cavities, e.g. paranasal sinuses.

If inductothermy, the cable may be applied as:

- a monode, minode, circuplode, diplode or drum-type electrode (see Figure 13.18)
- a coil wound as a flat spiral (see Figure 13.12)
- a coil, wound round the circumference of a limb (see Figure 13.11).

Position the electrodes or coils relative to the tissues with appropriate spacing. Protect other parts of the body from the field around connecting leads by placing towelling or felt spacers between them and the skin. Similarly, the leads must not be closer together than the terminals of the machine nor close to any conductor in which they could induce heating.

Instructions and warnings

Advise the patient of the level of any heating intended and give precise instructions and a warning that if it is hotter than is comfortably warm the therapist must be notified immediately, as failure to do so can result in a burn. Also advise the patient that they must report where they feel the heating and any concentration of it in a particular region. The only way the therapist can estimate the level of heating provided is by patient feedback. This requires that the patient can communicate, understand the risks of excessive heating and has an ability to reliably discriminate levels of heating. Instruct the patient not to move during the treatment nor to touch any part of the operating equipment.

Application

Switch the apparatus on and slowly adjust the heating to the appropriate intensity as indicated by the patient. Older machines may also require manual tuning to optimize their output, but this is rare nowadays. As vasodilation takes place, heat is dissipated and the intensity may have to be increased. The intensity should be increased only gradually, always remaining no more than comfortably warm. If any pain, aching or discomfort occurs during treatment the machine should be switched off at once.

Termination

At the end of treatment, which usually lasts 15 to 20 minutes, turn the equipment off and remove the coil or electrodes. Inspect the skin carefully for any changes, remembering that the presence and intensity of erythema on the skin and the increased surface temperature are not particularly reliable. Different ages and colours of skin will show more or less erythema and the skin temperature can vary considerably with the technique used.

DOSAGE

If energy is added to the tissues faster than it is being dissipated the temperature must rise, which causes vasodilation to increase heat removal until the heat gain and loss are once more in balance at a new, higher local temperature (see chapter 10 and Figure 13.14). It usually takes some 15 to 20 minutes for these vascular adjustments to occur and thus reach a steady state, but it can be longer. This is the reason for applying treatment for up to 30 minutes. The first 10 minutes or more are essentially wasted in heating the tissue up to therapeutically useful values.

Therapist knowledge of the extent of heating due to shortwave treatments is dependent on patient feedback. This means accurate and timely communication of the level of heating is essential. Since the shortwave field is strongest at the surface, any heat is detected by thermoreceptors in the skin. Dosage can be described as shown in Table 13.2. The terms 'subthermal' or 'athermal' for imperceptible

Practical point

Causes of pain during heating can include:

- an intensity which is too high
- heating areas of local inflammation
- heating collections of fluid, such as an inflamed bursa or a haemarthrosis or a haematoma (increased pressure due to heating a containing structure will cause pain)
- poor positioning.

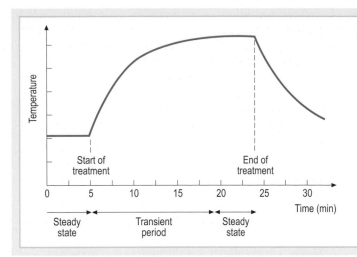

Figure 13.14 The temperature increase in tissue due to the thermoregulatory response to heating.

Table 13.2 Dosages of shortwave diathermy	
Dosage	**Description of heat to patient**
Moderate heating	Comfortable warmth
Mild heating	Mild gentle warmth
Minimal perceptible heating	So that you can only just feel the warmth
Imperceptible heating	No feeling of warmth at all

heating are best avoided as these words incorrectly imply that no local heating occurs as it cannot be felt. Most people can, however, identify heating threshold at quite low levels of intensity (Bricknell and Watson, 1995; Murray and Kitchen, 2000).

The minimum dose should be given that will achieve the required effect.

POTENTIAL DANGERS

All the potential dangers inherent in any heat treatment must be taken into account (see chapters 10 and 11). In addition, there are some considerations specific to shortwave diathermy, as described below.

Burns

Burns can be due to:

- the patient being unaware of the dangers of this type of heating because of poor therapist warnings and explanations, defective

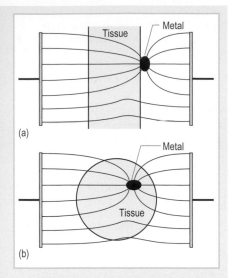

Figure 13.15 Metal touching the skin surface (a) and metal implanted in the tissues (b) will concentrate the electric field.

thermal sensation or an inability to communicate for whatever reason.

- concentration of the shortwave field happening so quickly that a burn occurs before the patient has time to react.

Concentration of the electric field

- A material of high dielectric constant/low impedance in the field, such as metal or moisture, will concentrate the electric field and a burn can result. All metals are relatively low-resistance conductors and even if enclosed in plastic, as in the armpieces of spectacles, will still concentrate the field. Similarly clothing contains many pieces of metal, often hard to distinguish from plastic equivalents, e.g. zips, hooks, buckles, all of which can have the same effect.

Figure 13.15a illustrates the effect of a wrist watch or other metal object near the skin surface. Field lines are concentrated on the metal, resulting in a high electric field intensity in tissues alongside. Figure 13.15b illustrates the effect of a metal implant in tissue. In each case, tissue adjacent to the metal undergoes a higher rate of heating due to the higher field intensity.

The metal itself in Figure 13.15 would not be heated appreciably as the metal has an extremely low resistance. The rate of heating is given by the formula:

$$P = I^2 R$$

Although I is large in the metal in Figure 13.15, R is extremely small so the rate of heating of the metal is small. The tissue adjacent to the metal has a much higher impedance. The combination of higher impedance and high induced current due to the high field intensity results in rapid heating of the tissue. Thus the situation depicted in Figure 13.15a could result in superficial burns while that shown in Figure 13.15b could produce deep tissue burns.

Whether a burn occurs or not will depend on local field strength, which depends on the output of the shortwave machine, the extent to which the field is concentrated, and the options available for dissipating heat. Something like an earring or a stud, although small, may cause burning as it has point contact with the tissues.

If a person in an electromagnetic field touches any conductor in the vicinity, such as the metal frame of a chair or couch, this can result in concentration of the electric field at the point of contact and consequent burns. For this reason a therapist must not attempt to feel the skin temperature of an area in between operating electrodes. The risk is a focal burn to the patient. Additionally, this approach could not accurately provide the therapist with any useful information about the output.

Implanted metal, from fixation of fractures and metal arthroplastic devices or if accidentally embedded in the tissues, can lead to burning at the junction of the metal with the tissues for the reasons

Whether small metal objects pose a hazard must be judged in terms of the size of the metal object and its distance from the area ostensibly being treated.

explained above. The problem is, the patient would not necessarily feel any heat as there are no thermoreceptors in the tissues and the evidence of damage would be deep, delayed onset pain. Small round pieces of metal such as tooth fillings and tongue studs have little or no effect but large wire dental splints may be a risk. An advantage with heating around the mouth is that saliva acts to dissipate rapidly any areas of local heating and help minimize all risks. Copper-bearing intrauterine contraceptive devices are usually regarded as not a problem during treatment of the pelvis or lower lumbar region. The temperature rise during heating with a diplode for 20 minutes (dosage unclear) was less than 1°C (Heick et al., 1991). This is considerably lower than the rise needed to reach the accepted therapeutic range of 42–45°C and well below that for tissue damage.

Water droplets on the skin, from sweat or wet dressings, can also provide areas of focus for the electric field and therefore carry risks.

- Inadequate spacing of electrodes or leads from the body part being treated or electrode or lead contact with tissue will also concentrate the field (note that it is the actual electrode distance which is important, not the plastic housing to skin distance). If the spacing is uneven so that the skin–electrode distance is smaller in a region, the field will also be concentrated.
- With the machine at high output, the field near the output cables will be extremely high. If the cable is touched by the patient or therapist, an electric arc breakdown of the insulation could occur. This method of damaging the cable insulation is probably less likely than that due to overheating caused by leads touching or lying on or under a metallic object. Leads should always be separated by the distance they exit the machine and if they have to lie on the couch or person, separated by towelling or felt spacers. They should never be compressed under the person.

Cardiac pacemakers and indwelling stimulators

Another possible danger is to those patients who have cardiac pacemakers or any other form of indwelling stimulator or electronic pump. The electronic circuitry of these types of equipment is designed so that they are safe from interference, i.e. will not malfunction when exposed to 'normal' (low intensity) electromagnetic fields, such as those produced by common household appliances such as computers, TV sets, hair dryers and electric razors. SWD fields are, however, thousands of times greater than 'normal' artificial fields. There is a significant risk for patients with indwelling devices if they are closer than a few metres from operating SWD apparatus. Thus, such patients should not only not be treated with SWD but should not be near operating SWD apparatus.

Although not as critical, electronic hearing aids can be affected by the shortwave diathermy field.

Synthetic materials

These may have the following disadvantages (personal communication (AR) with UK Department of Health; Mann, 1989):

- they do not absorb moisture as readily as natural materials
- they ignite more easily than natural materials and can produce large volumes of toxic fumes – there have been a number of cases where shortwave electrodes or cables have overheated and caught fire
- the material itself or any coating applied (e.g. for fire resistance) may alter the field either by absorbing energy or by concentrating the field.

Distance from the shortwave machine

These precautions are recommended by the Chartered Society of Physiotherapy (CSP UK, 1997) and the Australian Physiotherapy Association (Robertson et al., 2001).

To restrict exposure, it is recommended that operators should remain 1 m from continuous wave therapeutic diathermy equipment, 0.5 m from pulsed treatment with capacitive electrodes, and 0.2 m from pulsed inductive applicators (Lerman et al., 1996). Short excursions closer to the electrodes are permitted but only when necessary. Extra care should be exercised by pregnant operators. There is, however, no reason to suspect any long-term health risk to physiotherapists working with diathermy equipment (Martin et al., 1991).

Overweight or obese patients

As previously noted, the subcutaneous fat layer is heated to a similar extent as superficial muscle with capacitor field treatment. Capacitive electrodes should be avoided with overweight or obese patients (those who weigh 25% or more than normal body weight). A magnetic field output, e.g. a drum-type electrode (monode), is more suitable to produce deep tissue heating (Kloth et al., 1984).

The eye

Because of the poor dissipation of heat from the eye, more than a minimum exposure to shortwave diathermy, such as occurs during treatment to the sinuses or the cervical spine, should be avoided.

Pregnancy

When considering SWD and pregnancy, the pregnant patient or therapist must be considered. The issues are different, depending on whether the risks are assumed primarily to be thermally related or to other effects associated with exposure to high frequency, high intensity, electric or magnetic fields. Some women have inadvertently had SWD applied through their uterus in the early stages of pregnancy. The risk of teratogenic effects to the fetus from excess heating is negligible (particularly given the low temperature rises identified in studies with IUDs *in situ*). Less is known of whether exposure to SWD fields has any non-thermal, field intensity related, effects on the developing fetus.

Reviews of studies investigating the risks associated with exposure of pregnant therapists to SWD and having a spontaneous abortion or a higher incidence of congenital malformations find there is no statistically significant evidence of either (Shields et al., 2003). Despite the lack of evidence of any risk, for all therapists, male or female, avoiding extended periods of direct exposure to shortwave diathermy seems a reasonable precaution.

Earlier suggestions that SWD was a risk during pregnancy, typically ignored a range of issues including: the lack of a dose–response relationship, the very small number of cases and the risks in using unreliable exposure data based on therapist recall, often many years later (Cromie et al., 2002).

Implanted slow-release hormone capsules

It is sensible to avoid treating the area where the capsule is implanted.

CONTRAINDICATIONS TO SHORTWAVE DIATHERMY

From the foregoing a list of conditions and circumstances in which the application of shortwave might be dangerous or damaging can be deduced:

- Implanted pacemakers or other forms of stimulators or electronic pumps (within 3 m of SWD apparatus or as advised by the manufacturer).
- Metal in the tissues, surgically or otherwise implanted.
- Metal on the surface of the tissues that cannot be removed, such as external skeletal fixation or some dental splints.
- Impaired thermal sensation.
- Patients unable to control their movements or whose cooperation cannot be presumed. For example, the very young or mentally unstable patients or those with uncontrolled movements due to disease and those unable to communicate effectively and reliably.
- The pregnant uterus.
- Conditions in which haemorrhage is occurring or likely to occur. By increasing vasodilation and decreasing blood viscosity, heating might prolong haemorrhage. In the case of SWD, heating can occur in the deeper tissues, so the risk is greater than for superficial forms of heating. Additional bleeding may occur if pelvic SWD is applied during menstruation (a risk, not usually a contraindication).
- Conditions in which fluid is under tension, e.g. an acute bursitis, lymphoedema, haematoma or haemarthrosis.

Reflex heating of the proximal part is safe and may have therapeutic value since it will provoke reflex vasodilation of the affected distal part. However, this may only be moving a limited blood flow from one tissue to another and may have no long-term beneficial effect.

- Ischaemic tissues unable to respond to the need for an increased blood flow to assist with dissipating extra heat. Examples include the feet and lower legs of people with any vascular occlusions or obstructions. Heating ischaemic tissue is entirely inappropriate as it can lead to irreversible damage. A similar effect can occur if a capacitive pad is placed under a limb unless the weight of the part is supported.
- Malignant tumours should not be treated by any form of heat in case the increased metabolic rate leads to increased rates of growth or metastases. This is a particular risk with SWD given its effectiveness in heating at depth. Similarly, tissue damaged by radiation therapy should not be treated with SWD in the absence of advice to the contrary from the treating oncologist.
- Active tuberculous lesions should not be treated since heating may increase activity of the bacillus. In the absence of supporting evidence it seems reasonable to avoid such lesions.
- Sites of recent venous thrombosis should be avoided in case heating loosens the clot leading to pulmonary embolism (Scott, 1957). When the vessel is fibrosed it is safe to treat.
- While the patient is pyrexic or has an area of acute inflammation any form of extensive or intensive local heating should be avoided.

PULSED SHORTWAVE

The output of shortwave machines can be pulsed in the same way as ultrasound (see chapter 9). This modality is known by a profusion of different names.

Production of pulsed shortwave

Pulsed shortwave is sometimes called 'Pulsed electromagnetic field' or 'pulsed electromagnetic energy', and appropriate acronyms are used. Others know it by the manufacturers' names for the product.

The principles of production of the oscillating high-frequency 27.12 MHz continuous output have been described earlier. By incorporating a timing (gating) circuit, the output can be turned on and off, allowing bursts of current (pulses) to be emitted for any length of time. Some machines give fixed-length pulses, e.g. 65 or 400 µs, but others allow a choice.

Output

The output depends on the:

- peak (or pulse) power in watts
- pulse duration in µs
- pulse frequency (repetition rate) in Hz.

Each pulse is a burst of sinusoidal current (Figure 13.16). As the shortwave frequency is 27.12 MHz, in 1 second there are 27.12×10^6

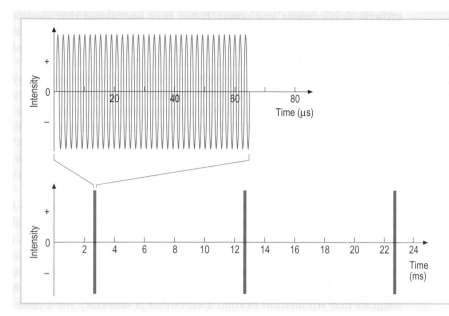

Figure 13.16 Pulsed high-frequency oscillations. The period is 10 ms and the pulse or burst duration is 65 μs so the duty cycle is 0.65%. If the peak power is 100 W, the average power is 0.65 W.

cycles, and in 1 μs there are 27.12 cycles. A 65 μs burst therefore contains 1762.8 cycles. At 100 pulses per second each complete period lasts 1/100 s (i.e. 10 ms or 10 000 μs). The first burst would therefore be separated from the next by an interval of 9935 μs. The duty cycle, i.e. the ratio of burst duration to total period, is in this case 0.65%. The mean power can be found by calculating the duty cycle and taking this proportion of the peak power.

Possible therapeutic mechanisms

Explanations advanced to explain the mechanisms by which pulsed shortwave might affect the tissues differently from continuous are speculative. This is also the case with other low-energy therapies such as pulsed ultrasound. An interesting and valuable review of this topic (Kitchen and Dyson, 1996) notes several cellular sites at which low-energy treatments might be active. A simple but reasonable explanation is that the electromagnetic energy 'stirs' ions, molecules, membranes and perhaps cells thus speeding up phagocytic activity, enzymatic activity, transport across membranes and so forth. This would account for the evident acceleration of inflammatory and healing processes.

The activities of all cells are related to their ionic environment. There is a characteristic potential difference across all cell membranes (see chapter 2). Some depolarization of the cell membrane is often associated with cell dysfunction and electrical potentials change during wound healing (see chapter 2). The membrane potential is also involved in the control of cell division and hence in the control of

An analogy might be drawn with hammering a nail into a piece of wood. Rapidly repeated gentle tapping has no effect but the same total energy delivered as a few stout blows can drive the nail firmly into the wood.

from the coil. The drum-type electrode is placed close to, or just touching, the skin over the area to be treated and the length of the casing ensures that the coil is well separated from the skin and superficial tissues. The difference between deep and superficial tissue exposure is reduced and more uniform effects would be expected.

A thermal sensation test should be carried out to ensure that there is no sensory deficit, especially when delivering pulsed shortwave at a mean power exceeding 5 W (Bricknell and Watson, 1995).

DOSAGE

There is little evidence and even less agreement concerning the treatment parameters that should be used for pulsed shortwave treatments.

One way of expressing the output is the average power in watts for each setting. The importance of average power is illustrated by comparing the three studies on sprained ankles mentioned above:

- treatment for 1 h per day with 600 bursts per second and 38 W mean power (Wilson, 1972). After 3 days the treated group had improved approximately twice as much as the controls
- 20-minute treatments at 38 W mean power and the treated ankles did marginally better than the controls (Pasila et al., 1978).
- 15-minute treatments at 20 W with no significant difference between treated and control groups (McGill, 1989).

Analysis of the energy applied per 24 h, in these and other clinical studies, showed that the threshold value for some success appeared to be 40 kJ/24 h, with the greatest success achieved with doses above 100 kJ/24 h. There were no effects at lower doses (Low, 1995). This meta-analysis conforms with the Arndt–Schultz law (see Figure 13.17) noted above, that an appropriate quantity of energy – 'not too little, not too much' – is needed over relatively long treatment durations for efficacy. This would account for the ineffectiveness noted in a number of the studies mentioned above (e.g. Grant et al., 1989).

A problem with any meta-analysis is that there are invariably confounding variables such as the peak power used, the extent of pathology and the stage at which treatment was applied.

CONTRAINDICATIONS

With the low average power of pulsed shortwave there is very little danger of a burn due to concentration of the field by metal or water. Thus it may be applied through wet dressings and in the presence of metal implants, but not implanted stimulators or other electronic equipment. However, it is very important to realize that the treatment is relatively, not absolutely, athermic as longer bursts of pulses delivered at higher frequencies can lead to heating and hence burning. This has been quantified in a study by Bricknell and Watson (1995) which found detectable heating at a mean power of 11 W delivered for some

7 minutes. In this case the potential dangers indicated for continuous shortwave are appropriate.

No damaging effects of any kind have been reported to date with pulsed shortwave. However, while the mode of action remains unknown, avoiding rapidly dividing tissues, such as the fetus or the uncontrolled growth of precancerous tissues or neoplasms is obviously prudent. Similarly treating encapsulated tubercular lesions and seriously hyperpyrexic patients should be avoided.

LOW-POWER PULSED HIGH-FREQUENCY ENERGY

A number of devices are available which generate pulses similar to those just described but at a tiny fraction of the power. They produce pulses of 27.12 MHz oscillations at various repeat rates but with about 0.5 W average power and 15 W peak power. The applicators are placed close to the skin. There are some reports of their effectiveness in treating a variety of conditions, e.g. Debelle et al. (1977). These results were not substantiated in a rigorous controlled trial by Barker et al. (1985) involving ligament sprains.

Oedema and bruising were found to be less on the treated side during a controlled study of recovery after bilateral blepharoplasty (Nicolle and Bentall, 1982). All these sources apply energy to the tissues by means of an induction coil aerial placed on the surface of the skin. It has been claimed that the proximity to the tissues compensated for their low output. (For the blepharoplasty study the aerials were fashioned into spectacle frames worn over the dressings.) There are several reports of these low-power pulses being used successfully to encourage healing of skin wounds. What is doubtful is that sufficient energy could reach deeper tissue to produce any therapeutic effect.

Foley-Nolan et al. (1990) applied low-power pulsed electromagnetic energy via a cervical collar for persistent neck pain and found an increase in range of movement and a decrease in pain. Methods of application vary but usually the small induction coil is held in contact with the skin over the lesion by a bandage or Velcro strap. Length of treatment times suggested also vary a good deal but are often quite long, 1–2 h or even up to 6 h per day. The small battery-operated devices have been used for 16 h each day, and some continuously.

Low power devices may be able to produce beneficial effects but only in tissue very close to the treatment coil. Again there is very limited clinical evidence that such treatment is of benefit.

KILOHERTZ FREQUENCY DEVICES

In the early 20th century, 'longwave diathermy' machines were used (Geddes, 1984). These are therapeutic sources generating alternating electric fields at frequencies of hundreds of kHz. Compared to shortwave diathermy, the effects are relatively superficial. This perhaps led to the abandonment of longwave diathermy by clinicians when shortwave machines were developed. Longwave machines are still commercially produced and their present-day incarnation is described as 'Indiba treatment'. These devices produce local heating through the application of a pair of metal electrodes to the skin (via a cream). Heating occurs throughout the intervening tissues, but is greatest close to the electrodes. If unequal size electrodes are used, greatest heating occurs under the smaller electrode. Longwave diathermy may have clinical advantages over, say, hot-pack treatment, but this has yet to be established.

Surgical diathermy units operate at high kHz frequencies. They have two electrodes. The smaller one is the 'knife' and the current density is much higher. The other electrode is large and connected to the skin with a highly conductive contact gel to ensure wide and even current dispersal (Vedovato et al., 2004).

Summary

Continuous shortwave diathermy:
- majority of sources 27.12 MHz frequency
- output up to a few hundred watts
- coupled to tissues inductively or capacitively
- can give clearly detectable heating
- usually applied for 20–30 minutes.

Pulsed shortwave:
- 27.12 MHz
- output up to a few tens of watts mean power, emitting very short pulse trains of up to 1000 W peak power
- coupled to tissues usually inductively, sometimes capacitively
- heating usually only detected with outputs above 7 W
- can be applied up to 60 minutes.

Low-power pulsed high-frequency energy:
- 27.12 MHz
- output often less than 1 W mean power, peak power of a few watts, various pulsing regimens
- coupled to tissues inductively
- no detectable heating
- often applied for hours a day.

Kilohertz devices:
- around 750 and 500 kHz frequency
- output a few hundred watts
- coupled to tissues via skin-contact electrodes
- detectable heating
- applied 20 to 30 minutes.

THE USE OF MAGNETISM IN THERAPY

The medical uses of electricity and magnetism have a long and fascinating history (Geddes, 1984). The early scientific study of electric and magnetic force was accompanied by speculation on the part of practitioners of the healing arts that electric and magnetic fields might have healing properties. Bar magnets were considered to have potential, thus early in the 16th century Theophrastus Bombastus Paracelsus von Honenheim had apparently used iron rodlets to 'heal fractures and ruptures, pull hepatitis out, and draw back dropsy' among other wonders (quoted by Cameron, 1983). Later Mesmer used iron magnets for treatment and ever since there have been therapies based on some form of permanent magnet.

While the static magnetic fields associated with permanent magnets are of dubious clinical value, low frequency alternating magnetic fields have a limited but well-established role.

Most readers would chuckle at the claims of von Honenheim and Mesmer, so it is a little surprising to see magnets still promoted as having healing properties in the 21st century.

Static magnetic fields

The most recent form of these therapies is based on the fact that modern permanent magnets are much more powerful than earlier magnets. The magnets are usually contained within a bracelet or sewn into a device that is worn over a painful area, usually a joint with osteoarthritis. Alternatively, a flexible material containing magnetic strips of alternating polarity and covered with a thin metal foil is bandaged or stuck to the skin over the lesion. The different configurations of the permanent magnets include a circular alternating polarity magnetic foil which can be used as a pad or a tunnel.

Existing studies of the effectiveness of using magnets to reduce the pain and loss of function of arthritis have mixed results. A recent randomized controlled trial compared the effectiveness of commercially available active magnetic bracelets with sham ones for treating hip or knee osteoarthritis (Harlow et al., 2004). The active magnetic bracelets were either strongly (134–197 milliTesla, abbreviated mT) or weakly (21–3 mT) magnetic and the non-magnetic ones had zero field strength. The results show all groups benefited, and those with the stronger magnetic field more so (difference between stronger and zero strength groups statistically significant). Since approximately half of those treated with the strong magnets and half with the dummy magnets correctly identified their treatment group, the blinding was of limited effectiveness. A lack of difference in results between the weak and dummy magnets, however, suggests a few options: a strong magnetic field is required (e.g. over 134 mT); there is no dose–response relationship; or that the effect is predominantly a placebo one.

One way of studying the effects of magnets on pain is by inducing delayed onset muscle soreness. A study that treated the affected elbow flexors with either a 0 mT or 35 mT magnet found no differ-

Modern magnets are alloys of cobalt, nickel and various rare earths such as yttrium, that can be up to 15 times the magnetic strength of the older steel magnets.

While one must always keep an open mind, it is difficult not to be sceptical of the largely unsubstantiated claims made for 'static magnetic field therapy'.

ences between the treated groups (Reeser et al., 2005). This result leaves open the question of the appropriateness of this model of testing when magnets are usually used to treat osteoarthritic joint pain and are worn in bracelets or other devices for many hours per day.

The mode of action of static magnetic fields is claimed, without supporting evidence, to be similar to pulsed shortwave, only much slower because the tiny induced electric currents must reach a threshold before any biological process is affected (Hayne, 1989). The main therapeutic uses are said to be for circulation, analgesia and wound healing.

Safety of static magnetic fields

As to the safety of static magnetic fields, there appears to be no evidence of any deleterious effects. The World Health Organization notes the absence of any adverse effects due to exposure to fields up to 2 tesla. The absence of deleterious effects, even at extremely high field intensities perhaps explains the lack of consistently identifiable therapeutic benefits and suggests a lack of any significant physiological effects, regardless of intensity.

Low-frequency pulsed magnetic fields

Magnetic force is inextricably linked to the movement of charges so that any electric current produces an associated magnetic field. If the magnetic field changes, this produces a force on charges in the vicinity and charge movement (current flow) is induced. In low frequency magnetic field therapy, a relatively powerful magnetic field is produced in a large coil into which the part can be placed. Current in the coil is pulsed at various frequencies up to about 150 Hz, producing a pulsed magnetic field. Other pulsed devices use higher pulsing frequencies but much weaker magnetic fields and a flat 'pancake' coil is placed in contact with the part to be treated. There is no objective evidence to support the therapeutic value of these therapies for many of the conditions for which they are recommended.

McMeeken (1992) found that the field settings of a pulsed magnetic field machine, specified as producing vasodilation, did not do so. There is, however, some evidence of the effectiveness of low-frequency pulses applied to the tissues by electromagnetic induction in the treatment of ununited fractures (Otter et al., 1998) and Perthes' disease (Harrison and Bassett, 1984). Similar low frequency pulses have been used successfully in the treatment of rotator cuff tendinitis in a double-blind trial (Binder et al., 1984). These therapies were applied for several hours each day, the patients often sleeping while the coils were active.

Safety of low-frequency magnetic fields

The safety of low frequency electromagnetic field exposure has been the subject of intense debate over many years. The concern has been engendered by the realization that exposure to all kinds of electromagnetic fields and radiation has greatly increased over the whole world during the past hundred years or so. This is especially so close to high-voltage electric power transmission lines where the magnetic field intensity can be much higher than the average static earth magnetic field of about 0.05 mT (Dowson, 1989).

There have been a number of studies examining whether there is any correlation between low frequency electromagnetic exposure and disease; mainly because exposure to the fields around mains power wiring is now almost universal, so if there is any effect it would be a major cause of concern. Studies can be classified into four groups:

- those in the laboratory on animals and cell cultures exposed to controlled, artificially produced electromagnetic fields
- similar studies of humans exposed to controlled electromagnetic fields
- epidemiological studies of human populations exposed to electromagnetic fields, for example those living near power transmission lines
- epidemiological studies of specific groups of people who are exposed to electromagnetic fields, e.g. in the electricity industry.

The biggest concern has been the apparent link between powerline fields and the incidence of certain forms of cancer (in particular, childhood leukaemia). The scientifically accepted view is that for powerline fields (or any other potentially harmful agent) to be classed as a 'definite' health hazard, the evidence must be sufficient to satisfy two criteria:

- epidemiological studies must shows a consistent, significant link between the disease and powerline fields
- a plausible biophysical mechanism for the systematic initiation or promotion of cancer by powerline fields must have been identified.

While it is impossible to prove that no deleterious health effects occur from exposure to any environmental factor, it is necessary to demonstrate a consistent, significant and causal relationship before one can conclude that such effects do occur.

A report by the National Institute of Environmental Health Sciences (NIEHS, 1999) concluded that the scientific evidence is weak. They state that:

the strongest evidence for health effects comes from associations observed in human populations with two forms of cancer: childhood leukemia and chronic lymphocytic leukemia in occupationally exposed adults. While the support from individual studies is weak, the epidemiological studies demonstrate, for some methods

The basic argument is that up to recent times living organisms had been exposed to natural background electric and magnetic fields over millions of years and would have evolved to tolerate and perhaps benefit from the resulting forces. Suddenly over the last century much greater intensity electric and magnetic fields have become a part of the environment.

of measuring exposure, a fairly consistent pattern of a small, increased risk with increasing exposure that is somewhat weaker for chronic lymphocytic leukemia than for childhood leukemia. In contrast, the mechanistic studies and the animal toxicology literature fail to demonstrate any consistent pattern across studies although sporadic findings of biological effects (including increased cancers in animals) have been reported. No indication of increased leukemias in experimental animals has been observed.

The NIEHS report also concluded that the lack of any apparent link between the human data and the experimental data (animal or in vitro) limits the interpretation of the reported findings. The human data seem to show an adverse effect of exposure to mains frequency electric and magnetic fields. The apparent increased risks, however, are small and could be due to some other factor or common source of error in the studies.

A review by the International Commission for Non-Ionizing Radiation Protection (ICNIRP, 2001) concluded that the body of evidence for a link between both childhood leukaemia and chronic lymphocytic leukaemia in adults demonstrated an association, but that this could be due to selection bias. The review also endorsed earlier conclusions that other links are yet to be established.

A later review by the UK National Radiological Protection Board (McKinlay et al, 2004), which weighed more recent evidence, came to similar conclusions.

The lack of conclusive findings, despite decades of investigative study, suggests that any deleterious effects are minimal or non-existent. A possible leukaemia link is yet to be confirmed.

> On the other hand, no consistent explanation other than exposure to low frequency electric and magnetic fields has been identified as a possible causal factor.

References

Barker, A., Barlow, P., Porter, J. et al. (1985). A double-blind clinical trial of low power pulsed shortwave therapy in the treatment of soft-tissue injury. Physiotherapy, **71**, 500–504.

Binder, A., Parr, G., Hayleman, B. et al. (1984). Pulsed electromagnetic field therapy of persistent rotator cuff tendinitis. Lancet, **344**, 695–698.

Bricknell, R., Watson, T. (1995). The thermal effects of pulsed shortwave therapy. Br J Ther Rehabil, **2**, 430–434.

Brown, M., Baker, R. (1987). Effects of pulsed shortwave diathermy on skeletal muscle injury in rabbits. Phys Ther, **67**, 208–213.

Cameron, B. (1961). Experimental acceleration of wound healing. Am J Orthop, **53**, 336–343.

Cameron, H. (1983). Electromagnetic therapy: fact or fiction. Mod Med NZ, **16**, 17.

Chartered Society of Physiotherapy (1997). Safe practice with electrotherapy (shortwave therapies). CSP, UK.

Collis, C., Segal, M. (1988). Effects of pulsed electromagnetic fields in Na+ fluxes across a stripped rabbit colon epithelium. J. Appl Physiol, **65**, 124–130.

Constable, J., Scapicchio, A., Opitz, B. (1971). Studies of the effects of Diapulse treatment on various aspects of wound healing in experimental animals. J Surg Res, **11**, 254–257.

Cromie, J., Robertson, V., Best, M. (2002). Occupational health in physiotherapy: general health and reproductive outcomes. Aust J Physiother, **48**, 287–294.

Debelle, M., Lorthier, J., Berghmans, M. et al. (1977). Therapeutic effect of very low powered hertzian wave transmissions. Brux-Med, **57**, 551–563.

Dowson, D. (1989). A review of epidemiological studies into the health effects of electromagnetic fields. Compl Hlth Res, **3**, 25–29.

Draper, D., Castro, J., Feland, B., Schulthies, S., Eggett.D. (2004). Shortwave diathermy and prolonged stretching increase hamstring flexibility more than prolonged stretching alone. J Orthop Sports Phys Ther, **34**, 413–420.

Fenn, J. (1969). Effects of pulsed electromagnetic energy (Diapulse) on experimental haematomas. Can Med Assoc J, **100**, 251–254.

Foley-Nolan, D., Barry, C., Coughlan, R. et al. (1990). Pulsed high frequency (27 MHz) electromagnetic therapy for persistent neck pains. Orthopaedics, **13**, 445–451.

Garrett, (2000). Heat distribution in the lower leg from pulsed shortwave diathermy and ultrasound treatments. J Athl Train, **35**, 50–55.

Garrett, C., Draper, D., Knight, K. (2005). The contribution of heating to tissue extensibility: a comparison of deep and superficial heating. Arch Phys Med Rehabil, **86**, 819–825.

Geddes, L. (1984). A short history of the electrical stimulation of excitable tissue including therapeutic applications. Physiologist (suppl.) **27**(1), s1–s47.

Grant, A., Sleep, J., McIntosh, J., Ashurst, A. (1989). Ultrasound and pulsed electromagnetic energy treatment for perineal trauma. A randomised placebocontrolled trial. Br J Obstet Gynaecol, **96**, 434–439.

Harlow, T., Greaves, C., White, A. et al. (2004). Randomising controlled trial of magnetic bracelets for relieving pain in osteoarthritis of the hip and knee. Br Med J, **329**, 1450–1454.

Harrison, M., Bassett, C. (1984). Use of pulsed electromagnetic fields in Perthes disease: report of a pilot study. J Paed Orthop, **4**, 579–584.

Hayne, C. (1984). Pulsed high frequency energy – its place in physiotherapy. Physiotherapy, **70**, 459–466.

Hayne, C. (1989). The healing fields. Ther Weekly, March 16.

Heick, A., Espersen, T., Pedersen, H., Raahauge, J. (1991). Is diathermy safe in women with copper-bearing IUDs? Acta Obstet Gynecol Scand, **70**, 153–155.

ICNIRP Standing Committee on Epidemiology (2001). Review of the Epidemiologic Literature on EMF and Health. Environ Hlth Perspect, **109** (Supp 6), 911–913.

Kitchen, S., Dyson, M. (1996). Low energy treatments: nonthermal or microthermal? In S. Kitchen, S. Bazin (eds), Clayton's Electrotherapy, 10th edn, pp. 110–115. Philadelphia: W. B. Saunders.

Kitchen, S., Partridge, C. (1996). A survey to examine the clinical use of ultrasound, shortwave diathermy and laser in England. Br J Ther Rehabil, **3**, 644–650.

Klaber Moffett, J., Richardson, P., Frost, H., Osborn, A. (1996). Placebo controlled, double-blind trial to evaluate the effectiveness of pulsed shortwave therapy for osteoarthritic hip and knee pain. Pain, **167**, 121–127.

Kloth, L., Morrison, M., Ferguson, B. (1984). Therapeutic Microwave and Shortwave Diathermy. HHS Publication FDA, 85-8237. US Dept of Health and Human Services.

Krag, C., Taudor, F., Siim, E., Bolund, S. (1979). The effect of pulsed electromagnetic energy (Diapulse) on the survival of experimental skin flaps. Scand J Plastic Reconst Surg, **13**, 377–380.

Lehmann, J., de Lateur, B. (1982). Therapeutic heat. In J. F. Lehmann (ed.), Therapeutic Heat and Cold, pp. 404–562. Baltimore: Williams & Wilkins,

Lerman, Y., Caner, A., Jacubovich, R., Ribak, J. (1996). Electromagnetic fields from shortwave diathermy equipment in physiotherapy departments. Physiotherapy, **82**, 456–458.

Low, J. (1978). The nature and effects of pulsed electromagnetic radiations. N Z J Physiother, **6**, 18–22.

Low, J. (1995). Dosage of some pulsed shortwave clinical trials. Physiotherapy, **81**, 611–616.

Ma, Y., Li, J., Liu, Y. (1997). Short-wave diathermy for small spontaneous pneumothorax. Thorax, **52**, 323–327.

Mann, J. (1989). Department of Health Procurement Directorate, London.

Marks, R., Ghassemi, M., Duarte, M., Van Nguyen, J. (1999). A review of the literature on shortwave diathermy as applied to osteo-arthritis of the knee. Physiotherapy, **85**, 304–316.

Martin, C. J., McCallum, H. M., Strelley, S., Heaton, B. (1991). Electromagnetic fields from therapeutic diathermy equipment: a review of hazards and precautions. Physiotherapy, **77**, 3–7.

McGill, S. (1989). The effect of pulsed shortwave therapy on lateral ligament sprain of the ankle. N Z J Physiother, **16**, 21–24.

McKinlay, A., Allen, S., R Cox, R. et al (2004). Review of the scientific evidence for limiting exposure to electromagnetic fields (0–300 GHz). UK National Radiological Protection Board (NRPB). Vol 15, document 3.

McMeeken, J. (1992). Magnetic fields: effects on blood flow in human subjects. Physiother Theory Pract, **8**, 3–9.

Murray, C., Kitchen, S. (2000). Effect of pulse repetition rate on the perception of thermal sensation with pulsed shortwave diathermy. Physiother Res Int, **5**, 73–85.

Nicolle, F., Bentall, R. (1982). Use of radio-frequency pulsed energy in the control of post-operative reactions in blepharoplasty. Aesth Plast Surg, **6**, 169–171.

NIEHS Report PR#9-99 (June, 1999). National Institutes of Environmental Health Sciences (USA).

Oliver, D. (1984). Pulsed electro-magnetic energy – what is it? Physiotherapy, **70**, 458–459.

Oosterveld, F., Rasker, J., Jacobs, J. et al. (1992). The effects of local heat and cold therapy on the intraarticular and skin surface temperature of the knee. Arth Rheum, **35**, 146–151.

Otter, M., McLeod, K., Rubin, C. (1998). Effects of electromagnetic fields in experimental fracture repair. Clin Orthop Rel Res, **355S**, S90–S104.

Pasila, M., Visuri, T., Sundholm, A. (1978). Pulsating shortwave diathermy: value in treatment of recent ankle and foot sprains. Arch Phys Med Rehabil, **59**, 283–286.

Peres, E., Draper, D., Knight, K., Ricard, M. (2002). Pulsed shortwave diathermy and prolonged long-duration stretching increase dorsiflexion range of motion more than identical stretching with diathermy. J Athl Training, **37**, 43–50.

Pope, G., Mockett, S., Wright, J. (1995). A survey of electrotherapeutic modalities: ownership and use in the NHS in England. Physiotherapy, **81**, 82–91.

Raji, A. (1984). An experimental study of the effects of pulsed electromagnetic field (Diapulse) on nerve repair. J Hand Surg, **9B**, 105–111.

Raji, A., Bowden, R. (1983). Effects of high-peak pulsed electromagnetic field on the degeneration and regeneration of the common peroneal nerve in rats. J Bone Joint Surg, **65B**, 478–492.

Reeser, J., Smith, D., Fischer, V. et al. (2005). Static magnetic fields neither prevent nor diminish symptoms and signs of delayed onset muscle soreness. Arch Phys Med Rehabil, **86**, 565–570.

Robertson, V. J., Chipchase, L., Laakso, E., Whelan, K., McKenna, L. (2001). Guidelines for the clinical use of electrophysical agents. Melbourne: Australian Physiotherapy Association.

Robertson, V., Spurritt, D. (1998). Electrophysical agents: Implications of EPA availability and use in undergraduate clinical placements. Physiotherapy, **84**, 335–344.

Robertson, V., Ward, A., Jung, P. (2005). The contribution of heating to tissue extensibility: a comparison of deep and superficial heating. Arch Phys Med Rehabil, **86**, 819–825.

Schwan, H. P. (1965). Biophysics of diathermy. In S. Licht (ed.), Therapeutic Heat and Cold. Baltimore, Maryland: Waverly Press Inc.

Scott, B. (1957). The Principles and Practice of Diathermy. London: Heinemann Medical Books.

Seaborne, D., Quirion-DeGiradi, C., Rousseau, M., Rivest, M., Lambert, J. (1996). The treatment of pressure sores using pulsed electromagnetic energy (PEME). Physiother (Can), **48**, 131–137.

Shields, N., Gormley, J., O'Hare, N. (2001a). Short-wave diathermy in Irish physiotherapy departments. Br J Ther Rehabil, **8**, 331–339.

Shields, N., Gormley, J., O'Hare, N. (2001b). Short-wave diathermy: A review of existing clinical trials. Phys Ther Rev, **6**, 101–118.

Shields, N., O'Hare, N., Gormley, J. (2003). Short-wave diathermy and pregnancy: What is the evidence? Adv Physiother, **5**, 2–14.

Tsong, T. (1989). Deciphering the language of cells. Trends Biol Sci, **14**, 89–92.

Van Nguyen, J., Marks, R. (2002). Pulsed electromagnetic fields for treating osteo-arthritis. Physiotherapy, **88**, 458–470.

Vedovato, J., Polvora, V., Leonardi, D. (2004). Burns as a complication of the use of diathermy. J Burn Care Rehabil, **25**, 120–123.

Wagstaff, P., Wagstaff, S., Downey, M. (1986). A pilot study to compare the efficacy of continuous and pulsed magnetic energy (shortwave diathermy) on the relief of low back pain. Physiotherapy, **72**, 563–566.

Whyte, H., Reader, S. (1952). Heating the knee joint. Ann Rheum Dis, **11**, 54.

Wilson, D. (1972). Treatment of soft tissue injuries by pulsed electrical energy. Br Med J, **2**, 269–270.

Wilson, D. (1974). Comparison of shortwave diathermy and pulsed electromagnetic energy in treatment of soft tissue injuries. Physiotherapy, **60**, 309–310.

Wilson, D., Jagadeesh, P. (1976). Experimental regeneration in peripheral nerves and the spinal cord in laboratory animals exposed to a pulsed electromagnetic field. In Proceedings of the Annual Scientific Meeting of the International Medical Society of Paraplegia. Part III: Paraplegia. pp. 12–20.

Electromagnetic radiation

The last four chapters of this book are concerned with the therapeutic uses of electromagnetic radiation of one kind or another. Heat and light are but two examples of electromagnetic radiation (EMR). The healing effects of heat and light were widely known to the ancients and repopularized during the scientific advances of the end of the seventeenth century and onwards to the present day. Nowadays, laser (visible and infrared) is increasingly popular. The aim of this chapter is to provide a general foundation for what follows by describing the nature and characteristics of radiant electromagnetic energy.

All forms of EMR have common features, which are described in the opening section. The interactions of EMR with matter are then considered, including reflection, refraction, scattering and, most importantly, absorption.

Historically, there has always been a powerful association between the rays of the sun and healing, and from earliest times the sun has been central to religious belief. The Latin *deus* (god) is said to derive from the sun-worshipping Aryans' name for the sun.

NATURE

Radio waves, microwaves, infrared, visible, ultraviolet, X-ray and gamma radiation are all examples of electromagnetic radiation. EMR is always in the form of a wave consisting of regular sinusoidal variations of an electric and a magnetic field at right angles to one another (Figure 14.1).

Electromagnetic waves are similar to sound and ultrasound waves, considered in chapter 9, in that they exhibit the features of wave motion including, importantly, energy transmission, but they differ from sonic waves in two important respects:

● the wave is a variation in the strength of both electric and magnetic fields and is thus independent of the atoms and molecules through which it passes, although it may give energy to them. Sonic waves, on the other hand, are oscillatory variations in compression of the material through which the wave passes (see chapter 9) which means changes in position of the atoms and molecules. A consequence is that sound waves can only exist in a material medium, made of atoms and molecules which can be squeezed together. Light and other electromagnetic radiation can travel

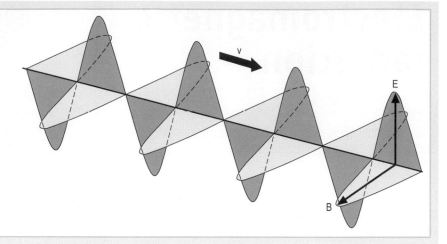

Figure 14.1 An electromagnetic wave consists of an alternating electric field (E) and an alternating magnetic field (B).

through a vacuum but sound waves cannot. So we can see the sun and bask in its visible and infrared electromagnetic radiation but we cannot hear its sounds. Sound waves cannot travel through the vacuum between the sun and earth as there are no (or too few) atoms to vibrate.

● electromagnetic waves are transverse waves, this means that the variations in electric and magnetic field intensities occur at right angles to the direction of travel. This is unlike the compressions and rarefactions of sonic waves which are longitudinal, i.e. in the direction of travel of the wave.

Wave velocity

To be more accurate, the velocity (the 'speed of light' in a vacuum) is $2.9979 \times 10^8 \, \mathrm{m\,s^{-1}}$.

All electromagnetic waves have the same velocity (v) in space. When no matter is present (a vacuum) they all travel at a speed of 300 million metres per second (written $3 \times 10^8 \, \mathrm{m\,s^{-1}}$) and in a straight line. When radiation passes through air, the velocity is decreased by a tiny amount. By contrast, the velocity is reduced markedly in a dense medium such as biological tissue.

The reduction in velocity is closely related to the rate of absorption of wave energy. Absorption results in the wave travelling more slowly. The process of absorption imposes, as it were, a frictional drag on the wave.

Wave frequency

As these waves are simply regular variations in amplitude of the electric and magnetic fields they can be described in terms of the number

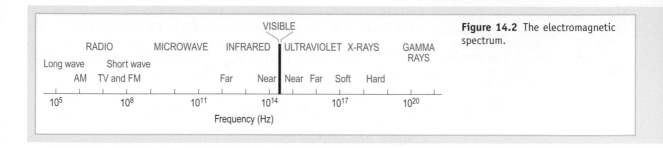

Figure 14.2 The electromagnetic spectrum.

of times in each second they repeat that change, that is the frequency (*f*) in hertz (Hz). Similarly, the distance between any point of the wave and the place where that point is repeated, say crest to crest, can be described as the wavelength (λ), in units of length such as metres, millimetres or nanometres. The waves vary sinusoidally with both time and distance.

The interaction of electromagnetic radiation with matter varies quite markedly with frequency. It is for this reason that different forms of electromagnetic radiation, such as radio waves, microwaves, infrared radiation, visible and ultraviolet radiation, X-rays, gamma and cosmic rays, are identified. The distinction is due to their different properties, which are in turn determined by their frequency. The list and spectrum of radiation is shown in the Figure 14.2.

The very small range of radiation which is able to stimulate the retinal cells of the eye is recognized as visible light and so, despite being the narrow band shown in Figure 14.2, is by far the most familiar and best studied. In fact, much of the behaviour of electromagnetic radiation is understood and illustrated by reference to experiments done with light.

The names given to the various radiations reflect their historical discovery and uses. Thus radio waves (also called hertzian waves) are divided into long-, medium- and shortwave bands in connection with radio and television broadcasting. Microwaves are also known as radar radiation. The naming of infrared, below the red, and ultraviolet, beyond the violet, is self-explanatory of their relationship to the colours of the visible spectrum. X-rays are also known as Röntgen rays, named after their discoverer.

There is only an arbitrary division between one kind of radiation and the next, except for the limits of the visible spectrum which can be defined fairly precisely by what the human eye can and cannot see. The naming covers wide bands of radiation so that different effects may be due to different frequencies of the same radiation.

The ultraviolet region of the spectrum is divided into three regions, designated ultraviolet A, B and C. Ultraviolet-C (UVC) is bactericidal, i.e. it destroys bacteria. The effect is, however, non-specific: UVC can also damage or destroy normal, healthy tissue cells. Ultraviolet-B

UVA penetrates more deeply through tissue than UVB or UVC. A consequence is that damage of the deeper (dermal) cells is greater with UVA than with UVC or UVB. The deeper damage produces tumours with cells of a kind which are more malignant, e.g. malignant melanoma, where melanocytes have mutated.

(UVB) is less damaging, but a consequence is that cell destruction is less likely while carcinogenesis is more likely. Ultraviolet-A (UVA) was thought to be less carcinogenic because the damage and destruction is less, due to the lower wave energy. This is not the case, because UVA penetrates biological tissue more efficiently and so produces more damage in deeper tissue.

Wave amplitude

The magnitude of any kind of wave (by analogy with water, the height of the wave) can vary. This is called the amplitude and, in the case of electromagnetic waves, is the strength of the electric and magnetic fields.

Wave energy

Photons act like little bullets, each having a fixed amount of energy. The photon energy is directly proportional to the wave frequency.

The energy of an electromagnetic wave depends not just on its amplitude but also on its frequency. Figure 14.2 shows that radiations which have the most vigorous and destructive effects on matter are those with the highest frequencies, like X-rays and gamma rays. This is because electromagnetic radiation comes in the form of discrete units, or quanta of energy, which cannot be subdivided. These quanta are called photons. A photon is a little bundle or packet of electromagnetic energy and its energy is proportional to the frequency. The photons in higher frequency radiation carry more energy and so interact more vigourously with matter.

A beam of radiation, whether visible light or some other form of electromagnetic radiation, can be thought of either as a beam of waves (see Figure 14.1) or a beam of particles (photons). The radiation has both wave-like and particle-like properties, so both views are valid: they are different perspectives of the same thing. If the frequency of the beam is increased, a 'wave' description would say that when higher frequency waves hit their target they accelerate the molecules more, because of the higher frequency of the disturbance. A 'particle' view would say that individual photons have higher energy at higher frequencies and so create more disturbance when they hit. Whichever view is used, the higher frequency radiation 'packs more punch' and is more damaging than lower frequencies.

Suppose the beam intensity is increased, with no change in the frequency. A 'wave' view would describe the wave amplitude (E and B in Figure 14.1) as increasing. A 'particle' view would describe this as an increase in the number of photons in the beam.

Electromagnetic waves are more wavelike at sub-optical frequencies and more particle-like at higher frequencies.

In most practical situations, the behaviour of electromagnetic radiation with frequencies lower than visible light is most easily explained using a wave description. To explain the behaviour of visible and higher frequency radiation, a particle view must often be invoked.

Ionizing radiation

Atoms can be thought of as having a positively charged nucleus with a number of rapidly moving electrons occupying fixed, discrete orbitals. Electrons occupying a particular orbital all have the same energy. Different orbitals have different energies associated with them so an electron can be described as occupying a particular orbital or occupying a particular energy level. By giving energy to the atom an electron can be 'kicked' to a higher energy level; in doing so, the atom absorbs a precise amount of energy. Similarly, when electrons drop from a high energy level to a lower one a precise amount of energy, equal to the difference in energy levels, is released. This is emitted in the form of a photon of electromagnetic radiation. The wavelength or frequency of the radiation depends on the energy difference.

When atoms are bombarded with high energy electromagnetic radiation, i.e. high frequency photons, it is possible to knock electrons from their orbitals and completely separate them from their parent atoms. If the electron is knocked so far from its parent atom that it cannot spontaneously return, the parent atom, deficient in electrons, is positively charged and is called an ion. Ionization means that an electron has been separated from its atom. Radiation that has this effect is called ionizing radiation.

The transition between two energy levels by one electron occurs by the absorption of one quantum of radiation at a particular frequency and causes the subsequent emission of one quantum of radiation when the electron drops to its original energy level.

Producing electromagnetic radiation

Electromagnetic radiation is produced whenever charges are accelerated or decelerated. Radio waves, for example, are produced by high-frequency alternating currents (accelerating electrons) in a wire.

Heat is molecular motion which includes rotational and vibrational movements of molecules. This means that the atoms (and the charges within them) are continually accelerating and this results in the emission of infrared radiation. Thus any object continually emits infrared radiation. If the object is heated, the frequency of molecular and atomic vibration will increase, leading to the emission of radiation with shorter wavelengths and higher frequencies which carry more energy. The emitted photons will have a range of different frequencies with the highest frequency produced depending on temperature. For example, at around 400°C the highest frequencies emitted from a heated solid are in the infrared region, but at about 700°C some radiation in the red visible region is emitted and the solid glows red-hot. Still further temperature rises lead to even more vigorous vibration of atoms with the emission of photons with still higher frequencies, including the whole of the visible spectrum so that the object appears white-hot; this can occur at temperatures around 1500°C.

A second way in which visible radiation can be produced occurs when, for example, atoms and ions are made to collide in a low pressure gas (in fluorescent tubes) giving energy to an outer-orbital

Although the physical means of producing, say, radio waves, infrared and X-rays appear very different, they are really just different means of accelerating charges.

The line spectrum acts as a 'fingerprint' for an atom. Copper, for example, has lines in the blue region of the spectrum. Strontium has lines in the violet region.

electron and causing it to jump to a higher energy orbital. When the electron subsequently drops back to its normal, lower energy orbital, a photon of energy characteristic of that particular transition is released. In this way, particular atoms produce a mixture of radiation of particular wavelengths. This forms a so-called 'line spectrum', a band of discrete frequencies in the visible range which is characteristic of the particular atoms. Sodium, for example, produces typical yellow lines in the spectrum. This is the familiar yellow light of sodium-vapour street lighting.

Ultraviolet radiation is produced in a similar way but involves higher energies and therefore shorter wavelengths.

X-rays are produced when high energy transitions are made to occur either when orbiting electrons jump between inner orbits or when rapidly moving electrons are abruptly decelerated.

Gamma radiation is emitted from the nuclei of radioactive atoms. When the atomic nucleus splits, the nuclear fragments are accelerated violently, producing gamma radiation.

Summary

Electromagnetic radiation is:

- emitted whenever charges are accelerated
- energy in the form of oscillating electric and magnetic fields perpendicular to one another and to the direction of travel (see Figure 14.1)
- named to encompass several bands but more precisely identified by frequency or wavelength
- able to travel at a constant velocity of 3×10^8 m s^{-1} in space
- both wave-like and particle-like. It is emitted as quanta whose energy is proportional to the frequency of the radiation
- able to induce ionization of atoms if their frequencies are high enough.

FEATURES OF ELECTROMAGNETIC RADIATION

The variation in intensity with distance

As with all waves, the velocity is the product of frequency and wavelength:

$$v = f.\lambda$$

Electromagnetic radiation travels in straight lines in space. This is called rectilinear propagation. It is clearly evident with visible radiation since shadows are formed where the light path is interrupted by an object. Radiation is emitted from its source in all directions so that if the source is relatively small the radiation will spread out equally in all directions with the result that the energy passing through a unit area per unit time – the intensity – will decrease with distance. This is illustrated in Figure 14.3.

The relationship between the distance from the source and intensity of radiation is expressed in *the inverse square law* which states

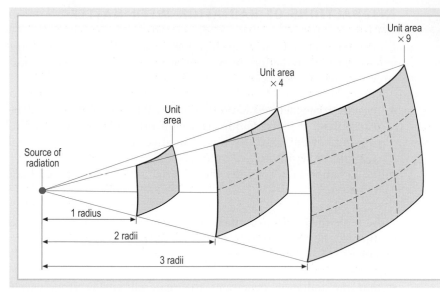

Figure 14.3 The inverse square law. The intensity of radiation from a point source is inversely proportional to the square of the distance from the source.

that the intensity of the radiation from a point source is inversely proportional to the square of the distance from the source:

$$I \propto \frac{1}{d^2}$$

where I = intensity and d = distance.

A consequence is that small changes of distance will cause large changes of intensity, as shown in Figure 14.3. Doubling the distance between the source and the irradiated surface will reduce the intensity to one-quarter because the area over which the wave energy is distributed is four times larger. Tripling the distance increases the area by a factor of nine and thus reduces the intensity to one-ninth and so on. Similarly, halving the distance will quadruple the intensity.

The inverse square law is only strictly true if there is no scattering or absorption of the radiation. For most radiation frequencies it is effectively true in air and of great practical importance. The relevance of the inverse square law to treatment using infrared and ultraviolet radiation will be discussed in later chapters.

Phase difference and coherence

Radiation emitted from a heated source consists of random bursts of waves (or photons, if we take a 'particle' view) because each atom or molecule of the source acts independently so that the varying electric and magnetic fields of the waves produced are not 'in time' or 'in step'. It is possible to make all the emitting atoms radiate in phase by stimulating light emission in a special way in a device called a laser (discussed in chapter 16). When this occurs the radiation is said to be coherent.

In a coherent beam, all the waves are in phase, i.e. the peaks and troughs of the waves are all synchronized.

INTERACTIONS OF RADIATION WITH MATTER

Electromagnetic radiation travels unhindered in space (and to a large extent, for most radiation, in air) but on meeting matter several possible interactions can occur:

- the electromagnetic radiation can pass into the material and be transmitted. If the radiation passes into the material it is said to *penetrate*. If the wave also travels unaffected through the material it is said to be *transmitted* unhindered.
- the radiation may not enter the material at all, being turned back or *reflected*.

In both these cases, as there is no energy lost to the material so there is no effect on the material. There is another possibility, however:

- that the radiation penetrates the material but is progressively absorbed as it travels. In this case the wave affects the medium. Wave energy is absorbed and the material will change its nature. For example, the material may heat up if molecules are given more movement energy, or may change its composition and properties if complex molecules are damaged or destroyed.

The (almost self-evident) notion that energy must be absorbed to have any effect was first proposed by Grotthus in 1820 and so it is sometimes called Grotthus' law.

In real situations all three will happen together so that some radiation is transmitted, some is reflected and some absorbed. The amount of each depends on the wavelength or frequency of the radiation and the nature and positioning of the material. Often one aspect predominates. For example, light will be mainly transmitted through panes of window glass but it is evident that some of the light is reflected (if this were not so the glass would be invisible), also some is absorbed (so ultraviolet radiation is filtered-out). In the case of a shiny metal, surface reflection of visible radiation predominates.

Radiation entering a new material, a new medium, may also be bent at the surface – a process called refraction – and transmitted at some angle to the original line.

In non-homogeneous materials, both reflection and refraction may occur in the bulk of the material – a process called *scattering*. This has a strong influence on where the radiation is absorbed in the material.

Reflection, refraction, absorption, penetration and scattering are our next topics.

Reflection and transmission of radiation

When electromagnetic radiation passes through matter it interacts with the electric fields of the atoms and molecules and this determines their velocity in that particular material. Generally speaking, the more

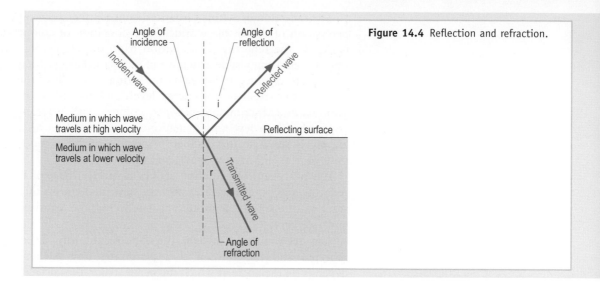

Figure 14.4 Reflection and refraction.

atoms and molecules are present, the slower the wave will travel. At the junction of two kinds of matter, the electromagnetic waves thus have to change velocity. The wave will not change in frequency so the wavelength must change.

For example, when electromagnetic radiation passes from air to glass, the wavelength is reduced. This is because the wave velocity is less in glass.

It is also true that if a wave strikes a boundary and is slowed, only part of the wave energy can be transmitted; the rest is turned back or reflected. When there is a change in the electrical nature of the medium through which the wave is travelling, some reflection is inevitable.

- *The amount* of reflection depends on the:
  - frequency of the radiation
  - angle of incidence
  - nature of the two media in contact.
- *The direction* of the reflected radiation depends on:
  - the angle of the incident radiation.
- *For a beam of radiation* impinging on a plane surface:
  - the angle of incidence is equal to the angle of reflection
  - the incident and reflected beam are in the same plane as the 'normal', a line perpendicular to the surface at the point of incidence (shown as a dashed line in Figure 14.4).

The last point states the two laws of reflection illustrated in Figure 14.4. They are well understood in connection with visible radiation, but are equally valid for other electromagnetic radiation, e.g. microwaves bouncing off a flat metal sheet in a microwave oven or, for that matter, any other wave system such as sonic waves, as described in chapter 9.

The wave equation:

$$v = f\lambda$$

tells us that if v is less and f is constant then λ the wavelength, must be less.

The reflection of visible radiation from matter is central to human perception of the visible world. The recognition of colour and form is due to the reflection of radiation from objects (except when the object is emitting visible radiation of its own). The eye focuses incoming light to produce an image on the retina. The cells of the retina are sensitive to extremely low energy levels and are able to detect a few photons and discriminate between colours with wavelength differences of only a few tens of nanometres. Thus the eyes provide an extremely sensitive and detailed perception of the outside world, but only over a very narrow wavelength range.

When a beam of radiation strikes a surface, part of the beam is reflected and part penetrates into the new medium; so there is a constant relationship – the more that is reflected, the less that penetrates and vice versa.

The relationship between the amount of any given radiation reflected and the amount that penetrates any particular surface depends on the angle at which the beam strikes the surface – the angle of incidence. The greater the angle of incidence, the greater the amount of wave energy reflected. Conversely, the smaller the angle of incidence, the less energy is reflected. If the angle of incidence is zero, the amount of wave energy reflected is least and the amount transmitted is greatest.

This has important implications for radiation striking a curved surface, such as an arm or leg or the trunk. Surfaces not at a right angle to the beam will reflect more radiation and so absorb less. Areas near the sides of a limb or the trunk will thus absorb much less energy. Areas where the surface is at right angles to the beam of radiation will receive the highest doses.

Penetration will diminish around the sides of a circular surface as the angle of incidence increases. To achieve more uniform irradiation it is necessary, at least, to apply radiation successively from two directions at about right angles to each other.

If the surface is elliptical in section, the angular changes between radiation and surface are small except at the very edge of the ellipse. Thus parallel beams applied to such surfaces give almost uniform penetration over much of the area. Since the trunk and some limb segments of the body are approximately ovoid in cross-section most of the body is more or less evenly irradiated in just two positions, i.e. lying prone and supine.

Energy spread – the cosine law

If a beam strikes a surface at right angles the area covered is the cross-sectional area of the beam but, if angled to the surface, the area covered increases so that the energy per unit area decreases.

The area increase can be easily demonstrated by shining a torch vertically down on to the floor and comparing the circle of light with the larger oval produced when the torch is shone at an angle (Figure

---

The lens in the eye refracts light, painting a picture of the outside world on the retina. The rod and cone cells of the retina fire-off signals (nerve impulses) to the brain where the pattern of pulses is reconstructed to produce the mental image.

The variation in the amount of reflection can be understood in terms of photons having a greater chance of penetrating if they meet the surface at right angles – as a dart is more likely to penetrate if it strikes the board at right angles and more likely to bounce off if it strikes a glancing blow.

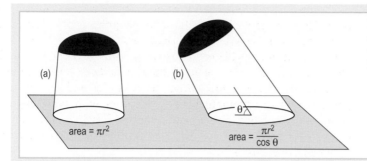

Figure 14.5 The cosine law: (a) a circular beam of radiation applied to a planar (flat) surface and (b) the same beam applied at an incident angle, θ.

14.5). When a beam of radiation strikes a boundary at an angle other than 90°, the intensity (energy per unit area) is less simply because the area of the incident beam is greater.

The *cosine law*, as it is called, relates the intensity of radiation falling on a surface to the cosine of the angle of incidence of the radiation. If the radiation is applied perpendicular to the surface the angle of incidence is 0°; the cosine of 0 is 1 and the area is a minimum, so the intensity (energy per unit area) is maximum (Figure 14.5a). If the radiation strikes at an angle θ which is not 90°, the area is greater so the intensity is less. At an angle of incidence of, say, 45°, cos 45° = 0.7, so the area is increased by 1/0.7. Hence the intensity is decreased by a factor of 0.7 and will be 70% of maximum. This has important implications clinically for users of ultraviolet and infrared radiation.

Summary

- Some reflection is inevitable if a wave strikes a boundary between two media with different electrical properties.
- The intensity of the transmitted radiation is greatest when the beam strikes at a right angle.
- When a beam of radiation strikes a surface at an angle, there is beam-spreading and the intensity (energy per unit area) is determined by the cosine law.

Refraction

When radiation meets a boundary with a medium in which it travels at a different velocity its velocity will be altered and it will be refracted or bent unless the radiation is perpendicular to the boundary (see Figure 14.4). The part of the wave front of any radiation entering a medium in which it travels more slowly will be delayed compared to the part of the wave front still in the high-velocity medium. This will cause the wave front to be turned through an angle which depends on its relative velocities in the two media.

Figure 14.6 Refraction at a boundary.

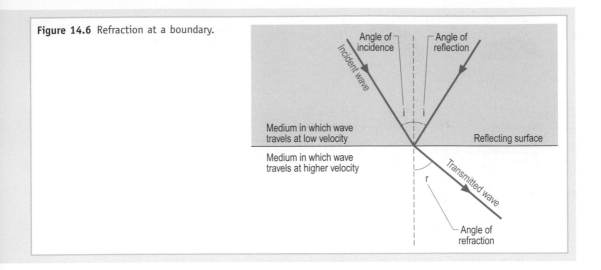

For more information on refraction, wave velocity and critical angle, see chapter 9 of the book 'Biophysical Bases of Electrotherapy' on the CD which comes with this book.

The relationship between the angle of incidence and the angle of refraction is given by the refraction equation:

$$\frac{\sin i}{\sin r} = \frac{v_1}{v_2}$$

where v_1 is the velocity of the incident wave and v_2 is the velocity of the transmitted wave.

The glass–air interface is used to bend visible radiation through lenses in all kinds of optical instruments, microscopes, magnifying lenses, cameras and so forth. The specialized transparent tissues forming the lens of the eye work in the same way. If a ray enters a medium in which it will travel more slowly, it is bent towards the normal as it enters (see Figure. 14.4). In this way, an image of the outside world is painted over the relatively small area of the retina.

If v_2 is bigger than v_1 (e.g. when light travels through glass into air), the refraction equation states that the angle of refraction will always be bigger than the angle of incidence (Figure 14.6). When this happens, there will be a 'critical angle' of incidence where the angle of refraction is 90°.

At the critical angle, the refracted wave travels parallel to the boundary. At any greater incident angle the radiation is completely reflected.

Reflection and refraction have been described largely in terms of visible radiation, but it must be understood that these are general principles which apply to all electromagnetic waves, albeit to different degrees with different frequency radiation and different media. For example, microwaves can easily be made to travel in tight beams which are reflected from metal surfaces, thus enabling the position of aircraft and ships to be monitored by radar and motorists to be 'booked' for speeding. Long radio waves can be reflected by the

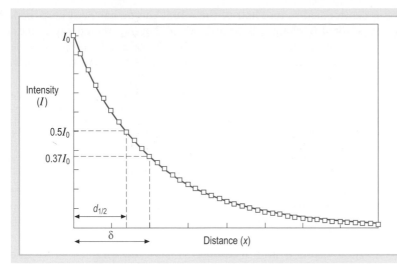

Figure 14.7 An exponential decrease in wave energy with distance.

ionized layer in the outer atmosphere (the ionosphere) and so can be beamed to parts of the world over the visible horizon. Visible light can be beamed through glass or plastic fibres, 'optical fibre', with negligible energy loss because of total internal reflection at the cylindrical wall of the fibre.

Absorption and penetration

The relationship between the amount of an electromagnetic radiation that is absorbed and the distance it penetrates any given material is of the greatest importance. Absorption is the reciprocal of penetration (i.e. the greater the penetration the less the absorption). For a homogeneous material the rate of absorption of wave energy is proportional to the energy present at that point. A consequence is that the amount of wave energy will fall exponentially with depth in the same way as sonic waves, described in chapter 9.

PENETRATION DEPTH

In order to describe the rate of absorption in a convenient way a single figure is used, either:

- the *penetration depth* – the depth at which 63% of the original radiation has been absorbed, or
- the *half-value depth* – the depth at which 50% has been absorbed.

This concept is illustrated in Figure 14.7. The half-value depth ($d_{1/2}$) is a simple and intuitive way of specifying the rate of absorption. At

For more information on penetration and exponential absorption, see chapter 9 of the book 'Biophysical Bases of Electrotherapy' on the CD which comes with this book.

a depth equal to $d_{1/2}$, half of the initial energy has been absorbed. As was noted in chapter 9, at a depth of $2 \times d_{1/2}$, the energy is reduced to half of one half or one quarter of the original energy. At a depth of $3 \times d_{1/2}$, the energy is reduced to half of one half of one half, or one eighth, of the original energy.

The 63% figure for the penetration depth (δ) comes about because the mathematical equation for an exponential decrease is:

$$I = I_o e^{-x/\delta}$$

where I_o is the initial intensity (at the surface), I is the intensity at a depth x and δ is a constant. The quantity δ is a number needed to describe the rate of decrease in energy with distance. When x, the distance penetrated, is equal to δ, the intensity is $I_o e^{-1}$ or $0.37 I_o$, meaning that 37% of the wave intensity remains so 63% must have been absorbed.

At a depth δ in a medium, 37% of the original wave energy remains. At a depth of $2 \times \delta$, the energy is reduced to 37% of 37% or about 14% of the original energy. At a depth of $3 \times \delta$, the energy is reduced to 37% of 37% of 37% or about 5% of the original energy.

Both $d_{1/2}$ and δ are thus different but equally valid measures of the rate of absorption of wave energy with distance. They are also valid measures of the penetration efficiency of the waves. The higher the value of $d_{1/2}$ or δ, the further the wave penetrates, i.e. the greater the energy remaining at depth and the less the rate of absorption.

Different frequencies/wavelengths of radiation have different penetration depths in any particular material, thus materials of a particular nature and thickness can be used as filters. This filtering effect is applied in many situations, e.g. filtering out the short ultraviolet (UVC) radiation but leaving the longer ultraviolet rays for some treatment or filtering out all the UVR but leaving visible radiation, as in protective ultraviolet goggles (see chapter 17).

The concepts of absorption and penetration depth are also important in considering the effect of radiation on the tissues. Some infrared and visible radiation has half-value depths of less than 1 mm while some microwaves have a half-value depth of several centimeters, so the physiological (and consequently the clinical) effects are quite different. It must, however, be emphasized that the tissues are not homogeneous so that absorption in the tissues is much more rapid and irregular than Figure 14.7 suggests. The rate of absorption with depth is greatly increased by the scattering of waves.

The penetration and absorption of the different modalities are considered in the relevant following chapters.

Scattering

Radiation passing through non-homogeneous matter may be partly scattered, i.e. the direction of some radiation is altered, effectively reducing the depth of penetration. The scattered radiation may travel in a different direction and be absorbed, over distance, in a direction away from the main beam. This is illustrated in Figure 14.8 where we envisage hard, reflective spheres in a transparent solid.

In this figure, we have assumed that waves hitting the spheres are completely reflected. This means that the wave energy is rapidly scattered in all directions. The result is a (rather dramatic) reduction in wave energy with depth, i.e. the effective penetration depth is reduced.

In biological tissues the reflecting surfaces are those of cells, fibres and tissue boundaries which are not completely reflective. Much energy is transmitted so the scattering effect and reduction in energy of the beam is not as pronounced as in Figure 14.8. Nonetheless, there is a more rapid decrease in wave energy with depth and the effective penetration depth is less than for a homogeneous medium with no reflecting surfaces.

The amount of scattering also depends on the wavelength of the radiation. Longer wavelengths are scattered less than shorter wavelengths. The reason is that waves are only reflected appreciably if their wavelengths are less than the size of the reflecting object. So if the waves in Figure 14.8 have short wavelengths, much energy will be reflected and so be scattered. If the wavelengths are longer than the spheres, a wave will simply span or 'ride-over' a sphere. The wave may push the sphere up or down, causing an oscillatory motion but it will not be reflected.

So, for example, ultraviolet radiation is scattered more than visible light and thus has a reduced penetration depth. Microwave radiation, with wavelengths much longer than cell or fibre dimensions, passes through tissues without being scattered.

Milk is white and translucent because it is a suspension of tiny fat droplets in water. The diameter of the droplets is much larger than light wavelengths so there is considerable scattering. A glucose solution is perfectly clear because glucose molecules are shorter than visible-light wavelengths so there is no scattering.

What, then, are the important conclusions for scattering of radiation which penetrates biological tissue? There are two:

- when radiation penetrates tissue, reflecting surfaces (e.g. of cells or fibres) will scatter the radiation, reducing the penetration depth
- shorter wavelength (higher frequency) radiation is scattered more than longer wavelength (lower frequency) radiation.

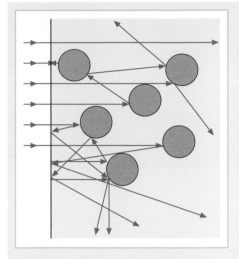

Figure 14.8 Scattering of radiation by reflecting surfaces in a medium.

The magnifying power of the light microscope is limited because objects smaller than the light wavelength do not reflect light and so cannot be seen.

Summary

Electromagnetic radiation interacts with matter by being:

- reflected – turned back from a surface with the angle of reflection being equal to the angle of incidence
- transmitted (penetrate) – with the line of travel of radiation altered at the junction of different materials (refraction)

- scattered – direction of radiation in material altered by numerous reflections (and refractions)
- absorbed – energy of the radiation is used or converted to some other form of energy (e.g. heat).

Further reading

Low, J., Reed, A. (1997). Physical Principles Explained. Oxford: Butterworth-Heinemann. (On the CD accompanying this text).

Ward, A. (2004). Biophysical bases of electrotherapy. Mount Waverley: Excell Biomedical Publications. (On the CD accompanying this text).

Microwave diathermy

With shorter wavelengths than the familiar radio waves but longer than infrared radiation, microwaves are, perhaps, one of the least well-recognized groups of electromagnetic waves. Figure 14.2 shows that they are sited between 1 m wavelength (300 MHz) and 1 cm wavelength (30 GHz), or as short as 1 mm (300 GHz). This unfamiliarity, coupled with their much increased commercial usage, has possibly engendered rather more frequent suspicions about their safety than seems justified by the evidence.

The nature and production of microwave radiation for therapeutic purposes are addressed briefly at the beginning of this chapter.

The interactions and effects of microwave radiation in the tissues are then considered, with the patterns of heating which may be expected. Comment is made on the therapeutic uses followed by the principles of application and dosage. Finally, some potential dangers are noted.

The microwave frequencies allotted for medical use are given in Table 15.1. The 2450 MHz frequency is the most widely available but is, perhaps, not the most satisfactory to achieve therapeutic muscle heating, for reasons considered below. In Europe, Australia and New Zealand, the three frequencies listed in Table 15.1 are approved for medical use; in the USA only the top two frequencies are approved.

The heating effect of microwaves is well known with microwave ovens (which also operate at a frequency of 2450 MHz). Microwaves are also used in telecommunications (including mobile phones) and in radar for tracking ships, aircraft, rockets and satellites.

The wavelengths shown in Table 15.1 are for microwaves in air (or a vacuum). In biological tissues, the wavelengths are reduced quite appreciably.

Microwave radiation behaves like other electromagnetic radiation, described in chapter 14, in that it is reflected and refracted at interfaces and will be absorbed or penetrate material to varying degrees depending on the nature of the materials and the microwave frequency. It can also be beamed, like a searchlight, a necessary feature for its use as radar.

Microwaves are particularly useful in therapy as they are more rapidly absorbed in tissues with a high water and ion content, such

Biological tissue slows electromagnetic radiation. The velocity, v, is reduced and the frequency, f, remains the same. The wave equation:

$$v = f\lambda$$

indicates that the wavelength, λ, must be reduced.

as muscle and less rapidly absorbed in fatty tissue and bone. This makes it an effective method of deep tissue heating, especially for muscle underlying fat.

PRODUCTION OF MICROWAVES

A high-frequency alternating current flowing through a wire (an antenna) will produce electromagnetic radiation. Radio and television transmissions work this way. At higher (microwave) frequencies, normal electronic circuits cannot produce sufficient amounts of current to energize an antenna and produce large amounts of electromagnetic radiation. At microwave frequencies a device called a magnetron is used which generates alternating current at a high power level which is fed to the antenna which radiates microwaves. The antenna, which is simply a suitable-sized and shaped piece of wire, is mounted in front of a metal reflector (like a car headlamp) so that a beam of microwaves is emitted (Figure 15.1).

The output of microwave energy can be controlled by varying the power supplied to the magnetron. Machines have an intensity control and the output is indicated on a meter which, of course, gives no reliable indication of the heating of the tissues. The frequency of the microwaves produced depends on the construction of the magnetron and is therefore fixed. There will also be a means of switching the mains power on and off and suitable indicator lights. On some machines a delay switch may be fitted to allow time for the magnetron to reach its proper working temperature.

Computers operate at GHz (microwave) frequencies but the power levels are low and the amount of associated microwave radiation is small.

Table 15.1 Frequency and wavelength of microwaves used in medicine	
Frequency (MHz)	Wavelength (cm)
2450	12.2
915	32.8
434	69.1

Figure 15.1 Production of microwaves: block diagram of a microwave diathermy generator.

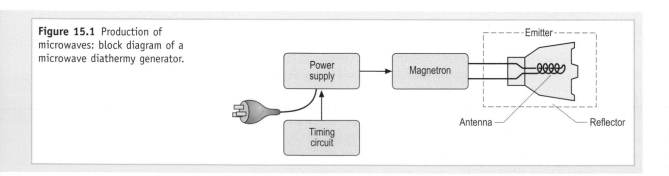

A standby switch may be provided. Thus successive treatments may be given or adjustment of the emitter made without having to switch off the magnetron and wait for it to warm up again. The emitter gives out a beam of microwaves which diverges somewhat because it is technically difficult to produce a completely uniform beam (Ward, 2004; chapter 11). The effect of this divergence is to reduce the intensity of radiation considerably with distance (see the inverse square law, chapter 14; Guy, 1982).

Microwave therapy can be in either continuous or pulsed mode.

THE PHYSIOLOGICAL EFFECTS OF MICROWAVES ON THE TISSUES

When the electromagnetic energy of microwave radiation is absorbed in the tissues it provokes ionic movement, rotation of dipoles and electron orbit distortion. The effects are similar to those described in chapter 13 for shortwave diathermy. A consequence is tissue heating. The amount of heating will be proportional to the amount of absorbed radiation.

The high-frequency alternating electric field which is part of an electromagnetic wave has a similar effect to the (lower frequency) fields produced with shortwave diathermy.

Since microwaves are strongly absorbed by tissues of high water and ion content, it would be expected that heating would be greatest in muscle and other tissues with a high water and ion content and less in fatty tissue and bone, which have a lower water and ion content. In each tissue layer, heating would be greatest at the surface and diminish exponentially with depth (see Figure 14.7). While this is a useful simple generalization it is too simplistic as it ignores reflection, which has some important consequences.

The pattern of microwave absorption in the tissues

In chapter 14 it was noted that when any radiation meets the surface of a different medium it may either be reflected or penetrate. Radiation that does penetrate will only have an effect if it is absorbed; thus it will be ineffective if it passes right through. In the case of microwaves there is little risk of it passing right through as the penetration depth is quite small (Ward, 2004; chapter 9). There is, however, considerable reflection at the air–skin boundary and at skin–fat, fat–muscle and muscle–bone boundaries and this has a major impact on the pattern of heat production in the tissues.

At 2450 MHz, the percentage of microwave radiation reflected varies with thickness of fat and skin from 50 to 75% (Scowcroft et al., 1977). Tissue thickness makes a great difference at this frequency. Some radiation that is reflected from the fat–skin interface and other interfaces in the tissues can be radiated out of the body. At the other lower frequencies in therapeutic use some 60–70% of the energy is reflected but it is much less affected by variations in skin tissue thickness (Ward, 2004; chapter 11).

While the generalizations described above are valid, it must be emphasized that the tissues are very irregular and microwave absorption is influenced by other factors, such as the thickness of the particular tissue layer. Consequently, absorption patterns cannot be predicted with certainty. Furthermore, the heating in the tissues depends not only on microwave absorption but also on the rate of heat transfer within and between the tissues.

Effect of emitter shape

The distribution of energy over the body surface will depend on the size and shape of the emitter. Circular emitters usually give a somewhat ring-shaped pattern (but if close it may be more or less circular). Other emitters are available which are rather longer in one direction and give an oval pattern; still other emitters of apparently similar shape may give the greatest output at the central axis, diminishing outwards. This is often the situation in practice since many body areas are convex so that the centre of the area is nearest to the emitter. Some emitters are designed to focus the radiation into the tissues and thus achieve a better depth of heating. Alternatively, special sandbags can be used with some distance emitters effectively to increase the intensity by preventing the microwave radiation diverging so far. All the emitters described so far are distance emitters, i.e. they are applied to the tissues with an air gap. It is also possible to have contact emitters.

> Manufacturers normally supply information describing the distribution of energy produced by their particular microwave emitters.

Contact emitters

Microwaves are markedly reflected from skin and in chapters 9 and 14 it was explained that reflection depends on the different impedances encountered when waves, whether sonic or electromagnetic, pass from one medium to another. To achieve better transmission to skin and to enable the emitter to be made much smaller a suitable ceramic dielectric material is used. This enables a better match to be made between the applicator and the tissues and, as the emitter is in contact with the skin the amount of scattered radiation is also reduced.

Contact emitters can be quite small, 1.5 or 3.5 cm diameter, and will radiate microwaves directly into the tissues away from the surface of the emitter. Other small emitters can be placed in body cavities – rectum, vagina and external auditory meatus – emitting radially to heat the walls of the cavity.

As microwave transmission is better with contact emitters and the radiating area is smaller, the power that can be applied may be limited to a low level (25 W). Alternatively, if the skin is water or air cooled a higher output can be applied and the risk of burning the skin and superficial tissues is decreased. This method is considered by some to

> It is important to remember that if the thermal receptors in the skin are deliberately cooled there is the risk of a deep burn so caution is required when using a cooled contact emitter.

be an efficient way of generating even heating in the deep tissues and a higher power, up to 100 W output, can be used.

Heating effect

The heating effects from microwaves, even at 2450 MHz can be considerable. Clinical levels of 2450 MHz frequency microwaves will, within 15 minutes of applying it to a normal human forearm, increase the local skin temperature by approximately 10°C and the blood flow by 250% (McMeeken, 1994). The increased flow lasts for up to 20 minutes after the machine has been turned off (McMeeken and Bell, 1990). The researchers attributed this prolonged effect to a local increase in metabolic rate in the heated tissues and commented that microwave was particularly effective in heating deep muscle and increasing the blood flow to both the hand and forearm. Heating the hand did not produce changes in forearm blood flow but did increase finger flow by approximately 200% and also increased the finger skin temperature.

A comparison of the effects on blood flow produced by hot packs and microwaves (2450 MHz) applied to the hindlegs of anaesthetized dogs showed that microwave was much more effective at increasing tissue temperature at a depth of 2 cm (McMeeken, 1994). The machine had an output of 40 W, the emitter was placed 3 cm from the skin and turned on for 10 minutes. For a comparable rise in tissue temperature the hot packs needed to have increased the skin temperature by double that required for microwave. Also, at the same tissue depth, microwave produced nearly twice the increase in blood flow. This indicates that microwave, even at 2450 MHz can be a very effective method of increasing local blood flow, a change that does not stop immediately the heat is turned off.

Another way of evaluating the effectiveness of heating with microwave is to compare the changes in blood flow it produces with that following voluntary muscle activity in humans. Fifteen squeezes of a hand dynamometer produced forearm blood flow increases from 6.0 ml/100 g/minute at rest to 16.3 ml/100 g/minute (McMeeken and Bell, 1990). By contrast, microwave increased the flow rate to 44.9 ml/100 g/minute. This change was greater in females than males but in both it was more effective than an active exercise, gripping.

Summary

- Much radiation is reflected from the skin
- The theoretical absorption pattern indicates absorption in skin, fat, muscle (especially at interfaces) and very little in bone
- Refraction in the tissues could influence the degree and depth of absorption

- The widely used 2450 MHz has a less satisfactory absorption pattern for therapeutic purposes than lower frequencies
- The shape and size of the emitter influences the energy distribution onto the tissues
- Higher levels of transmission to the skin can be achieved with contact emitters
- Generally, microwave heating occurs in the first few centimetres of tissue traversed, especially in muscle
- Microwave heating at 2450 MHz increases blood flow much more effectively than local muscle activity or hot packs.

THERAPEUTIC USES

The indications are those of heating. The therapeutic effects of heat were considered in chapter 10, with further discussion on low-energy heating due to pulsed applications of energy in chapter 13.

Like shortwave, some debate surrounds the issue of whether there are any specific therapeutic effects due to microwave. There is no clear supporting evidence of any effect except heat. Microwaves can be pulsed and the effects are claimed to be those of pulsed shortwave (see chapter 13). Again, there is little supporting evidence for this.

Microwave is suitable for deep tissue heating, both muscle and other soft tissue with a high water and ion content. Articular structures close to the surface, such as the wrist joint or anterior aspect of the knee, might also be heated effectively, but it is not likely to affect deeply placed structures covered with muscle tissue like the hip joint. Perhaps it should be emphasized that heating patterns are highly irregular and probably vary considerably along with the individual's distribution of fat and muscle.

Consistent with the earlier comments regarding the unpopularity of microwave for clinical treatments following injury, there are relatively few studies evaluating its effectiveness. One that did (Giombini et al., 2001) found 434 MHz frequency microwave was more effective than 1 MHz frequency ultrasound for treatment 72 hours after a muscle injury. Giombini et al. (2001) reported a randomized controlled trial with 40 subjects which used, as outcome measures, pain and haematoma size. Pain was recorded using a visual analogue scale, and haematoma size was determined by ultrasonographic scanning. Baseline measures appear similar for both groups. Each patient was treated three times a week for 3 weeks, with 15 minutes ultrasound per treatment (continuous, $1.5 \, W \, cm^{-2}$) or with 30 minutes of 434 MHz microwave with a water cooled contact emitter (maximum temperature, 30 to 42°C). One difference was possibly the volume of tissue affected by heating. With ultrasound it would have been smaller, assuming a $5 \, cm^2$ applicator, than the effective field size of $96 \, cm^2$ of

A comparison might be made with ultrasound (see chapter 9) which has similar penetration to microwave but is usually applied with a continuously moving treatment head which evens out the distribution of energy in the tissues.

A clinical trial by Weinberger et al. (1989), using 915 MHz microwave, found that pain from articular effusions reduced and walking time increased following exposure.

the microwave unit. Given the average size of haematoma was approximately 3 to $4\,cm^2$, this alone is unlikely to explain the outcomes. More research is necessary to identify the most effective dosages and the range of conditions for which different frequencies of microwave might be clinically effective.

Similar results were obtained by the same group when treating 44 patients with a patella or Achilles tendinopathy with 434 MHz frequency microwave or 3.2 MHz frequency ultrasound (Giombini et al., 2002). Subjects were randomly assigned to one or other treatment group and the assessor was blinded to their group assignment. Each subject had a tendinosis for 6 to 72 weeks, confirmed clinically by pain and palpation. Those treated with microwaves had better clinical outcomes (reduced pain on palpation and contraction) suggesting that 434 MHz microwave is preferable to ultrasound for treating some musculoskeletal conditions. However, except for age, the initial statistical homogeneity of subject groups is not specified.

Both studies by Giombini et al. highlight the need for more clinical research on similar musculoskeletal problems by other researchers, using both 434 MHz and other frequencies of microwave to establish when it is most effective and dosage guidelines, including treatment duration and frequency.

The effectiveness of 434 MHz for treating deeper tissue is likely to be greater than 2450 MHz frequency microwave. Despite the more limited depth of heating using 2450 MHz microwave, one case report identified clinically significant changes in pain in a patient treated with microwave for her primary dysmenorrhoea (Vance et al., 1996). A range of conventional treatments over the preceding 13 years made little difference to the patient's monthly pain. Her pain reduced considerably after a series of applications of 2450 MHz frequency microwave applied with an emitter over her abdomen on days in which she had severe pain. Replications of this procedure are clearly desirable.

Another use of microwaves in the clinical context is to produce hyperthermia selectively to ablate tissue. This requires purpose designed microwave eqiupment to destroy tumours and selected tissue, such as the endometrium following excessive bleeding. These uses and the equipment, techniques used and outcomes will not be discussed in the present chapter where the focus is on lesser levels of heating and on using microwave heating to promote healing and tissue repair.

Method of application

The following stages apply to most forms of microwave treatment.

Stages

Patient

Explanation: describe the nature of the treatment to the patient, perhaps including how the microwave energy is dissipated in the body so that only a small temperature rise will occur, unlike the situation of a microwave oven in which the temperature can be made to rise to cooking levels because the heat and reflected microwaves cannot escape.

Examination: test the thermal sensitivity of the skin to which the microwaves are to be applied; inspect the skin for evidence of any inflammatory skin conditions as they should be avoided.

Protection: give the patient a pair of microwave goggles (see below) if radiation could enter the eye.

Apparatus

The choice of emitter is dictated by the size of tissue area to be treated. The power should be switched on and the machine given time to warm up, if necessary (consult the manufacturer's instructions).

Preparation of part

Position the patient so the part to be treated is comfortably supported and sufficiently exposed. Microwave should not be applied through clothing or where there is metal in the field. Use wooden furniture and take care that the emitter (treatment head) does not irradiate any large metal surfaces that could reflect the beam.

Setting up

Position the emitter so that the radiation strikes the surface at right angles, bearing in mind that as distance emitters have diverging beams, only the axial radiation will be strictly at right angles, while the peripheral radiation will strike at small incident angles. While this may not make much difference (see cosine law, chapter 14) when the emitter is 'square on', slight angling of the emitter increases the already considerable reflection from the skin surface, making the treatment ineffective.

Instructions and warnings

Describe the degree of heating required to the patient, as for short-wave (see chapter 13). Similarly, most information about the intensity and site of heating in the tissues is derived from reports from the patient of their sensations. The meter only indicates the output of the machine so it is essential to have the patient's full cooperation and they must have accurate cutaneous thermal sensations. He or she must also be warned to call the therapist immediately if the heating becomes more than a comfortable warmth or if discomfort or pain is felt, and to remain still throughout the application.

Application

Switch the microwave output on for the predetermined length of time.

Practical point

The distance between the emitter and the skin determines both the area treated and the intensity because of the diverging beam. Thus, if a small area is to be treated the emitter should be placed close to the skin, say 2–5 cm, and the appropriate heating regulated with the intensity control on the machine. If larger areas are to be heated, increase the spacing to 10 or 15 cm and increase the intensity to ensure sufficient heating. Distances of about 4 cm are commonly used for most treatments.

Termination

After switching off and removing the apparatus, the treated area is examined and the skin surface temperature and presence of any erythema are noted and recorded.

DOSAGE

Treatment is usually applied for 15 to 20 minutes to provide sufficient time for the vascular adjustments to stabilize. Deeper tissues will take longer to heat than more superficial and for that reason some users apply microwave for up to 30 minutes.

The intensity applied is regulated according to the patient's reports of the level of heating they are experiencing. It seems to take an absorbed dose of some $200 \, mW \, cm^{-2}$ to give detectable heating (Knauf, 1968). What matters is the rate of energy that is absorbed per unit of tissue mass in both microwave and shortwave heating. This can be quantified as the specific absorption rate (SAR) in $W \, kg^{-1}$. SARs of $50–170 \, W \, kg^{-1}$ are used therapeutically, the upper limit being close to the tolerable maximum (Kloth, 1986).

POTENTIAL DANGERS

Microwave absorption leads to heating and if the heating is excessive it can cause a burn. Investigation of microwave burns in living tissue, in piglets, showed a characteristic pattern called 'layered tissue sparing' in which the skin and muscle tissues were burned but the intervening subcutaneous fat was relatively spared (Surrell et al., 1987). This is consistent with the pattern of microwave heating described earlier and with what would be expected.

Some points need to be considered specifically in connection with microwaves. The first two are that the patient must have accurate thermal sensation and they must be able to communicate effectively. Other issues are raised below.

Effects of metal

Microwaves are strongly reflected from metal surfaces. This means any metal between the target tissues and the microwave emitter will shield the underlying tissues from the radiation. Metal may also distort and concentrate a microwave field and cause local overheating, which can be dangerous. For example, metal embedded in the tissues, either by accident or surgically, might reflect microwave energy back into the tissues and cause a local concentration and overheating. As there are no heat receptors in the deep tissues the patient

If, for example, the hand is rested on a metal surface and microwave radiation applied to the other surface some will pass through the hand and be reflected by the metal back into it again. With normal sensory awareness there is no reason why this should lead to burning but users need to be aware of this effect.

will only be aware of deeper damage if pain occurs subsequently, after the damage has occurred. No reports of this have been identified and it is most probable only with superficially placed metal. Despite this, it is generally advisable to avoid treating with microwaves in the region of metal implants.

Note that the reason for avoiding metal in or near the area being treated by microwaves is rather different from that when using short-wave (chapter 13).

Effects of changed blood flow

If there is a reduction in the normal level of perfusion to an area, treating with microwaves can be a serious risk. Unless a sufficient increase in local blood flow is possible, enough to dissipate the heat, there is a serious risk of local tissue damage and burns. A reduced local perfusion might occur with arterial disease and emboli (high risk) or damage to the autonomic nerve supply (high risk).

Following an acute tissue bleed, such as after muscle damage, applying local heat may cause bleeding to recommence.

Heating any collections of fluid, such as an acute haematoma, a tense haemarthrosis, bursitis or joint effusion, may cause considerable pain. This is especially important with microwave treatment due to the high rate of absorption and restricted heat dissipation.

Applying heat to an area with an acute inflammation increases the risk of causing local tissue damage. The extent of any damage will depend on the extent of inflammation and the capacity of the local circulation to limit the temperature increase due to externally applied microwave heating.

Effects of surface moisture

Perspiration must be allowed to evaporate freely. If moisture appears on the surface from any source, e.g. open wounds or wet dressings, it will absorb radiation, so treatment should be stopped and the moisture removed.

Implanted electronic equipment

Direct applications of microwaves to implanted electronic equipment, such as pacemakers, should be avoided as the equipment might malfunction. However, there is little, if any, risk from scattered radiation.

The eyes

Avoid exposing the eyes directly to microwave radiation. Microwaves are reflected from the curved, bony orbit and focused in the eye. Its structure, a water-filled sphere, also ensures the eye will selectively absorb microwaves and, since it cannot easily dissipate heat, it can become overheated. Although cataracts have been produced in laboratory animals with high doses of microwaves there is no evidence that they have been caused in humans (Lehmann and de Lateur, 1982). If radiation may enter an eye during a treatment, when treating the anterior aspect of the shoulder with a distance emitter for example, the patient should be given goggles which are impervious to microwaves. Such goggles are of two kinds – either a metal mesh which reflects practically all microwave radiation but allows sufficient light between the mesh to see clearly, or a thin layer of metal supported on glass which again reflects microwave radiation but interferes little with visible light. Closing the eyes would diminish but not prevent the transmission of microwaves.

It is important that microwave goggles are not confused with ultraviolet or laser goggles. In a busy clinic some may look similar but their functions are very different.

The testes

Quite small temperature rises can interfere with spermatogenesis in mammals, which is why the testes are located outside the abdominal cavity. There is, however, no evidence that mild heating has any damaging effect, although marked heating can cause damage, albeit reversible. It is suggested that heating of $100\,\mathrm{mW\,cm^{-2}}$ could possibly produce testicular damage in humans (Watson, 1971); therefore direct irradiation of the testes should be avoided and care taken to prevent large amounts of reflected or scattered radiation reaching the region.

The testes are more susceptible than the ovaries because of their exposed position and possibly their structure. Ovaries are deeply placed and therefore unlikely to be heated by microwave treatment.

Pregnancy

Pregnancy is an accepted contraindication to the use of microwaves over the uterus. However, especially early in pregnancy, the risk is possibly considerably lower than with shortwave given the depth in the pelvis of the uterus and the lower specific absorption rate of microwave, especially with a frequency of 2450 MHz (Hocking and Joyner, 1995). Despite this, treating pregnancy as a contraindication is always advisable given the implications of an adverse outcome.

Other local pathologies

Heat treatments are not advised following radiotherapy for two reasons: the reduced capacity of the skin to manage an increased local temperature, and a possible effect of local heating on any remaining malignant cells.

It is worth noting that a recent study (Lönn et al., 2004) found an increased risk of acoustic neuroma in individuals using a mobile phone for 10 or more years. This indicates the need for further long-term studies of this kind.

due to microwave exposure, there was still no sound evidence of any harmful effects (Sienkiewicz and Kowalczuk, 2005). The effects identified were associated with mild heating of superficial tissues close to the handset. A subequent review by the NRPB (National Radiation Protection Board, 2004b) came to a similar conclusion.

References

Australian Radiation Protection and Nuclear Safety Agency. (2002). Maximum exposure levels to radiofrequency fields 3 kHz to 300 GHz. Radiation protection series #3. Australia, ARPNSA.

Brown, B., Johnson, S. (1975). Microwave diathermy (treatment note). Physiotherapy, **61**, 117.

Giombini, A., Casciello, G., Di Cesare, M. et al. (2001). A controlled study on the effects of hyperthermia at 434 MHz and conventional ultrasound upon muscle injuries in sport. J Sports Med Phys Fitness, **41**, 521–527.

Giombini, A., Dei Cesare, A., Sorrenti, D. et al. (2002). Hyperthermia at 434 MHz in the treatment of overuse sport tendinopathies: A randomised controlled clinical trial. Int J Sports Med, **23**, 207–211.

Guy, A. (1982). Biophysics of high frequency currents and electromagnetic radiation. In J. Lehmann (ed.), Therapeutic Heat and Cold, pp. 199–277. Baltimore: Williams & Wilkins.

Health Equipment Information (1980). No. 188, September. London: DHSS.

Hocking, B., Joyner, K. (1995). Re: Miscarriages among female physical therapists who report using radio- and microwave-frequency electromagnetic radiation [Letter]. Am J Epidemiol, **141**, 273–274.

ICNIRP (1998). Guidelines for limiting exposure to time-varying electric, magnetic and electromagnetic fields (up to 300 GHz). Health Phys, **74**, 494–522.

IEGMP (2000). Mobile phones and health. Report of an independent expert group on mobile phones (Chairman: Sir William Stewart). Chilton, NRPB. Available at http://www.legmp.org.uk/report/index.htm.

Kloth, L. (1986). Shortwave and microwave diathermy. In S. Michlovitz (ed.), Thermal Agents in Rehabilitation. Philadelphia: Davis.

Knauf, G. (1968). Biological effects of microwave radiations. Arch Ind Hlth, **17**, 48.

Lehmann, J., de Lateur, B. (1982). Therapeutic heat. In J. Lehmann (ed.), Therapeutic Heat and Cold, pp. 404–562. Baltimore: Williams & Wilkins.

Lönn, S., Ahlborn, A., Hall, P., Feychting, M. (2004). Mobile phone use and the risk of acoustic neuroma. Epidemiology, **15**, 653–659.

Matsche, D. (2004) The ICNRPB Guidelines: Risk assessment built on a house of cards. Paper presented at the Radiation Research Trust scientific meeting, Liverpool, September 24.

McMeeken, J. (1994). Tissue temperature and blood flow: a research based overview of electrophysical modalities. Aust J Physiother, **40**, 49–57.

McMeeken, J., Bell, C. (1990). Microwave irradiation of the human forearm and hand. Physiother Theory Pract, **6**, 171–177.

National Radiological Protection Board (NRPB, UK). (2004a). Advice on limiting the exposure to electromagnetic fields (0–300 GHz). Documents of the NRPB, Vol 15, #2.

National Radiological Protection Board (NRPB, UK). (2004b). Mobile phones and health 2004: report of the NRPB. Documents of the NRPB, Vol 15, #5.

Scowcroft, A., Mason, A., Hayne, C. (1977). Safety with microwave diathermy: preliminary report of the CSP working party. Physiotherapy, **63**, 359–361.

Sienkiewicz, Z., Kowalczuk, C. (2005) A summary of recent reports on mobile phones and health. publication NRPB-W65. Chilton, NRPB.

Surrell, J., Alexander, R., Cohle, S. et al. (1987). Effects of microwave radiation on living tissues. J Trauma, **27**, 935–939.

Vance, A., Hayes, S., Spielholz, N. (1996). Microwave diathermy treatment for primary dysmenorrhea. Phys Ther, **76**, 1003–1008.

Ward, A. (2004). Biophysical Bases of Electrotherapy. Mt Waverley, Vic, Australia: Excell Biomedical Publications. [On the CD which comes with this book]

Watson, P. (1971). Microwaves – their effects and safe use. N Z J Physiother, **4**, 20–24.

Weinberger, A., Fadilah, R., Lev, A. et al. (1989). Treatment of articular effusions with local deep microwave hyperthermia. Clin Rheumatol, **8**, 461–466.

Infrared and visible radiation

Of all forms of electromagnetic radiation, perhaps the two most 'natural' kinds from a human perspective are visible and infrared radiation. Infrared radiation is constantly emitted and absorbed by any warm object including the human body. Sensory receptors detect infrared through its heating effect. Light reflected or emitted by objects enables us to construct an exquisitely detailed view of our surroundings. Thus both forms of radiation produce sensory stimulation, albeit of a different kind.

Both visible and infrared radiation are used therapeutically, but only the shorter infrared wavelengths (near infrared, having relatively small wavelengths). Traditionally, infrared lamps and light bulbs have been used as the energy source. More recently, lasers have been introduced as a source of infrared or visible radiation.

In this chapter, the nature and definition of infrared (IR) and visible radiation is described, also the way the radiation is produced for therapy. Discussion of the absorption and penetration of IR and visible radiation in the tissues follows.

The physiological effects and therapeutic uses of these radiations are then described and considered. This is followed by the therapeutic application and dangers.

INTRODUCTION

Visible light is electromagnetic radiation with wavelengths between 400 and 760 nm. The spectrum can be described scientifically as a range of wavelengths or subjectively as a range of colours. Infrared radiation has no colour: its wavelengths are longer than that of visible red light and it is only detected via a feeling of warmth. Infrared extends to the microwave region, i.e. from 760 nm to 1 mm (Harlen, 1982). Other authorities suggest that the longer radiation only extend to wavelengths of 0.1 or 0.4 mm, but the distinction is of questionable importance.

Infrared radiation is subdivided into three regions or bands, A, B and C (Harlen, 1982). They are approximately distinguished by their absorption characteristics. A and B are utilized therapeutically and

Lasers used therapeutically produce visible or infrared radiation. They are thought by some to have special effects which depend on the unique properties of laser radiation. Lasers are therefore discussed separately, towards the end of this chapter.

Table 16.1 Classification of infrared radiation

Type	Wavelength
IRA	760–1400 nm
IRB	1400–3000 nm
IRC	3000 nm–1 mm (not used in therapy)
Former classification:	
near or short IR	760–1500 nm
far or long IR	1500–15 000 nm

correspond roughly to an older classification of 'near' and 'far' infrared (Table 16.1). A is near or short wavelength radiation and B is at the short end of the far infrared.

Infrared radiation is produced in all matter by various kinds of molecular vibration. When atoms within a molecule vibrate and move further apart or closer together without breaking free from one another, the charges within the molecules are accelerated and infrared radiation is emitted. Any given molecule is already in a state of vibration and rotation and so emits its own IR 'fingerprint' of radiation across a range of frequencies. This can be altered by absorbing heat which leads to an increase in the vibration frequencies of the molecules and a corresponding increase in the frequency of emitted radiation.

The result is that any heated object emits infrared radiation and the hotter the object, the higher is the frequency (and shorter the wavelength) of the emitted radiation. Although the radiation will comprise a whole range of different frequencies, the frequency at which the maximum intensity of radiation is emitted is proportional to temperature. The higher the temperature the higher the frequency and hence the shorter the wavelength. At the higher temperatures generated by a tungsten filament light bulb the peak emission is about 960 nm, i.e. in the near infrared, with plenty of emission in the visible region (see Figure 16.6). The human body also emits a whole range of infrared radiation, mainly type C, with a peak around 10 000 nm. Absorption of infrared radiation causes similar kinds of molecular vibrations regardless of the wavelength.

Shorter wavelength visible electromagnetic radiation causes molecular and atomic motion and can also break chemical bonds when absorbed. Our sight, for example, is dependent on a visible light-induced chemical change. Visible radiation splits the pigment molecules (rhodopsins) embedded in the membranes of retinal cells. The splitting changes the membrane potential and triggers an action potential which travels via the optic nerve to the central nervous system. This response, together with the input from many other retinal cells, produces the detailed and informative sensation we call sight. Unlike the heat induced by infrared, visible light produces relatively little or no heat.

As noted in chapter 14, the visible part of the spectrum is a narrow region separating radiation which can only produce heat (IR) and radiation which is sufficiently energetic to damage molecules by breaking them (ultraviolet and higher frequencies). Visible light is considered safe, providing the power levels are low enough not to pose a hazard through heating. By contrast, ultraviolet and higher frequency radiation are classified as hazardous as they can produce irreversible molecular damage at any power level. This is because at ultraviolet and higher frequencies the smallest 'package' of energy, one photon, has sufficient punch to break indiscriminately the bonds between atoms.

Summary

Infrared radiation:

- is emitted from any heated body
- is divided into long and short wavelengths for therapeutic purposes
- produces heat when absorbed.

Visible radiation:

- produces generally non-damaging chemical changes as well as heat when absorbed.
- can stimulate beneficial physiological effects.

PRODUCTION OF INFRARED

Heated materials produce infrared radiation, the wavelength being determined by the temperature. Higher temperatures are associated with shorter wavelength and higher frequency radiation. If short infrared is to be produced efficiently the material must not be oxidized (burnt) by the higher temperatures used. The most convenient method is to heat a resistance wire by passing an electric current through it. An ordinary household electric heater can be made of a coil of suitable resistance wire, such as nickel-chromium alloy, wound on a ceramic insulator.

Various kinds of infrared lamps are used for therapy. They are classified as either luminous or non-luminous generators.

Non-luminous generators

One type is constructed in a similar way to an ordinary household electric heater: the infrared source is a coil of wire wrapped around a cylindrical ceramic insulator. In these heaters the wire glows red thus giving some radiation in the visible region but peak emission is in the

Nickel-chromium alloy has a relatively high resistance for a metal. Consequently when current flows, the electrical energy is rapidly converted to heat energy. It also resists the oxidation which often results if metals are heated in air.

short infrared range. The ceramic material, being heated to a lower temperature than the wire, gives mainly infrared and little visible radiation. Some infrared lamps for therapy have the wire embedded in the insulating ceramic (or porcelain or fireclay) so that little or no visible radiation is emitted.

The heater wire can also be mounted behind a metal plate or inside a metal tube which does not become red hot but emits infrared in the same way. As such a lamp becomes hotter, all the parts – the emitter, the metal plate on the end of the emitter, the protective wire mesh and the reflector – are heated, giving off a range of wavelengths from near to far infrared.

The infrared emitter is placed at the focus of a reflector to produce an approximately uniform beam (Figure 16.1). However, the emitter is large compared to the size of the reflector and this means that not all parts of the emitter are located at the focus. Consequently, parts of the beam will converge and hot spots will be produced if the reflector is parabolic in shape. If the reflector shape is more spherical, beam convergence is avoided but the penalty is beam divergence. This is the compromise that is usually adopted clinically.

The reflector and emitter are mounted on a mobile metal stand which can be adjusted to alter the height and angle of the reflector/emitter. When such lamps are switched on they require time to warm up because of the thermal inertia of the mass of metal and insulating material that has to be heated; thus small lamps may take about 5 minutes but larger ones may take up to 15 minutes to reach maximum emission (Forster and Palastanga, 1985).

Although lamps with an exposed coil give off a red glow they are collectively designated as 'non-luminous' sources to distinguish them from those that emit strong visible radiation; these are called 'luminous' lamps.

For more information on beam shape and 'hot-spots' see chapter 11 of the book 'Biophysical Bases of Electrotherapy' on the CD which comes with this book.

Practical point

Because of thermal inertia, switch this type of lamp on for a sufficient time (at least 5 minutes) before it is needed for treatment.

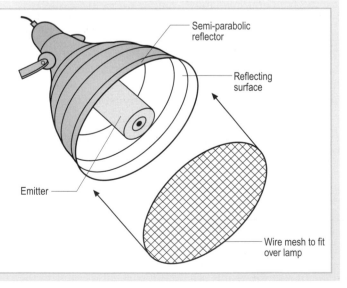

Figure 16.1 A non-luminous infrared lamp with a semi-parabolic reflector.

Semi-parabolic reflector

Reflecting surface

Emitter

Wire mesh to fit over lamp

Luminous generators

Luminous generators (incandescent lamps) consist of a tungsten filament in a large glass envelope which contains inert gas at low pressure. Part of the inside of the glass bulb is often silvered to provide a reflector. These lamps work on the same principle as a simple electric light bulb; the filament is heated to a high temperature (around 3000 C) by the current passed through it and so gives off a continuous spectrum in the infrared and visible regions. Oxidation of the filament does not occur because there is no oxygen present, only a trace of some inert gas. The peak emission occurs at near 1000 nm, but radiation extends from the long infrared throughout the visible to the ultraviolet (see Figure 16.6). The ultraviolet radiation is absorbed by the glass and therefore not transmitted by the lamp (Ward, 2004). Sometimes the glass is reddened, absorbing some of the green and blue rays to give a red visible emission; this is believed to make little difference therapeutically (Lehmann and de Lateur, 1982). Luminous generators are sometimes called 'radiant heat' generators, indicating that heating is by both infrared and visible radiation.

Power

The power of infrared sources can broadly be described as:

- small lamps (luminous and non-luminous), usually 250–500 W
- large, non-luminous, 750–1000 W.
- large, luminous, 650–1500 W.

Generally, the larger lamps are used to treat extensive areas, but the same effect can be achieved by mounting three smaller luminous bulbs in one holder. Some large lamps are fitted with wire-mesh screens over the front of the reflector to prevent accidental contact with the hot emitter. The screen also reduces the very remote risk of the hot emitter element falling out.

Emission

Non-luminous:

- mainly 3000–4000 nm (long IR), with about 10% between 1500 nm and visible (short IR)

Luminous:

- approximately 70% short IR
- 5% visible
- 24% long IR
- 1% UVR absorbed by glass of bulb

(Wadsworth and Chanmugan, 1980).

Summary

Infrared sources for therapy are categorized as luminous or non-luminous.

Non-luminous lamps:
- have electrically heated wire embedded in ceramic and backed by an external reflector
- produce long IR radiation around 3000 or 4000 nm (some give off a little red visible radiation)
- if small have a power of 250–500 W
- if large have a power of 750–1000 W.

Luminous lamps:
- have electrically heated filament in an evacuated glass bulb, often with silvered inner surface to provide a reflector
- produce both IR and visible radiation mostly in the short IR band (peak around 1000 nm)
- if small have a power of 250–500 W
- if large have a power of 600–1500 W.

ABSORPTION AND PENETRATION OF INFRARED AND VISIBLE RADIATION

Some radiation striking the surface of the skin will be reflected and some will penetrate, to be scattered, refracted and ultimately absorbed in the tissues. The amount of reflection of visible radiation varies with skin colour but, for therapeutic infrared, is negligible. Close to 95% of the radiation applied perpendicular to the skin is transmitted rather than reflected (Ward, 2004). The transmitted energy is rapidly absorbed so only small amounts of radiation penetrate to the subcutaneous tissues; most is absorbed in the skin. Skin (epidermis and dermis) is not, of course, a single homogeneous tissue but a complicated multilayered structure full of irregular forms, such as hair follicles and sweat glands. In general, water and proteins are strong absorbers of infrared. What happens, therefore, to any radiation entering the skin is highly complex, depending on the:

- structure
- vascularity
- pigmentation of the skin and, most crucially
- wavelength of the radiation.

This complexity accounts for the difficulty in determining the pattern of penetration and absorption of radiation in the skin; see, for example, Van Breugel (1992) and also the discrepancies in the quoted figures (Table 16.2).

Penetration

The usual method used to describe the overall penetration of radiation is to give the penetration depth (Table 16.2). Confusion

Table 16.2 Penetration depths of infrared from different authors

Source	Penetration depth (mm)	Wavelength (nm)
King (1989)	2–4	800–900
Harlen (1982)	3	'short IR'
Ward (2004)	'few'	1200
Nightingale (1959)	0.36	1100
Gourgouliatos (1990)	5–10	1200
Laurens (1933)	1–2.5	'near IR'

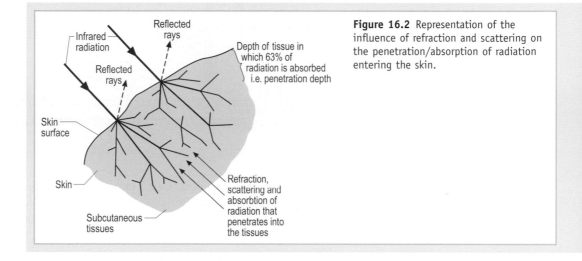

Figure 16.2 Representation of the influence of refraction and scattering on the penetration/absorption of radiation entering the skin.

sometimes arises from a failure to appreciate that this term has a specific, clearly defined meaning (see chapter 14 and Figure 14.7). It should be stressed that the penetration depth is the depth at which approximately 63% of the radiation energy has been absorbed and 37% remains. It is neither the depth to which all radiation penetrates nor the depth beyond which none penetrates.

Figure 16.2 shows what happens to IR once it penetrates the skin, how scattering and refraction decrease the penetration depth and can modify the pattern of absorption.

Looking at the whole spectrum of infrared and visible radiation from the microwave to the ultraviolet (Figure 14.2), some very different patterns of penetration/absorption emerge. Very long wavelength infrared (around 40 000 nm) behaves like microwave and penetrates several centimetres. However, the long infrared used therapeutically is absorbed at the surface, much of it by the water on the skin surface. At around 3000 nm, the penetration depth is about 0.1 mm (Ward, 2004). There is increasing penetration with decreasing wavelength in the short infrared region, to a maximum penetration depth of about 3 mm around the 1000 nm wavelength region (Table 16.2). Very short infrared and red visible radiation have

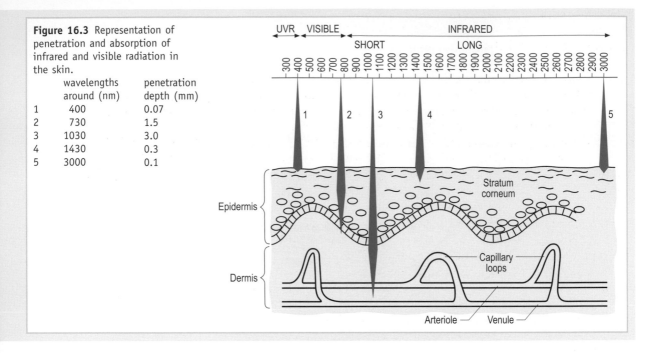

Figure 16.3 Representation of penetration and absorption of infrared and visible radiation in the skin.

	wavelengths around (nm)	penetration depth (mm)
1	400	0.07
2	730	1.5
3	1030	3.0
4	1430	0.3
5	3000	0.1

penetration depths of about 1 or 2 mm, while those of the rest of the visible spectrum penetrate much less (Figure 16.3). In fact, at the blue end of the visible spectrum, the penetration depth is about 0.07 mm and decreases uniformly with wavelength through the ultraviolet region. The much greater penetration of red light is easily demonstrated by putting a small torch in the mouth and seeing that only red light emerges through the cheek. Only a tiny proportion of the original radiation is being transmitted, but it is evident because the eyes are such highly efficient photon detectors.

The effect of infrared is therefore marked heating of the skin. Some of this heat will be conducted more deeply into the subcutaneous tissues, due both to simple conduction and to increased local circulation of heated blood. This is the same as the situation of surface conduction heating, described in chapter 11 and distinct from the diathermies (shortwave, microwave and ultrasound) which are directly able to heat subcutaneous tissues.

Summary

- Infrared radiation is strongly absorbed near the skin surface.
- Little infrared is reflected from the surface if it is applied perpendicular to the skin.
- The only infrared radiation to penetrate the tissues to any significant extent is a band approximately between 650 nm in the red visible and 1500 nm in the short infrared.

PHYSIOLOGICAL EFFECTS

Cutaneous vasodilation

Heating with infrared radiation causes local cutaneous vasodilation to occur. This is due to the liberation of chemical vasodilators, histamine and similar substances, as well as a possible direct effect on the blood vessels (mediated through polymodal nociceptors by an axon reflex mechanism). The vasodilation starts after a short latent period of 1 to 2 minutes (Crockford and Hellon, 1959) and appears to be largely due to arteriolar vasodilation. This is evident from the nature of the erythema which develops with an irregular patchy appearance (quite unlike the erythema due to ultraviolet irradiation in which the capillaries are directly affected). The irregular margin of the erythema shows where some arterioles have dilated, engorging the capillaries they supply while adjacent ones are unaffected. The rate at which the erythema develops and its intensity are related to the rate and degree of heating. For normal individuals, heating the skin to about core temperature (37°C) over some 20 minutes will lead to very mild erythema; heating to around 42°C will lead to marked erythema. The local erythema lasts for about 30 minutes after irradiation has stopped (Crockford and Hellon, 1959).

Reflex dilation of other (not directly irradiated) cutaneous vessels will also occur in order to maintain a normal body heat balance, as discussed in chapter 10. With mild heating the vasodilation of other parts, detectable only by a skin thermometer, is likely to begin after some 10 minutes or so.

Sweating

With prolonged or intense cutaneous heating, sweating will start to occur. This will absorb some of the applied infrared radiation and leads to surface cooling as it evaporates; see chapters 10 and 11 for discussion on thermal control. This does not necessarily lead to inefficiency since cooling the surface may allow better heating at depth (Figure 16.4).

Sensation

Thermal heat receptors will be stimulated in the skin so that the patient is aware of the heating.

Increase in metabolism

Where the temperature is raised there will be an increase in local tissue metabolism.

Figure 16.4 Temperature gradient in the tissues due to heating with long and short infrared radiation. (Modified from Nightingale, 1959.)

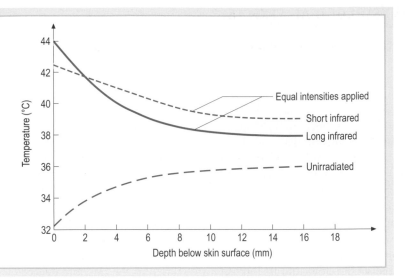

Summary

Physiological changes due to heating (discussed in chapters 10 and 11):

● increased metabolic rate
● decreased viscosity
● stimulation of sensory nerves
● vascular changes.

Chronic changes

Excessive and prolonged infrared application can cause the destruction of erythrocytes, releasing pigments and causing brown discoloration of the skin. This rarely occurs as a sequel to normal treatment; it usually results from prolonged exposure of the legs to domestic fires.

Premature ageing of skin (photoageing) is principally associated with ultraviolet (UV) exposure but there is a substantial body of evidence that infrared and visible radiation also cause photoageing (Schieke et al., 2003). Epidemiological studies also indicate a link between infrared exposure and skin cancer. Although infrared radiation is not in itself carcinogenic, it has long been known that a spectrum including UV, visible and infrared is more carcinogenic than UV exposure alone (Bain et al., 1943). The increased carcinogenicity is likely due to the higher temperatures induced by infrared radiation.

THERAPEUTIC USES OF INFRARED

Therapeutically, infrared has been used as a form of heat for the purposes discussed in chapter 11. These include:

- pain relief
- reduction of muscle spasm
- acceleration of healing and repair.

There is considerable anecdotal evidence that infrared is useful for relieving pain and muscle spasm and it is widely used, non-clinically, for these purposes. Perhaps for this very reason, no controlled scientific studies have been carried out. Surveys in a number of countries suggest infrared is used relatively infrequently in clinics (Lindsay et al., 1995; Pope et al., 1995; Robertson and Spurritt, 1998). This pattern is consistent with infrared being safe for home use and ownership and likely to have been used prior to clinical consultation.

Infrared continues, however, to be used as a form of heat prior to stretching, mobilization, traction, massage and exercise therapy, as discussed in chapter 11. This type of use continues despite the lack of evidence that muscle temperature or blood flow is increased to any significant extent by infrared radiation, unlike the diathermies (SWD, MW and ultrasound). Infrared can also be used prior to electrical stimulation or biofeedback to warm the skin, making it a more effective conductor.

A previous role of infrared in treating fungal infections such as paronychia by drying the skin is of limited value given existing fungicides and changes in clothing and footwear. Similarly for drying wounds to promote healing; optimum conditions for most wounds are not achieved by infrared exposure, a form of intermittent heating which dries out the wound.

EFFECTS AND USES OF VISIBLE RADIATION

Visible radiation is, by definition, able to stimulate the retinal cells of the eye. Simple exposure to light, light therapy, is used to treat a range of conditions including seasonal affective disorder. Previous reviews show that light alone is effective in treating this condition in approximately 50% of patients. This level appears to rise when supplemented with other methods of psychological treatment (Rohan et al., 2004). In patients with dementia there is little evidence that light therapy reduces mood disturbances, depression or sleep disorders (Forbes et al., 2004; Skjerve et al., 2004).

Another use for visible light is in the treatment of neonatal hyperbilirubinaemia (a form of neonatal jaundice). The bile pigment, bilirubin, formed by the breakdown of haemoglobin, can reach high levels in the blood of newborn babies leading to brain damage. This condition is successfully treated by exposing the baby to light in the 420–480 nm region. Bilirubin is converted by the visible light to compounds which can be easily excreted. A choice of lighting systems exist, one being halogen spotlights that can be used directly or directed through a fibreoptic mat. Another is fluorescent tubes, white or a set of some blue and some white. Any ultraviolet radiation is screened out. Whichever system is used it must have sufficient power to be effective. For further details of dosages see an appropriate paediatric textbook.

Colour therapy, in which particular colours are applied or viewed for particular conditions, has a long history as alternative medicine in various forms. While there is no direct evidence of significant therapeutic effect an interesting association has been shown, using electromyographic activity, between viewing red light and greater maximum voluntary (hand-grip) contraction (Hasson et al., 1989). It is speculated that seeing red light leads to arousal in the central nervous system and/or sympathetic stimulation (red for danger). Although blue light has been considered to have a calming effect, the study quoted above found no significant difference between the blue light group and the controls.

> Red light has been used to stimulate healing since ancient times. Karu (1989) discusses the experimental evidence for this effect.

Summary

Infrared and visible radiation are used therapeutically to:

- relieve pain and muscle spasm
- promote superficial healing and repair
- promote tissue extensibility and reduce stiffness
- reduce the severity of some mood disturbances and sleep disorders.

These effects have been more convincingly demonstrated with infrared, rather than visible, radiation.

CHOICE OF LUMINOUS (RADIANT HEAT) OR NON-LUMINOUS SOURCES

- The luminous heat source is a more efficient tissue-heating source since it penetrates further (because peak emission is in the short infrared) and therefore the energy is distributed in a larger volume of tissue.
- Non-luminous radiation, with peak emission around 4000 nm, is absorbed almost entirely in the skin.

If the desired effects are due to:

- heating – the luminous shorter infrared source is preferred
- sensory stimulation – the non-luminous is more satisfactory.

It is possible to achieve more even, deeper penetration by cooling the surface with a draught of cool air but the risks of burning may also be greater. Compare the similar mechanism for microwave (chapter 15).

Technique of application of infrared radiation

Stages

Patient

Position: position the patient in a suitable, well supported position with the area to be treated exposed.

Explanation: explain the nature and effects of the treatment to the patient.

Examination and testing: examine the skin to be treated and test the thermal sensation.

Apparatus

If a non-luminous lamp is chosen, switch it on at least 5 minutes before treatment to allow time for it to warm up and reach its maximum emission. A luminous lamp needs no warm-up time and can be switched on once the patient is ready for the treatment.

Setting up

Expose the skin to be irradiated with infrared and cover or shield the eyes. A towel is sufficient to limit the exposure of eyes. Position the lamp so that the radiation strikes the surface at or near right angles to achieve maximum penetration, as described in chapter 14. Set the lamp at an appropriate distance: about 60–75 cm for large 750 or 1000 W lamps and about 45–50 cm for the smaller ones.

Instructions and warnings

Advise the patient of the required level of heat and that it must not be hot as it can burn. Ask them to indicate the level of heat they can feel and where. Advise the patient not to touch any part of the lamp or to move during treatment and to alert the therapist if it is more than a comfortably warm level of heating.

Application

The intensity of heating in most infrared lamps is controlled by the distance of the lamp from the skin. In some lamps it is by altering a resistance and hence the current to the element. Despite the reflector, radiation diverges considerably so that small changes of distance lead to quite large changes of intensity on the skin surface. For example, doubling the lamp-to-skin distance reduces the intensity ($W\,cm^{-2}$) to one quarter. Tripling the lamp-to-skin distance reduces the intensity to one ninth, and so on. This is predicted by the inverse square law, described in chapter 14, but is only a rough guide as it strictly only applies to sources which emit radiation in all directions, not to sources mounted in reflectors.

Adjacent areas can be protected from heating by judicious placement of a layer of towelling. The therapist should check the level of heating on completion of the set up and again after 5 to 8 minutes and, if required, adjust the distance of the lamp to the skin. Infrared is usually only applied for 10 to 15 minutes as it is only part of a treatment, not a treatment in itself.

Termination

On completion of the treatment the skin should be carefully checked. On palpation it may feel mildly or moderately warm and a moderate erythema should be evident. Note, the intensity of erythema tends to vary with skin colour, not just temperature.

POTENTIAL DANGERS WITH INFRARED TREATMENT

Burns

The main danger of infrared treatment is a burn. Burns are always a potential risk if heat is too intense, the patient is not fully aware of the level of heating for one or other reasons, or they are unable to communicate effectively. Burns can also be due to the method of applying heating.

The risk of burns can be reduced considerably by:

- careful applications that involve testing the patient's ability to differentiate heat levels. If their accuracy or communication skills are limited, ensure sufficient distance of the lamp from the skin so that a burn is not possible
- adequate warnings to the patient regarding the level of heating required
- checking the effects on the skin during the application. The therapist can feel the skin or place their own hand under the lamp at the appropriate distance.

Metal (e.g. jewellery) should be removed from the skin areas being treated or covered with towelling. However, burns from overheated superficial metal are unlikely with the intensity and duration of most infrared treatments.

Reduced or altered peripheral blood flow

Do not use heating if the vascular response is insufficient because of the risk of tissue damage. The increased local flow during heating must be sufficient to dissipate the heat applied. Areas affected by arterial disease, such as atherosclerosis, arterial injury or after skin grafting, should not normally be treated with infrared. Similarly, skin treated with irradiation should be not be treated with infrared for at

Harley and Dziewulski (2003) report the example of a woman with full thickness burns on her abdomen caused when she fell asleep lying on an operating infrared massaging device.

In a related case report, a patient with a successfully replanted thumb self-treated with infrared to his thumb (Madura et al., 2002). This treatment resulted in a full thickness burn to the digit although heat was reported as applied at a subthermal dosage.

least 2 months following radiotherapy or until advised by the relevant medical practitioner that it is safe.

Infection

As a general rule avoid applying heat over local infections or previously known tumour sites. The level of risk of spreading infection or promoting tumour growth is possibly very low given the superficial nature of infrared.

Skin inflammatory conditions

Heating typically makes many acute inflammatory skin conditions worse and so should be avoided when relevant.

Eye damage

Prolonged and extensive exposure to infrared, such as occurs in furnace men and those working in glass blowing factories, can cause eye damage. The main problem is the formation of cataracts (Sisto et al., 2000). The infrared radiation penetrates the eye and is focused by the lens. In addition, heat absorbed by the iris seems to be transferred to the lens by a process of conduction. The net result can be the formation of cataracts.

The usual clinical treatment times and intensity mean there is only a very low level risk of eye damage. However, for patient comfort, and to avoid eye surface drying, and possible irritation, eyes should be either covered with a light towel or the head averted during an exposure.

CONTRAINDICATIONS

- Defective cutaneous circulation.
- Acute skin disease, e.g. dermatitis or eczema.
- Following radiotherapy.
- Superficial infections or tumours.

LASERS

The acronym 'laser' stands for 'light amplification by stimulated emission of radiation'. Lasers are electromagnetic wave amplifiers which can produce pencil-like beams of electromagnetic waves with special properties.

The divergence of a laser beam is so small that a beam pointed at the moon could illuminate a target less than a metre across.

The pencil-like beam of the laser means that the wave energy is always concentrated on the same area: the intensity (which is the energy per unit area) does not decrease appreciably with distance due to beam spreading.

The roots of the laser mechanism are relatively modern. In 1900 the great German physicist Max Planck presented an explanation of why the colours of a glowing hot body change with temperature. He proposed that radiation comes in discrete quantities ('quanta'). So radiation was not only wave-like but, at one and the same time, behaved like a stream of particles ('photons') which can be visualized as tiny bundles of energy. By 1917, Einstein had outlined the principles underlying the production of laser radiation as part of what is now known as quantum theory.

The earliest medical lasers, developed in the 1960s and 1970s, were relatively high powered and utilized the concentration of energy in a tiny, pencil-like beam for tissue destruction and coagulation. Some beneficial effects were noted in sites adjacent to the coagulated tissue, at which low energy had been applied. This led to the therapeutic use of low-energy lasers.

Laser radiation differs from ordinary light in the following ways:

- *monochromaticity*: lasers are of a single specific frequency and hence have a defined wavelength. In the case of visible lasers, a single pure colour is produced, e.g. ruby lasers give a red light at exactly 694.3 nm wavelength (see Table 16.3). The specific frequency of a gallium/aluminium arsenide laser is set (within the range shown) by varying the proportions of gallium and aluminium arsenide.

- *coherence*: laser radiation is not only of the same wavelength but also in phase, that is to say the peaks and troughs of the electric and magnetic fields all occur at the same time. This is called 'temporal coherence'. Furthermore, they are all travelling in the same direction; this is called 'spatial coherence' (Figure 16.5). The distance over which the wavelengths stay in phase is called the coherence length. It can be thousands of metres in air, but much less (as low as a fraction of a millimetre) in biological tissues.

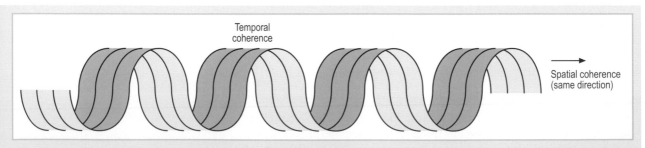

Figure 16.5 Coherent waves follow parallel paths and are synchronized.

- *collimation*: as a consequence of spatial coherence lasers remain in a parallel beam. Because the radiation does not diverge the energy is propagated over very long distances. This property makes it invaluable for measurement and aiming purposes.

An analogy: ordinary visible (non-coherent) radiation is like a crowd of people all in different clothing, walking in different directions out of step. Laser radiation is like a column of soldiers all marching in step (in phase) in the same direction (spatial coherence) and wearing the same uniform (monochromatic).

When laser radiation interacts with matter the effects are the same as any other electromagnetic radiation – reflection, refraction and absorption occur. Hence, the radiation is both scattered and absorbed and this means the collimation is diminished and coherence is lost. The extent to which this happens will depend on the nature and density of matter present, so that laser radiation will pass unaffected through space and be only slightly altered in air (at least for visible radiation) but be markedly altered on entering a more dense material such as the tissues. In biological tissue, coherence will be lost in a fraction of a millimetre so the beam will no longer be coherent but it will still be monochromatic, i.e. it will still have a precise frequency.

Lasers can be both pulsed and focused. They can therefore be used to deliver large amounts of energy to a small region in a very short time. When laser radiation is absorbed by the tissues it will cause heating if it is of sufficient intensity, but it is also claimed to have specific biological effects due to the special nature of laser radiation, i.e. its monochromaticity, coherence and lack of beam divergence (collimation).

For more information on lasers and production of laser radiation see chapter 11 of the book 'Biophysical Bases of Electrotherapy' on the CD which comes with this book.

Summary

Laser radiation:

- is monochromatic, i.e. of a single wavelength
- is coherent in both
  - phase – temporal coherence
  - direction – spatial coherence
- is collimated, i.e. a parallel beam
- behaves like all radiation
  - reflected
  - refracted, hence can be focused or scattered
  - absorbed
- is the emission of large numbers of identical, coherent, collimated photons.

Two types of laser are worth special mention because of their common clinical usage: helium-neon and diode lasers.

Figure 16.6 Comparison of laser output with that of a typical infrared lamp.

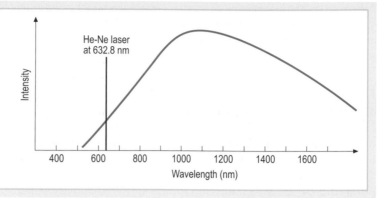

Table 16.3 Examples of lasers		
Laser type	**Wavelength (nm)**	**Radiation**
Ruby	694.3	Red light
Helium–neon	632.8	Red light
Gallium/aluminium arsenide	630 to 1550	Red to infrared
Carbon dioxide	10 600	Infrared

Helium–neon (He–Ne) lasers produce radiation in the red visible region at 632.8 nm. Figure 16.6 compares helium–neon laser output with an infrared lamp. Infrared and visible radiation are emitted from typical luminous infrared lamps giving radiation over a range of wavelengths and peak emission around 1000 nm.

Diode lasers are commonly made from the semiconductive materials gallium and aluminium arsenide (GaAlAs). As with any diode, electrons can flow more readily in one direction than in the other. The special property of diode lasers is that when current flows through the diode, the electrical energy is converted into laser radiation energy. The wavelength of the radiation (Table 16.3) depends on the proportions of gallium and aluminium.

Making diode lasers fully coherent is difficult in practice. It is cheaper to produce *superluminous diodes* (SLDs) which are fully monochromatic and collimated but non-coherent. It is argued that coherence is therapeutically superfluous (Karu, 1987) and, in any case, is rapidly lost when radiation enters the tissues. While SLDs are 'unconventional lasers' in that they do not produce coherent radiation, they are widely used in therapy.

Due to their small size, semiconductor lasers can be applied directly to the tissues in a hand-held applicator. Sometimes several laser diodes of assorted wavelengths are mounted together to form an emitter, which can be used to treat a larger area. These are known as 'cluster probes'. They may also contain SLDs. For all these forms of low-power laser a suitable electronic circuit is provided to generate

Table 16.4 Classification of lasers

Class	Power	Effect	Usage
1	Low	None on eye or skin	Laser pointer Barcode reader
2	Low up to 1 mW	Safe on skin. Eyes protected by aversion response	Therapeutic lasers Laser pointer
3A	Low-medium up to 5 mW	Viewing with optical aids may be hazardous	Therapeutic lasers Laser pointer
3B	Medium up to 500 mW	Viewing may be hazardous	Therapeutic lasers
4 & 5	High over 500 mW	Hazardous to skin and eye	Destructive – surgical

appropriate currents to power the diodes. Pulsing and timing are also controlled electronically.

LASER CLASSIFICATION

The different types of lasers are divided into classes according to their power, effect on the eye given the blink reflex time and the duration of the on-time if pulsed. Table 16.4 lists the classes, their power, effect on the eye and how they are generally used. Those used for therapy are generally class 2, 3A or 3B. Some He–Ne lasers that are used therapeutically have a very low power rating (less than 0.5 mW) and so are class 1 lasers. Eye protection is not required for class 1 lasers.

Class 2 lasers are low power lasers and are safe for momentary viewing and for extended skin exposure. Despite this, they should never be pointed at an eye. By contrast, class 3A and 3B lasers do represent a potential hazard to the eyes but little to exposed skin. They include both low and mid-power lasers (1 mW to 500 mW). Class 3B, in particular, should be used only by experienced personnel and with an enclosed beam in a restricted area.

Laser protective goggles must be worn with class 3B lasers and are advisable with 3A lasers. These are purpose designed goggles to block specific wavelengths and must not be interchanged with other types of protective goggles, such as sunglasses or welders' goggles.

Class 4 and 5 lasers are high power lasers and represent a high level of risk to both eyes and unprotected skin. Surgical lasers, CO_2, Nd:YAG and argon lasers are in these classes. The levels of care required for users of classes 4 and 5 lasers include use only behind locked doors, laser goggles for all in the vicinity and warning signs. This level of precaution is not necessary for the lasers used clinically by therapists, typically class 2, 3A or 3B lasers.

Laser pointers are commonly from class 2 or 3A. Most have a low power rating (1 to 5 mW) but, despite this, they can cause some, usually temporary, visual disturbances and so should never be pointed directly at an eye. The extent of risk will depend on the power and the type of laser pointer.

Maintenance

For example, the Nussbaum et al. (1999) study found that 60% of the laser diodes and 31% of the superluminous diodes were within 1 to 79% of the expected levels of power output.

Maintenance of all types of laser equipment used clinically is an important issue. As with other items of electromedical equipment, a regular electrical safety test is necessary. The frequency of testing will depend on the local legal requirements and on the usage per month but at least annual tests are recommended. In addition, the output should be calibrated. Some equipment offers a test diode to ascertain the intensity of the output from a single probe. However, this is a guide and testing and calibration by a qualified electromedical technician is recommended for accuracy. Also, cluster probes and scanners need testing and this must be done using specialized photodiode equipment. One study which reported the outputs of lasers being used clinically found the performance of many was not as indicated by their manufacturer (Nussbaum et al., 1999). As with ultrasound (chapter 9), this lack of reliability of output is a possibly very important source of the widely different findings in many research studies.

MEASUREMENT OF LASER ENERGY

- The amount of energy falling on a surface is expressed in joules per square metre ($J m^{-2}$) or joules per square centimetre ($J cm^{-2}$). It is often called *energy density*.
- The rate at which energy is produced or absorbed is measured in joules per second, i.e. in watts ($1 W = 1 J s^{-1}$) and called *power*.
- Most lasers used by therapists have output powers of milliwatts (see Table 16.4). The average power per unit area can be expressed as irradiance or *power density* in $W cm^{-2}$.
- The level of power can describe the temporal peak power or temporal average power. The temporal peak power is that of each pulse but the temporal average (or mean) power depends on the pulse length and the pulse frequency. This means that very short individual pulses may be a few watts (peak power), but the average power will be a few milliwatts if a low frequency and pulse length.
- The laser beam is not perfectly collimated and the divergence may be expressed in terms of an angle.

EFFECTS OF LASER RADIATION ON THE TISSUES

Like all radiation, laser may:

- be reflected from the surface
- penetrate the tissues in proportions that depend on the:
  - wavelength
  - nature of the tissue surface
  - angle of incidence.

Having entered the tissues laser radiation is diffused, scattered and spread by:

- divergence
- reflection
- refraction

and further attenuated by absorption (see Figure 16.2).

The penetration depth of red visible and short infrared radiation is only a few millimetres, 1–2 mm for He–Ne lasers (red light) and 2–4 mm for GaAlAs lasers (IR lasers) of 800–900 nm in soft tissue (King, 1989).

Due to this marked scattering in the tissues, it is considered that areas between the diodes of a cluster probe are also treated (Gourgouliatos, 1990). This is questionable as the individual beams are only a millimetre or so in diameter and would need to spread and cover an area about 50 times larger. Were this true, penetration would be severely compromised as most of the energy would be going sideways.

Absorption in the tissues

As noted previously, the passage of light through the skin is complex (see Figure 16.2 and Lipper and Anderson, 2003). Most is scattered by the dermis back through the epidermis as the dermis is thick. The dermis is also punctuated by light absorbing blood vessels and hair follicles. The patterns of light absorption in skin relate to the melanin and haemoglobins within the dermis. The optical properties of the dermis are quite different from those of the epidermis, basically because of the large proportion of collagen fibres which predominate in the extracellular connective tissue matrix. Collagen scatters light strongly, blue more than red and this is what makes freshly exposed tendon a bluish-white colour. A consequence is that longer wavelength light penetrates further into the dermis than shorter, the maximum happening at near 1200 nm.

Most biological macromolecules and tissue structures absorb visible and infrared radiation quite strongly. As a consequence, the penetration depths, as noted above, are quite small. Some biological molecules are particularly strong absorbers: haemoglobin and melanin are examples. Infrared is strongly absorbed by water (Diamantopoulos, 1994), which predominates in all tissue and is often present on the skin surface as perspiration. The superficial nature of visible and infrared absorption is thus unquestionable. What is questionable is whether with laser the energy remaining at depth is sufficient to produce beneficial effects. This depends on whether the biological process stimulated is sufficiently sensitive and discriminatory, able to respond to the specific wavelength applied and whether a low intensity level is sufficient to trigger a positive effect. A more likely scenario, based on known biochemical/physiological mechanisms is that the responsiveness is broad spectrum, in which case the precise wavelength is less important than the total energy delivered over a range of wavelengths.

Scientific evidence shows that beneficial radiation does not need the wavelength precision of lasers. It is true that biological effects are stimulated at certain optimum frequencies, but frequencies either side are also effective. The reason is an 'effectiveness' graph resembles the broad curve shown in Figure 16.6 more than a precise line for laser radiation. This is fortunate as the chances of the laser wavelength happening to coincide with a sharply peaked effectiveness graph is negligibly small. Thus lasers might be effective despite, rather than because of, their monochromaticity.

It has been argued that red light is absorbed by cytochromes in the mitochondria of the cell and that all cells have mitochondria, so all may be stimulated by red light. This is a better argument for red-light therapy than laser treatment as the optimum absorption wavelength is not the same as that of a He–Ne laser, but higher at 810 to 904 nm (closer to GaAs or GaAlAs lasers).

Another argument is that laser radiation could affect cell membrane permeability. The hypothesis is that various types of cells have different photoreceptors in their membranes and that these photoreceptors control membrane permeability. Because of this, different wavelengths could have an all-or-none effect on specific cells, which may provide a way, in future, of targeting these cells. This hypothesis does not seem to be supported by any scientific evidence.

As with ultrasound, the transport of calcium ions across the cell membrane has been invoked to support claims of healing. The claim is that exposure sets in train a whole sequence of events (not identified) which are necessary to restore the cell to its normal function. As long as an energy threshold at cellular level is reached, it is claimed, an effect can occur. Mester et al. (1985) suggest that $4\,J\,cm^{-2}$ is an appropriate dose, but a range of $1–48\,J\,cm^{-2}$ has been used clinically. As described in the next section, the higher end of this range has been shown to be effective in some studies. Also, while calcium ion imbalance is an important indicator of cell damage and dysfunction, the effects on this of laser therapy have yet to be demonstrated.

It has also been claimed that there is a 'window' for effective photobiostimulation; above threshold, beneficial effects are produced but, if the intensity is too high, the beneficial effects do not occur. This argument would be sustainable if 'too high' were at levels which produce biological damage but the levels identified are not. The windows are hypothesized to be narrow. This concept has been invoked to account for the conflicting results of laser studies (Baxter, 1994). A possible alternative explanation for the conflicting results derives from simple statistics. The more comparative tests that are made, the greater the probability of obtaining a false positive and, if the studies are split and grouped, the chances of false positives dominating in any group must increase. Evidence as currently presented for the 'magic window' hypothesis is thus not convincing.

Were the Arndt-Schultz law to explain the hypothetical narrow 'windows', the effects would be appreciable and positive above some threshold but negative at increasingly higher doses. The absence of a negative effect above the 'windows' except at destructively high power levels suggests that the 'narrow window' effects are probably illusory and due to random chance.

THERAPEUTIC USES OF LASERS

The types of laser used clinically to promote healing provide what is sometimes called 'low level laser therapy' (LLLT) and includes different types of lasers from classes 1 to 3B. Their level of power output is part of what distinguishes them from the class 4 and 5 lasers that are used to cut the skin in surgery or for the ablation of tumours or skin lesions of different types. Sometimes the terms 'photobiomodulation' and 'photobiostimulation' are used with therapeutic lasers to indicate the claimed method of action. This section will discuss what is known about the therapeutic effectiveness of laser from existing clinical studies.

The two major uses of laser therapy are for tissue healing and pain control. Within these two broad categories, laser therapy is used to promote wound healing and in the treatment of different types of soft tissue injuries, such as muscle tears, haematomas and tendinopathies. Treating these problems is expected to reduce pain and laser is also used specifically for this effect.

Tissue healing

Tissue healing is one of the main claimed clinical effects of laser and the focus of a varied body of research. Specific studies include systematic reviews of its effectiveness for treating venous ulcers and a range of studies conducted on both animals and humans.

A Cochrane review of the effect of laser on venous leg ulcers identified four randomized controlled trials that met the inclusion criteria (Flemming and Cullum, 2004). Two studies used a He–Ne laser with a dosage of $4\,\mathrm{J\,cm^{-2}}$, one a GaAs laser at $2\,\mathrm{J\,cm^{-2}}$, and one provided no details of the laser used. Each study used at least a sham laser or another form of phototherapy as a control. The results do not indicate any evidence of benefit on venous ulcers in humans from low level laser therapy.

Other ways of evaluating the effects of laser on wounds are *in vitro* studies and ones that use animals. One such review identified 36 animal studies which met their inclusion criteria (Lucas et al., 2002). The initial results show that for the 49 outcomes in the studies, 30 were positive. However, when the methodologically poor studies were excluded, 13 of the 21 outcomes from the methodologically 'good and moderate' studies were negative. That is, the findings generally do not

While the findings of Flemming and Cullum (2004) are not atypical of Cochrane collaborations where the body of methodologically-acceptable studies is small, it is consistent with those of other large reviews of laser and wound healing.

support the notion that laser promotes wound healing in animals. The topic is complicated by differences in skin between humans and some animals. If studies on loose skinned animals whose healing might not be relevant are excluded and pig studies retained the answer is still not clear cut. The reason is, of the pig wounds in their review one study supported and one did not the use of laser for wound healing.

Individual studies have contradictory outcomes and there are issues of the relevance to human clinical conditions. For example, rabbit tendo achilles surgically cut and treated for 14 days with He–Ne (632.8 nm) laser and a dosage of 1.5 J cm^{-2} had better outcomes than those sham treated (Reddy et al., 1998). A study in rats following blunt trauma to muscle identified increases in collagenous proteins in all groups irrespective of treatment (Fisher et al., 2000). The authors concluded that there was no benefit in the 3 to 12 day period following the trauma.

Another issue is the dosage. The use of too low a dosage was used to provide a possible explanation for a non-significant change in surgical wounds in horses following treatment with sham or real 830 nm laser at 2 J cm^{-2} (Petersen et al., 1999). By contrast, considerably higher dosages (up to 50 J cm^{-2}, 685 nm or 830 nm) to experimentally created wounds in rats produced more advanced wound healing from day 3 to day 7 (Mendez et al., 2004). In particular, the results for both lasers were best at 20 J cm^{-2}. One human study that used a very much higher dosage than usual had positive findings. Low level laser (48 J cm^{-2} for 10 minutes) was found to be effective in increasing the duration of non-recurrence of oral herpes simplex lesions in humans (Schindl and Neumann, 1999).

Treatment of pressure ulcers in humans with different frequencies of laser (4.5 J cm^{-2}, GaAlAs) showed no significant differences in time to healing (Taly et al., 2004). Those with more severe ulcers treated with laser had shorter healing times but, overall, those in the sham treated group healed faster.

In summary, there is little evidence to support the use of laser for wound healing at present. Despite this, there is a considerable level of support for it among some groups. In one survey it was ranked as more effective for promoting wound healing than other electrophysical agents, such as particular types of electrical stimulation and ultrasound (Cambier and Vanderstraeten, 1997).

Musculoskeletal pain

Anecdotally, low level laser is sometimes reported to reduce musculoskeletal pain. However, there is little methodologically adequate research to support this. A review of a number of older studies found the evidence contradictory (Fargas-Babjak, 2001). As is usual with many laser studies, they report on treatment of a range of different conditions, the use of different outcome measures and quite different

The Schindl and Neumann (1999) study found that the median recurrence-free period of herpes simplex lesions in those treated with laser was 37.5 weeks (95% CI, 24–42) and 3 weeks in those sham treated (95% CI, 2–4 weeks).

treatment protocols. Another review investigated 11 trials of laser directly over the joint to reduce the pain of chronic joint disorders (Bjordal et al., 2003). Their findings suggest that low level laser does reduce pain and improve the health status of patients with these disorders. However, the reviewers advised caution in accepting these results because of the extent of heterogeneity in patient groups and in the treatments used.

Systematic reviews on the use of laser to treat musculoskeletal problems include the Cochrane Collaboration reviews on the topic of the effectiveness of classes 1, 2 and 3 laser to treat osteoarthritis (Brosseau et al., 2004a) and rheumatoid arthritis (Brosseau et al., 2004b). The conclusions from seven trials for osteoarthritis are that there is a need for standardized and validated outcome measures plus studies of the effects of dosage factors (Brosseau et al., 2004a). Rheumatoid arthritis was treated with laser in five placebo-controlled trials with a total of 204 patients (Brosseau et al., 2004b). Laser reduced pain by 70% and morning stiffness by 27.5 minutes (95% CI: 2.9–52 minutes). Both hands improved raising the possibility of a systemic effect, a strong placebo response or a statistical coincidence. Also, less subjective outcomes such as function, range of movement and swelling did not change, suggesting that the placebo effect might be quite important with laser.

The effects of low level laser and exercise on outcomes for patients with painful osteoarthritis of the knee were investigated in a double-blinded randomized controlled trial (Gur et al., 2003). Those treated with laser all improved more than those in the sham treatment group.

Laser also appears to reduce pain and increase function in patients with cervical osteoarthritis (Ozdemir et al., 2001). The results show less pain in those treated with laser (GaAlAs, 830 nm, $0.9\,J\,cm^{-2}$ to each of 12 points in the paravertebral muscle midline) than sham laser. Similar results were obtained with patients with chronic low back pain with laser (GaAlAs, 904 nm, $4\,J\,cm^{-2}$ per point in pain area) (Soriano and Rios, 1998). Another study treated chronic low back pain with sham or real laser (Nd:YAG) and reported those treated with laser had better outcomes, albeit small changes that lessened with time (Basford, 1999).

A more acute pain, experimentally induced delayed onset muscle soreness (DOMS) was treated with laser (Glasgow et al., 2001). The results show no significant differences in pain or tenderness between the placebo and treatment groups, although there was a slight trend favouring laser. A randomized controlled trial of the effects of low level laser on pain following a dental extraction found less pain and swelling in those treated with laser (Ong and Ho, 2001).

Studies that have not identified differences in pain following treatment with laser include one of acute ankle sprains (904 nm; $5\,J\,cm^{-2}$, $0.5\,J\,cm^{-2}$, or $0\,J\,cm^{-2}$) (de Bie et al., 1998). Another treated experimentally induced ischaemic arm pain in humans (830 nm, sham, $1.5\,J\,cm^{-2}$ or $9\,J\,cm^{-2}$) (Lowe et al., 1997). Similarly, another treated DOMS with laser using a range of frequencies (660–950 nm) and

Brosseau et al. (2004a) also stressed the need for studies which investigate the effect of dosage factors including the dosage, treatment duration and site of application of laser.

The use of a non-coherent light source in the Glasgow et al. (2001) study is unlikely to explain the negative findings as once within tissue the radiation loses its coherence. Also, existing research suggests the effects produced by coherent and non-coherent light do not differ (Lucas et al., 2002).

found the pain may have even lasted longer and been greater than in the groups not treated with laser (Craig et al., 1999). No changes were identified in subjects with lateral epicondylitis treated with Nd:YAG lasers at $12\,\mathrm{J\,cm^{-2}}$ (Basford et al., 2000).

Differences in outcome highlight the problems in evaluating the effectiveness of low level laser for treating pain; the reasons for the differences in outcomes are not easily explained and most systematic reviews have inconclusive findings.

Trigger/acupuncture points

Different types of electrophysical agents are applied to trigger and acupuncture points to relieve pain. These include laser, cold and electrical stimulation. One study investigated the effects on pain of treatment of myofascial trigger points with sham, 670 nm and 820 nm laser (Laakso et al., 1997). This well conducted randomized controlled trial identified some statistically significant changes in all groups treated with $1\,\mathrm{J\,cm^{-2}}$, including the placebo group, and all bar those treated with the 670 nm laser at $5\,\mathrm{J\,cm^{-2}}$. Given the small size of the groups and the variability in pain ratings across the 6 days this suggests little difference in effect whether sham or real laser was used at those dosages. Another randomized controlled trial used laser (780 nm) and stretching exercises to treat 62 patients with trigger points associated with pain in their neck or upper back (Hakguder et al., 2003). Those in the sham laser group improved but not as much as those treated with laser ($5\,\mathrm{J\,cm^{-2}}$). The outcomes were evaluated using a visual analogue pain scale, a pressure algometer over the treated trigger point and infrared thermography.

A related study of the effect of laser on myofascial trigger points showed changes in plasma ACTH and β-endorphin levels in response to applications of sham and real laser (Laakso et al., 1994). The variability across time, combined with the differences between sham and laser type and level of dosage, makes the results hard to interpret. However, there is no clear physiological explanation, except for subject variability over time, why the level of β-endorphin should rise in response to sham laser but drop with near monochromatic red (660 nm). The study controls were thorough and included time of day of treatment to reduce diurnal variations. More research is needed to investigate the effect of treating trigger or acupuncture points with laser to reduce pain.

Carpal tunnel syndrome

Studies of the effect of laser on nerve conduction have produced conflicting findings, but particularly careful and valuable work (Baxter et al., 1991) has shown that laser irradiation over the median nerve of normal subjects increases nerve conduction latencies. Such an effect

Although a quite different light source, dosage and patient group, the use of light therapy has been shown to decrease the levels of thyroid stimulating hormone (TSH) in patients with seasonal affective disorder (Martiny et al., 2004). This is one of few studies that appear to show systemic effects of externally applied light.

can hardly be due to heating, which would decrease nerve latency. The possible clinical relevance of this finding is in treating carpal tunnel syndrome. One study applied laser (GaAlAs, 830 nm, 9 J per point over five points) over the median nerve to treat patients with carpal tunnel syndrome (Weintraub, 1997). This altered the physiological responsiveness and improved clinical symptoms in 23 of the 30 hands treated this way. When, in another study, a sham laser group (860 nm, 6 J cm^{-2}) was included there were no differences between the groups (Irvine et al., 2004). This study also investigated the effectiveness of blinding and found that the therapist and most patients (6/7 in control group and 3/7 in treatment) wrongly identified the sham as the real laser.

Oedema

A study of 47 soccer players with a second degree ankle sprain investigated the contribution of laser (820 nm, 7.5 J cm^2) to oedema reduction in the acute stage (Stergioulas, 2004). Laser was compared to rest, ice, compression and elevation (RICE, see chapter 12) with no laser, with sham laser or with real laser. Statistically significant differences in volume (displacement measurement) were apparent at 24, 48 and 72 hours after treatment in the laser group. Further studies are needed, but this suggests laser did affect the volume of oedema in the ankles treated with laser.

Lymphoedema

Laser has been used to treat limbs affected by post-mastectomy lymphoedema (Carati et al., 2003). Treatment with 904 nm laser (1.5 J cm^{-2}) reduced the volume of lymphoedema affected limbs and softened the tissues only after two cycles of nine treatments (three per week for three weeks). Neither sham for two cycles nor one cycle of sham and one of real laser was as effective. How or why laser might have been effective is not clear as the results suggest considerable changes must have occurred in a limb to improve drainage sufficient to produce the results reported.

Raynaud's phenomenon

The results of a randomized controlled trial using a sham and a real laser (670 nm, continuous wave, energy density unclear) suggests that laser can decrease the severity of the symptoms of Raynaud's phenomenon (Al-Awami et al., 2004). Laser was applied to the palms of hands and soles of feet in 10 sessions over a 5-week period. Both groups improved, the laser group more and the effects were evident 3 months after treatment.

Tuberculosis

One claimed effect of laser is its value in treating tuberculosis. Lasers of many different types are used this way, including He–Ne, He–Cd and GaAs, particularly in Russia and in India. They are applied either to the skin over an affected area or, during a procedure, intrabronchially or intravenously. A Cochrane review on this topic (Vlassov et al., 2002) found no randomized or quasi-randomized trials on the topic and concluded that this use is not supported by any reliable evidence. Further, the reviewers noted the need for future studies to document the anti-tuberculous drugs used concurrently with the laser treatment.

EFFECTIVENESS OF LOW-INTENSITY LASER THERAPY

Basic biophysical principles indicate that if lasers are effective then coloured light should be even more effective, particularly if the appropriate filters are used. No studies have been identified which compare laser and coloured light exposure.

A few years ago the clinical usage of laser was reported as increasing in parts of Europe (Cambier and Vanderstraeten, 1997). The reasons why are not clear from the findings of the range of systematic reviews and individual studies described above. At best there is possibly an effect on pain and oedema reduction in humans. The size of the effect, the dosage parameters required and the durability of the effect are unclear. Also, no studies have been identified which compare the effectiveness of laser for treating types of pain with that of other electrophysical agents such as electrical stimulation or deep or superficial heating, or with commonly available analgesic medications. Nor have there been any comparisons between laser, which has a precise wavelength and ordinary coloured light, which has a broad spectrum of wavelengths.

The other issue is, there is considerable variation in the findings concerning the dosage and other parameters. This suggests that considerably more research is required on laser, especially research aimed at identifying a dose–response relationship. Identifying one and confirming the conditions under which it exists is very important to justify the continuing usage of low level laser in clinical practice.

Literature reviews of the effectiveness of low level laser therapy are either non-commital or slightly positive in their findings. There is also a possible publication bias, which means that positive findings are overrepresented in the set of studies available in the research literature.

Another problem with accepting the effectiveness of laser while the research findings remain mixed is the lack of an understood mechanism of action. This is especially so when the depth of penetration is low and the metabolic or systemic effects are little more than can be induced in other everyday ways.

The question of whether laser therapy works is thus unanswered. However, the use of light therapy for some mood and sleep disorders is known to be effective. No studies comparing the effect of laser and similarly coloured light or even white light on pain, using comparable dosages, have been identified. This is regrettable as it would help answer the question of whether the coherence and mono-chromaticity of laser beams are clinically important.

PRINCIPLES OF APPLICATION

Most low- or medium-power laser sources are applied to the skin by one of three methods:

- probe
- cluster probe
- scanning system.

A probe is a hand-held applicator the size of a large marker pen. It has one laser diode, close to the tip, which is a small lens. This is used in direct contact with the skin and can treat only a small area, less than $1 \, mm^2$, but its area of effect is usually accepted as being larger, up to $0.5 \, cm^2$ ($50 \, mm^2$) (Gourgouliatos, 1990). Whether this is justified remains unknown.

A cluster probe, as explained earlier, is a collection of individual laser diodes which all emit at different wavelengths. This takes advantage of any effects that may ensue from the use of different wavelengths. The advantage of a cluster diode is that it can be used to treat a larger area, approximately $25 \, cm^2$. This will depend on the size of an individual probe, but in a single application it can treat a considerably larger area than a probe with its single diode.

The third type of system used to apply laser is a scanning system. A laser applicator is attached to a stand up to 30 cm away from the skin. The applicator can have several sources of laser output and is moved either mechanically or manually in a systematic path over the area to be treated.

Technique of application

Stages

Patient

Explanation: explain the nature of the treatment and the need to wear wavelength specific goggles throughout the treatment to obviate any risk of accidental application of the laser beam into the eye (see below).

Apparatus

Position the laser apparatus and have goggles ready for the patient and operator (and anyone else in the immediate vicinity).

Preparation of the part

Clean the surface of the skin to be treated with an alcohol wipe to remove any material that might absorb or reflect the radiation. Support the part being treated so the patient is comfortable throughout and not likely to need to move.

Application

To obtain an output from a class 3B and sometimes a class 2 or 3A machine usually requires turning a key as well as switching on the power. This is a safety mechanism designed to ensure that unauthorized people do not accidentally switch the laser on, given the possible risk of eye damage.

The laser applicator is then applied to the skin surface before switching on the output. The applicator also usually has a switch and an indicator light to show when there is an output as this is not visible when using an infrared laser. The laser applicator is kept in contact with the tissues and held so that the beam is applied at right angles to achieve maximal penetration. There is usually also a switch in the timer so that the output ceases once the preset time is reached.

If contact by the probe (single or cluster) is not desirable, for example directly over a wound, the applicator may be held just above the surface or covered with transparent non-reflective film. In all other circumstances firm contact should be maintained throughout treatment but not so it causes pain if the area is tender. The position of the probe is maintained for the selected time.

The actual methods of application are as follows:

- single point or spotting
- gridding
- scanning.

As explained above, for the single point or spotting method of application the single or cluster probe is held on or immediately over the site. This might be along the edges of a wound (see Figure 16.7) or directly over a wound, over an acupuncture point or over a joint or an area of pain.

Gridding is typically used systematically to cover a larger area. The single or cluster probe is moved and repositioned on a new site after each single dosage is completed. This is done prior to setting the timer each time to ensure there is no output while the probe is moved. As Figure 16.7 shows, the probe is moved as though a grid were over the area being treated. A grid is marked, or visualized, on the skin or on a transparent cover used over a wound. The distance between grid spots may be varied but is usually no more than 1 cm for a single probe, depending on the size of the probe tip. A similar system may be used with a cluster probe if a large area is being treated, or a scanning system might be used.

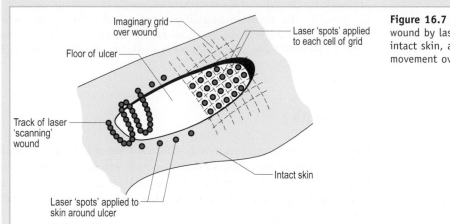

Imaginary grid over wound

Floor of ulcer

Track of laser 'scanning' wound

Laser 'spots' applied to each cell of grid

Laser 'spots' applied to skin around ulcer

Intact skin

Figure 16.7 The treatment of an open wound by laser 'spots' on a grid and on intact skin, as well as continuous movement over the lesion.

Scanning is used for a larger area again, such as the anterior surface of a limb. The laser applicator is moved systematically to cover the surface of the limb.

Termination

Switch the device off before removing the applicator from skin contact. The dosage parameters (including date, time, energy density, if gridding or other system used to treat, size and location of area) and any patient response, such as an immediate increase or decrease in pain, are noted and recorded.

DOSAGE

Dosage issues with low level laser have been canvassed by many researchers. Most reviews of laser effectiveness conclude that a major problem with many existing studies is the lack of dosage details provided. Further, one such review reported that dosages are often calculated wrongly and the methodological problems in studies range from heterogeneity of subjects to the use of inappropriate placebos and raises questions of clinical relevance of using laser to treat wounds in healthy tissue (Tuner and Hode, 1998). Until more methodologically and scientifically acceptable research is conducted and published, knowing how and when laser is effective will remain unknown, as will optimal dosage. This means the element of guesswork in laser dosages remains.

Despite this, it is important to discuss the variables that contribute to laser dosage. In general:

- the wavelength and
- the size of the area of application

are fixed by the type of laser apparatus used. The energy density can be varied by the duration of a single application of the probe and by varying the pulsing parameters. The size of the area treated is adjusted by the number of discrete applications made and also by the choice of probe (single or cluster).

Wavelength

Currently there is no research justification for selecting a particular wavelength to obtain a particular response. However, from physical principles we know that wavelength affects depth of penetration and can use that as a basis for wavelength selection. Consistent with that, GaAlAs lasers are probably used more commonly now because of their greater depth of penetration (810–940 nm, 3 to 4 mm) than He–Ne lasers (632.8 nm, 1 to 2 mm). Also, they typically have a higher power output. They can therefore be used to treat a greater variety of lesions at different depths. This is a benefit even with superficial skin lesions where the aim is to affect the cells in the floor of the wound and those a few millimetres deeper.

Energy density

The treatment dose is usually given in $J\,cm^{-2}$ (or $mJ\,cm^{-2}$) and called energy density or sometimes radiant exposure.

- The mean power output in milliwatts is usually fixed (it can be varied on some machines by altering the pulsing regimen).
- When divided by the (fixed) area of the beam it gives the power density or irradiance in $mW\,cm^{-2}$.
- When multiplied by the number of seconds for which the treatment is applied, it gives the number of $J\,cm^{-2}$ or energy density.

The recommended dosages typically range from 1 to $10\,J\,cm^{-2}$ but doses as low as $0.5\,J\,cm^{-2}$ and up to $48\,J\,cm^{-2}$ have been suggested. Initially $4\,J\,cm^{-2}$ was widely accepted as the upper level with a therapeutic 'window' for laser dosage between $0.5\,J\,cm^{-2}$ and $4\,J\,cm^{-2}$ (Laakso et al., 1993). However, as noted above, the evidence for specific 'windows' is questionable. Further, the lack of a clearly identified dose–response relationship suggests the following principles as the basis for establishing a dosage:

- initial treatment – start with a dosage less than $4\,J\,cm^{-2}$, adjust in next treatment according to patient response
- acute lesion – start with a lower dosage, less than $4\,J\,cm^{-2}$ and adjust in next treatment according to patient response
- chronic lesion – use a dosage between 4 and $50\,J\,cm^{-2}$
- deeper structures – use a higher dose to ensure some energy is remaining at the required depth of treatment.

Example:

Mean power = 10 mW

Beam area = $0.125\,cm^2$

Therefore power density = 10/0.125 = $80\,mW\,cm^{-2}$

If the treatment is applied for 50 s, the energy density = $80\,mW\,cm^{-2} \times 50\,s$ = $4000\,mJ\,cm^{-2} = 4\,J\,cm^{-2}$.

The final point on this aspect of dosage is there is a need for clinicians to keep reading current research to optimize dosage selection.

Pulsed output

On some machines the mean power output is always the same regardless of pulse frequency. This is achieved by adjusting the pulse duration so that the low pulse rates have long pulse lengths and the high rates have shorter pulse lengths. It is accepted practice that low pulse frequencies and long pulse durations are used for acute conditions and higher pulse repetition rates and short pulse durations for chronic conditions, but there is no scientific justification for this. On machines where the mean power output is constant the energy applied will not be altered by changing the pulsing.

The arguments presented for pulsed versus continuous beam lasers are similar to those for ultrasound but the evidence base is limited. The best evidence for this probably comes from the responses of bacteria of different types to pulsed and continuous laser. A laser (810 nm) applied to different types of bacterium, either continuously or pulsed at a frequency of 26 Hz, 292 Hz, 3.8 kHz or 1 kHz produced different rates of growth (Nussbaum et al., 2002). With the same energy density, between 1 and 10 J cm^{-2}, a frequency of 1 kHz and continuous laser consistently increased the number of *E. coli*. However, the extent of variability in the data, combined with decreases at 1, 5 and 10 J cm^{-2} when using a frequency of 3.8 kHz means the answer to questions of the effects of pulsed or continuous laser, or of different intensities of laser is still uncertain. Given the study appears to be a well controlled and systematic investigation, but that the responses of similar types of bacterium varied, the results are difficult to explain. Another study investigated the effects of He–Ne (632.8 nm) and InGaAlAs (670 nm) lasers on *Staphylococcus aureus* and *Pseudomonas aeruginosa* (DeSimone et al., 1999). Although the results were inconsistent, the higher dosages of the InGaAlAs laser, 2.5 to 10 J cm^{-2} produced greater growth inhibition.

Where the duty cycle (percentage of time the laser is on) varies, the mean power will also vary as the same proportion of peak power.

Area of treatment

Discrete lesions should be treated directly by applying laser over them. For wounds and large areas, the part is divided into centimetre squares (a grid) and each area is separately stimulated, or a scanning technique may be used in which the laser is moved continuously over the wound surface. Alternatively, the healthy skin at the edge of the wound can be stimulated with a series of applications (spotting) at usually 1 cm distances (see Figure 16.7). While the applicator is pressed firmly onto normal skin, for the treatment of open wounds it is held just above the wound or on a sterile clear plastic wrap over the wound. For painful areas, apply laser directly over the most tender or painful spots or over a trigger or acupuncture point (which may be one and the same).

Progression of treatment

If there is no response after one treatment the dose should be increased. No response after two or three treatments usually suggests that selecting an alternative method of treatment is appropriate.

There is no consensus about the optimum frequency of treatment.

Summary of dosage parameters

- Wavelength
  - fixed for a given laser
  - choice can affect the depth of penetration (note: 1–2 mm for He–Ne versus 3–4 mm for GaAlAs)
- Area treated
  - cross-section of single beam
  - repeated applications of single beam
  - continuous movement of single beam (scanning)
  - collection of laser diodes (cluster diode probes)
- Mean power (in mW)
  - fixed
  - variable by laser control
  - by pulsing
- Duration of application (in seconds)
  - determines the energy density in $J\,cm^{-2}$
- Pulsing (in Hz) – may have special effects
- Frequency of treatment – unknown and should be regulated by results.

DANGERS AND CONTRAINDICATIONS

The retina is especially vulnerable to absorbing light at 400 to 1400 nm (retinal hazard region) because it is melanin rich.

The main danger involving low level laser therapy is a risk of damage if the beam is applied directly into the eye. As therapeutic lasers have very little power there is normally no thermal effect when it is applied to the skin. However, if it passes through the cornea and lens of the eye, the beam can become focused on a very small area (as small as 10 to 20 µm) and cause local intense heating and even total loss of vision in that eye. Although the risk to humans posed by therapeutic lasers (especially classes 2 and 3A) is small, shining a laser into the eye or looking directly into the laser beam should always be strictly avoided. With rabbits, the threshold for corneal damage appears to be $56 \, J \, cm^{-2}$ for 1540 nm laser, a type used most commonly for range finding and in military systems (Clarke et al., 2002). Rabbits' eyes are similar to humans but not identical.

Extended exposure of skin to laser is unlikely to be a risk in humans. A study evaluated the effect of laser on pigs (Jensen-Waern and Ekman, 2000). Laser was applied daily for 2 weeks using a 30-diode probe with either 956 nm (12 minutes) or 637 nm laser (18 minutes). The dosage was $6.3 \, J \, cm^{-2}$. No morphological changes other than the minor abnormalities found in treated and untreated pigs were identified. Pigs were used as their skin structure is similar to that of humans. This finding is consistent with the accepted wisdom that low level laser does not produce adverse effects in the skin of humans.

Reasonable precautions

Eye protection

Although any risk to the eye is small, the following are often advised:

- use laser devices in specially designated areas
- avoid reflecting the laser beam from shiny surfaces
- switch the laser on only when the applicator is in contact with the skin.

Wear appropriate protective glasses or goggles: the therapist and patient should always wear protective eye wear when using class 3B and it is advisable to do so for classes 2 and 3A. Some authorities require a notice is on display outside the immediate treatment area warning that a laser is in use. However, this is unusual for a laser below class 4.

Tumours

Avoid treatment over known tumours or recently irradiated areas. The level of risk of effecting malignant cell growth or metastasization is unknown.

Infection

Always clean the contact area of any probe immediately after use with a recommended method such as an alcohol wipe and air drying. This is especially critical if treating wounds.

Contraindications

These include treatment directly over:

- tumours and recently irradiated areas
- the pregnant uterus. The level of risk to the fetus is likely to be very low but, as adverse consequences could be serious, is probably currently justified.

References

Al-Awami, M., Schillinger, M., Maca, T. et al. (2004). Low level laser therapy for treatment of primary and secondary Raynaud's phenomenon. VASA, **33**, 25–29.

Bain, J., Rusch, H., Kline, B. (1943). The effect of temperature upon ultraviolet carcinogenesis with wavelength 2,800–3,400 Å. Cancer Res, **3**, 610–612.

Basford, J. (1999). Laser therapy: a randomised controlled trial of the effects of low-intensity NdYAG laser irradiation on musculoskeletal back pain. Arch Phys Med Rehabil, **80**, 647–652.

Basford, J., Sheffield, C., Cieslak, K. (2000). Laser therapy: a randomized, controlled trial of the effects of low intensity Nd:YAG laser irradiation on lateral epicondylitis. Arch Phys Med Rehabil, **81**, 1504–1510.

Baxter, G. D. (ed.) (1994). Therapeutic Lasers: Theory and Practice. Edinburgh: Churchill Livingstone.

Baxter, G., Bell, A., Allen, J., Ravey, R. (1991). Laser mediated increases in nerve conduction latencies: long term effects. WCPT 11th Int Congress Proc, Book II, London: World Confederation for Physical Therapy, 747–749.

Bjordal, J., Couppe, C., Chow, R. et al. (2003). A systematic review of low level laser therapy with location-specific doses for pain from chronic joint disorders. Aust J Physiother, **49**, 107–116.

Brosseau, L., Welch, V., Wells, G. et al. (2004a). Low level laser therapy (Classes I, II and III) for treating osteoarthritis. The Cochrane Library, 4.

Brosseau, L., Welch, V., Wells, G. et al. (2004b). Low level laser therapy (Classes I, II and III) for treating rheumatoid arthritis. The Cochrane Library, 4.

Cambier, D., Vanderstraeten, G. (1997). Low level laser therapy: the experience in Flanders. Eur J Phys Med Rehabil, **7**, 102–105.

Carati, C., Anderson, S., Gannon, B., Piller, N. (2003). Treatment of postmastectomy lymphedema with low-level laser therapy. Cancer, **98**, 1114–1122.

Clarke, T., Johnson, T., Burton, M. et al. (2002). Corneal injury threshold in rabbits for the 1540 nm infrared laser. Aviation Space Environ Med, **73**, 787–790.

Craig, J., Bradley, J., Walsh, D., Baxter, G., Allen, J. (1999). Lack of effect of combined low intensity laser therapy/phototherapy (CLICT) on delayed onset muscle soreness in humans. Lasers Surg Med, **24**, 223–230.

Crockford, G., Hellon, R. (1959). Vascular responses of human skin to infra-red radiation. J Physiol, **149**, 424–432.

de Bie, R., de Vet, H., Lenssen, T. et al. (1998). Low-level laser therapy in ankle sprains: a randomized clinical trial. Arch Phys Med Rehabil, **79**, 1415–1420.

DeSimone, N., Christiansen, C., Dore, D. (1999). Bactericidal effect of 0.95-mW helium-neon and 5-mW indium-gallium-aluminum-phosphate laser irradiation at exposure times of 30, 60, and 120 seconds on photosensitized *Staphylococcus aureus* and *Pseudomonas aeruginosa* in vitro. Phys Ther, **79**, 839–846.

Diamantopoulos, C. (1994). Bioenergetics and tissue optics. In G. D. Baxter (ed.), Therapeutic Lasers: Theory and Practice, pp. 67–88. Edinburgh: Churchill Livingstone,

Fargas-Babjak, A. (2001). Acupuncture, transcutaneous electrical nerve stimulation, and laser therapy in chronic pain. Clin J Pain, **17**, S105–113.

Fisher, B., Rennie, S., Warren, S. et al. (2000). The effects of low power laser therapy on muscle healing following acute blunt trauma. J Phys Ther Sci, **12**, 49–55.

Flemming, K., Cullum, N. (2004). Laser therapy for venous leg ulcers. The Cochrane Library, 4.

Forbes, D., Morgan, D., Bangma, J. et al. (2004). Light therapy for managing sleep, behaviour, and mood disturbances in dementia. Cochrane Database Syst Rev, 2.

Forster, A., Palastanga, N. (1985). Clayton's Electrotherapy: Theory and Practice, 9th edn. London: Baillière Tindall.

Glasgow, P., Hill, I., McKevitt, A. et al. (2001). Low intensity monochromatic infrared therapy: a preliminary study of the effects of a novel treatment unit upon experimental muscle soreness. Lasers Surg Med, **28**, 33–39.

Gourgouliatos, Z. (1990). Application of the Monte Carlo model in the investigation of the direct penetration of light produced by single and multiple wavelength diode cluster probes. 4th Int Biotherapy Laser Assoc. Seminar on Laser Biomodulation, Guy's Hospital, London.

Gur, A., Cosut, A., Sarac, A. et al. (2003). Efficacy of different therapy regimes of low-power laser in painful osteoarthritis of the knee: a double-blind and randomized-controlled trial. Lasers Surg Med, **33**, 330–338.

Hakguder, A., Birtane, M., Gurcan, S. et al. (2003). Efficacy of low level laser therapy in myofascial pain syndrome: an algometric and thermographic evaluation. Lasers Surg Med, **33**, 339–343.

Harlen, F. (1982). Physics of infrared and microwave therapy. In M. F. Docker (ed.), Physics in Physiotherapy, p. 18. London: Hospital Physicists Association Conference report series 35.

Harley, O., Dziewulski, P. (2003). Accidental burns caused by domestic infra-red muscle massaging device. Burns, **29**, 173–174.

Hasson, S., Williams, J., Gadberry, W., Henrich, T. (1989). Viewing low and high wavelength light. Effect on EMG activity and force production during maximal voluntary handgrip contraction. Physiother Can, **41**, 32–35.

Irvine, J., Chong, S., Amirjani, N., Chan, K. (2004). Double-blind randomized controlled trial of low-level laser therapy in carpal tunnel syndrome. Musc Nerve, **30**, 182–187.

Jensen-Waern, M., Ekman, S. (2000). Effects of a 2-week treatment with pulsed monochromatic light in healthy pigs: a clinical and morphological study. Photodermatol Photoimmunol Photomed, **16**, 178–182.

Karu, T. (1989). Photobiology of low-power laser effects. Health Phys, **56**, 691–704.

King, P. (1989). Low level laser therapy – a review. Laser Med Sci, **4**, 141–150.

Laakso, E., Cramond, T., Richardson, C., Galligan, J. (1994). Plasma ACTH and beta-endorphin levels in response to low level laser therapy (LLLT) for myofascial trigger points. Laser Ther, **6**, 133–142.

Laakso, E., Richardson, C., Cramond, T. (1997). Pain scores and side effects in response to low level laser therapy (LLLT) for myofascial trigger points. Laser Ther, **9**, 67–72.

Laakso, L., Richardson, C., Cramond, T. (1993). Factors affecting low level laser therapy. Aust J Physiother, **39**, 95–99.

Laurens, H. (1933). The Physiological Effects of Radiant Energy. New York: Chemical Catalog.

Lehmann, J., de Lateur, B. (1982). Therapeutic heat. In J. F. Lehmann (ed.), Therapeutic Heat and Cold, pp. 404–562. Baltimore: Williams & Wilkins.

Lindsay, D., Dearness, J., McGinley, C. (1995). Electrotherapy usage trends in private physiotherapy practice in Alberta. Physiother Can, **47**, 30–34.

Lipper, G., Anderson, R. (2003). Lasers in dermatology. In I. Freedberg, A. Eisen, K. Wolff, K. Austen, L. Goldsmith, S. Katz (eds), Fitzpatrick's Dermatology in General Medicine, 6th edn, Vol. 2, pp. 2493–2515. New York: McGraw-Hill.

Lowe, A., McDowell, B., Walsh, D. et al. (1997). Failure to demonstrate any hypoalgesic effect of low intensity laser irradiation (830 nm) of Erb's point upon experimental ischaemic pain in humans. Lasers Surg Med, **20**, 69–76.

Lucas, C., Criens-Poublon, L., Cockrell, C., de Haan, R. (2002). Wound healing in cell studies and animal model experiments by low level laser therapy; were clinical studies justified? A systematic review. Lasers Med Sci, **17**, 110–134.

Madura, T., Kubo, T., Yano, K., Hosokawa, K. (2002). Thermal injury to replanted finger caused by infrared rays. Ann Plastic Surgery, **48**, 448–449.

Martiny, K., Simonsen, C., Lunde, M. et al. (2004). Decreasing TSH levels in patients with Seasonal Affective Disorder (SAD) responding to 1 week of bright light therapy. J Affect Disord, **79**, 253–257.

Mendez, T., Pinheiro, A., Pacheco, M. et al. (2004). Dose and wavelength of laser light have influence on the repair of cutaneous wounds. J Clin Lasers Med Surg, **22**, 19–25.

Mester, E., Mester, A., Mester, A. (1985). The biomedical effect of laser application. Lasers Surg Med, **5**, 31–39.

Nightingale, A. (1959). Physics and Electronics in Physical Medicine. London: G. Bell.

Nussbaum, E., Van Zuylen, J., Baxter, G. (1999). Specification of treatment dosage in laser therapy: unreliable equipment and radiant power determination as confounding factors. Physiother Can, **51**, 159–167.

Nussbaum, E., Lilge, L., Massulli, T. (2002). Effects of 810 nm laser irradiation on in vitro growth of bacteria: comparison of continuous wave and frequency modulated light. Lasers Surg Med, **31**, 343–351.

Ong, K., Ho, V. (2001). Pain reduction by low level laser therapy: a double-blind, controlled, randomized study in bilaterally symmetrical oral surgery. Am J Pain Management, **11**, 12–16.

Ozdemir, F., Birtane, M., Kokino, S. (2001). The clinical efficacy or low-power laser therpay on pain and function in cervical osteoarthritis. Clin Rheumatol, **20**, 181–184.

Petersen, S., Botes, C., Olivier, A., Guthrie, A. (1999). The effect of low level laser therapy (LLLT) on wound healing in horses. Equine Vet J, **31**, 228–231.

Pope, G., Mockett, S., Wright, J. (1995). A survey of electrotherapeutic modalities: ownership and use in the NHS in England. Physiotherapy, **81**, 82–91.

Reddy, G., Stehno-Bittel, L., Enwemeka, C. (1998). Laser photostimulation of collagen production in healing rabbit Achilles tendons. Lasers Surg Med, **22**, 281–287.

Robertson, V., Spurritt, D. (1998). Electrophysical agents: Implications of EPA availability and use in undergraduate clinical placements. Physiotherapy, **84**, 335–344.

Rohan, K., Lindsey, K., Roecklein, K., Lacy, T. (2004). Cognitive-behavioral therapy, light therapy, and their combination in treating seasonal affective disorder. J Affect Disord, **80**, 273–283.

Schieke, S., Schroeder, P., Krutmann, J. (2003). Cutaneous effects of infrared radiation: from clinical observations to molecular response mechanisms. Photodermatol Photoimmunol Photomed, **19**, 228–234.

Schindl, A., Neumann, R. (1999). Low-intensity laser therapy is an effective treatment for recurrent herpes simplex infection. Results from a randomized double-blind placebo-controlled study [see comments]. J Invest Dermatol, **113**, 221–223.

Sisto, R., Pinto, I., Stacchini, N., Giuliani, F. (2000). Infrared radiation exposure in traditional glass factories. J Sci Occ Environ Hlth Safety, **61**, 5–10.

Skjerve, A., Bjorvatn, B., Holsten, F. (2004). Light therapy for behavioural and psychological symptoms of dementia. Int J Geriatr Psychiatr, **19**, 516–522.

Soriano, F., Rios, R. (1998). GA laser treatment of chronic low back pain: a prospective, randomised and double blind study. Laser Therapy, **10**, 175–180.

Stergioulas, A. (2004). Low-level laser treatment can reduce edema in second degree ankle sprains. J Clin Laser Med Surg, **22**, 125–128.

Taly, A., Nair, K., Murali, T., John, A. (2004). Efficacy of multiwavelength light therapy in the treatment of pressure ulcers in subjects with disorders of the spinal cord: a randomized double-blind controlled trial. Arch Phys Med Rehabil, **85**, 1657–1661.

Tuner, J., Hode, L. (1998). It's all in the parameters: a critical analysis of some well-known negative studies on low-level laser therapy. J Clin Laser Med Surg, **16**, 245–248.

Van Breugel, H. (1992). A Monte Carlo model for laser light distribution in tissue: effects of intensity profile and divergence of the laser beam [abstract]. 2nd Meeting of the International Laser Therapy Association, London: International Laser Therapy Association, 18–20 September, 33.

Vlassov, V., Pechatnikov, L., MacLehose, H. (2002). Low level laser therapy for treating tuberculosis. Cochrane Database Syst Rev 4.

Wadsworth, H., Chanmugan, A. (1980). Electrophysical Agents in Physiotherapy: Therapeutic and Diagnostic Use. Marrickville, NSW: Science Press.

Ward, A. (2004). Biophysical Bases of Electrotherapy. Mt Waverley, Vic, Australia: Excell Biomedical Publications. (On the CD which comes with this book).

Weintraub, M. (1997). Noninvasive laser neurolysis in carpal tunnel syndrome. Musc Nerve, **20**, 629–631.

Young, S., Bolton, P., Dyson, M. et al. (1989). Macrophage responsiveness to light therapy. Lasers Surg Med, **9**, 497–505.

Ultraviolet radiation

Invisible radiation beyond the violet end of the visible spectrum was termed 'ultravioletten' by Johann Ritter in 1801. This type of radiation causes sunburn and tanning of the skin on exposure to the sun and has wavelengths smaller than those of visible light.

The benefit of natural sunlight for healing has been documented over many years. It can, perhaps, be traced to the worship of sun gods in almost all ancient cultures (Licht, 1983). However, there is a distinct paucity of accounts of the therapeutic usage of sunlight emanating from the period of the Middle Ages. Licht (1983) ascribes this to the rise of Christianity which suppressed 'all pagan practices including sun worship and sun bathing' in many European cultures. About the middle of the 19th century a great interest developed in the use of heliotherapy. Later, therapeutic usage increased as artificial sources of ultraviolet radiation (UVR) were developed.

In the early 20th century the relative success of UVR treatment for tuberculosis, rickets and infections led to therapeutic applications for a plethora of pathologies. By the middle of the 20th century the advent of antibiotic and other drug treatments had superseded many uses of UVR therapies and usage of UVR diminished. Also, knowledge of the long-term risks associated with using UVR increased. At the same time the drug options available to treat conditions previously treated only with UVR increased in number and effectiveness. This has meant that, in some countries, the use of UVR outside dermatology practices and suntan parlours is no longer as widespread as previously.

More recently, it has been recognized that the situation is not so unequivocal. UVR exposure is ultimately harmful and the damage is cumulative. Nonetheless it is essential for normal body function. The therapist must balance the longer-term hazards against the shorter-term benefits. UVR still has an important role in the management of some conditions, sometimes alone and sometimes in association with drugs such as photosensitizers and anti-inflammatories.

In this chapter, the nature and production of therapeutic UVR is considered along with a brief description of skin structure and of the physiological effects on it of UVR. An outline of the therapeutic uses is followed by a discussion of skin responses to treatment using UVR,

Using UVR therapy involves a risk/benefit analysis which, in many instances, favours its use. Dosage (both immediate and cumulative) is the important factor in the analysis.

Table 17.1 Classification of ultraviolet radiation

Region	Wavelength (nm)	Other names
Biotic		
UVA	400–315	Long UV, blacklight
UVB	315–280	Medium UV, erythemal UV
Abiotic		
UVC	280–100	Short UV, germicidal UV

treatment principles and then the contraindications. Finally, comment is added on the use of heliotherapy and sunbeds.

THE NATURE OF ULTRAVIOLET RADIATION

Ultraviolet radiation (UVR) behaves in a similar way to visible light in the way it is reflected, refracted or absorbed, except that it is more strongly absorbed, both in air and in biological tissue. Shorter wavelength ultraviolet radiation is most strongly absorbed. Another difference is that UVR transmits much more energy than visible radiation (see chapter 14) and can provoke chemical changes, and not simply heat, at sites where it is absorbed.

The ultraviolet spectrum is divided into three regions: A, B and C. The wavelength ranges of these regions are internationally agreed and are those endorsed by the National Radiological Protection Board in the UK (Table 17.1). Some variations are given in other sources (Walker et al., 2003).

As already noted, UVR is usually described in terms of its wavelength, extending down from the violet end of the visible spectrum at 390–400 nm to the soft X-ray region, which is below 100 nm.

The UV wavelength range corresponds to a frequency range from 0.75×10^{15} Hz at 400 nm to 3×10^{15} Hz at 100 nm. UVA borders the visible spectrum and has the lowest of UV frequencies, UVB is shorter wavelength (and higher frequency) and UVC has shorter wavelengths (and higher frequencies) still.

Radiation of wavelengths between 200 and 100 nm, and sometimes below, are often called 'vacuum UV' because, being rapidly absorbed in air, they can only be effectively passed in a vacuum. Consistent with this, oxygen and ozone in the stratosphere screen out UVC and much UVB from the sun's radiation. At the earth's surface approximately 95 to 98% of solar UV is UVA, 2 to 5%, UVB and no UVC (Walker et al., 2003).

The meaning and derivation of certain terms used in the description of UVR are summarized in Table 17.2.

Ultraviolet, like any other form of electromagnetic radiation, is progressively absorbed in matter. It has a very low penetration depth in biological tissues and so is absorbed superficially (in the skin).

Table 17.2 The meaning and derivation of certain terms

Term	Derivation	Meaning
Radiation	Probably from Aton Ra, Egyptian Sun god	Emission of any waves or particles; usually applied to EM spectrum
Heliotherapy	Helios: Greek god of the Sun	Treatment by means of the sun's radiation
Actinic radiation	*Aktis* = a ray (Greek)	Radiation that can cause a photochemical reaction: visible, UVR, X-ray and near IR
Actinotherapy		Treatment with actinic radiation
Phototherapy	*Phos* = light (Greek)	Treatment with UVR and visible radiation
Photobiomodulation		Biological effects of light on tissues

PRODUCTION OF UVR

Incandescent sources like the sun can produce UVR if their temperature is high enough. However, clinically, UVR is usually produced by the passage of a current through an ionized vapour – normally mercury vapour. To conduct current in gases requires a high temperature and/or low pressure in the containing tube.

Principle of working of a mercury vapour lamp

Applying a voltage across a pair of electrodes sealed into a UV transmitting quartz tube containing a little mercury vapour (Figure 17.1) will cause free electrons to accelerate. Collisions between electrons and mercury atoms cause the formation of free mercury ions and more electrons. The electrons, in turn, are accelerated and collide with more mercury atoms, producing an avalanche of accelerated electrons and mercury ions – an (increasing) electric current is produced. This process needs a high voltage to start (to produce the first few ions and free electrons) but, once started, the current flow must be controlled and limited. Current flow, once initiated, will continue with a lower voltage and a current-limiting power supply is used to reduce the voltage and so limit the amount of current.

When free electrons are being accelerated in the tube, many collisions with neutral mercury vapour atoms will occur:

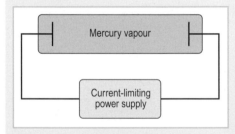

Figure 17.1 Schematic diagram of a mercury-vapour lamp.

Figure 17.2 Spectrum of electromagnetic radiation emitted by UVA and UVB fluorescent lamps and occuring naturally in sunlight.

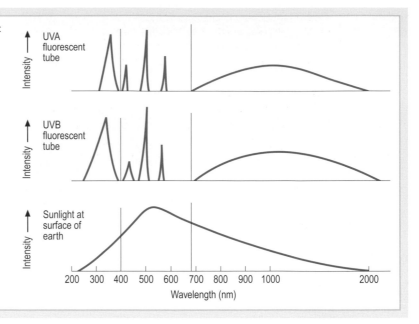

- by elastic collisions not affecting the atom's electrons
- by knocking an electron out of its orbital, completely separating it from the atom – ionization
- by kicking an electron into a higher orbital (energy level) – excitation.

The elastic collisions heat up the mercury vapour, causing it to emit a broad range of infrared radiation (Figure 17.2). The jumping of electrons from one orbital to another is responsible for the peaks in the visible and UV parts of the spectrum. Molecular vibration is responsible for the broad peak at longer wavelengths.

When excited electrons return to their normal energy level, the energy they lose is emitted as a photon of a characteristic wavelength for that particular transition (see chapter 14). The photon wavelengths given off by mercury atoms are in the green-blue-violet end of the visible spectrum and in the ultraviolet. The spectrum produced and its intensity may be modified by using different lamp pressures and by the addition of traces of metal halides, such as lead iodide. It is also filtered by the quartz or special glass envelope of the tube. Figure 17.2 shows the spectrum of electromagnetic radiation emitted by UVA and UVB fluorescent tubes. The spectrum of natural sunlight is shown for comparison.

Fluorescent lamps

These are low-pressure mercury discharge tubes with a phosphor coating on the inside. This layer absorbs short UVR and causes excitation of the phosphor atoms and re-emission at a longer wavelength, i.e. fluorescence. The particular wavelengths and the amount of each emitted will depend on the composition of the phosphor used. (The phosphor coatings are mixtures of phosphates, borates and silicates.)

The output of these lamps also varies with their operating temperature. Most give an optimal output with the outside of the tube at about 40°C. Such tubes are familiar as standard fluorescent lighting tubes. The tubes used clinically for ultraviolet treatments are identical in size and shape but the special phosphor coating in the tube means it produces a continuous spectrum between 250–280 nm and 380 nm (with a peak at 313 nm) and specific frequencies in the blue and green visible part of the spectrum (see Figure 17.2; see also Diffey, 1982), i.e. the output contains UVA and UVB and no UVC.

The same type of tube is used to produce large amounts of UVA radiation for use in the treatment of psoriasis. In this case, UVA is used in conjunction with a sensitizer called a psoralen, which makes the skin extremely sensitive to UVA radiation.

Psoralen-UVA or PUVA treatment is described in more detail later in this chapter.

For UVA tubes, the phosphor coating is different and the emission is from 315 to 400 nm. There are also several emission lines (particular frequencies) in the blue and green visible region (see Figure 17.2).

A reflecting layer is normally applied between the glass envelope and the phosphor layer over more than half the circumference of the tube along its length. This ensures that the radiation is largely directed forwards and when several of these tubes are packed together side by side they provide an almost uniform emission; a 'wall of light'. A number of tubes (48 in one type) are fixed in the walls of a treatment cabinet in which the patient stands to receive all-round body irradiation.

Another more recent development is the availability of narrow band fluorescent tubes. These have a wavelength of 311 nm (UVB) and are used in a similar way to the older types of tubes. The difference is that the specificity helps reduce the overall dose of UVR required to treat a range of skin disorders including those currently treated using the PUVA regimen (Krutmann and Morita, 2003). The wavelength is the same as that known as the 'action spectrum' for psoriasis. The output does include some UVA (20%) but is predominantly UVB (80%) (Kochevar and Taylor, 2003).

For whole body treatments long fluorescent tubes of the selected wavelength are mounted in semi-cylindrical tunnels, bed and canopy arrangements or cylindrical cubicles. Shorter tubes are mounted in other configurations for local treatments.

These fluorescent lamps also all emit visible radiation when operating. The visible bluish-white light has no relation to the level of ultraviolet being emitted.

All fluorescent tubes also have a slight fall in output during their working lives. This is trivial for fluorescent lighting tubes but the ultraviolet lamps use less stable phosphors so their useful life is usually limited to about 1000 hours.

One such option is the 'Theraktin tunnel', consisting of four 120 cm length tubes mounted in a semicircular assembly. This can be wheeled into position and raised or lowered over a couch. However, the small number of tubes results in low irradiance and uneven skin exposure, especially at the sides of the trunk.

Table 17.3 The major spectral lines emitted by medium-pressure mercury vapour arc lamps (from Diffey, 1982)

Wavelength (nm)	Radiation
578	Visible
546	Visible
436	Visible
405	Visible
365	UVA
334	UVA
313	UVB
302	UVB
297	UVB
265	UVC
254	UVC

Medium-pressure mercury arc lamps – the Alpine sunlamp

By analogy with the UV-rich sunlight in high altitude parts of the world (regions normally above any cloud cover, which absorbs UV) these lamps are called 'high-altitude' lamps (*Höhensonne* in German), hence the name Alpine sunlamp. The spectral line frequencies emitted are in the UV and visible regions as shown in Table 17.3. As with fluorescent lamps (see Figure 17.2), a broad range of infrared radiation is also produced. The amount of infrared is greater than that produced by low-pressure tubes because of the higher gas density which results in more frequent collisions with, and between, atoms. The temperatures produced are higher and the broad band of infrared radiation extends into the visible region of the spectrum because of the higher operating temperature. One consequence of the higher temperature is that there is a risk of burns: the amount of infrared radiation ('radiant heat') precludes placement close to the skin unless the lamp is cooled.

In addition, short wavelength UVR is produced and it reacts with oxygen in the air to produce small amounts of ozone (O_3). This is evident from the smell, which is noticeable even at very low concentrations. Since ozone is toxic at high concentrations, the ventilation must be adequate around these lamps. Some lamps are designed not to emit ozone-producing ultraviolet below 270 nm.

The Alpine lamp has a U-shaped tube. The U-tube is set inside a parabolic reflector. This is supported on an adjustable stand and is usually applied at a distance of 45 or 50 cm. The parabolic reflector is used to produce a beam of radiation which can be directed at the part of the patient to be treated. The reflector directs the radiation but the intensity across the beam is not uniform.

A UVR beam is not like that of a searchlight, which has relatively uniform intensity across the beam. Like a car headlamp, it spreads and is weaker in the periphery than at the centre.

All mercury vapour lamps require a 'kick-start' (a brief high-voltage pulse) to the tube to get them started. This causes argon atoms present in the mercury-vapour tube to become ionized. The high charge displaces an outer orbital electron from several argon atoms, leaving them as positive ions. The presence of sufficient free positive ions and electrons allows the flow of current. The small quantity of mercury – a drop of liquid at normal temperature – is rapidly vaporized due to the heat generated by the passage of current. Over the 5 minutes or so it takes for the mercury atoms to ionize fully, the spectral emission output changes to that described above.

There are marked ageing changes in the output of Alpine lamps. For this reason the correct exposure time with one lamp will be quite different to that of another lamp which is ostensibly the same.

For more information on reflectors and beam shape, see chapter 11 of the book 'Biophysical Bases of Electrotherapy' on the CD which comes with this book.

The Kromayer lamp

The Kromayer lamp is a hand-held gun which emits a beam of UVR. It is designed for use in direct contact with tissue; either the skin surface or body cavities. The lamp is a medium-pressure, mercury-vapour tube. The tube is normally coiled or U-shaped, and of small diameter, so as to occupy a small volume. The UVR emitting tube is mounted in, and so surrounded by, a water jacket which traps and absorbs infrared radiation. The jacket allows the visible and UVR to pass while cooling the handpiece applicator and filtering out the infrared radiation which would otherwise cause a heat burn.

Many uses of the Kromayer lamp have been replaced by treatment with local and systemic antibiotics but it may be that this treatment will become more popular as antibiotics lose their effectiveness.

Summary

UVR for therapy is produced by excitation of mercury atoms in:

- fluorescent tubes – the output is determined by the nature of the phosphor coating. There are various lamp configurations, usually for whole body irradiation in vertical cabinets or horizontal 'beds'. Vertical cabinet irradiation is more efficient as the whole body can be exposed.
- medium-pressure mercury arc lamps:
  - the Alpine sunlamp. These lamps are well suited for treatment of smaller areas of tissue (smaller than the whole body), e.g. the leg or the forearm.
  - the Kromayer lamp is water-cooled and so can be used in direct contact with body tissue. It is best suited for localized treatment involving small areas, such as a particular region of the skin, which have treatable lesions.

MEASUREMENT OF UVR

The output of a UV lamp is normally specified in terms of its irradiance, which is the output power per unit area. The standard unit of irradiance is the watt per square metre ($W\,m^{-2}$) but UV lamp irradiance is normally stated in watts per square centimetre ($W\,cm^{-2}$). Both the irradiance and the wavelength outputs of UVR lamps are quantifiable. A device called a photometer is used to measure irradiance and by using filters the output over specific wavelength ranges can be measured.

The 'radiant exposure' is the irradiance ($W\,cm^{-2}$) multiplied by the time of exposure (in seconds). The units of radiant exposure are thus joules per square centimetre ($J\,cm^{-2}$):

$$\text{Radiant exposure } (J\,cm^{-2}) = \text{Irradiance } (W\,cm^{-2}) \times \text{Time of exposure (s)}$$
$$\text{Irradiance} = \text{Power delivered per unit area } (W\,cm^{-2})$$

NORMAL SKIN – A REVIEW OF STRUCTURE AND ACTIVITY

Epidermis

The epidermis and dermis overlie the subcutaneous fat layer which provides the body with thermal insulation and protection against some types of mechanical trauma, such as blunt penetration. The epidermis is itself avascular but cells near the base receive oxygen and nutrients by diffusion from the (vascular) dermis which provides a strong and flexible base (see Figures 10.3 and 17.3). As cells are displaced towards the skin surface, their nutrient supply is reduced and the cells eventually die.

The epidermis is a dynamic structure in which cells are constantly dividing and maturing as they migrate towards the skin surface. As Figure 17.3 shows, the epidermis has four layers: basal, spinous (mid

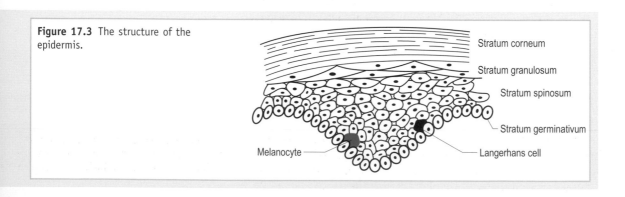

Figure 17.3 The structure of the epidermis.

epidermis), granular and stratum corneum. The basal layer, the stratum germinativum, is where cell division, or mitosis, continuously takes place. After mitosis in the basal layer the daughter keratinocytes are displaced towards the skin surface and proceed through their life cycle until eventually lost from the skin surface as hard dry keratin flakes. The continual process of skin flaking-off the stratum corneum is called desquamation.

At least 80% of epidermal cells are keratinocytes which synthesize and store the fibrous protein, keratin. The others include melanocytes (pigment-producing cells), Langerhans cells (cells of the immune system) and stem cells (undifferentiated cells with the potential to develop into any kind of specialized cell).

The average time for a cell to pass from the basal layer to be shed as a keratin flake at the surface, the stratum corneum, is called the epidermal transit time and takes about 28 days (Chu et al., 2003) but can be longer, up to 45–70 days. If the transit time remains constant but the rate of mitosis speeds up, i.e. the cell turnover time is decreased, the skin will be thickened. The rate of basal cell division is controlled by a variety of factors including friction on the skin surface. Also, the loss of skin integrity provokes keratinocyte activity, as does UVR.

Fingernails and hair are almost pure keratin. The specialized cells which produce these structures extrude keratin to form an extracellular matrix, unlike keratinocytes which store keratin in the cytosol.

Stratum corneum

The outer layer of the epidermis is the stratum corneum, a layer of dead keratinocytes. As indicated in chapter 10, its principal role is to prevent water loss from the body. A secondary role is to act as a defence against infection, preventing entry of bacteria and viruses. The stratum corneum also protects the body against some mechanical forces, repels water and filters UVR.

As a keratinized epithelium it is pliable while wet but becomes harder and more brittle on drying. Hydrating it by trapping moisture in the surface by putting oils or grease on the skin, as described in connection with wax treatment in chapter 11, will make it soft and pliable. The sebaceous glands which pass through the stratum corneum produce sebum. This helps with waterproofing and has a mild fungicide function. Also, the hairs and hair follicles which pass through the stratum corneum have sensory functions, adding to the considerable importance of the epithelium to a body.

Pigmentation

The pigment melanin determines hair, skin and eye colour and absorbs UVR. It is produced by melanocytes in the basal layer of the epidermis. This means that skin colour is determined by the normal level of activity of melanocytes. Their number varies with location in the

Melanocytes, like keratinocytes, are pushed towards the skin surface and suffer death by starvation followed, eventually, by desquamation.

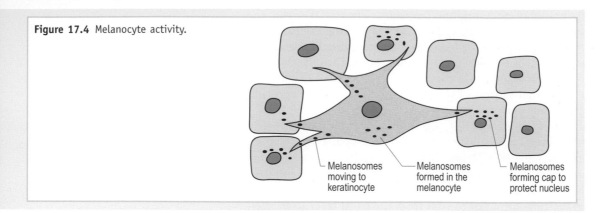

Figure 17.4 Melanocyte activity.

Melanosomes moving to keratinocyte

Melanosomes formed in the melanocyte

Melanosomes forming cap to protect nucleus

body, but not with racial background. In fair-skinned individuals, the melanocyte activity is down-regulated.

Melanin is formed in special organelles, called melanosomes, which can pass along dendritic processes of the melanocytes to enter the neighbouring keratinocytes. Melanocytes thus distribute pigment (in the basal layer in particular) and help protect the keratinocytes from potentially harmful UVR. In the keratinocytes, melanosomes cluster over the nucleus forming a protective cap – a sort of umbrella – which absorbs UVR before it can reach the DNA of the nucleus (Figure 17.4).

Melanocyte activity is stimulated by UVR (290–400 nm). The mechanism is not fully understood but involves enzymic activity and hormones, melanocyte-stimulating hormone from the pituitary, adrenocorticotrophic hormone and oestrogen.

The extent of tanning depends on the type of UVR, the dose of ultraviolet applied and the pigmentation proclivity of the individual. It is the outcome of the formation of melanin in the epidermis and the migration of existing melanin into more superficial layers. This process is usually noticeable about 2 days after exposure. Immediate tanning occurs in some individuals, as a result of effects on pre-existing melanin precursor molecules after exposure to UVA.

Pigmentation is strongly stimulated by erythema-producing UVB at about 300 nm and also, to a lesser extent, by longer wavelengths in UVA and even into the visible spectrum (Diffey, 1982). Thus sunbeds, which emit UVA and visible radiation, can induce a tan without the erythema, although an erythema will occur at sufficiently high doses or if the patient has taken a sensitizer (see section on PUVA). The increased melanin content of the skin affords protection by preventing UVR reaching the lower layers of the epidermis where the dividing keratinocytes are situated. This protective effect is aided by the skin thickening that also occurs.

Summary

- The epidermis has four main layers: basal, spinous, granular and stratum corneum.
- Most epidermal cells are keratinocytes.
- It is a dynamic structure, constantly responding to environmental stimuli such as UVR.
- Pigmentation is partly due to genetic factors and partly a response to UVR.
- The responses to UVA and UVB are different.

PHYSIOLOGICAL EFFECTS OF ULTRAVIOLET

The distribution and intensities of the different wavelengths of visible and invisible radiation absorbed in the skin cause a range of outcomes. The obvious acute effects of UVR in sunlight are sunburn (erythema) and tanning (melanogenesis). Other effects include vitamin D production, immunosuppression and cell damage. When the cell damage includes damage to DNA molecules, a possible result is tumour formation (Halaban et al., 2003).

With UVR exposure, a range of photoproducts are produced, the amounts depending on the endogenous and exogenous agents present. One photoproduct is a precursor to vitamin D: it forms in the skin in response to UVB (Kochevar and Taylor, 2003). Exogenously administered (oral or topical) substances, such as some antibiotics (e.g. sulphonamides, tetracyclines), anticancer drugs (e.g. methotrexate), antidepressants (e.g. tricyclics), cardiac medications (e.g. amiodarone) and diuretics (e.g. furosemide), increase the level of photosensitivity (Lim, 2003).

Stimulation of vitamin D production has been described as the single apparent benefit of UVR (Walker et al., 2003).

Acute effects of UVR

UVR is largely absorbed in the outer layer of the skin so that the direct effects are limited to those on the skin and the eyes. Sunburn is the most obvious cutaneous response. The classic signs of inflammation occur: pain, swelling, redness and warmth. The severity depends on the skin type and dosage (Table 17.4). These changes are accompanied by a depletion of Langerhans cells and, consequently, immunosuppression (Walker et al., 2003).

The erythema, or reddening is uniform and not mottled and it usually appears immediately after or within hours of an application of UVR. This time is called the latent period. Over some hours the erythema increases and then fades during the subsequent hours or days. Oedema and irritation of the skin also occur if the application

Table 17.4 Description of degrees of erythema

Degree of erythema	Approximate latent period	Appearance	Approximate duration	Skin discomfort	Desquamation	Relation to E_1	Other features
E_1	6–12 h	Mildly pink	<24 h	None	None	×1	
E_2	6 h	Definite pink-red	2 days	Slight soreness	Powdery	×2.5	Blanches on compression
E_3	3 h	Very red	3–5 days	Hot and painful	In thin sheets	×5	Does not blanch on compression
E_4	<2 h	'Angry' red	1 week	Very painful	In thick sheets	×10	Blistering

Suberythemal doses are exposures each insufficient to provoke visible reddening.

of UVR is sufficiently intense, as well as desquamation (peeling) of the superficial epidermis.

If the same dose of UVB is repeated after these changes have recovered it provokes a less strong reaction due to the pigmentation (tanning) and skin thickening that occurs. This protective pigmentation and skin thickening can last 30–40 days following either a single erythematous exposure or a series of suberythemal doses (Nonaka et al., 1984). The degree to which these effects occur depends on the amount of UVB energy applied, the duration of exposure and the reactivity or sensitivity of the skin of the subject. Thus a fair-skinned person will exhibit a more marked reaction than a dark-skinned one given the same exposure. These changes are summarized in Table 17.4.

Longer-term effects of UVR

The longer-term cutaneous response to UVR exposure is the initiation of tanning or melanogenesis. This visible and UVR protective response, in which an increased melanin production becomes obvious in the days after exposure to UVB, was described above. This contrasts with the immediate 'tanning' after exposure to UVA, which is not UVR protective.

Pigmentation changes and immunosuppression, discussed above, are two longer-term effects of UVR on the skin. Another is increased skin growth or hyperplasia of the dermis, epidermis and stratum corneum. UVR exposure provokes an increased keratinocyte cell turnover so that the skin grows more rapidly for a time, a type of photoprotection. This can result in a 20 to 40% increase in the number of cell layers in the stratum corneum, particularly in fairer skinned people (Walker et al., 2003). Both protective effects (pigmentation and hyperplasia) fade over 4–6 weeks if there are no further UVR applications. The cumulative longer-term effect of frequent UVR exposure, especially to UVB, is called photoageing (Walker et al., 2003). The skin becomes dry, deeply wrinkled, inelastic and leathery. This is associated with the collagen fibrils degrading and becoming disorganized.

UVR is needed for the production of vitamin D in the skin. The conversion from cholesterol requires a minimal amount of regular exposure of skin to sunlight or a UVR lamp. Insufficient vitamin D, especially if coupled with undernourishment leads to rickets in babies and osteomalacia in adults as it is essential to facilitate the absorption of calcium from the intestine. Those living in locations with little sunlight or in institutions or wearing clothing that precludes or severely limits exposure can be at risk, for example, of pathological fractures if their UVR exposure is too low.

DNA damage and skin cancer

The connection between sun exposure and the genesis of skin cancers is well known and accepted. UVR has been implicated not only as a tumour initiator but also as a promoter (Walker et al., 2003). UVB is especially implicated in the genesis of skin cancers. The precursor appears to be damage to epithelial DNA. Repeated exposures can lead to the development of an actinic keratosis which may, in turn, become a squamous cell carcinoma (SCC). Similarly, the UVR mediated cell mutations are associated with the development of basal cell carcinomas (BCC).

The other type of skin cancer is cutaneous melanomas, the malignant transformation of melanocytes. Sun exposure is again implicated as a major cause. Supporting evidence includes sex-based distribution patterns, distribution by latitude and race, and migration studies (Langley et al., 2003).

Recent evidence (Agar et al., 2004) suggests that it is the UVA component of sunlight, rather than UVB, which poses the greatest malignant melanoma risk. This is likely because of the greater penetration depth of UVA which allows greater wave energy to reach the more deeply located melanocytes.

What is probably less well known and accepted is that tanning salon exposures can also produce the type of changes that are accepted as essential in the process of developing skin cancers (Whitmore et al., 2001). This observation is entirely consistent with the findings of Agar et al. (2004).

Abnormal effects of UVR

UVR can also cause a number of abnormal responses of the skin. Clinical users of UVR must be aware of these. The four categories are acquired idiopathic responses (e.g. actinic prurigo, solar urticaria); DNA repair-defective photodermatoses (e.g. xeroderma pigmentosum); photosensitization by exogenous drugs or chemicals (e.g. eczematous reactions); and dermatoses exacerbated by UVR (e.g. acne, herpes simplex, psoriasis) (Hawke et al., 2003). Consult a dermatology textbook for further information (for example, Freedberg et al., 2003).

The effects of UVR on the eye

Strong doses of UVB and UVC to the eyes can cause conjunctivitis (inflammation of the tissue over the cornea and lining of the eyelids) and photokeratitis (inflammation of the cornea). These produce watering, a feeling of grit in the eye and an aversion to light (photophobia). In severe cases intense pain and spasm of the eyelid may also occur. This condition is also known as 'snow blindness' and is due to solar UVB reflection from the snow (or sand, or from using welding arcs without eye protection). Although all UVB and UVC will produce these effects, the most damaging wavelength seems to be 270 nm. The condition usually recovers in about 2 days without permanent damage but the eye, unlike the skin, does not develop a tolerance to UVR.

While UVB and C are absorbed in the cornea, UVA can pass through to be absorbed mainly in the lens of the eye. High doses of UVA have been implicated in the formation of cataracts but this is not evident in studies of patients who wore protective goggles during PUVA exposures (Honigsmann et al., 2003).

THERAPEUTIC USES AND INDICATIONS

The principal therapeutic clinical use of UVR is to treat skin diseases, particularly psoriasis and vitiligo. These are described below, followed by mention of some of the other conditions presently and historically treated with UVR (see later section for an explanation of PUVA, psoralen and UVA).

> The eye, unlike the skin, does not develop a tolerance to UVR. In fact, subsequent applications seem to provoke conjunctivitis more readily. This may be because initial recovery is apparent but not complete for several days longer.

Table 17.5 Summary of physiological effects of UVR

Acute effects	Acute effects	Chronic effects

On skin
  Erythema
  Pigmentation
  Thickening (hyperplasia)
  Vitamin D production
  Cell DNA damage
  Immunosuppression
	On eyes
	  Conjunctivitis
	  Photokeratitis
		On skin
		  Photoageing
		  Tumour initiation and
		    promotion

Psoriasis

Psoriasis is a chronic relapsing skin disease of unknown cause affecting 2% of the population (Christophers and Mrowietz, 2003). Psoriasis vulgaris, or plaque-type psoriasis, is the commonest form. Its sharply demarcated lesions (plaques) have a homogeneous, glossy, erythematous (red) appearance and are covered with silvery scales. The other types include eruptive psoriasis (guttate), with small lesions scattered over the trunk and pustular psoriasis, with sterile pustules. With psoriasis the epidermal transit time is reduced to about 36 hours, and there is a near doubling of the epidermal proliferative cell number (Christophers and Mrowietz, 2003).

The methods of treating psoriasis are still imperfect but they have changed considerably over recent years. They include topical treatments (e.g. local applications of tar, vitamin D and analogues, and glucocorticosteroids), UVR (e.g. PUVA and 311/312 nm UVB), and systemic treatments (e.g. methotrexate, ciclosporin, retinoids and fumaric acid esters). Laser (in UVB range, 308 nm) is a possible future treatment (Christophers and Mrowietz, 2003).

Figure 17.5 shows the action spectrum for erythema compared with a graph of therapeutic efficacy for psoriasis.

Explanations of the possible mechanism by which UVR affects psoriasis suggest it is, at least in part, systemically mediated and related to the immunosuppressive effect. The PUVA effect is most probably a phototoxic effect on lymphocytes in the skin or an effect on an abnormal immune function (Honigsmann et al., 2003). This means psoriasis can improve following treatment of unaffected skin and, in areas not directly treated by UVR (e.g. the scalp following treatment of the trunk).

The predisposition to psoriasis appears to be inherited and 10% of people with it will also have psoriatic arthritis (Winchester, 2003).

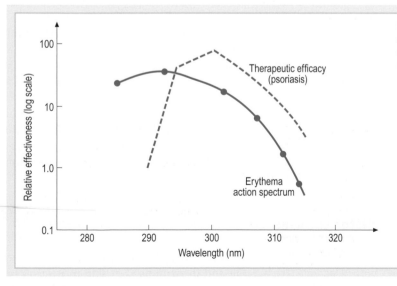

Figure 17.5 Action spectrum for erythema compared with graph of therapeutic efficacy for psoriasis. (After Parrish and Jaenicke, 1981.)

Vitiligo

Vitiligo is a common skin condition characterized by the absence of melanocytes. White patches appear on the skin either locally, segmentally or more generally. For those with a darker coloured skin vitiligo can be a serious cosmetic problem. Treatment options include topical glucocorticoids and PUVA or narrow band UVB at a wavelength of 311 nm (Orotonne et al., 2003). During UVR treatment the surrounding normally pigmented area should be protected to avoid darkening the contrasting area.

Other uses

UVR is used to treat a mild deficiency of vitamin D. Suberythemal doses of UVB are thought to be adequate to promote vitamin D synthesis while minimizing the harmful effects of UVR. Note that too high an exposure can result in a depletion of folate, which can increase the risk of congenital abnormalities, particularly neural tube defects such as spina bifida. UVA and psoralen (PUVA) are also used to treat miscellaneous dermatoses, cutaneous T cell lymphomas, atopic dermatitis, lichen planus and cutaneous mastocytosis (Honigsmann et al., 2003). Uses of narrow band UVB include for atopic dermatitis, some photodermatoses, scleroderma and urticaria pigmentosa (Krutmann and Morita, 2003) and seborrhoeic dermatitis (Pirkhammer et al., 2000).

Chronic infection

UVR is an effective and convenient way of controlling surface bacterial infections. This may be of use when antibiotics cannot reach the area in adequate proportions, if the infection is antibiotic resistant or if their use is contraindicated.

Infected open wounds such as pressure sores are sometimes treated with high doses of UVR. An E_4 dose (see later) is required (High and High, 1983; Burger et al., 1985). The reduction in colony numbers correlates with the exposure dose, an E_4 being required to inhibit totally colony growth (High and High, 1983). Also, swabs cultured from some pressure sores before and after an E_4 ultraviolet dose given with a Kromayer lamp showed a dramatic and extensive reduction in bacterial numbers (Burger et al., 1985).

While the lethal effects of UVC on bacteria, especially the 254 nm peak, have been well known for many years, the effect of clinically used doses given with a standard Kromayer lamp have only been quantified in the last 20 years.

Historical uses

Historically, UVR has had many uses. These include treating patients with acne vulgaris, eczema and those in need of skin protection prior to extended UVR exposures. The known risks of using UVR and the

Table 17.6 Summary of therapeutic uses of UVR

UVA	UVB	UVA and UVB
Cutaneous T cell lymphomas	Vitamin D deficiency	Psoriasis
Lichen planus	Some photodermatoses	Vitiligo
Cutaneous mastocytosis	Scleroderma	Dermatitis
Miscellaneous dermatoses	Urticaria pigmentosa	
	Atopic dermatitis	

absence of evidence of the effectiveness of these treatments suggests they are no longer justified. For example, acne vulgaris was treated with UVR at the E_2 level. Only anecdotal evidence exists to justify this use of UVR. The known risks, as with those of superficial X-ray therapy (which has been shown to be effective in treating acne) outweigh the possible advantages. A large range of other treatment options exist, including local and systemic drug regimens. These generally have a known level of risk and a higher success rate than does using UVR (Thiboutot and Strauss, 2003). Deliberate prior exposure using low level UVR to increase tolerance and reduce the risk of sunburn is also questionable, given the availability of effective sunscreen lotions.

SKIN RESPONSES TO TREATMENT USING UVR

This section discusses factors affecting the response of the skin to treatment using UVR.

The skin response to UVR depends on:

- the quantity of ultraviolet energy applied to unit area of the skin
- the biological responsiveness (sensitivity) of the skin to which it is applied.

The first can be measured, or at least controlled to keep it constant, but the second can only be adequately assessed by trial applications of UVR.

The quantity of energy applied

Typically about $20\,mJ\,cm^{-2}$ of UVB at a wavelength of 300 nm will produce minimal erythema on the moderately fair-skinned (Diffey, 1982; Nonaka et al., 1984). This figure is not, however, generalizable to other wavelengths as the response of skin varies quite dramatically.

At 300 nm the skin is one hundred times more sensitive than at 320 nm (Diffey, 1994; see also Figure 17.5).

So it is not enough to specify a UV intensity in mJ cm^{-2}, it is also necessary to specify the wavelength or wavelength range concerned.

Setting aside, for the moment, the effect of wavelength on the physiological response, consider the question of how to describe the actual dosage. The actual dose received, the exposure dose, depends on a number of factors including the output of the lamp, the distance between the lamp and the skin, the angle at which radiation falls on the skin and the time for which the radiation is applied. Each factor is considered below.

The lamp output. A statement of the output intensity is not sufficient. Any description of the output of the source must include the specific wavelengths emitted and their relative intensity.

Even if the same make and type, lamps usually have slightly different outputs. This is mainly due to the effect of the ageing of the tube (hours of use). For this reason it is very important to use the same source throughout a course of treatment. If this is not possible, a new test dose should be completed and a new treatment regimen planned.

The lamp distance from the skin. The distance between the ultraviolet source and the skin is critical. An inverse square relationship (see chapter 14) is used to calculate the relationship of intensity and distance when using lamps with small burners and large parabolic reflectors.

An inverse square relationship means that if the distance is doubled the intensity is reduced to one-quarter, so, to achieve an equivalent effect, the time of application must be four times the original. For example, if the desired effect was achieved in 1 minute at a distance of 50 cm, the time needed at a distance of 100 cm would be four times that (4 minutes).

The exposure dose or effect depends on the intensity of the irradiation (I) and the time for which it is given (t), as noted above.

$$\text{Exposure dose} = It$$

From the inverse square law:

$$I \propto \frac{1}{d^2} \quad \text{so} \quad \text{Exposure dose} \propto \frac{t}{d^2}$$

If the same effect is required, but either time or distance is altered:

$$\frac{t_1}{d_1^{\,2}} = \frac{t_2}{d_2^{\,2}}$$

For example, if an E_2 is produced in 60 s (t_1) at 50 cm (d_1), at 30 cm (d_2) it is produced in 22 s (t_2):

$$\frac{60}{50 \times 50} = \frac{t_2}{30 \times 30} \quad \text{so } t_2 = 22\,\text{s}$$

An ultraviolet emitter is not a point source, however, and is backed by a reflector, which reduces the loss in intensity with distance. At the

The use of an inverse square relationship is questionable. The inverse square law only applies to a point source of radiation without a reflector. The use of a reflector lessens the drop in intensity with distance.

same time, wave energy is lost by absorption and scattering in air, which increases the loss in intensity with distance. The effects fortuitously cancel each other so an inverse square law can be used as a good first-approximation. For the Alpine sunlamp, the intensity at distances between 50 and 150 cm conforms with that predicted by the inverse square law (Goats, 1988). At distances of less than 50 cm the intensity is less accurately predicted.

The angle of radiation on the skin. The intensity of radiation on the skin depends on the cosine of the angle of incidence of the radiation due to spreading of the beam over a greater area (see chapter 14). This means that the intensity of radiation will 'fall off' around curved body surfaces and if the lamp is not parallel to the skin. Thus the lamp should be applied at or near a right angle to the skin to achieve maximum and consistent effects.

The duration of exposure. This is strictly controlled in therapeutic applications of UVR. If the intensity of UVR falling on the skin is constant then the effects are directly proportional to the time of exposure. This is in accordance with the Bunsen–Roscoe reciprocity law, which states that the same photochemical effect will occur if the product of the intensity and time are constant; thus a low intensity exposure for a long time can produce the same effect as a short duration high intensity exposure. Although the reciprocity law is not generally applicable, it does seem to apply to UVR exposure where the effects are often damaging and the extent of damage accumulates with the exposure duration. Guidelines on how to establish the duration of the initial test dose and subsequent treatments will be considered shortly, as will the frequency of subsequent treatments and the dosage increases needed to compensate for the skin's protective responses following an exposure to UVR.

> The 'Bunsen–Roscoe reciprocity law' is not actually a law as it is not always true. For example, a large amount of heat delivered for a short time can produce a burn. The same amount of heat delivered at a lower intensity for a longer period could be harmless.

The biological response

The extent of the biological response to UVR depends on three main factors:

- skin type
- skin sensitivity
- recent exposures of skin to UVR.

Skin type

Skin types can be graded according to their expected responses to UVR (Table 17.7).

These distinctions between skin types and their expected tolerances of UVR are only guides. The response to UVR can be so variable that it is extremely difficult accurately to predict it. Sayre et al. (1966), for example, were unable to find significant relationships between the energy needed to produce erythema and the skin colour of the subject.

Table 17.7 Classification of skin types based on response to UVR exposure (Wolff et al., 1977)

Type I	White skin, always burns, never tans
Type II	White skin, always burns, tans slightly
Type III	White skin, sometimes burns, always tans
Type IV	Olive skin, rarely burns, always tans
Type V	Brown skin, never burns, always tans
Type VI	Black skin, never burns, always tans

One possible reason concerns the next two variables that also affect skin responses to UVR.

Skin sensitivity

While the photoprotective effects of skin colour are undoubted, it is likely that skin sensitivity has a genetic component apart from that which determines skin colour. Thus some individuals will be more (or less) UV sensitive than others with similar skin pigmentation.

The presence of a number of different types of topical or systemic substances will change the response of the skin to UVR. A photosensitizing effect is used deliberately with PUVA and Re-PUVA treatment (both explained below) to reduce the dosage of UVA or UVB required to treat conditions such as psoriasis.

Recent exposures of skin to UVR

Recent exposures of skin to UVR changes the rate of cell transit from the basal layer to the stratum corneum (see Figure 17.3), thus changing responses to UVR in the near future. The rate of cell production and transit are increased, resulting in a thickening of the epidermis. A clinical implication of this skin hyperplasia is that the duration of all subsequent treatment doses will need to be increased to obtain the same effect. See below in progression of UVR treatment.

Summary of factors determining the skin response to UVR treatment

The quantity of UV energy applied per unit area of skin, this depends on the:

- lamp output
- distance of lamp from the skin
- angle of lamp radiation to the skin
- duration of exposure to UVR.

The biological response of the skin which, in turn, depends on the:

- skin type (category I to VI)
- current level of photosensitivity
- recent exposures of skin to UVR.

TREATMENT PRINCIPLES USING UVR

Using UVR treatments safely and effectively requires knowledge not only of the condition being treated but also of the usual skin response to UVR and the principles discussed below. In planning to use UVR for treatment a therapist must be aware of the following:

- grades of erythema
- erythema testing
- skin photosensitizers
- progression of treatment.

Grades of erythema

Four grades of erythema are commonly used (E_1, E_2, E_3, E_4). Their descriptions are based on the following:

- the duration of the latent period in hours – the time for the erythema (reddening) to become evident
- the intensity of erythema – how red it is
- the duration of the erythema in hours or days – how long it lasts
- the severity of any irritation
- the presence of oedema or blistering
- the extent and type of desquamation.

The grading of skin reaction is a subjective judgement that applies to the individual *patient* in the test conditions used. Referring to 'the E_1 of the lamp' is meaningless. Instead, an E_1 indicates the observed erythemal response on an area of a patient's skin for a particular lamp at a given distance after a specified time of exposure. That is, the terms 'first-degree erythema' (E_1) and 'minimal erythemal dose (MED)' refer to the *response* used to define a dose. They also are used to define the subsequent treatment doses.

The four grades of erythema doses are related. As Table 17.4 shows, there is an approximately log/linear relation between the grade and the dosage multiple which must be used to achieve it. There is also an approximately log/linear relation between the grade and the time required to produce a higher or lower erythema dose (Low, 1986). Light reflectance spectrophotometry has confirmed the relationship between the grades and the duration of their latent periods by measuring the changing erythemal intensity by light reflectance (Farr and Diffey, 1984).

Another point to note is the range of names used for the first grade of erythema (E_1). The following are all equivalent terms:

E_1, first-degree erythema
MED, minimal erythemal dose – widely used
MPD, minimal perceptible dose or minimal phototoxic dose
MPE, minimal perceptible erythema.

The four grades of erythema are described in Table 17.4, earlier.

A log/linear relationship between, say, the dosage multiple and the erythema grade means that the dose must be doubled from the previous value to produce a linear (stepwise) increase in the grade.

Technically, this last term (MPE) is the most precise as even low levels of UVR applications can have an effect that may not be visible or perceptible to the recipient or the observer.

Principles of erythema testing

Erythemal testing provides essential information for UVR treatment. The test is a way of reliably ascertaining the effect of a particular UVR dosage level on a given individual. The test can identify the dosage required to produce an E_1 (or MED) response or to produce the level of erythema determined as appropriate for treatment.

Stages

Patient

Check for any contraindications to using UVR.

Check and record any use of photosensitizers – topical applications or systemic medications.

Check skin is freshly washed to remove surface grease, perfumes and skin lotions.

Explain the test carefully, including how the results are obtained and get patient consent. Include a warning that two or three red marks may be visible for a day and for those who tan readily, a slight pigmented mark for a week or so.

Provide patient with UVR blocking goggles and explain why they must be worn.

UVR source

If using a lamp, turn it on 5 minutes prior to test to stabilize the output, also, fully screen the output with a tightly woven fabric. A single thickness of lint allows 13% of the UVR to be transmitted, increasing to 23% if the lint is wet (Wood and Reed, 1990). Tightly woven fabrics offer the best protection (Robson and Diffey, 1990). Fluorescent tubes do not require significant warm-up time and can be used immediately.

Estimate the time to produce the erythema at the intended distance with a given lamp. The following factors are used:

- the skin classification (see Table 17.7) and extent of recent exposures
- the specific lamp characteristics. If not known, with the Alpine sunlamp an E_1 typically takes about 30–90 s at 50 cm from the burner and a typical Theraktin about 4–5 minutes at 50 cm. But remember that lamps can vary considerably so this is only a very, very rough guideline.

- distance (usually 50 cm).
- any topical applications or systemic medication they are taking that may alter photosensitivity.

Estimate the time to irradiate each template hole, aiming to have the E_1 dose in the middle to avoid either under- or overdosing an area.

Template

Decide which test area to use. The anterior forearm or an area of the body not usually exposed to sunlight, or the area of body to be treated, is usual. Make a template to cover this area. Use a piece of lint or other light-blocking material. Cut three (or four or five) separate holes of at best $2\,cm^2$ and at least $1\,cm^2$ in the template. The area chosen must be easily and conveniently visible to the patient.

Fix the template firmly to the skin so that only deliberately exposed holes will be irradiated and none are over a joint line.

Applying the test dose

The therapist and patient put on their UVR goggles.

Cover the exposed areas of the patient with a suitable material to screen them from the UVR.

Check the distance of UVR source to skin (usually 50 cm) and ensure the radiation is at right angles to the test area.

Uncover the UVR source and time the exposure to each template hole. Usually the first hole is exposed for the entire time, the second for one time period less, the third for two time periods less etc. This means the test can be conducted more quickly in a controlled manner as long as the exposures have been precalculated. The therapist should minimize exposing themselves during this process.

Post test

Advise the patient to check their skin at 4 or 6 h intervals for any signs of reddening, pain or swelling and provide them with a card to help them record their observations (Figure 17.6).

Alternatively, have the patient return in 24 h to check the area. By definition, the E_1 or minimal erythemal dose (MED) is the hole that appeared last and disappeared first, i.e. the least visible (minimally perceptible) response.

Repeat tests

A repeat test will be required if the patient's medications are changed or a topical sensitizer or a new lamp has to be used.

Figure 17.6 An example of a card given to a patient to record the result of a UVR test dose.

Test applied 11.00 a.m. Monday	Monday			Tuesday	
	3 p.m.	7 p.m.	11 p.m.	7 a.m.	11 a.m.
○					
◇					
▭					

Look at the areas at the time shown and place a tick in a box if any reddening is seen. If no reddening is seen, put a cross.

Skin photosensitizers

List of commonly encountered systemic and topical photosensitizers

Systemic photosensitizers include:

furocoumarins – including the psoralens
retinoids – used in conjunction with UVR treatment
antibiotics – e.g. sulphonamides, tetracyclines
antipsychotics – e.g. phenothiazine
cardiac medications – e.g. amiodarone, quinidine
diuretics – e.g. furosemide
anticancer drugs – e.g. methotrexate
antidepressants – e.g. tricyclics
antifungals – e.g. griseofulvin
antimalarials – e.g. chloroquine, quinine
NSAIDs – e.g. ibuprofen, naproxen, celocoxib

Topical photosensitizers include:

coal tar – used as a sensitizer to UVR
psoralens and other furocoumarins

(See Lim, 2003 for more extensive lists.)

Skin develops an increased sensitivity to UVR following the ingestion or topical applications of a number of different substances. This has two important implications. First, prior to erythema testing the therapist must record all current medications and clean the skin of any topical substances not required for the test or treatment. For example, sunscreen and perfume or aftershave may alter skin sensitivity. Second, care needs to be exercised if a patient's drug regimen has been altered during a course of ultraviolet treatments. Deleting or adding some medications may necessitate a new erythemal test if their photosensitivity may have changed.

Listed in the margin are some of the commonly encountered systemic and topical substances that can alter sensitivity. This is not a comprehensive list as that would be prohibitively long and need constant updating. See a drug compendium or dermatology textbook for further details.

The furocoumarins are a particularly interesting group of compounds which occur naturally in plants including lemons, parsley and parsnip. They are found in perfumes, cosmetics and fragrances, and act as sensitizers to UVA and UVB. They are photomutagenic, meaning that when used in conjunction with UVR, greater genetic damage is produced than would occur with the UV exposure alone. They are thus associated with an increased risk of malignancy and carcinogenesis.

Table 17.8 Increased dose of UVR to compensate for increased tolerance

Initial dose	Earliest time at which the dose can be repeated	Increase (%)
E_0 (suberythemal)	24 h	12.5
E_1 (MED dose)	1 or 2 days	20 to 25
E_2	3–4 days	50
E_3	7–10 days	75

MED = minimal erythemal dose.

Because of their natural occurence, furocoumarins are found in some sun-protection and bronzing lotions. Recognition of their phototoxicity has led the European Commission to limit the allowable content in these products to 1 part per million. The limit has recently been reviewed and reconfirmed (SCCNFP, 2003).

Progression of ultraviolet dosage

Even the smallest dose of UVR, one which has no evident effect, causes skin changes. One such change is an increased tolerance of UVR. This means, if the same erythemal effect is to be achieved repeatedly the dose must be increased to compensate each time.

Table 17.8 provides guidance for progression of the dosage. The increased dose needed is only an approximate guide as it depends on skin pigmentation and thickening. This means that patients who tan easily will need the full increase whereas those who do not will need less. An essential point is that these figures only apply if the erythema has faded completely before a further dose of UVR is given. Repeat doses are not normally given before the erythema disappears as the skin response is too unpredictable.

Advice on the increases used to repeat suberythemal doses varies: 10, 12.5 and 15% of the E_1 have all been suggested. This probably reflects different perceptions of what is a suberythemal dose: half, five-eighths, three-quarters and just less than an E_1. Each has been suggested. Two-thirds is perhaps a reasonable figure.

Note that there is no reason for ever applying an E_4 dose to the skin. An E_4 should be used only to treat the floor and walls of an open wound. Surrounding normal skin must be fully protected from the UVR and the application can be daily.

Proportion of body surface irradiated

High doses of UVR involving large areas are not justified. This can cause considerable patient distress, even systemic illness. Table 17.9

Table 17.9 Usual size of body area treated for different erythemal levels	
Level of erythema	**Size of area treated**
E_0	Whole body
E_1	Half or whole body
E_2	20 to 25% of body surface
E_3	4% of body surface (no more than $600\,cm^2$)
E_4	Area in wound only

lists the usual guidelines for the maximum proportion of body surface to be irradiated with UVR.

Summary

Treatment requires knowledge of:

- grades of erythema
- how to do erythemal testing
- effects of skin photosensitizers
- principles of treatment progression.

PRINCIPLES OF UVR APPLICATION

The principles of application are like those for the erythemal test. The main differences are due to:

- treatment options (see PUVA and UVB below)
- the need to adjust dosage (progress, but if treatments are missed, regress) for subsequent treatments
- the implications of size of area treated
- evaluating the outcome.

The following section outlines the general points a therapist must consider when applying UVR treatments. This is followed by separate sections describing special features of PUVA and UVB treatments.

General application of UVR

Stages

Patient

A test dose having been completed, the nature and effects of the treatment are explained.

Apparatus

A suitable plinth is usually kept in position so that the Theraktin tunnel or the lamp can be placed a standard distance (usually 50 cm) from the area to be treated.

Setting up

If a general body treatment, the patient undresses completely, puts on protective ultraviolet goggles and stands in the UV cabinet or lies down on the plinth with their arms and legs straight and a little abducted. Limbs must not shade one another or the trunk. If using a tunnel, the head and feet protrude, thus receiving a somewhat lower dose. The tunnel is then lowered and the distance from patient to tubes is measured. The position of the patient must be repeatable from one treatment to the next. If the patient starts in prone lying with the palms facing upwards the position of the head must be made comfortable, usually turned to one side.

Instructions and warnings

The patient is warned to keep still and not to touch the tunnel or lamp.

Application

The UVR source is switched on for the appropriate time for the required dose. If a lamp is used it must have been turned on for at least 5 minutes prior to this to stabilize the output. After this time the source is switched off or covered and the patient turns over, this time with the palms facing downwards and the head turned to the same side, to give an equivalent dose to the opposite side of the face. The source is again switched on for the required time and then off or covered, and the treatment is completed.

Progression

This has four separate components: duration of subsequent treatments, size of area treated, total number of treatments and adjustments for missed treatments.

- *Duration of subsequent treatments.* The dose is increased by prolonging the duration (time) of successive treatments. In part this depends on the response to the previous treatment. If, for example, an erythema occurs after a suberythemal treatment the next dose should obviously be reduced. See Table 17.8 for recommended progressions. Note that increasing by exactly 12.5% (one-eighth) at each treatment to repeat a suberythemal dose would be absurdly pedantic. It is more sensible to increase by convenient fractions of a minute.

Table 17.10 Regression of general UVB treatments	
If no treatments have been given for	**Dose**
Up to 4 days	Usual progression
5–7 days	Repeat previous dose
8–13 days	Use the dose given at 4 treatments before this one
14–20 days	Use the dose given at 8 treatments before this one
21–27 days	Use the dose given at 12 treatments before this one
28 days or more	Use the original dose

- *Size of area treated*. The size of the area treated depends on the level of E given. Treatment may be given each day for an E_0 for the whole body, or an E_1, half the body (i.e. one side only), or the whole body with an E_1 on alternate days (see Tables 17.8 and 17.9).
- *Total number of treatments*. This is usually limited as it is a balance between the benefits of UVR and the risks (see section on PUVA). Progression cannot be continued indefinitely since the protective changes will reach their maximum at some stage, the time differing primarily with the patient's skin type. With successive treatments the E_1 (or MED) is raised to many times the original E_1 with most UVB treatment regimens to between 3 and 5 times the original. The usual practice is to limit treatment progression in terms of multiples of the E_1 rather than using an arbitrary length of course in weeks or a maximum dosage in minutes. Alternative options would be something such as 4-week courses or 20-minute maximum applications.
- *Adjusting for missed treatments*. If for any reason regular treatments are missed for a time some of the protective pigmentation and skin thickening is lost. It is usual to presume all protective effect is lost over 4 weeks. If less, the therapist must decide what the appropriate dose to use is. Table 17.10 offers guidance only, as the responses of individual patients vary widely.

PUVA treatment

PUVA originally meant Psoralen and UVA. A more recent option is to use narrow wavelength UVB (311 nm) instead of UVA.

Psoralens are UV sensitizers which can be applied topically or systemically. The rationale for PUVA treatment is that the UVA dose can be reduced while producing the same therapeutic effect. An assumption is that the lower dose represents less risk. This may not be the case. The 'sensitization' seems to be more general in that therapeutic effects are achieved at lower UVR levels, but so are biologically damaging mutagenic effects. It is yet to be established whether the benefits outweigh the penalties.

Practical point

If desired, a suitable cloth can be used to cover the genitalia and removed by the patient as treatment begins. Alternatively, if the patient prefers to wear a pair of briefs they must be the same at each treatment. Otherwise a previously untreated region of skin may become exposed late in the course, possibly giving the patient an E_2 or E_3 in a very inconvenient site!

This calls into question whether psoralens are of any real value in clinical applications of UVR.

Other options concern the photosensitizer regimen used with the selected UVR. The treatment may follow 14 days (or so) of a patient taking another systemic photosensitizer such as methotrexate, ciclosporin or one of the retinoids.

Treatment is provided in a PUVA unit or cabinet. Some are like the Theraktin tunnel – the patient is treated lying – others are in vertical cabinets in which the patient stands.

PUVA erythema differs from that produced by sunburn or UVB alone. The effects take 24 to 36 hours to appear and they peak at 72 to 96 hours or later (Honigsmann et al., 2003). The treatment dose is usually at the E_1 (MPD or MED) level. This means a barely perceptible but well defined skin erythema is produced in areas exposed to an appropriate dose during the erythemal test.

To maintain this level in successive treatments requires systematically increasing the duration of the UVA exposure. Treatment is typically given twice a week, progressively increasing the dose at weekly intervals for several weeks. The UVA dosage is measured in $J\,cm^{-2}$ and increases of $0.5-1\,J\,cm^{-2}$ are a usual progression. The principle of basing the dosage on the response of the patient and progressing the dose is the same as for UVB, the difference being that the response to UVA is slower than to UVB. Each PUVA method is briefly described below.

> The tubes in PUVA units traditionally produce UVA but they can be replaced with UVB tubes. This is because UVB tubes produce appreciable amounts of UVA which, with UVB, is also therapeutically effective.

Topical psoralen applications

For a small area of psoriasis or a resistant area, a topical preparation of 8-methoxypsoralen is applied. Using a topical application produces a higher local concentration of the drug in the skin than a systemic application. The UVR dose required is therefore much lower (Klaber, 1980).

Alternatively, a PUVA bath can be used. This limits the photosensitivity of the body to 2 h, considerably less than if an oral (systemic) dose is used (Honigsmann et al., 2003).

Systemic psoralens

Patients are given 8-methoxypsoralen by mouth some 1–3 h before exposure to the UVR. They are given grey or green glasses to wear while sensitized, i.e. from the time of taking the tablets until 8 h afterwards. They are also warned not to expose themselves to the sun for at least 8 h from ingestion (Fusco et al., 1980).

Re-PUVA (retinoid PUVA)

This has been shown to clear those plaques not cleared with either PUVA or retinoids alone at normal dosages (Kuenzli and Saurat, 2003). This means that a lower total dose of UVR is required than with PUVA treatment alone, where the normal dose would have to be exceeded. Although the treatment is undoubtedly effective, whether

> Kuenzli and Saurat (2003) claim that Re-PUVA treatment reduces the carcinogenic effect of the large number of PUVA treatments that would otherwise be required.

the lowered dose is less mutagenically harmful when the skin is sensitized with retinoids is questionable.

Dangers of PUVA

Recent longitudinal studies have shown an increased risk of melanoma in association with long-term repeated treatments using PUVA (Stern et al, 1997; Wolff, 1997; Stern, 2001). The incident risk ratio is 2.0 (95%CI 0.9 to 9.5) for all melanomas in patients who have had more than 200 PUVA treatments. If more than 15 years have passed since the first PUVA treatment, the incident rate ratio for all melanomas is 5.9 (95%CI 2.2 to 15.9: Stern, 2001). These results mean that patients having PUVA, on average, have an approximately fivefold risk of developing a melanoma compared to the rest of the population. An inevitable conclusion is that the risks of PUVA must be weighted very carefully when treatment options are considered.

After 2 or 3 weeks of PUVA treatment marked pigmentation can develop. UVA stimulates the production of melanin, but the melanosomes are not transferred to the more superficial layers of the epidermis, as with UVB. This, plus the fact that UVA does not result in a thicker stratum corneum, explains why exposure to UVA results in minimum or no protection against UVB (Black et al., 1985). It is important for therapists to recognize this since patients who are deeply tanned by PUVA or from commercial sunbeds may not be as well protected as their colour might suggest.

The epidemiological studies of the dangers of PUVA are backed by recent histological studies which indicate that UVA may be more damaging than previously assumed because of its greater penetration depth in tissue (Agar et al., 2004). While UVB predominantly damages keratinocytes, UVA is more readily able to damage dermal cells. The most life-threatening malignancies are those of the skin's sub-epidermal layers (e.g. malignant melanoma and other basal cell carcinomas).

UVB

UVB is increasingly replacing the use of PUVA. Evidence suggests it is cheaper and more practical. UVB can be used on pregnant women, in childhood, is possibly less carcinogenic than UVA and, as it does not require the use of psoralen as a sensitizer, means the use of post-treatment eye protection is not required (Krutmann and Morita, 2003).

The tubes used to treat with UVB have an output at 311/312 nm. This means they are optimal for treating psoriasis as they are in its action spectrum (Krutmann and Morita, 2003). Other conditions are also treated using narrow band UVB, although less is known about their action spectrum than for psoriasis.

Topical and systemic sensitizers

As with PUVA, sensitizers can be applied topically or taken prior to treatment to increase the response to UVR. As with UVA the aim is to increase the rate of healing while reducing the carcinogenic risks of repeated UVR exposures. Also as with UVA, the topical sensitizers

As noted previously, reducing the mutagenic risk while increasing the therapeutic benefit may not be possible in practice.

include tar, vitamin D analogues, retinoids, saltwater baths and glucocorticoids (Krutmann and Morita, 2003). The systemic ones include retinoids.

UVB treatment

The stages in applying UVB are those described in the erythemal test above, except for the section on the template and post-test. Treatments should ideally be at 70% of E_1 (MED) test dose and increased on subsequent exposures by 20%, assuming no erythema at the time of the next treatment (Krutmann and Morita, 2003). This dose is altered according to the response of the last treatment. If minimal erythema developed, the dose is repeated, if more than that then clinical judgement is required.

Some regimens for both UVB and PUVA continue as maintenance, i.e. a moderate dose applied at weekly, fortnightly or monthly intervals in an attempt to prevent the recurrence of psoriasis. The value of this method is difficult to quantify and now most feel that treatment should not be prolonged unless there is good evidence that cessation leads to further development of psoriasis.

Records of UVR treatment

Records of all UVR treatments must be precise and complete both for safety and to ensure adequate treatment planning. For all ultraviolet treatments the following should always be recorded:

- *date* – knowing the exact date of a given treatment is essential for calculating progression etc.
- *lamp used* – the particular lamp should be clearly identified
- *distance* at which treatment is applied; this must be accurate and precise
- *exact area treated* – and precisely where and how untreated regions were screened. Use bony landmarks as reference points. The position of the patient should be noted in the case of the Theraktin tunnel
- *time* for which the treatment was applied
- *reaction obtained* – this should be recorded at the subsequent attendance.

Other information may also be needed, such as any change in the condition (the size of the ulcer, perhaps, or the condition of the psoriatic plaques etc.).

If treatment is to be repeated, it is particularly important that the lamp to patient distance is measured accurately as any changes in distance will have a major effect on the dose through the 'inverse square' relation discussed earlier in this chapter.

Practical point

Curvature of an exposed skin surface creates a problem. Some areas will be underexposed, e.g. the shoulders during treatment of the upper back. To produce a more gradual shading, the screening is moved slightly during treatment. Thus after, say, a quarter of the treatment time the cover is rolled down 2 or 3 cm; after half the time a further 3 cm; after three quarters of the time it is completely removed. The result is a gradual change over the area of skin at the edge of the treatment area which is both safer for subsequent treatments and cosmetically more acceptable. The alternative is to screen the skin to the same exact line each time. This becomes easier if the line is subsequently marked by pigmentation.

DANGERS

Since the results of ultraviolet treatment are not immediately evident, there is no sensation and visible erythema appears only later, mistakes can easily occur. (Remember, any sensation of heat is due to infrared from the lamp, not the UVR.)

Eyes

The eyes of the patient and therapist must be protected at all times from direct as well as reflected and scattered radiation. The patient should wear goggles even when not facing the source of radiation. So should a therapist who must also be aware of the possible cumulative effects in a day of UVR on themselves, e.g. six treatments of 20 s in a day = 2 minute exposure.

Overdose

- *Too long an exposure*. An accurate timing device is essential and it should have an alarm if used for longer periods.
- *Too close to the lamp*. This occurs either because of inaccurate measurement or because the patient moves. Patients may move closer to the lamp in the hope of receiving a more effective treatment.
- *Previously protected skin* being irradiated at subsequent treatments. This can be caused by alterations in screening, different clothes, a haircut or even removal of a watch strap.
- *Sensitizers*, e.g. change in medications or even skin perfume or aftershave used.
- *Change of lamp*. Using a different lamp is not an option unless an erythemal test is done first.

A failure of the therapist to recognize the implications of the inverse square law is possibly the most frequent cause of excessive exposure when positioning the lamp, e.g. if an E_1 at 50 cm is 2 minutes, at 30 cm an E_1 is obtained in under 45 s.

Ozone

Because ozone is formed it is important to ensure adequate ventilation in the area.

CONTRAINDICATIONS

- Acute skin conditions – acute eczema, dermatitis and an existing ultraviolet erythema.
- Skin damage due to ionizing radiation – radiation therapy.
- Conditions that can be triggered or exacerbated by UVR such as systemic lupus erythematosus.

- Photoallergy – allergic reaction to UVR (see earlier section on abnormal responses to UVR).
- Acute febrile illness – whole-body treatment should be avoided.
- Recent skin grafts.

HELIOTHERAPY

Heliotherapy is treatment by natural sunlight and has been used since Greek and Roman times. Early in the twentieth century heliotherapy was widely used for the treatment of tuberculosis.

A more recent form of heliotherapy, balneotherapy, involves the treatment of psoriasis at the Dead Sea in Israel (Krutmann and Morita, 2003). It is argued that the lower UVB spectrum of the sun in this region, 400 m below sea level, allows patients to receive more ultraviolet without burning; i.e. the spectrum contains relatively more UVA. Recent evidence, however, suggests that higher UVA levels are detrimental rather than beneficial (Agar et al., 2004). The high salt concentration of the Dead Sea (much higher than in normal seawater) is also argued to contribute, though there is no credible evidence for any beneficial effects.

A randomized controlled trial comparing the efficacy of saline spa baths, UVB or a combination of the two found the baths made only a very minimal contribution to the outcome (Leaute-Labreze et al., 2001)

Sunburn from solar UVB typically occurs only in the summer in temperate zones. The UVB component of solar radiation is particularly dependent on the angle of the sun to the surface of the earth, so although visible and UVA radiations increase in summer, the UVB increases proportionally much more. The UVB is about 100 times more intense in summer than in winter (Diffey, 1982).

In some areas of the world, e.g. New Zealand and the southern parts of Australia, ozone depletion in the upper atmosphere is causing a marked increase of UVB and UVA. The UN Environmental Program (1999) reported a 12% increase in summer peak levels in New Zealand in the previous decade.

There are claims that heliotherapy at the Dead Sea is a highly effective treatment for psoriasis, but no evidence from controlled trials has been reported.

SUNBEDS

Various types of sunbeds exist but most have panels containing a number of fluorescent tubes giving UVA and visible radiation. An individual may lie under, and sometimes on, such a panel of tubes and it is claimed that pigmentation without erythema will occur: 'tanning without burning'. Those who already have some pigmentation tend to pigment further but for others the effect may not be marked (Rivers et al., 1989). Also, the pigmentation induced is not a very efficient protection against later exposure to UVB from the sun.

The main risk of using sunbeds for tanning is that of skin cancers. Exposures in a tanning salon have been shown to produce the pre-

The use of UVA-emitting sunbeds for cosmetic tanning has increased enormously in the past few years despite the demonstrated risks.

cursors to skin cancers (Whitmore et al., 2001). This suggests the long-term risks are perhaps greater than many current users realize (Agar et al., 2004). Basal cell carcinomas are more likely to be fatal than those in more superficial layers so, although UVB is more intrinsically mutagenic than UVA, the greater penetration depth of UVA allows greater damage at depth and makes UVA more of a hazard.

References

Agar, N., Halliday, G., Barnetson, R. et al. (2004). The basal layer in human squamous tumours harbors more UVA than UVB fingerprint mutations: a role for UVA in human skin carcinogenesis. Proc Natl Acad Sci U S A, **101**, 4954–4959.

Black, G., Matzinger, E., Gange, R. (1985). Lack of photoprotection against UVB induced erythema by immediate pigmentation induced by 382 nm radiation. J Invest Dermatol, **85**, 448–449.

Burger, A., Jordaad, M., Schombee, G. (1985). The bacteriocidal effect of ultraviolet light on infected pressure sores. S Afr J Physiother, **41**, 55–57.

Christophers, M., Mrowietz, U. (2003). Psoriasis. In I. Freedberg, A. Eisen, K. Wolff, K. Austen, L. Goldsmith, S. Katz (eds), Fitzpatrick's Dermatology in General Medicine, 6th edn, Vol. 1, pp. 407–427. New York: McGraw-Hill.

Chu, D., Haake, A., Holbrook, K., Loomis, C. (2003). The structure and development of skin. In I. Freedberg, A. Eisen, K. Wolff, K. Austen, L. Goldsmith, S. Katz, (eds), Fitzpatrick's Dermatology in General Medicine, 6th edn, Vol. 1, pp. 58–88. New York: McGraw-Hill.

Diffey, B. (1982). Ultraviolet Radiation in Medicine. Bristol: Adam Hilger.

Diffey, B. (1994). The physics of ultraviolet phototherapy. Paper presented at the The Chartered Society of Physiotherapy and the Institute of Physical Sciences in Medicine; Electrotherapy: A Multi-disciplinary Conference, Manchester 12–13 April 1994.

Diffey, B., Oakley, A. (1987). The onset of ultraviolet erythema. Br J Dermatol, **116**, 183–187.

Farr, P., Diffey, B. (1984). Quantitative studies on cutaneous erythema induced by ultraviolet radiation. Br J Dermatol, **111**, 673–682.

Freedberg, I., Eisen, A., Wolff, K., Austen, K., Goldsmith, L., Katz, S. (eds) (2003). Fitzpatrick's Dermatology in General Medicine, 6th edn, Vol. 1. New York: McGraw-Hill.

Fusco, R., Jordan, P., Kelley, A., Samuel, M. (1980). PUVA therapy for psoriasis. Physiotherapy, **66**, 39–40.

Goats, G. (1988). Appropriate use of the inverse square law. Physiotherapy, **74**, 8.

Halaban, R., Hebert, D., Fisher, D. (2003). Biology of melanocytes. In I. Freedberg, A. Eisen, K. Wolff, K. Austen, L. Goldsmith, S. Katz (eds), Fitzpatrick's Dermatology in General Medicine, 6th edn, Vol. 1, pp. 127–148. New York: McGraw-Hill.

Hawke, J., Norris, P., Honigsmann, H. (2003). Abnormal responses to ultraviolet radiation: Idiopathic, probably immunologic and photoexacerbated. In I. Freedberg, A. Eisen, K. Wolff, K. Austen, L. Goldsmith, S. Katz (eds), Fitzpatrick's Dermatology in General Medicine, 6th edn, Vol. 1, pp. 1283–1298). New York: McGraw-Hill.

High, A., High, J. (1983). Treatment of infected skin wounds using ultraviolet radiation – an in vitro study. Physiotherapy, **69**, 359–360.

Honigsmann, H., Szeimes, R., Knobler, R. et al. (2003). Photochemotherapy and photodynamic therapy. In I. Freedberg, A. Eisen, K. Wolff, K. Austen, L. Goldsmith, S. Katz (eds), Fitzpatrick's Dermatology in General Medicine, 6th edn, Vol. 2, pp. 2477–2493. New York: McGraw-Hill.

Klaber, M. (1980). Ultraviolet light for psoriasis. Physiotherapy, **66**, 36–38.

Kochevar, I., Taylor, C. (2003). Photophysics, photochemistry, and photobiology. In I. Freedberg, A. Eisen, K. Wolff, K. Austen, L. Goldsmith, S. Katz (eds), Fitzpatrick's Dermatology in General Medicine, 6th edn, Vol. 1, pp. 1267–1275. New York: McGraw-Hill.

Krutmann, J., Morita, A. (2003). Therapeutic photomedicine: Phototherapy. In I. Freedberg, A. Eisen, K. Wolff, K. Austen, L. Goldsmith, S. Katz (eds), Fitzpatrick's Dermatology in General Medicine, 6th edn, Vol. 2, pp. 2469–2477. New York: McGraw-Hill.

Kuenzli, S., Saurat, J. (2003). The retinoids. In I. Freedberg, A. Eisen, K. Wolff, K. Austen, L. Goldsmith, S. Katz (eds), Fitzpatrick's Dermatology in General Medicine, 6th edn, Vol. 2, pp. 2409–2420. New York: McGraw-Hill.

Langley, R., Barnhill, R., Mihm, M. et al. (2003). Neoplasms: Cutaneous melanoma. In I. Freedberg, A. Eisen, K. Wolff, K. Austen, L. Goldsmith, S. Katz (eds), Fitzpatrick's Dermatology in General Medicine, 6th edn, Vol. 1, pp. 917–947. New York: McGraw-Hill.

Leaute-Labreze, C., Saillour, F., Chene, G. et al. (2001). Saline spa water or combined water and UV-B for psoriasis vs conventional UV-B: lessons from the Salies de Bearn randomized study. Arch Dermatol, **137**, 1035–1039.

Licht, S. (1983). History of ultraviolet therapy. In K. Stillwell (ed.), Therapeutic Electricity and Ultraviolet Radiation, 3rd edn. London: Williams & Wilkins.

Lim, H. (2003). Abnormal responses to ultraviolet radiation: Photosensitivity induced by exogenous agents. In I. Freedberg, A. Eisen, K. Wolff, K. Austen, L. Goldsmith, S. Katz (eds), Fitzpatrick's Dermatology in General Medicine, 6th edn, Vol. 1, pp. 1298–1308. New York: McGraw-Hill.

Low, J. (1986). Quantifying the erythema due to UVR. Physiotherapy, **72**, 60–64.

Nonaka, S., Kaidley, K., Kligman, A. (1984). Photoprotective adaptation – some quantitative aspects. Arch Dermatol, **120**, 609–613.

Orotonne, J., Bahadoran, P., Fitzpatrick, T. et al. (2003). Hypomelanoses and hypermelanoses. In I. Freedberg, A. Eisen, K. Wolff, K. Austen, L. Goldsmith, S. Katz (eds), Fitzpatrick's Dermatology in General Medicine, 6th edn, Vol. 1, pp. 836–881. New York: McGraw-Hill.

Parrish, J., Jaenicke, K. (1981). Action spectrum of phototherapy for psoriasis. J Invest Dermatol, **76**, 359–362.

Pirkhammer, D., Seeber, A., Honigsmann, H., Tanew, A. (2000). Narrow-band ultraviolet B (ATL-01) phototherapy is an effective and safe treatment option for patients with severe seborrhoeic dermatitis. Br J Dermatol, **143**, 964–968.

Rivers, J., Norris, P., Murphy, G. (1989). UVA sunbeds: tanning, photoprotection, acute adverse effects and immunological changes. Br J Dermatol, **120**, 767–777.

Robson, J., Diffey, B. (1990). Textiles and sun protection. Photodermatol Photoimmunol Photomed, **7**, 32–34.

Sayre, R., Olson, R., Everett, M. (1966). Qualitative studies on erythema. J Invest Dermatol, **46**, 240–244.

Scientific Committee on Cosmetic Products and Non-Food Products (SCCNFP) (2003). Furocoumarins in sun protection and bronzing products. Statement to the European Commission. SCCNFP/0765/03.

Stern, R. (2001). The risk of melanoma in association with long-term exposure to PUVA. J Am Acad Dermatol, **44**, 755–761.

Stern, R., Nichols, K., Vakeva, L. (1997). Malignant melanoma in patients treated for psoriasis with methoxsalen (psoralen) and ultraviolet A radiation (PUVA). N Engl J Med, **336**, 1041–1045.

Thiboutot, D., Strauss, J. (2003). Diseases of the sebaceous glands. In I. Freedberg, A. Eisen, K. Wolff, K. Austen, L. Goldsmith, S. Katz (eds), Fitzpatrick's Dermatology in General Medicine, 6th edn, Vol. 1, pp. 672–687. New York: McGraw-Hill.

United Nations Environmental Program (UNEP). (1999). Environmental effects of ozone depletion: Interim summary. http://www.gcrio.org/ozone/unep1999summary.html

Walker, S., Hawk, J., Young, A. (2003). Acute and chronic effects of ultraviolet radiation on the skin. In I. Freedberg, A. Eisen, K. Wolff, K. Austen, L. Goldsmith, S. Katz (eds), Fitzpatrick's Dermatology in General Medicine, 6th edn, Vol. 1, pp. 1275–1282. New York: McGraw-Hill.

Whitmore, E., Morison, W., Potten, C., Chadwick, C. (2001). Tanning salon exposure and molecular alterations. J Amer Acad Dermatol, **44**, 775–780.

Winchester, R. (2003). Psoriatic arthritis. In I. Freedberg, A. Eisen, K. Wolff, K. Austen, L. Goldsmith, S. Katz (eds), Fitzpatrick's Dermatology in General Medicine, 6th edn, Vol. 1, pp. 427–436). New York: McGraw-Hill.

Wolff, K. (1997). Should PUVA be abandoned [Editorial]. N Engl J Med, **336**, 1090–1091.

Wolff, K., Gschnait, F., Honigsmann, H. et al. (1977). Phototesting and dosimetry for photochemotherapy. Br J Dermatol, **96**, 1–10.

Wood, K., Reed, A. (1990). A study of the intensity of ultraviolet radiations transmitted through a variety of screening materials. Physiotherapy, **76**, 720–724.

Some 'basic science' ideas

Electrophysical agents can be broadly categorized as involving either electric current, electric or magnetic fields, or waves (whether sound or electromagnetic waves). This appendix aims to summarize the important features of each of these three forms of energy. It is important to distinguish them as their different clinical effects are due to the different physical and biophysical properties of electricity, fields and waves.

Electric current

An electric current is a flow of electric charges. Electrons and ions are the charges involved. In metals, current flow takes the form of electron movement. In conducting solutions (and human tissues), current flow is due to movement of positive and negative ions.

Metallic conductors are materials in which the outer shell electrons are free to move between constituent atoms. Normally this movement is random but if a voltage (an 'electric pressure') is applied to the material electrons will move away from the negative towards the positive electrode. Although the motion of electrons is very rapid the movement of electrons from atom to atom (the electron drift) is quite slow. This is a conduction current and it is how charges move in metals and carbon and hence in electrical apparatus. Current is a rate of flow, the quantity of electrons per unit time. A rather large number of electrons (6.25×10^{18}) is the unit of quantity called a coulomb and when this quantity passes a point in $1\,s$ the rate of flow, or current, is called 1 ampere.

It is important to recognize that random electron movement occurs constantly at normal temperatures and that the electric current is superimposed on this. It is analogous to the arrivals channel of a large international airport; aircraft deliver passengers who pass through passport control, customs etc. and eventually leave by car, bus or train. Looked at over a time period of, say, a day the number of passengers leaving the airport is the same as the number arriving – the rate of flow may be expressed as so many thousand passengers per day – yet individual passengers have followed different pathways and

At an atomic level a metal has a rigid framework of positive metal ions with a sea of negative electrons moving freely through the crystal lattice.

For more information on current flow and conductors see chapter 1 of the book 'Biophysical Bases of Electrotherapy' on the CD which comes with this book.

spent different lengths of time at the airport. Some have been delayed by customs, some have had to wait for friends to meet them, some have gone to the restaurant for a meal and so forth, while others have passed through as quickly as they could. On a normal working day the airport is full of people as a conductor is full of electrons.

In a metal conduction occurs by movement of electrons. The relatively large, heavy, positive metal ions are firmly held in crystalline structures while there are many small, light, negative electrons which are free to move around in and through the crystal lattice. In fluids, liquids and gases, the atoms and molecules are free to move and therefore can take part in the flow of charges if they become charged. When an atom gains or loses an electron – hence it becomes negatively or positively charged – it is called an ion. Thus when common salt, sodium chloride, is dissolved in water it does not exist as sodium chloride molecules (NaCl) but as positive sodium (Na^+) and negative chloride (Cl^-) ions. Electrolytes are solutions containing ions. Body fluids are electrolytes and current can flow by the movement of these ions. Positive ions move towards the negative electrode, the source of additional electrons, while negative ions move to the positive electrode where electrons are being removed. Thus there is a two-way motion of ions which constitutes the current.

In any given conductor, current intensity will depend on the electric pressure or electric force, known as the voltage. It is ultimately due to the attraction of electrons for protons; the fundamental force of attraction between things negative and things positive. This is measured in volts and is known, descriptively, as an electromotive force. The difficulty electrons have in moving within a solid conductor, or ions have in moving in an electrolyte, will also determine the rate of flow and this is described as the resistance, measured in ohms. Thus a conductor with a greater resistance will allow a smaller flow of electrons. These concepts are expressed in Ohm's law which states that the current intensity (I) in amperes is directly proportional to the electromotive force (V) in volts and inversely proportional to the resistance (R) in ohms. $I = V/R$. This is analogous to the flow of water from a tap which depends on the pressure driving it (height of the tank) and the resistance offered by the tap (how far it is turned on). Thus if the voltage and resistance are known, the current can be calculated using Ohm's law. More generally, if any two of the three quantities, I, V or R are known, the third can be calculated using Ohm's law.

For more information on voltage, resistance and Ohm's law see chapter 1 of the book 'Biophysical Bases of Electrotherapy'.

Electrolysis

Electrolytes are solutions containing ions. When crystalline substances dissolve in water some separation into ions always occurs. If an electric field is applied by means of a pair of metal electrodes the ions will move through the solution, as shown in figure A1. Thus positive ions move towards the negative electrode or cathode and are sometimes, rather confusingly, called cations. Negative ions move to the positive electrode or anode, hence these are called anions. When the ions reach the metal plate or electrode they lose their charge. Positive ions gain an electron from the negatively charged metal plate and the negative ions give up their extra electron to the positive plate.

The current in the solution is transmitted as ions (charges) moving in both directions. Sodium chloride solutions are utilized in transmitting current to and from the tissues for treatment purposes and will be considered, but similar effects occur where other salts, acids or bases are involved. The sodium chloride and water molecules dissociate into sodium and chloride ions, and hydrogen and hydroxyl ions respectively:

$$NaCl \rightarrow Na^+ + Cl^-$$

and $\qquad H_2O \rightarrow H^+ + OH^-$

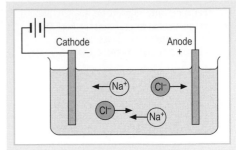

Figure A1 Current flow in a solution of ions

The positive ions move to the negative electrode, the cathode, where they receive electrons. The negative ions move to the positive electrode, the anode, where they give up electrons.

At the cathode:

$$H^+ + e^- \rightarrow H \quad and \quad 2H \rightarrow H_2$$

So hydrogen gas is given off. The hydrogen ion concentration falls (the pH value rises), therefore the reaction is alkaline. Hydrogen gas is also produced from the sodium ion movement:

$$Na^+ + e^- \rightarrow Na \quad and \quad 2Na + 2H_2O \rightarrow 2NaOH + H_2$$

NaOH, a strong base, is the end product and this can cause a chemical burn.

At the anode:

$$OH^- - e^- \rightarrow OH \quad and \quad 4OH \rightarrow 2H_2O + O_2$$

Also $\qquad Cl^- + e^- \rightarrow Cl \quad and \quad 4Cl + 2H_2O \rightarrow 4HCl + O_2$

Thus hydrochloric acid is formed and oxygen gas given off. HCl, a strong acid, is the end product and this can cause a chemical burn.

These effects of altered pH and release of oxygen and hydrogen will occur whatever the salt, acid or base in solution with inert electrodes. The amount of gas produced is small in therapeutic situations and tends to remain dissolved in the water. However, if the current density is made high – say by passing a large current between two electrodes placed in a bowl of water – gas bubbles can be seen. These are especially evident at the cathode because of the larger quantity of hydrogen produced; in fact this can be used to determine the polarity as can the acidity/alkalinity tested with litmus paper.

Electric and magnetic fields

A consequence of matter being made of positive and negative particles (protons and electrons) is that charges can be separated and, as a consequence an electric field is produced. When dry hair is combed

For more information on electric and magnetic fields see chapter 6 of the book 'Biophysical Bases of Electrotherapy' on the CD which comes with this book.

Induced current is discussed in chapter 7 of 'Biophysical Bases of Electrotherapy'.

with a plastic comb, the hair becomes charged. The comb becomes equally and oppositely charged. The result is that the hair 'stands on end', being attracted towards the oppositely charged comb. The fundamental idea is that when charges are separated, an electric field is produced between them. The concept of an electric field is discussed briefly in chapter 13.

When current flows though a conductor, a magnetic field is produced. This is also discussed briefly in chapter 13. Some concern has been expressed that we might all be at some risk by being exposed to the magnetic fields around power lines and power wiring in the home or work environment. This is also discussed in chapter 13. There are two important ideas:

- magnetic fields are produced whenever charges move (current flows)
- if the current is alternating, the magnetic field will alternate and an alternating current will be induced in anything nearby (whether metal, human tissue or 'other').

Shortwave treatment (chapter 13) involves applying high-frequency alternating electric or magnetic fields to induce a high-frequency alternating current, i.e. charge movement, in tissue. The principal effect of this treatment is heat production but there may be other, less directly thermal, effects.

Waves

A wave is any repetitive (i.e. regularly repeated) oscillation. Examples are waves in a pond when a rock is thrown in and the blurred vibration of a guitar string when it is plucked. It is the regular repeated nature of the oscillation which characterizes the wave. A simple wave, described as a sinusoidal wave or sinewave, is represented in figure A2 which is a graph of amplitude versus time. From a graph like this the period can be measured. The **period** is the time for one complete oscillation or repeat. This might be measured in seconds (s), milliseconds (ms) or microseconds (µs).

The **frequency** is the number of complete cycles in a second, given in hertz (Hz). Thus if the period is 20 ms or 1/50th of a second, there are 50 periods (cycles) in one second so the frequency is 50 Hz. These cycles or repeats could be pulses (electrical or cardiac), waves, nerve impulses etc. Whichever, the number of cycles or repeats per second is the frequency in Hz. Higher frequencies are expressed in multiples e.g. kilohertz (kHz), megahertz (MHz) and gigahertz (GHz).

The distance through which the wave motion repeats itself – the distance from, say, one wave peak to the next – is called the **wavelength** and is often denoted by λ (lambda). If figure A2 were replotted as amplitude versus distance rather than time, the distance between two peaks would be the wavelength (instead of the period).

The wavelength is measured in metres (m) or some multiple or sub-multiple e.g. millimetres (mm), micrometres (μm) or nanometres (nm). In the case of longitudinal waves passing in a medium (e.g. ultrasound, chapter 9) it is the distance from, say, the central point of one compression of molecules to the next.

Consider the familiar experience of standing knee-deep in the sea. A photograph taken looking out to sea would show a series of waves spaced apart. That is, the height of the surface of the sea varies with distance at a single instant of time. The cold seawater regularly falling to the ankles and rising, breathtakingly, up the thighs makes the observer vividly aware of the variation over time in one place.

Any wave travelling through a particular medium (gas, liquid or solid) will travel with a certain velocity. The wave will also have a particular frequency and wavelength. The three quantities describing the wave – wavelength, frequency and velocity – are not independent. They are related by the **wave equation**:

$$v = f\lambda$$

which states that the wave **velocity**, v (in $m\,s^{-1}$), is equal to the frequency, f (in Hz or s^{-1}), multiplied by the wavelength, λ (in m).

For any given velocity the wave could travel with either a high frequency and short wavelength or a low frequency and high (long) wavelength. This relationship is obvious when it is realized that the speed of travel of any cyclical motion depends on the length of the cycle and the number of repetitions per unit time. Consider a 5-year-old boy walking hand in hand with his father; both travel at the same velocity, covering the same distance in the same time; the boy takes many small steps (of high frequency, short length) while the father takes fewer longer strides (of low frequency, large length).

Energy and power

Frequent reference is made to energy and power in this text, so it may be helpful to look at their relationship. The concept of energy is not easily explained, because it only becomes evident when one form of energy is converted to another, such as when electrical energy is converted to heat energy in the wire of an infrared lamp, or in the tissues during the application of shortwave diathermy. Perhaps even more evident is the action of some mechanical force, such as a pull or push on a solid piece of matter, causing it to move. Here mechanical energy is converted to kinetic (movement) energy.

Energy can be considered in two forms; kinetic energy, by virtue of motion, and potential energy, which is a stored form by virtue of structure, weight, charge, position etc.

The unit of energy is the joule (J); it represents the ability to do work. Work is also measured in joules. One joule is the energy (E) that results, or the work done (W), when a force (*F*) of 1 newton acts through a distance (*d*) of one metre. The relationship is thus:

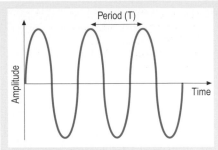

Figure A2 A simple sinusoidal waveform where the amplitude varies with a regular repeat.

If a graph of seawater height up the limb versus time was plotted, the graph would resemble figure A2 as would a graph of seawater height versus distance from the observer. The graphs would not be as smooth, but they would show a characteristic regular periodicity.

For more information on waves see chapter 9 of the book 'Biophysical Bases of Electrotherapy' on the CD which comes with this book.

$$\text{Energy} = \text{Work done} = \text{Force} \times \text{distance} \quad \text{or}$$
$$E = W = Fd$$

A joule is 1 newton metre i.e. J = Nm as indicated by the energy equation.

In many practical situations the important factor is the rate of energy conversion or rate of work done, i.e. the number of joules per second or watts. One joule of energy expended per second is a power dissipation of one watt. This can be written:

$$1 \, \text{J} \, \text{s}^{-1} = 1 \, \text{W}$$

This rate of energy use is called power and its units are watts (W). Thus if an ultrasound transducer is delivering a power output of 5 W, it means that electrical energy is being converted to sonic energy and 5 joules of sonic energy are produced every second. Similarly a 60 W light globe consumes electrical energy at the rate of 60 joules per second (or over 200 kJ per hour).

To work out how much energy has been delivered, multiply watts by seconds:

$$1 \, \text{J} = 1 \, \text{W} \, \text{s}$$

For example: 1 watt hour = 3600 J. Because the numbers are often large, kilojoules (kJ) and kilowatt hours (kWh) are frequently used.

Often it is helpful to know the amount of power per unit area. This is called power density and is measured in $\text{W} \, \text{cm}^{-2}$. With ultrasound, this value is often called intensity, and for lasers and light is termed brilliance or irradiance. In the same way it is sometimes convenient to describe energy density ($\text{J} \, \text{cm}^{-2}$).

Whatever conversions occur, the principle of conservation of energy applies. This states that energy can neither be created nor destroyed.

Quantities and units

As might be apparent from the above discussion of electricity, fields and waves, quantities and units can be a stumbling block to understanding electrophysical agents. Table A1 lists the quantities used in this book, which are briefly explained as they are introduced. They are explained in more detail in the book 'Biophysical Bases of Electrotherapy' (on the CD which comes with this book). See especially Appendix 2 of the book, which provides a more comprehensive list of quantities.

Note that the symbol 'E' can mean either electric field strength or energy. In context, there is little risk of confusion. Similarly 'I' is used both for electric current and wave intensity. Again, in context, there is little risk of confusion though it would certainly be better if separate symbols were used.

Although the unit of temperature is the kelvin, the degree Celsius (symbol °C) is an acceptable alternative. Temperatures in degrees

Table A1 Some fundamental quantities and their units

Electricity:

Quantity	Symbol	Unit
Charge	q	coulomb (C)
Voltage	V	volt (V)
Current	I	ampere (A)
Resistance	R	ohm (Ω)
Capacitance	C	farad (F)
Impedance (electrical)	Z	ohm (Ω)
Current density	i	$A\,m^{-2}$

Fields:

Quantity	Symbol	Unit
Electric field strength	E	$V\,m^{-1}$
Magnetic flux density	B	tesla (T)

Waves:

Quantity	Symbol	Unit
Frequency	f	hertz (Hz)
Wavelength	λ	m
Velocity	v	$m\,s^{-1}$
Intensity (wave)	I	$W\,m^{-2}$
Penetration depth	δ	m

General/other:

Quantity	Symbol	Unit
Length	L	metre (m)
Mass	m	kilogram (kg)
Time	t	second (s)
Temperature	T	kelvin (K)
Force	F	newton (N)
Energy	E	joule (J)
Power	P	watt (W)
Intensity	I	$W\,m^{-2}$
Heat capacity	c	$J\,kg^{-1}\,K^{-1}$

Celsius are converted to kelvins by adding 273.15. The size of the degree Celsius is equal to the size of the kelvin so a temperature increase of 10 K is the same as an increase of 10°C.

Magnetic field intensity (more correctly called magnetic flux density) is measured in units of teslas. Sometimes an older unit, the gauss is used. 1 tesla is 10 000 gauss.

Prefixes (multiples and submultiples)

The quantities described in this book are often stated in multiples or submultiple of the base unit and this is indicated with a prefix (e.g. milli-, micro-, etc). Table A2 lists the more important prefixes. A more comprehensive list is provided in Appendix 1 of 'Biophysical Bases of Electrotherapy'.

Table A2 Prefixes used to specify multiples and submultiples of units

Prefix	Symbol	Multiple
nano	n	10^{-9}
micro	μ	10^{-6}
milli	m	10^{-3}
centi	c	10^{-2}
kilo	k	10^{3}
mega	M	10^{6}
giga	G	10^{9}
tera	T	10^{12}

Some examples

10^9 hertz (Hz) = 1 gigahertz (GHz)
10^6 ohms (Ω) = 1 megohm (MΩ)
10^6 hertz (Hz) = 1 megahertz (MHz)
10^3 joules (J) = 1 kilojoule (kJ)
10^{-2} metre (m) = 1 centimetre (cm)
10^{-3} watt (W) = 1 milliwatt (mW)
10^{-6} sec (s) = 1 microsecond (μs)
10^{-9} metre (m) = 1 nanometre (nm)

Index

ELSEVIER CD-ROM LICENCE AGREEMENT

PLEASE READ THE FOLLOWING AGREEMENT CAREFULLY BEFORE USING THIS PRODUCT. THIS PRODUCT IS LICENSED UNDER THE TERMS CONTAINED IN THIS LICENCE AGREEMENT ('Agreement'). BY USING THIS PRODUCT, YOU, AN INDIVIDUAL OR ENTITY INCLUDING EMPLOYEES, AGENTS AND REPRESENTATIVES ('You' or 'Your'), ACKNOWLEDGE THAT YOU HAVE READ THIS AGREEMENT, THAT YOU UNDERSTAND IT, AND THAT YOU AGREE TO BE BOUND BY THE TERMS AND CONDITIONS OF THIS AGREEMENT. ELSEVIER LIMITED ('Elsevier') EXPRESSLY DOES NOT AGREE TO LICENSE THIS PRODUCT TO YOU UNLESS YOU ASSENT TO THIS AGREEMENT. IF YOU DO NOT AGREE WITH ANY OF THE FOLLOWING TERMS, YOU MAY, WITHIN THIRTY (30) DAYS AFTER YOUR RECEIPT OF THIS PRODUCT RETURN THE UNUSED PRODUCT AND ALL ACCOMPANYING DOCUMENTATION TO ELSEVIER FOR A FULL REFUND.

DEFINITIONS As used in this Agreement, these terms shall have the following meanings:

'Proprietary Material' means the valuable and proprietary information content of this Product including without limitation all indexes and graphic materials and software used to access, index, search and retrieve the information content from this Product developed or licensed by Elsevier and/or its affiliates, suppliers and licensors.

'Product' means the copy of the Proprietary Material and any other material delivered on CD-ROM and any other human readable or machine-readable materials enclosed with this Agreement, including without limitation documentation relating to the same.

OWNERSHIP This Product has been supplied by and is proprietary to Elsevier and/or its affiliates, suppliers and licensors. The copyright in the Product belongs to Elsevier and/or its affiliates, suppliers and licensors and is protected by the copyright, trademark, trade secret and other intellectual property laws of the United Kingdom and international treaty provisions, including without limitation the Universal Copyright Convention and the Berne Copyright Convention. You have no ownership rights in this Product. Except as expressly set forth herein, no part of this Product, including without limitation the Proprietary Material, may be modified, copied or distributed in hardcopy or machine-readable form without prior written consent from Elsevier. All rights not expressly granted to You herein are expressly reserved. Any other use of this Product by any person or entity is strictly prohibited and a violation of this Agreement.

SCOPE OF RIGHTS LICENSED (PERMITTED USES) Elsevier is granting to You a limited, non-exclusive, non-transferable licence to use this Product in accordance with the terms of this Agreement. You may use or provide access to this Product on a single computer or terminal physically located at Your premises and in a secure network or move this Product to and use it on another single computer or terminal at the same location for personal use only, but under no circumstances may You use or provide access to any part or parts of this Product on more than one computer or terminal simultaneously.

You shall not (a) copy, download, or otherwise reproduce the Product or any part(s) thereof in any medium, including, without limitation, online transmissions, local area networks, wide area networks, intranets, extranets and the Internet, or in any way, in whole or in part, except for printing out or downloading nonsubstantial portions of the text and images in the Product for Your own personal use; (b) alter, modify, or adapt the Product or any part(s) thereof, including but not limited to decompiling, disassembling, reverse engineering, or creating derivative works, without the prior written approval of Elsevier; (c) sell, license or otherwise distribute to third parties the Product or any part(s) thereof; or (d) alter, remove, obscure or obstruct the display of any copyright, trademark or other proprietary notice on or in the Product or on any printout or download of portions of the Proprietary Materials.

RESTRICTIONS ON TRANSFER This Licence is personal to You, and neither Your rights hereunder nor the tangible embodiments of this Product, including without limitation the Proprietary Material, may be sold, assigned, transferred or sublicensed to any other person, including without limitation by operation of law, without the prior written consent of Elsevier. Any purported sale, assignment, transfer or sublicense without the prior written consent of Elsevier will be void and will automatically terminate the Licence granted hereunder.

TERM This Agreement will remain in effect until terminated pursuant to the terms of this Agreement. You may terminate this Agreement at any time by removing from Your system and destroying the Product and any copies of the Proprietary Material. Unauthorized copying of the Product, including without limitation, the Proprietary Material and documentation, or otherwise failing to comply with the terms and conditions of this Agreement shall result in automatic termination of this licence and will make available to Elsevier legal remedies. Upon termination of this Agreement, the licence granted herein will terminate and You must immediately destroy the Product and all copies of the Product and of the Proprietary Material, together with any and all accompanying documentation. All provisions relating to proprietary rights shall survive termination of this Agreement.

LIMITED WARRANTY AND LIMITATION OF LIABILITY Elsevier warrants that the software embodied in this Product will perform in substantial compliance with the documentation supplied in this Product, unless the performance problems are the result of hardware failure or improper use. If You report a significant defect in performance in writing to Elsevier within ninety (90) calendar days of your having purchased the Product, and Elsevier is not able to correct same within sixty (60) days after its receipt of Your notification, You may return this Product, including all copies and documentation, to Elsevier and Elsevier will refund Your money. In order to apply for a refund on your purchased Product, please contact the return address on the invoice to obtain the refund request form ('Refund Request Form'), and either fax or mail your signed request and your proof of purchase to the address indicated on the Refund Request Form. Incomplete forms will not be processed. Defined terms in the Refund Request Form shall have the same meaning as in this Agreement.

YOU UNDERSTAND THAT, EXCEPT FOR THE LIMITED WARRANTY RECITED ABOVE, ELSEVIER, ITS AFFILIATES, LICENSORS, THIRD PARTY SUPPLIERS AND AGENTS (TOGETHER 'THE SUPPLIERS') MAKE NO REPRESENTATIONS OR WARRANTIES, WITH RESPECT TO THE PRODUCT, INCLUDING, WITHOUT LIMITATION THE PROPRIETARY MATERIAL. ALL OTHER REPRESENTATIONS, WARRANTIES, CONDITIONS OR OTHER TERMS, WHETHER EXPRESS OR IMPLIED BY STATUTE OR COMMON LAW, ARE HEREBY EXCLUDED TO THE FULLEST EXTENT PERMITTED BY LAW.

IN PARTICULAR BUT WITHOUT LIMITATION TO THE FOREGOING NONE OF THE SUPPLIERS MAKE ANY REPRESENTATIONS OR WARRANTIES (WHETHER EXPRESS OR IMPLIED) REGARDING THE PERFORMANCE OF YOUR PAD, NETWORK OR COMPUTER SYSTEM WHEN USED IN CONJUNCTION WITH THE PRODUCT, NOR THAT THE PRODUCT WILL MEET YOUR REQUIREMENTS OR THAT ITS OPERATION WILL BE UNINTERRUPTED OR ERROR-FREE.

EXCEPT IN RESPECT OF DEATH OR PERSONAL INJURY CAUSED BY THE SUPPLIERS' NEGLIGENCE AND TO THE FULLEST EXTENT PERMITTED BY LAW, IN NO EVENT (AND REGARDLESS OF WHETHER SUCH DAMAGES ARE FORESEEABLE AND OF WHETHER SUCH LIABILITY IS BASED IN TORT, CONTRACT OR OTHERWISE) WILL ANY OF THE SUPPLIERS BE LIABLE TO YOU FOR ANY DAMAGES

System Requirements for 'ELECTROTHERAPY EXPLAINED Principles and Practice.'

This CD will run on both PCs and Macs:

To function properly, the computer utilizing this collection should support at least an 800×600 pixels screen resolution, 256 colors, 128 MB RAM and operate on the Windows 98 SE, 2000 or XP operating system or the MAC OS 9 and MAC OS 10+ operating system.

Microsoft Windows Users

The recommended Software Acrobat Reader 7.0.

Instructions

1. If your system does not support Autorun, then please explore the CD contents click on 'EEPP.exe' to start.
2. Acrobat Reader 7.0 can be installed from the CD.

Macintosh Users

Mac OS 9:

The recommended Software Acrobat Reader 5.0.

Your computer should meet the following minimum requirements: 800×600 pixels screen resolution, 256 colors, 128 MB RAM, and MAC OS 9+ operating system.

Instructions

1. Acrobat Reader 5.0 can be installed from the CD.
2. The CD auto runs on the Mac OS 9.

Mac OS 10+:

The recommended Software Acrobat Reader 7.0.

Your computer should meet the following minimum requirements: 800×600 pixels screen resolution, 256 colors, 128 MB RAM, and MAC OS 10+ operating system.

Instructions

1. Click on the CD icon that appears on your desktop, then select EEPP to open the application.
2. Acrobat Reader 7.0 can be installed from the CD.

The CD does not auto run on the Mac OS 10+.

Minimum Software Requirements

Adobe Acrobat Reader / Acrobat Reader
Some of the content in this product is available in PDF format. To view these contents you will need a copy of Adobe Acrobat Reader / Acrobat Reader or any other product that can read the PDF file format.

Technical Support

Technical support for this product is available between 7.30 a.m. and 7.00 p.m. CST, 8.00 a.m. and 1.00 a.m. UK, Monday through Friday.
Before calling, be sure that your computer meets the minimum system requirements to run this software.
Inside the United States and Canada, call 1-800-692-9010.
Inside the United Kingdom, call 0-0800-6929-0100.
Outside North America, call +1-314-872-8370.
You may also fax your questions to +1-314-997-5080,
or contact Technical Support through e-mail: technical.support@elsevier.com.